Lookingbill and Marks'
PRINCIPLES OF DERMATOLOGY

FIFTH EDITION

For additional online content visit
expertconsult.com

Senior Content Strategist: Russell Gabbedy
Senior Content Development Specialist: Nani Clansey
Senior Content Coordinator: John Leonard
Senior Project Manager: Beula Christopher/Vinod Kumar
Design: Miles Hitchen
Illustration Manager: Jennifer Rose
Illustrator: Richard Tibbits
Marketing Manager: Shaun Miller

Lookingbill and Marks'
PRINCIPLES OF DERMATOLOGY

FIFTH EDITION

James G. Marks Jr MD
Professor of Dermatology
Chair, Department of Dermatology
Pennsylvania State University College of Medicine
Penn State Hershey Medical Center
Hershey, PA, USA

Jeffrey J. Miller MD
Professor of Dermatology
Vice Chair, Department of Dermatology
Pennsylvania State University College of Medicine
Penn State Hershey Medical Center
Hershey, PA, USA

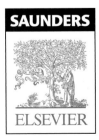

SAUNDERS

ELSEVIER

LONDON · NEW YORK · OXFORD · ST LOUIS · SYDNEY · TORONTO

ELSEVIER
SAUNDERS

An imprint of Elsevier Inc.

ISBN: 978-1-4557-2875-6
Ebook ISBN: 978-1-4557-5014-6

your source for books, journals and multimedia in the health sciences
www.elsevierhealth.com

Working together to grow libraries in developing countries

www.elsevier.com • www.bookaid.org

The publisher's policy is to use paper manufactured from sustainable forests

Printed in China
Last digit is the print number: 9 8 7 6 5 4 3 2 1

Contents

Preface

The primary goal of this fifth edition has not changed from that of the first edition; it is to facilitate dermatologic diagnosis through a morphologic approach to skin disease. Unlike most other introductory manuals, each chapter in our text is based on the appearance of the primary skin process (e.g., pustules) rather than on the etiology (e.g., infection). This arrangement helps to reflect the way in which most patients present in the clinical setting.

We are grateful to our many students and residents who have used our previous editions and provided us with thoughtful feedback over the years. Their suggestions have been incorporated into this new 5th edition of *Lookingbill and Marks' Principles of Dermatology*. It includes more color illustrations, more diseases, key points, abstracts, and initial and alternative treatments that should be of use to medical students , primary care physicians, and physician extenders who peruse this book.

Preface to the First Edition

Skin diseases affect virtually everyone sometime during life. Because changes in the skin are so easily recognized by the patient, medical attention is frequently sought. Skin reacts in a limited number of ways, but the neophyte is often bewildered by the appearance of rashes that superficially look alike. This text is meant to be an introduction to cutaneous disorders. It is aimed toward medical students so that they may develop a logical approach to the diagnosis of common cutaneous diseases with an understanding of the underlying clinicopathologic correlations. It has been a most rewarding experience for us to see students on our clinical service at the M.S. Hershey Medical Center grasp the basic principles of skin disease in the short time they spend with us. Their questions, learning experience, and suggestions have been incorporated into this book.

We have purposely not tried to make this an encyclopedia of skin diseases, but have chosen those diseases that are most commonly seen. Uncommon diseases are discussed only to illustrate dermatologic principles or important diseases that should not be missed. There are several up-to-date large textbooks available for those who want to delve into the field more deeply.

We are grateful for the contribution of artwork and clinical slides from audiovisual programs in the series A Brief Course in Dermatology, produced and distributed by the Institute for Dermatologic Communication and Education, San Francisco, California, as follows: From Skin Lesions Depicted and Defined, Part One, Primary Lesions, and Part Two, Secondary and Special Lesions, by Richard M. Caplan, M.D., Alfred W. Kopf, M.D., and Marion B. Sulzberger, M.D., and from Techniques for Examination of the Skin, by David L. Cram, M.D., Howard I. Maibach, M.D., and Marion B. Sulzberger, M.D.

We wish to acknowledge those people whose efforts contributed greatly to producing this book. Our secretaries, Dianne Safford, Joyce Zeager, and Sharon Smith, spent many hours typing the drafts and final manuscript. Nancy Egan, M.D., and Ronald Rovner, M.D., proofread much of the book and gave many worthwhile suggestions. Schering Corporation supported the cost of the illustrations which were so handsomely drawn by Debra Moyer and Daniel S. Beisel. Lastly, and most importantly, our families gave us the support and time necessary to write this volume.

Dedication

To Donald P. Lookingbill, M.D., Friend, colleague, mentor, and inspiration for this text.

Acknowledgments

We acknowledge our families for again giving us the time to produce this book.

Introduction   1

Key Points

1. Many outpatient visits are for dermatologic complaints
2. The patient's chief complaint can be divided into two diagnostic skin diseases: growths and rashes

Skin diseases are common and a significant number of outpatient visits are for dermatologic complaints. A minority of these patients are seen by dermatologists; most of the remainder are seen by primary care physicians and physician extenders. In a survey of the family practice clinic at the Pennsylvania State University College of Medicine, we found that dermatologic disorders constituted 8.5% of diagnoses. The incidence is higher in a pediatric practice, in which as many as 30% of children are seen for skin-related conditions.

Although thousands of skin disorders have been described, only a small number account for most patient visits. The primary goal of this text is to familiarize the reader with these common diseases. Some uncommon and rare skin disorders are covered briefly in this book to expand the readers' differential diagnosis.

Our diagnostic approach divides skin diseases into two large groups: growths and rashes. This grouping is based on both the patient's presenting complaint (often a concern about either a skin growth or a symptom from a rash) and the pathophysiologic process (a growth represents a neoplastic change and a rash is an inflammatory reaction in the skin).

Growths and rashes are then subdivided according to the component of skin that is affected. Growths are divided into: epidermal, pigmented, and dermal proliferative processes. Rashes are divided into those with and those without an epidermal component. Furthermore, the correlation between the clinical appearance of the disorder and the pathophysiologic processes responsible for the disease facilitates making the diagnosis and selecting the proper treatment.

2   Structure and Function of the Skin

Key Points

1. The major function of the skin is as a barrier to maintain internal homeostasis
2. The epidermis is the major barrier of the skin

ABSTRACT

The skin is a large organ, weighing an average of 4 kg and covering an area of 2 m^2. Its major function is to act as a barrier against an inhospitable environment – to protect the body from the influences of the outside world. The importance of the skin is well illustrated by the high mortality rate associated with extensive loss of skin from burns.

The major barrier is provided by the epidermis. Underlying the epidermis is a vascularized dermis that provides support and nutrition for the dividing cells in the epidermis. The dermis also contains nerves and appendages: sweat glands, hair follicles, and sebaceous glands. Nails are also considered skin appendages. The third and deepest layer of the skin is the subcutaneous fat. The functions of all these components are listed in **Table 2.1**.

Components of skin:
1. Epidermis
2. Dermis
3. Skin appendages
4. Subcutaneous fat

Skin disease illustrates structure and function. Loss of or defects in skin structure impair skin function. Skin disease is discussed in more detail in the other chapters.

EPIDERMIS

Key Points

1. Keratinocytes are the principal cell of the epidermis
2. Layers in ascending order: basal cell, stratum spinosum, stratum granulosum, stratum corneum
3. Basal cells are undifferentiated, proliferating cells
4. Stratum spinosum contains keratinocytes connected by desmosomes
5. Keratohyalin granules are seen in the stratum granulosum
6. Stratum corneum is the major physical barrier
7. The number and size of melanosomes, not melanocytes, determine skin color
8. Langerhans cells are derived from bone marrow and are the skin's first line of immunologic defense
9. The basement membrane zone is the substrate for attachment of the epidermis to the dermis
10. The four major ultrastructural regions include: the hemidesmosomal plaque of the basal keratinocyte, lamina lucida, lamina densa, and anchoring fibrils located in the sublamina densa region of the papillary dermis

The epidermis is divided into four layers, starting at the dermal junction with the basal cell layer and eventuating at the outer surface in the stratum corneum. The dermal side of the epidermis has an irregular contour. The downward projections are called *rete ridges*, which appear 3-dimensionally as a Swiss cheese-like matrix with the holes filled by dome-shaped dermal papillae. This configuration helps to anchor the epidermis physically to the dermis. The pattern is most pronounced in areas subject to maximum friction, such as the palms and soles.

The cells in the epidermis undergo division and differentiation. Cell division occurs in the basal cell layer, and differentiation in the layers above it.

Cell division occurs in the basal cell layer.

2

TABLE 2.1 Skin functions

Function	Responsible Structure
Barrier	Epidermis
Physical	Stratum corneum
Light	Melanocytes
Immunologic	Langerhans cells
Tough flexible foundation	Dermis
Temperature regulation	Blood vessels
	Eccrine sweat glands
Sensation	Nerves
Grasp	Nails
Decorative	Hair
Unknown	Sebaceous glands
Insulation from cold and trauma	Subcutaneous fat
Calorie reservoir	Subcutaneous fat

STRUCTURE
Basal Cell Layer
The basal cells can be considered the 'stem cells' of the epidermis. They are the undifferentiated, proliferating cells. Daughter cells from the basal cell layer migrate upward and begin the process of differentiation. In normal skin, cell division does not take place above the basal cell layer. It takes about 2 weeks for the cells to migrate from the basal cell layer to the top of the granular cell layer, and a further 2 weeks for the cells to cross the stratum corneum to the surface, where they finally are shed. Injury and inflammation increase the rate of proliferation and maturation (**Fig. 2.1**).

Stratum Spinosum
This layer lies above the basal layer and is composed of *keratinocytes*, which differentiate from the basal cells beneath them. The keratinocytes produce keratin, a fibrous protein that is the major component of the horny stratum corneum. The stratum spinosum derives its name from the 'spines,' or intercellular bridges, that extend between keratinocytes and are visible with light microscopy. Ultrastructurally, these are composed of desmosomes, which are extensions from keratin within the keratinocyte; functionally, they hold the cells together (**Fig. 2.2**).

Keratinization begins in the stratum spinosum.

Stratum Granulosum
The process of differentiation continues in the stratum granulosum, or granular cell layer, in which the cells acquire additional keratin and become more flattened. In addition, they contain distinctive dark granules, seen easily on light microscopy, that are composed of keratohyalin. Keratohyalin contains two proteins, one of which is called profilaggrin, the precursor to filaggrin. As its name suggests, filaggrin plays an important role in the aggregation of keratin filaments in the stratum corneum. The other protein is called *involucrin* (from the Latin for 'envelope'), and plays a role in the formation of the cell envelope of cells in the stratum corneum. Ichthyosis vulgaris (*ichthys*, Greek for 'fish') is an inherited dry skin condition secondary to deficient filaggrin production, as noted on light microscopy of a skin biopsy by a reduced or absent granular layer (**Fig. 2.3**).

Granular cells also contain lamellar granules, which are visualized with electron microscopy. Lamellar granules contain polysaccharides, glycoproteins, and lipids that extrude into the intercellular space and ultimately are thought to help form the 'cement' that holds together the stratum corneum cells. Degradative enzymes also are found within the granular cells; these are responsible for the eventual destruction of cell nuclei and intracytoplasmic organelles.

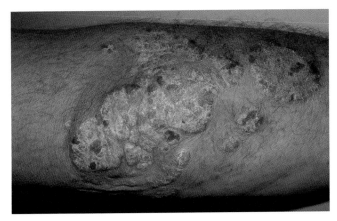

FIGURE 2.1 Psoriasis – an autoimmune disorder characterized by thickened epidermis and increased scale.

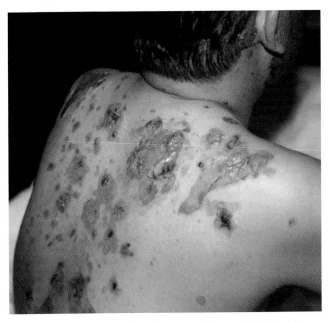

FIGURE 2.2 Pemphigus vulgaris – an autoimmune blistering disease wherein antibodies directed against desmosomes result in keratinocyte separation in stratum spinosum.

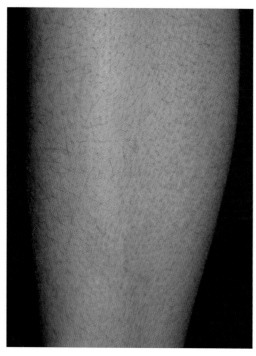

FIGURE 2.3 Ichthyosis vulgaris – a common autoimmune inherited dry skin condition secondary to deficient filaggrin production. Note 'fish-like' scale on the anterior shin.

Granular cells contain keratohyalin and lamellar granules.

Stratum Corneum

A remarkably abrupt transition occurs between the viable, nucleated cells at the top of the granular cell layer and the dead cells of the stratum corneum (**Fig. 2.4**). The cells in the stratum corneum are large, flat, polyhedral, plate-like envelopes filled with keratin. They are stacked in vertical layers that range in thickness from 15 to 25 layers on most body surfaces to as many as 100 layers on the palms and soles. The cells are held together by a lipid-rich cement in a fashion similar to 'bricks and mortar.' The tightly packed, keratinized envelopes in the stratum corneum provide a semi-impenetrable layer that constitutes the major physical barrier of the skin.

The stratum corneum is the major physical barrier.

The epidermis, then, is composed of cells that divide in the basal cell layer (basal cells), keratinize in the succeeding layers (keratinocytes), and eventuate into the devitalized, keratin-filled cells in the stratum corneum.

OTHER CELLULAR COMPONENTS

In addition to basal cells and keratinocytes, two other cells are located in the epidermis: melanocytes and Langerhans cells.

Melanocytes

Melanocytes are dendritic, pigment-producing cells located in the basal cell layer (**Figs 2.4, 2.5**). They protect the skin from ultraviolet radiation. Individuals with little or no pigment develop marked sun damage and numerous skin cancers. The dendrites extend into the stratum spinosum and serve as conduits, through which pigment granules are transferred to their neighboring keratinocytes. The granules are termed *melanosomes*, and the pigment within is melanin, which is synthesized from tyrosine. Melanosomes are preferentially situated above the nucleus to protect the DNA.

People of all races have a similar number of melanocytes. The difference in skin pigmentation depends on (1) the number and size of the melanosomes and (2) their dispersion in the skin. In darkly pigmented skin, melanosomes are larger in size and more numerous compared with melanosomes in lightly pigmented skin. Sunlight stimulates melanocytes to increase pigment production and disperse their melanosomes more widely.

Langerhans Cells

Langerhans cells are dendritic cells in the epidermis that have an immunologic function (**Fig. 2.4**). They are derived from the bone marrow and constitute about

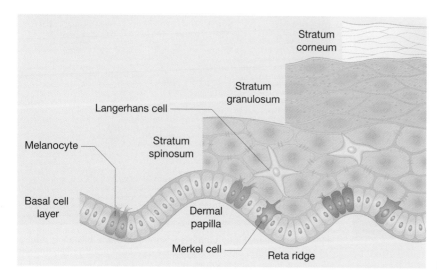

FIGURE 2.4 Epidermis.

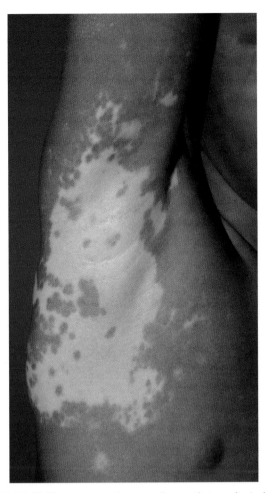

FIGURE 2.5 **Vitiligo** – an autoimmune disease that results in loss of melanocytes.

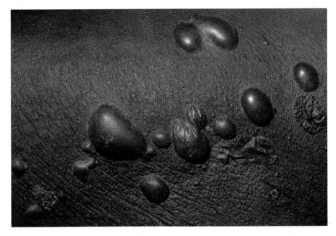

FIGURE 2.6 **Bullous pemphigoid** – the most common autoimmune blistering disease in the elderly secondary to immune disruption of the hemidesmosome. Note bullae on inner thigh, a characteristic location.

5% of the cells within the epidermis. On electron microscopic examination, characteristic 'tennis racket'-shaped granules are seen. Langerhans cells are identical to tissue macrophages and present antigens to lymphocytes, with which they interact through specific surface receptors. As such, Langerhans cells are important components of the immunologic barrier of the skin.

> Langerhans cells are the first line of immunologic defense in the skin.

Merkel Cells

Merkel cells are located in the basal cell layer. They are more numerous on the palms and soles and are connected to keratinocytes by desmosomes. Merkel cells function as mechanoreceptors. Merkel cell carcinoma is a rare skin cancer with a high mortality rate, as discussed in Chapter 5.

DERMAL–EPIDERMAL JUNCTION – THE BASEMENT MEMBRANE ZONE

The interface between the epidermis and dermis is called the *basement membrane zone*. With light microscopy, it is visualized only as a fine line. However, electron microscopic examination reveals four regions: (1) keratin filaments in the basal keratinocytes attach to hemidesmosomes (electron-dense units), which in turn attach to anchoring filaments in (2) the *lamina lucida*. The lamina lucida is a relatively clear (lucid) zone traversed by delicate anchoring filaments that connect hemidesmosome of basal cells to (3) the *lamina densa*; the lamina densa is an electron-dense zone composed primarily of type IV collagen derived from epidermal cells and (4) *anchoring fibrils*, which are thick fibrous strands, composed of type VII collagen, and located in the sublamina densa region of the papillary dermis. The basement membrane zone serves as the 'glue' between the epidermis and dermis, and is the site of blister formation in numerous diseases (**Fig. 2.6**). Hence, its structure, composition, and immunologic make-up continue to be investigated intensely.

DERMIS

> ### Key Points
>
> 1. Provides structural integrity and is biologically active
> 2. The primary components of the dermal matrix are collagen, elastin, and extrafibrillar matrix
> 3. Collagen is the principal component of the dermis and represents 70% of skin's dry weight

The dermis is a tough, but elastic, support structure that contains blood vessels, nerves, and cutaneous appendages. It provides structural integrity and is biologically active by interacting and regulating the functions of cells (i.e., tissue regeneration). The dermis ranges in thickness from 1 to 4 mm, making it much thicker than the epidermis, which in most areas is only about as thick as this piece of paper (**Fig. 2.7**). The dermal matrix is composed primarily of collagen fibers (principal component), elastic fibers, and ground substance (now called extrafibrillar matrix), which are synthesized by dermal fibroblasts. Collagen accounts for 70% of the dry weight of skin. Collagen and elastic fibers are fibrous proteins that form the strong, yet compliant skeletal matrix. In the uppermost part of the dermis (papillary dermis), collagen fibers are fine and loosely arranged. In the remainder of the dermis (reticular dermis), the fibers are thick and densely packed (**Fig. 2.8**). Elastic fibers are located primarily in the reticular dermis, where they are thinner and more loosely arranged than collagen fibers. The extrafibrillar matrix fills the space between fibers. It is a non-fibrous material made up of several different mucopolysaccharide molecules, collectively called proteoglycans or glycosaminoglycans. The extrafibrillar matrix imparts to the dermis a more liquid quality, which facilitates movement of fluids, molecules, and inflammatory cells.

Structural components of the dermis:
1. Collagen
2. Elastic fibers
3. Extrafibrillar matrix

Nerves and blood vessels course through the dermis, and a layer of subcutaneous fat lies below it (**Fig. 2.9**).

Free nerve endings are the most important sensory receptors.

Nerves

The skin is a major sensory receptor. Without the sensations of touch, temperature, and pain, life would be less interesting and more hazardous. Sensations are detected in the skin by both free nerve endings and more complicated receptors that are corpuscular in structure. The free nerve endings are the more widespread and appear to be more important. The nerve supply of the skin is

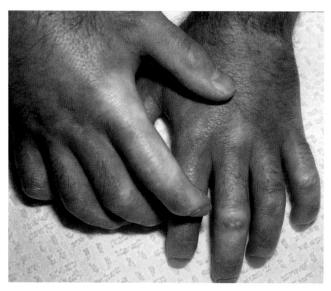

FIGURE 2.7 **Systemic scleroderma** – an increase in the number and activity of fibroblasts produces excessive collagen and results in dermal thickening.

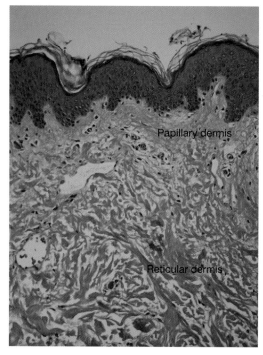

FIGURE 2.8 **Papillary dermis** – fine and loose collagen strands. Reticular dermis – thick and dense collagen strands.

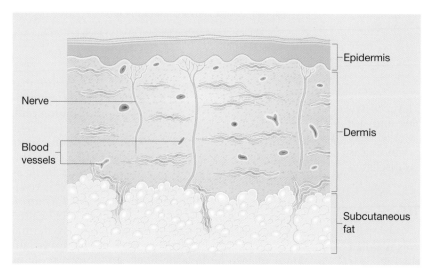

FIGURE 2.9 **Dermis and subcutaneous fat.**

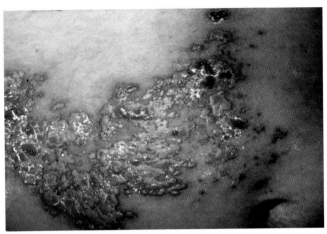

FIGURE 2.10 **Herpes zoster** – reactivation of varicella-zoster virus in sensory nerve ganglia results in a painful, vesicular, dermatomal eruption.

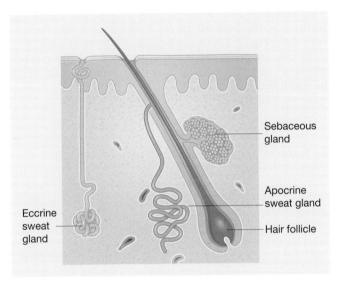

FIGURE 2.11 **Sweat gland, apocrine gland, and hair follicle with sebaceous gland.**

segmental (dermatomal), with considerable overlap between segments (**Fig. 2.10**).

Blood Vessels

The blood vessels in the skin serve two functions: nutrition and temperature regulation. The epidermis has no intrinsic blood supply and therefore depends on the diffusion of nutrients and oxygen from vessels in the papillary dermis. Blood vessels in the dermis also supply the connective tissue and appendageal structures located therein.

> Functions of blood vessels:
> 1. To supply nutrition
> 2. To regulate temperature

The vasculature of the skin is arranged into two horizontal plexuses that are interconnected. The superficial plexus is located at the lower border of the papillary dermis, and the deep plexus is located in the reticular dermis. Temperature regulation is achieved through shunts between the plexuses. Increased blood flow in the superficial plexus permits heat loss, whereas shunting of blood to the deep plexus conserves heat.

SKIN APPENDAGES

> ### Key Points
>
> 1. Eccrine glands help to regulate body temperature
> 2. Apocrine sweat glands depend on androgens for their development
> 3. The stem cells of the hair follicle reconstitute the non-permanent portion of the cycling hair follicle
> 4. Sebaceous glands are under androgen control
> 5. Nails, like hair, are made of keratin

The skin appendages are the eccrine and apocrine sweat glands, hair follicles, sebaceous glands, and nails. They are epidermally derived but, except for nails, are located in the dermis.

Eccrine Sweat Glands

For physically active individuals and for people living in hot climates, the eccrine sweat glands are physiologically the most important skin appendage. They are activated by emotional and thermal stimuli. Cholinergic innervation is responsible for physiologic eccrine secretion. Botulinum toxin type A (Botox) injected intradermally can treat axillary hyperhidrosis by blocking acetylcholine action. Eccrine sweat glands help to regulate body temperature by excreting sweat onto the surface of the skin, from which the cooling process of evaporation takes place. Two to three million eccrine sweat glands are distributed over the entire body surface, with a total secretory capacity of 10 L of sweat per day. The secretory portion of the sweat apparatus is a coiled tubule located deep in the dermis. The sweat is transported through the dermis by a sweat duct, which ultimately twists a path through the epidermis (**Fig. 2.11**). Sweat secreted in the glandular portion is isotonic to plasma but becomes hypotonic by the time it exits the skin as a result of ductal reabsorption of electrolytes. Hence, the sweat apparatus is similar to the mechanism in the kidney, that is, glandular (glomerular) excretion is followed by ductal reabsorption.

> Eccrine sweat glands help to regulate temperature and are under cholinergic innervation.

Apocrine Sweat Glands

In humans, apocrine sweat glands are androgen dependent for their development and serve no known useful function, although they are responsible for body odor. The odor actually results from the action of surface skin bacteria on excreted apocrine sweat, which itself is odorless. Apocrine sweat glands are located mainly in the axillary and anogenital areas. The secretory segment of an apocrine gland is also a coiled tubule located deep in the dermis. However, unlike in eccrine glands, in which the secretory cells remain intact, in apocrine glands the secretory cells 'decapitate' their luminal (apical) portions as part of the secretory product (**Fig. 2.11**). The apocrine duct then drains the secreted sweat into the midportion of a hair follicle, from which it ultimately reaches the skin surface.

Bacterial action on apocrine sweat causes body odor.

Hair Follicle

In most mammals, hair serves a protective function, but in humans it is mainly decorative.

Hair follicles are distributed over the entire body surface, except the palms and soles. Hair comes in two sizes: (1) vellus hairs, which are short, fine, light colored, and barely noticed; and (2) terminal hairs, which are thicker, longer, and darker than the vellus type. Terminal hairs in some locations are hormonally influenced and do not appear until puberty, e.g., beard hair in males, and pubic and axillary hair in both sexes.

Types of hair:
1. Vellus (light and fine)
2. Terminal (dark and thick)

A hair follicle can be viewed as a specialized invagination of the epidermis (**Fig. 2.11**), with a population of cells at the bottom (hair bulb) that are replicating even more actively than normal epidermal basal cells. These cells constitute the hair matrix. As with basal cells in the epidermis, the matrix cells first divide and then differentiate, ultimately forming a keratinous hair shaft. Melanocytes in the matrix contribute pigment, the amount of which determines the color of the hair. As the matrix cells continue to divide, hair is pushed outward and exits through the epidermis at a rate of about 1 cm per month. Hair growth in an individual follicle is cyclical, with a growth (anagen) phase, a transitional (catagen) phase, and a resting (telogen) phase. The lengths of the phases vary from one area of the body to another. On the scalp, e.g., the anagen phase lasts for about 3 years, the catagen phase for about 3 weeks, and the telogen phase for about 3 months. The length of anagen phase varies from individual to individual, explaining why some persons can grow hair longer than others.

Hair growth cycles through growth (anagen), transitional (catagen), and resting (telogen) phases.

At the end of the anagen phase, growth stops and the hair follicle enters the catagen and telogen phase, during which the matrix portion and lower two-thirds of the hair follicle shrivels and the hair within the follicle is shed. Subsequently, through mesenchymal interaction

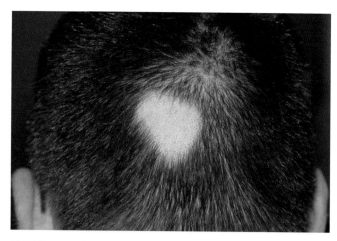

FIGURE 2.12 Alopecia areata – autoimmune condition resulting in nonscarring circular patches of alopecia.

with the hair follicle stem cells, a new hair matrix is formed at the bottom of the follicle, and the cycle is repeated (**Fig. 2.12**). At any time, 80–90% of scalp hair is in the anagen phase and 10–20% is in the telogen phase, thus accounting for a *normal* shedding rate of 25 to 100 hairs per day.

Normally, 25–100 hairs are shed from the scalp each day.

As shown in **Figure 2.11**, the hair follicle is situated in the dermis at an angle. Not shown is an attached arrector pili muscle. When this muscle contracts, the hair is brought into a vertical position, giving a 'goose flesh' appearance to the skin. The stem cells of the hair follicle are located in the 'bulge' area of the follicle, where the arrector pili muscle inserts into the hair follicle. The stem cells are important for reconstituting the non-permanent portion of the cycling hair follicle.

Sebaceous Glands

Sebaceous glands produce an oily substance termed *sebum*, the function of which is unknown. In fact, the skin of children and the palmar and plantar skin of adults function well without sebum.

Sebaceous glands are part of the *pilosebaceous unit* and so are found wherever hair follicles are located. In addition, ectopic sebaceous glands are often found on mucous membranes, where they may form small yellow papules called *Fordyce spots*. In the skin, sebaceous glands are most prominent on the scalp and face, and are moderately prominent on the upper trunk. The size and secretory activity of these glands are under androgen control. The sebaceous glands in newborns are enlarged owing to maternal hormones, but within months, the glands shrink (**Fig. 2.13**). They enlarge again in preadolescence from stimulation by adrenal androgens and reach full size at puberty, when gonadal androgens are produced.

Sebaceous glands are androgen dependent.

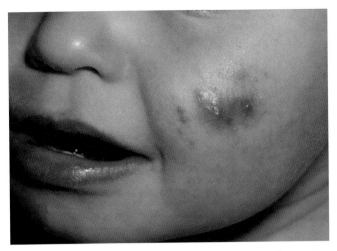

FIGURE 2.13 **Infantile acne** – a common disorder affecting the pilosebaceous unit. Maternal androgens are influential.

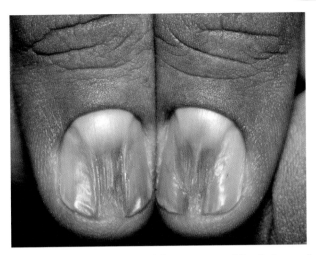

FIGURE 2.15 **Lichen planus** – an inflammatory condition that normally affects the skin and mucous membranes, but can affect the nail matrix and cause dystrophic nails.

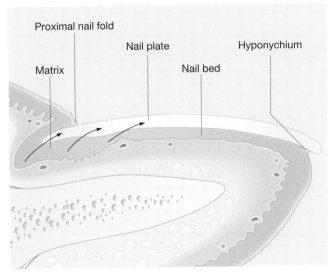

FIGURE 2.14 **Normal nail.**

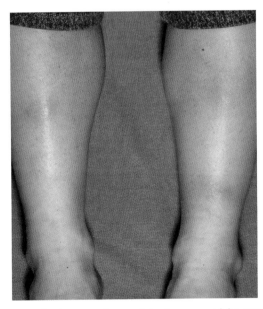

FIGURE 2.16 **Erythema nodosum.** Subcutaneous nodules most commonly seen on shins of women after starting birth control pills which results from inflammation concentrated in the fibrous septa that separate the aggregated fat cells or lobules.

The lipid-laden cells in the sebaceous glands are wholly secreted (holocrine secretion) to form sebum. Triglycerides compose the majority of the lipid found in sebaceous gland cells. From the sebaceous glands, sebum drains into the hair follicle (**Fig. 2.11**), from which it exits onto the surface of the skin.

Nails

Nails, like hair, are made of keratin, which is formed from a matrix of dividing epidermal cells (**Fig. 2.14**). Nails, however, are hard and flat, and lie parallel to the skin surface. Located at the ends of fingers and toes, they facilitate fine grasping and pinching maneuvers.

Nail is made of keratin produced in the matrix.

The *nail plate* is a hard, translucent structure composed of keratin. It ranges in thickness from 0.3 to 0.65 mm.

Fingernails grow at a continuous rate of about 0.1 mm/day, and toenails at a slightly slower rate.

Four epithelial zones are associated with the nail:

1. The *proximal nail fold* helps to protect the matrix. The stratum corneum produced there forms the cuticle.
2. The *matrix* produces the nail plate from its rapidly dividing, keratinizing cells. Most of the matrix underlies the proximal nail fold, but on some digits (especially the thumb) it extends under the nail plate, where it is grossly visible as the white lunula. The most proximal portion of the matrix forms the top of the nail plate; the most distal portion forms the bottom of the nail plate (**Fig. 2.15**).

3. The epithelium of the *nail bed* produces a minimal amount of keratin, which becomes tightly adherent to the bottom of the nail plate. The pink color of a nail is due to the vascularity in the dermis of the nail bed.
4. The epidermis of the *hyponychium* underlies the free distal edge of the nail plate. Stratum corneum produced there forms a cuticle to seal the junction of the distal nail bed and nail plate.

SUBCUTANEOUS FAT

A layer of subcutaneous fat lies between the dermis and the underlying fascia. It helps to insulate the body from cold, cushions deep tissues from blunt trauma, and serves as a reserve source of energy for the body. Biologically active fat cells play a role in hormone messaging, as evidenced by metabolic disturbances in obese children and adolescents with peripheral insulin resistance. Within the subcutaneous fat layer, aggregates of fat cells (lipocytes) are separated by fibrous septa that are traversed by blood vessels and nerves (**Fig. 2.16**).

Subcutaneous fat:
1. Insulates
2. Absorbs trauma
3. Is a reserve energy source
4. Is biologically active

Principles of Diagnosis 3

Chapter Contents

Key Points

1. Morphologic appearance is critical in making the diagnosis
2. Skin diseases can be divided into growths and rashes

ABSTRACT

The approach to a patient with skin disease does not differ markedly from the approach to any other patient. Data are collected from a history and physical examination (and sometimes from the laboratory), a differential diagnosis is generated, and the best diagnosis is selected.

Steps in dermatologic diagnosis:
1. History
2. Physical – identify the morphology of basic lesion
3. Consider clinicopathologic correlations
4. Configuration or distribution of lesions (when applicable)
5. Laboratory tests

In history taking, a modified format is suggested. Instead of beginning with an exhaustive interrogation, it is more efficient to divide the history into a preliminary and a follow-up format. You should sit, face the patient, let the patient talk, listen, show empathy, and then clarify with questions.

The most important part of the physical examination is inspection. Dermatology is a visual specialty, and diagnosis rests heavily on skin inspection. Unfortunately, although the skin is the most visible organ of the body, in a routine physical examination it often is the one most overlooked. Skin lesions need to be looked *for*, not *at*. Just as the examiner hears only the subtle heart sounds for which he or she listens, so will a clinician see on the skin only the lesions for which he or she searches. We need to train our eyes to see the skin lesions before us and ultimately be able to recognize them.

Dermatologic diagnosis depends on the examiner's skill in skin inspection.

We have divided skin disorders into two broad categories: growths and rashes. A *growth* is a discrete lesion resulting from proliferation of one or more of the skin's components. A *rash* is an inflammatory process that usually is more widespread than a growth. For both skin growths and rashes, the most important task is to characterize the clinical appearance of the basic lesion, that is, to identify its morphology. The pathophysiologic processes responsible for the clinical lesion must then be considered. These clinicopathologic correlations are emphasized in the diagnostic approach presented in this book. For skin rashes, important diagnostic information can sometimes also be obtained by noting the manner in which the lesions are arranged or distributed.

After the history and physical examination have been completed, laboratory tests may be indicated. In dermatology, these are usually simple office procedures that can provide valuable information needed either to confirm or to establish a diagnosis in selected disorders.

11

HISTORY

> ## Key Points
>
> 1. Let the patient talk uninterruptedly in the beginning
> 2. Clarify duration, symptoms, distribution, and prior treatment
> 3. Expand the history based on the differential diagnosis

In medicine, the traditional approach is to take the history before doing the physical examination. Some dermatologists prefer to reverse this order. We find it most useful to ask questions both before and after the examination. With this approach, a preliminary history is taken, in which several general questions are asked of all patients. Depending on the physical findings, more selective questions may be asked subsequently. For example, a history of sexual contacts would be inappropriate for an 82-year-old invalid complaining of an itching scalp, but would be indicated for a patient with an indurated ulcer on the penis.

PRELIMINARY HISTORY

In addition to its diagnostic value, a preliminary history also helps to establish rapport with the patient. The short-cut of examining the skin without expressing an interest in the person will often be found wanting, especially by the patient. This initial history is composed of two parts that correlate with the chief complaint and the history of the present illness in the standard history format.

> The initial history can be abbreviated by asking four general questions:
> 1. How long?
> 2. Where affected?
> 2. Does it itch or other symptoms?
> 3. How have you treated it?

Chief Complaint

In eliciting the chief complaint, one can often learn much by asking an open-ended question, such as, 'What is your skin problem?' This is followed by four general questions regarding the history of the present illness.

History of the Present Illness

The general questions concern onset and evolution of the condition, distribution, symptoms, and treatment to date.

Onset and Evolution. 'When did it start? Has it gotten better or worse?' Answers to these questions determine the duration of the disorder and how the condition has evolved over time. For most skin conditions, this is important information.

Symptoms. 'Does it bother you?' is an open-ended way of asking about symptoms. For skin disorders, the most common symptom is itching. If the patient does not respond to the general symptom question, you may want to ask specifically, *'Does it itch?'* Questions concerning systemic symptoms (e.g., 'How do you feel otherwise?') are not applicable for most skin diseases and are more appropriately reserved until after the physical examination.

Treatment to Date. The question, 'How have you treated it?' results in an incomplete response from almost all patients. For skin disease, one is particularly interested in learning what topical medications have been applied. Many patients do not consider over-the-counter preparations important enough to mention. The same applies for some systemic medications. Providing the patient with specific examples of commonly used topical and systemic medications, such as calamine lotion and aspirin, may jog a patient's memory enough to recall similar products that they may have used. It is important to inquire about medications, not only because they cause some conditions, but also because they may aggravate many others. For example, contact dermatitis initially induced by poison ivy may be perpetuated by contact allergy to an ingredient in one of the preparations used in treatment.

After the skin examination, one may need to return to the treatment question if any suspicion exists that a medication is causing or contributing to the disorder. Interestingly, a patient often recalls using pertinent medication only when he or she is asked the question again.

> Persistence is often required in eliciting a complete medication history.

Finally, at the end of the visit, when one is ready to prescribe medications for the patient, it is helpful to know what medications have already been used. This approach avoids the potentially awkward situation in which a patient replies to your enthusiastic recommendation of your favorite therapy with, 'I've already tried that and it didn't work!'

FOLLOW-UP HISTORY

After the initial history and physical examination, it is hoped that a diagnosis, or at least a differential diagnosis, has been formulated. With a diagnosis in mind, more focused questions may be necessary. This questioning may include obtaining more details about the history of the present illness or may be directed toward eliciting specific information from other categories of the traditional medical history, including past medical history, review of systems, family history, and social history. The following serve only as examples for the use of focused questions.

Past Medical History

After the physical examination, one may want to learn more about the patient's general health. For example, in a patient with suspected herpes zoster, a past history of chickenpox would be of interest. We have discussed how topically applied and systemically administered medications often contribute to skin conditions. Skin findings may encourage further pursuit of these possibilities. For example, in a patient with a generalized erythematous rash or hives, systemic drugs should be high on the list of possible causes. Because drugs can cause virtually any type of skin lesion, it is useful to consider drug eruptions in the differential diagnosis of almost any skin disease. It may also be helpful to ascertain whether the patient has any known allergies, in order to determine whether any medications are currently being used that could produce a cross-reaction.

> Drugs can cause all types of skin rash.

Review of Systems

In a patient with a malar rash, a diagnosis of systemic lupus erythematosus should be considered, and the examiner will want to question the patient further for symptoms of additional skin or other organ involvement, including Raynaud's phenomenon, photosensitivity, hair loss, mouth ulcers, and arthritis. In a patient with a generalized maculopapular eruption, the two most common causes are drugs and viruses, so the physician will want to inquire about both medication use and viral symptoms such as fever, malaise, and upper respiratory or gastrointestinal symptoms.

Family History

In certain cutaneous conditions, some knowledge of the family history may help in diagnosis. Innumerable inherited disorders have dermatologic expression. The following serve only as examples:

- In a child with a chronic itching eruption in the antecubital and popliteal fossae, atopic dermatitis is suspected. A positive family history for atopic diseases (atopic dermatitis, asthma, hay fever) supports the diagnosis.
- In a youngster with multiple café-au-lait spots, a diagnosis of neurofibromatosis is considered. A positive family history for this disorder, substantiated by examination of family members, helps to support the diagnosis of this dominantly inherited disease.

Knowledge of the family's present health is also important when considering infectious diseases. For example, impetigo can occur in several family members, and this knowledge may help in considering the diagnosis; it would certainly be important for treatment. Likewise, in a patient with suspected scabies, it is important to know, for both diagnostic and therapeutic purposes, whether other family members are itching.

Social History

In some disorders, knowledge of the patient's social history may be important. For example, a chronic skin ulcer from persistent herpes simplex infection is a sign of immunosuppression, particularly acquired immune deficiency syndrome (AIDS). Therefore, a patient with such an ulceration should be asked about high-risk factors for acquiring AIDS, including sexual behavior, intravenous drug abuse, and exposure to blood products.

> For persistent skin infections, consider the possibility of AIDS.

Another common occasion for probing into a patient's social history is when the patient is suspected of having contact dermatitis; this aspect of the social history could be subtitled the *skin exposure history*. Patients encounter potentially sensitizing materials both at work and at play. Industrial dermatitis is a leading cause of workers' disability. For chronic hand dermatitis, questions about occupational exposure are important and should be directed particularly to materials and substances the patient contacts either by handling or by immersion. Similarly, a patient presenting with an acute eruption characterized by streaks of vesicles should be queried regarding recent outdoor activities resulting in exposure to poison ivy or poison oak. Contact dermatitis is a common and challenging problem. On the part of the physician, it often requires painstaking efforts in a detective-type search to elicit from the patient an exposure history that fits the dermatitis.

> A complete 'skin exposure history' is required whenever contact dermatitis is suspected.

Some harbor the misconception that in dermatology, one needs only to glance at the skin to arrive at a diagnosis and that talking with the patient is superfluous. Although this is occasionally true, we hope that the previous examples serve to illustrate that this frequently is not the case. In fact, in some instances (and contact dermatitis is a good example), detailed historical information is essential to establish a diagnosis.

PHYSICAL EXAMINATION

Key Points

1. Complete skin examination is recommended at the first visit
2. Good lighting is critical
3. Describe the morphology of the eruption

The physical examination follows the preliminary history. For the skin to be inspected adequately, three essential requirements must be met: (1) an undressed patient, clothed in an examining gown; (2) adequate illumination, preferably bright overhead fluorescent lighting; and (3) an examining physician prepared to see what is there.

You should examine the entire mucocutaneous surface, but patients will be more firmly convinced of your sincere interest in their particular problems if you start by examining the affected areas before proceeding with the more complete examination.

At least for the initial examination, the patient needs to be disrobed so that the entire skin surface can be examined. Busy physicians who tend to overlook this rule will miss much. An occasional patient may be reluctant to comply, saying, 'My skin problem is only on my hands; why do you need to look at the rest of my skin?' We tell such patients that we have at least two reasons:

1. Other lesions may be found that 'go along with' the lesions on the hands, and help to confirm the diagnosis. For example, in a patient with sharply demarcated plaques on the palms, the finding of a few scaling plaques on the knees or a sharply marginated intergluteal plaque will help to substantiate a suspicion of psoriasis.
2. An important incidental skin lesion may be found. The finding of a previously undetected malignant melanoma on a patient's back is an example. We studied the yield from a complete skin examination in 1157 consecutive new dermatology patients and found an incidental skin malignancy in 22. Some 20 of these patients had basal cell carcinoma, one had melanoma, and one had Kaposi's sarcoma that served as the presenting manifestation of AIDS. A subsequent study of 874 patients reported an incidental skin cancer detection rate of 3.4%.

> The entire skin surface is examined for:
> 1. Lesions that may accompany the presenting complaint
> 2. Unrelated but important incidental findings

For the skin to be examined adequately, it must be properly illuminated. Natural lighting is excellent for this purpose but is difficult to achieve in most offices and hospital rooms. The alternative is bright overhead fluorescent lighting, supplemented with a movable incandescent lamp that is usually wall mounted. One additional illuminator that is often useful is a simple penlight. Either this or the movable incandescent lamp can be used as side-lighting to detect whether a lesion is subtly elevated. For this technique, the light is directed onto the lesion from an angle that is roughly parallel to the skin. If the lesion is elevated, a small shadow will be thrown, and the relief of the skin will be appreciated. The penlight also is useful for examining the mouth, an area that is sometimes overlooked but in which one may detect lesions that are helpful in diagnosing a cutaneous disorder.

> 'Side-lighting' helps to detect subtle elevations.

Another piece of examination equipment that is occasionally useful is the Wood's light, a long-wavelength ultraviolet 'black' light. Contrary to some popular misconceptions, this light does not enable one to diagnose most skin fungal infections; it detects fluorescence of affected hairs only in some, now uncommon, types of tinea capitis. The Wood's light is, however, still used to accentuate pigmentary alterations in the skin, such as vitiligo.

Except for provision of adequate illumination, minimal equipment is needed for examining the skin. A simple hand-held lens can be helpful. Enlarging the image may improve diagnostic accuracy. However, on some occasions, such as clarifying a burrow in scabies or detecting Wickham's striae in a lesion of lichen planus, a hand-held lens can be useful. For diagnosing pigmented growths, some dermatologists employ a dermatoscope. This is an illuminated hand-held magnifying device intended to help the clinician to diagnose melanoma clinically.

An adequate examination of the skin should actually be called a mucocutaneous examination so that one is reminded to include an examination of the mouth. Similarly, the scalp and nails should not be overlooked. Because both cutaneous and systemic diseases may be expressed in the nails and nail beds as well as in the mouth, inspection of these areas should be included in every cutaneous examination.

> The scalp, mouth, and nails should not be overlooked.

Physical examination depends largely on inspection, but one should not neglect the opportunity to palpate the skin as well. One should do hand hygiene prior to and after touching the patient. The two major purposes for this are: (1) to assess the texture consistency and tenderness of the skin lesions; and (2) to reassure patients that we are not afraid to touch their skin lesions – that they do not have some dreadful contagious disease. Nothing is more disquieting to a patient than to be cautiously approached with a gloved hand. For anogenital, mucosal, and all weeping lesions, gloving is necessary and expected, but for most other lesions, the physician learns more and the patient is less frightened if the touching is done without gloves. Palpation is the major method by which we evaluate not only the consistency (e.g., softness, firmness, fluctuance) but also the depth of a lesion.

> Palpation helps to:
> 1. Assess texture and consistency
> 2. Evaluate tenderness
> 3. Reassure patients that they are not contagious

After the patient is properly gowned and perfectly illuminated, for what do we inspect and palpate? The first and most important step is to characterize the appearance (i.e., identify the morphology) of each skin lesion. After the morphology of a lesion is identified, its clinicopathologic correlation can be considered.

> The most important task in the physical examination is to characterize the morphology of the basic lesion.

TERMINOLOGY OF SKIN LESIONS

Key Points

1. Primary lesions include macule, patch, papule, plaque, nodule, cyst, vesicle, pustule, ulcer, wheal, telangiectasia, burrow, and comedo
2. Secondary lesions include scale, crust, oozing, lichenification, induration, fissure, and atrophy

A special vocabulary is used in describing the morphologic appearances of skin lesions. These terms are illustrated and defined in **Figure 3.1**.

CLINICOPATHOLOGIC CORRELATIONS

Key Points

1. Envisioning the gross and microscopic morphology together helps to make the diagnosis
2. Rash or growth?
3. Epidermal, dermal, or subcutaneous?

The lesions defined in **Figure 3.1** result from alterations in one or more of the skin's structural components. For clinical diagnostic purposes, we try to envision what pathologic changes are associated with each clinical lesion (**Table 3.1**). Scale, lichenification, vesicles, bullae, pustules, and crusts represent epidermal alterations, whereas erythema, purpura, and induration reflect changes in the dermis. Such clinicopathologic correlations form the basis of the diagnostic approach. For example, scaling of a nodule suggests hyperkeratosis of the stratum corneum and, thus, an epidermal growth.

> Determine which of the skin components are involved in the clinical lesion.

TABLE 3.1 Clinicopathologic correlations

Skin Component	Pathologic Alteration	Clinical Manifestation
Epidermis		
Stratum corneum	Hyperkeratosis	Scale
Subcorneal epidermis	Hyperplasia Hyperplasia Disruptive inflammatory changes Dried serum	Lichenification Papules, plaques, and nodules Vesicles, bullae, and pustules Crusts
Melanocytes	Increased number or function Decreased number or function	Pigmented macules, papules, and nodules White spots
Dermis		
Blood vessels	Hyperplasia or inflammation Vasodilatation Hemorrhage Vasodilatation with edema	Macules, papules, and nodules Erythema Purpura Wheals
Nerves	Hyperplasia	Papules, nodules
Connective tissue	Hyperplasia Loss of epidermis and dermis	Induration, papules, nodules, and plaques Ulceration
Dermal appendages		
Pilosebaceous units	Hyperplasia Atrophy Hyperplasia or inflammation	Hirsutism Alopecia Comedones, papules, nodules, and cysts
Sweat glands	Hypersecretion Hyperplasia or inflammation	Hyperhidrosis Vesicles, papules, pustules, and cysts
Subcutaneous fat	Hyperplasia or inflammation	Induration and nodules

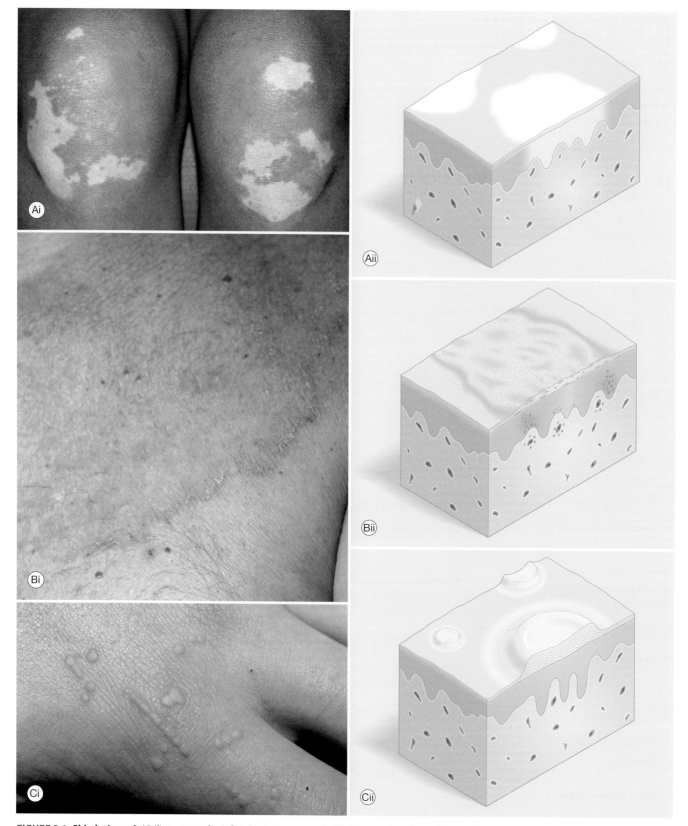

FIGURE 3.1 Skin lesions. A. Vitiligo – **macule**. A flat skin lesion recognizable because its color is different from that of the surrounding normal skin. The most common color changes are white (hypopigmented), brown (hyperpigmented), and red (erythematous and purpuric). **B.** Tinea corporis – **patch**. A macule with some surface change, either slight scale or fine wrinkling. **C.** Flat warts – **papules**. Small elevated skin lesions <0.5 cm in diameter.

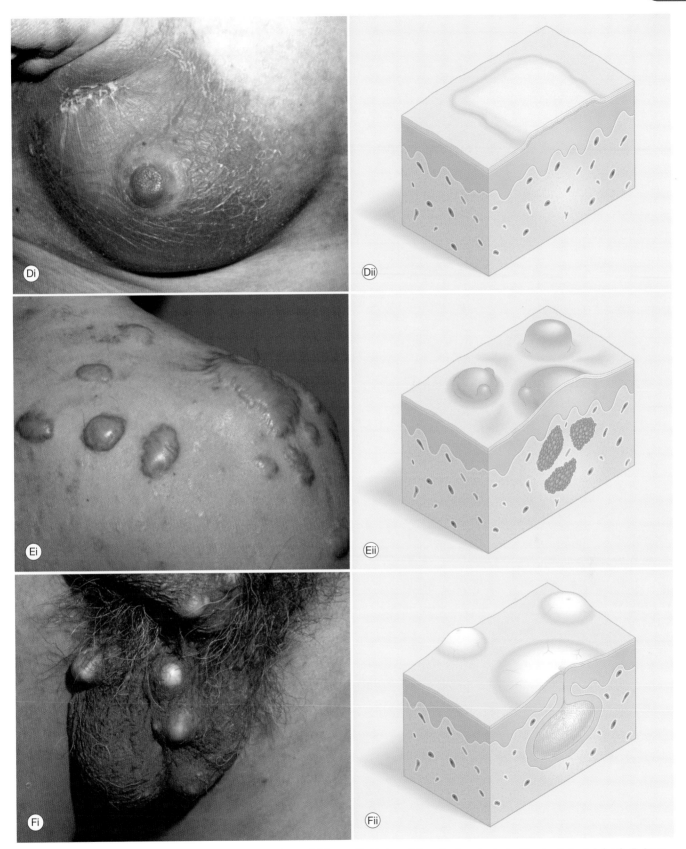

FIGURE 3.1 *Continued* **D.** Breast carcinoma – **plaque.** An elevated, 'plateau-like' lesion >0.5 cm in diameter but without substantial depth. **E.** Scars – **nodules.** Elevated, 'marble-like' lesions >0.5 cm in both diameter and depth. **F.** Epidermal inclusion **cysts.** Nodules filled with expressible material that is either liquid or semi-solid.

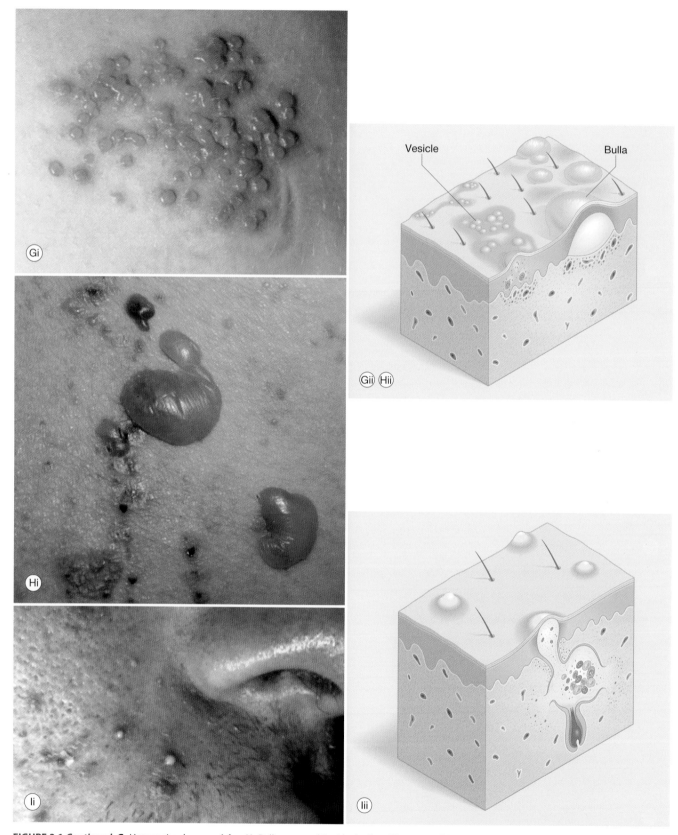

FIGURE 3.1 *Continued* G. Herpes simplex – **vesicles**. **H.** Bullous pemphigoid – **bullae**. Blisters are filled with clear fluid. Vesicles are <0.5 cm and bullae are >0.5 cm in diameter. **I.** Acne – **pustules**. Vesicles filled with cloudy or purulent fluid.

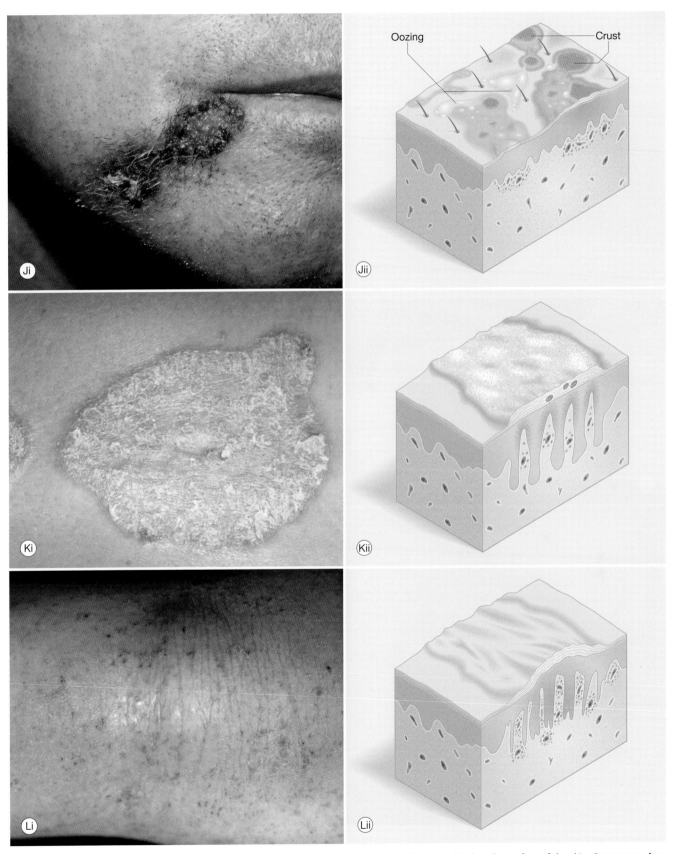

FIGURE 3.1 *Continued* **J.** Chronic herpes simplex – **crust**. Liquid debris (e.g., serum or pus) that has dried on the surface of the skin. Crust most often results from breakage of vesicles, pustules, or bullae. **K.** Psoriasis – **scale**. Visibly thickened stratum corneum. Scales are dry and usually whitish. These features help to distinguish scales from crusts, which are often moist and usually yellowish or brown. **L.** Atopic dermatitis – **lichenification**. *Epidermal thickening* characterized by (i) visible and palpable thickening of the skin with (ii) accentuated skin markings.

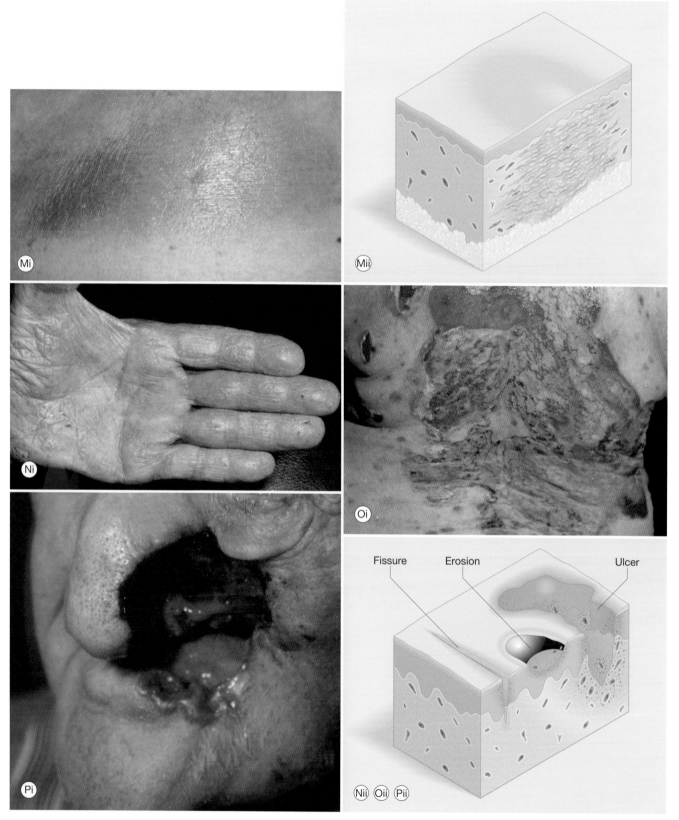

FIGURE 3.1 *Continued* **M.** Localized scleroderma (morphea) – **induration**. *Dermal thickening* resulting in the skin that *feels* thicker and firmer than normal. **N.** Hand dermatitis – **fissure**. **O.** Pemphigus vulgaris – **erosion**. **P.** Basal cell carcinoma – **ulcer**. A fissure is a thin, linear tear in the epidermis. An erosion is wider but is limited in depth, confined to the epidermis. An ulcer is a defect devoid of epidermis, as well as part or all of the dermis.

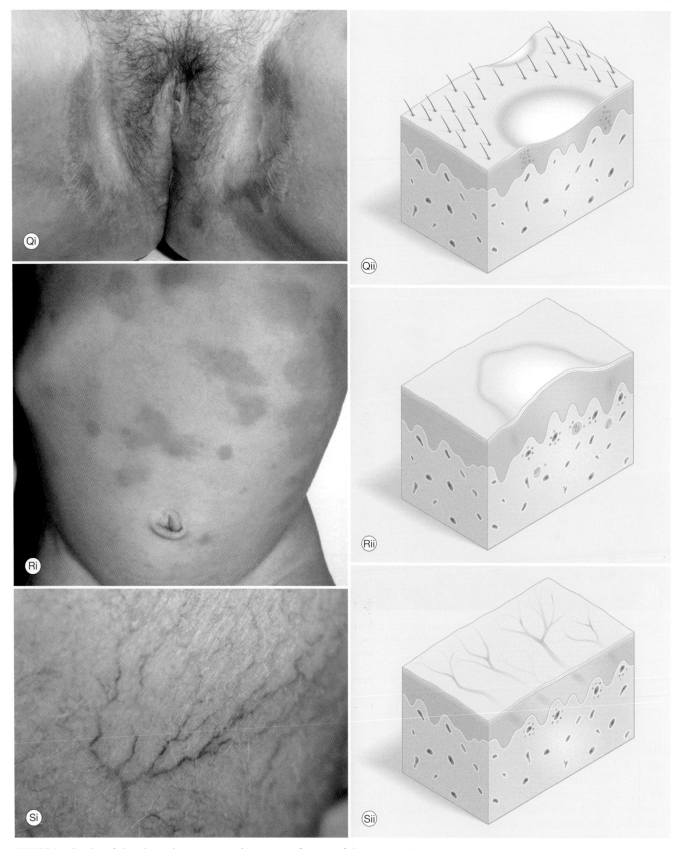

FIGURE 3.1 *Continued* Q. Lichen sclerosus et atrophicus – **atrophy**. Loss of skin tissue. With epidermal atrophy, the surface appears thin and wrinkled. Atrophy of the much thicker dermal layer results in a clinically detectable depression in the skin. **R.** Urticaria – **wheal**. A papule or plaque of dermal edema. Wheals (or *hives*) often have central pallor and irregular borders. **S.** Sun damage/aging – **telangiectasia**. Superficial blood vessels enlarged sufficiently to be clinically visible.

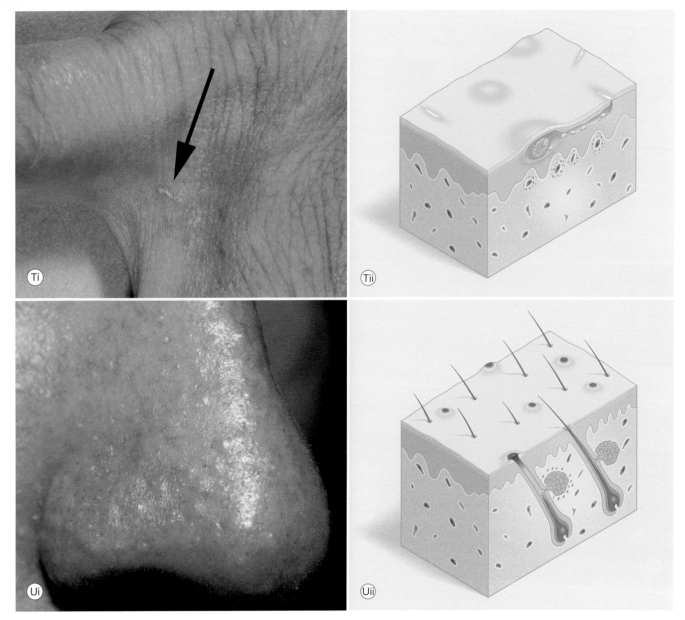

FIGURE 3.1 *Continued* **T.** Scabies – **burrow**. Serpiginous tunnel or streak (arrow) caused by a burrowing organism. **U.** Acne – **comedo** (plural, *comedones*). The non-inflammatory lesions of acne that result from keratin impaction in the outlet of the pilosebaceous canal.

Table 3.2 presents an algorithm for this approach and outlines the organization of the remainder of this book. Most skin disorders can be categorized first as proliferative 'growths' (neoplasms) or inflammatory 'rashes' (eruptions). The growths and rashes are then subdivided, depending on how they appear clinically and which structural component is involved pathologically.

> Growths are hyperplastic lesions; rashes are inflammatory.

GROWTHS

Growths are subdivided into epidermal, pigmented, and dermal or subcutaneous proliferative processes.

> Growths are subdivided into one of three categories:
> 1. Epidermal
> 2. Pigmented
> 3. Dermal or subcutaneous

TABLE 3.2 Schematic for diagnosis of skin diseases

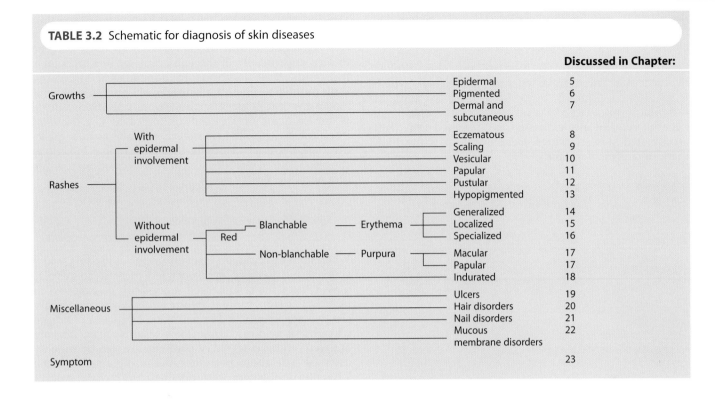

Epidermal growths result from hyperplasia of keratinocytes; many of these neoplasms have scaling surfaces. *Scale* accumulates when the rate of stratum corneum production exceeds the rate of shedding. *Hyperkeratosis* is another term used to describe excessive accumulation of keratin, the fibrous protein that makes up the stratum corneum. The term 'hyperkeratosis' is most often used with skin growths (e.g., seborrheic keratoses); 'scaling' is used to describe both growths and rashes.

> Scale and hyperkeratosis are both terms for excess stratum corneum.

Because the normal function of the epidermis is to produce the keratotic stratum corneum, hyperkeratosis may be expected in epidermal neoplasms. These proliferative processes may be benign (e.g., seborrheic keratoses), premalignant (e.g., actinic keratoses), or malignant (e.g., squamous cell carcinoma).

Hyperplasia of the subcorneal epidermis results in elevated lesions of the skin papules, plaques, and nodules. Benign growths originating in the epidermis often appear superficial. Malignant epidermal growths, by definition, have invaded the dermis, and they therefore feel *indurated*, a term used to designate thickening of the dermis.

> Malignant epidermal growths usually feel indurated, except for superficial basal and squamous cell carcinomas, which are patches.

Pigmented lesions result from increased melanin production or increased numbers of melanin-producing cells, and so may be either macular or papular. Freckles are common examples of hyperpigmented macules that result from increased melanin production. Nevi and melanomas are examples of growths characterized by increased numbers of melanin-producing cells. Nevi that are sufficiently cellular to impart a mass effect are elevated, and so appear clinically as hyperpigmented papules, plaques, or even nodules.

Dermal and subcutaneous growths result from *focal* proliferative processes in the dermis or subcutaneous fat. They appear most often as nodules, which are most fully appreciated by palpation. The proliferative elements that form nodules may be either endogenous (e.g., a dermatofibroma that results from the proliferation of dermal fibroblasts) or exogenous (e.g., a metastasis from an internal malignant disease) to the skin. Because often no surface markers exist to differentiate one dermal nodule from another, the definitive diagnostic test frequently must be a biopsy. This clinical point deserves emphasis: for undiagnosed skin nodules, particularly firm lesions, malignancy must be suspected, and a biopsy must be performed.

> A skin biopsy is often required for the diagnosis of a dermal nodule.

RASHES

For rashes, the first diagnostic step is to determine whether the epidermis is involved. Types of epidermal involvement are listed in **Table 3.2**. Although some rashes produce several epidermal changes, usually one change is distinctive or predominant.

Eczematous dermatitis is histologically characterized by epidermal intercellular edema (spongiosis), which is manifested clinically by vesicles, 'juicy' papules, or lichenification. *Lichenification* represents epidermal hyperplasia clinically expressed as thickened skin with accentuated skin markings. Lichenification is the hallmark of chronic dermatitis.

> Lichenification is the hallmark of chronic eczematous dermatitis.
>
> Epidermal rashes:
> 1. Eczematous
> 2. Scaling
> 3. Vesicular
> 4. Papular
> 5. Pustular
> 6. Hypopigmented
>
> Scale must be distinguished from crust

Scaling eruptions are the result of thickened stratum corneum. Scaling rashes can involve either focal areas or the entire cutaneous surface. Examples of the former are more common and are represented by the so-called papulosquamous diseases. These disorders are characterized by scaling (squamous) papules and plaques and patches. Psoriasis and fungal infections serve as examples. Ichthyosis ('fish skin') is an example of generalized scaling.

Scale is usually white or light tan and flakes off rather easily. These features help to distinguish scale from crust. *Crust* is dried serum and debris on the skin surface and is usually darker, most often yellow or brown; it is adherent and, when removed, a weeping base is revealed. The distinction between scale and crust is important because the differential diagnoses are entirely different. Crusts are associated with vesicles, bullae, pustules, and malignant growths.

Vesicles and bullae occur when fluid accumulates within or beneath the epidermis. They characterize a relatively small number of important dermatologic disorders, so are extremely helpful diagnostic findings. Vesicles and bullae occur either intraepidermally or subepidermally. The differential diagnoses are different for intraepidermal and subepidermal blisters, so it is important to try to distinguish them. Clinically, one clue is the fragility of the blister. Because of their more substantial roof, fresh subepidermal blisters are tense and less easily broken, whereas intraepidermal bullae are flaccid and easily ruptured. A biopsy of the *edge* of an early lesion confirms the clinical impression.

> Vesicles and bullae are important diagnostic findings.

Pruritic papules are produced by inflammation, predominantly in the dermis. Pustules occur when inflammatory cells aggregate within the epidermis. Pustules may be located superficially in the epidermis, or they may arise from superficial locations in appendageal structures. With purulence, one usually thinks of bacterial infection. This is an appropriate reflex, and Gram-staining or culture of the contents of a pustule is indicated if a bacterial infection is suspected. However, not all pustular processes are bacterial in origin; viral and fungal infections can also result in pustules, and acne is a common example of a non-infectious cause.

> Pustules often (but not always) indicate infection.

When melanin pigment is lost from the epidermis, white spots result. Because no associated increase in cellular mass occurs, hypopigmented lesions can be expected to be macular (not papular) white spots. Hypopigmentary changes are accentuated under Wood's light examination, whereby previously unnoticed lesions may become apparent and the degree of pigment loss can be roughly assessed. The more pronounced the pigment loss, the whiter the lesion appears under the scrutiny of the Wood's light.

> Hypopigmentary changes are accentuated with Wood's light examination.

Dermal rashes without epidermal involvement are either inflammatory or infiltrative; most are inflammatory. Inflammatory eruptions appear red because of vasodilatation of *dermal* blood vessels (the epidermis is devoid of vasculature). Redness in skin lesions can be due to either *erythema* or *purpura*. It is extremely important to differentiate between the two. With erythema, the increased blood in the skin is contained within dilated blood vessels. Therefore, erythema is *blanchable* (**Fig. 3.2**). With purpura, blood has extravasated from disrupted blood vessels into the dermis, and the lesion is non-blanchable

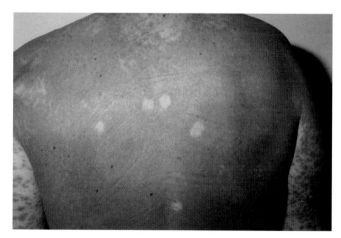

FIGURE 3.2 Erythema is blanchable, as demonstrated with fingertip pressure on the midback in this patient with a drug eruption.

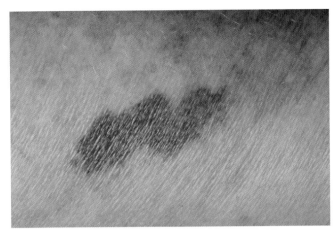

FIGURE 3.3 **Purpura is purple** and was not blanchable in this patient with fragile skin that had been injured.

(Fig. 3.3). The test for blanchability is called *diascopy*. It is performed by simply applying pressure with a finger or glass slide and observing color changes.

Erythematous rashes are subdivided into generalized, localized, and specialized (e.g., hives) types. A *wheal*, or hive, is a special type of blanchable, transient, erythematous lesion of the skin. Blood vessels in a wheal are dilated, and fluid leaks from them, causing edema in the surrounding dermis. This fluid is not compartmentalized as in vesicles or bullae, but rather is dispersed evenly throughout the dermal tissue. The result is an elevated erythematous lesion, often with central pallor that is due to the intense edema.

Purpuric rashes are subdivided into macular and papular categories. *Macular purpura* is flat and non-palpable, whereas *papular purpura* is elevated (sometimes subtly) and palpable. This clinical distinction is important because the differential diagnoses and clinical implications are different for the two types. Macular purpura occurs in two settings: (1) conditions associated with increased capillary fragility and (2) bleeding disorders. Macular hemorrhage is not accompanied by inflammation. In papular or palpable purpura, inflammatory changes are present in the vessel walls and are responsible for the elevation of the lesions. Disruption and necrosis of the blood vessels caused by an inflammatory reaction are called *necrotizing vasculitis*. This condition is usually immunologically mediated and can occur in numerous settings, such as sepsis, collagen vascular diseases, and, occasionally, drug reactions. In diagnosis of a patient with palpable purpura, such systemic processes must be excluded.

> Macular purpura is usually a sign of a bleeding disorder or vascular fragility; papular purpura indicates a necrotizing vasculitis, often systemic.

Rashes resulting from *infiltrative processes* in the dermis are much less common than inflammatory disorders. Clinically, they feel indurated. Induration, resulting from

increased amounts of collagen, is also called *sclerosis*. Scleroderma, an idiopathic disorder of increased collagen deposition, is an example.

MISCELLANEOUS CONDITIONS

Skin ulcers and disorders of hair, nails, and mucous membranes are easily recognizable and grouped as miscellaneous.

An *ulcer* is totally devoid of epidermis, and some or all of the dermal tissue is missing. Ulcers may extend down to underlying bone, as, e.g., in advanced decubitus ulcers. Malignant processes can result in ulcerations that do not heal. For this reason, all chronic ulcers should be biopsied.

> Chronic skin ulcers should undergo biopsy to rule out malignancy.

Too little hair is a much more common dermatologic complaint than too much hair. *Alopecia* means hair loss. For diagnostic purposes, it is helpful to classify alopecia as either *non-scarring* or *scarring*. Clinically, the distinction depends on whether follicular openings are visible. The differential diagnoses are different for each of these two categories.

> For alopecia, first determine whether it is scarring or non-scarring.

Most nail disorders are inflammatory and can affect the nail matrix, nail bed, or periungual skin (paronychia). Inflammation and scaling in the nail bed result in separation of the nail plate from the bed (onycholysis). Fungal infection and psoriasis are the most common causes.

The two most common manifestations of mucous membrane disorders are: (1) erosions and ulcerations; and (2) white lesions. On mucous membranes, whiteness represents hyperkeratosis, which is white because of maceration from continuous wetness.

CONFIGURATION OF SKIN LESIONS

Key Points

1. Configuration can help make the diagnosis
2. Morphology is more important than configuration

The diagnosis of rash is often aided by considering the configuration of the lesions or their distribution on the body surface. *Configuration* refers to the pattern in which skin lesions are arranged. The four most common patterns are listed in **Table 3.3**, along with examples of

TABLE 3.3 Some examples of configuration

Configuration	Morphology	Disease	Illustration
Linear	Vesicles Papules	Contact dermatitis[a] Psoriasis[b] Lichen planus[b] Flat warts	See **Fig. 3.4**
Grouped	Vesicles Papules	Herpes (simplex and zoster) Insect bites	See **Fig. 3.5**
Annular	Scaling	Tinea corporis	See **Fig. 3.6**
		Secondary syphilis	
		Subacute cutaneous lupus erythematosus	
	Dermal plaque	Granuloma annulare	
Geographic	Wheals Plaques	Urticaria Mycosis fungoides	See **Fig. 3.7**

[a]Typical for contact dermatitis from a plant resin (e.g., poison ivy).
[b]The Koebner reaction.

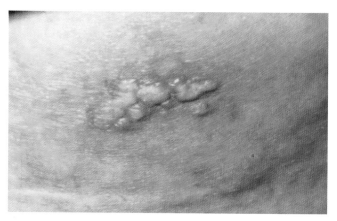

FIGURE 3.5 **Herpes simplex** – grouped vesiculopustules.

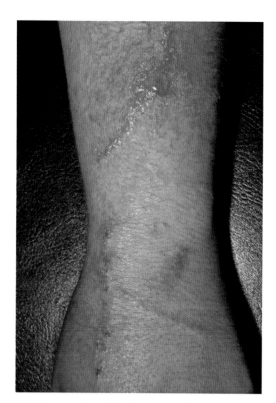

FIGURE 3.4 **Contact dermatitis** from poison ivy, demonstrating linear streaks of vesicles.

diseases that most often present in these configurations. Occasionally, a configuration is specific for a disease. For example, streaks of vesicles are characteristic of contact dermatitis from poison ivy or poison oak. More often, a configuration is not completely specific for a given disease, but may still be helpful in the diagnosis. For example, in psoriasis, scaling papules sometimes develop in streaks as a result of the Koebner reaction, in which lesions of a disorder develop after trauma, such as scratching.

As can be seen from **Table 3.3** (**Figs 3.4–3.7**), configuration considerations are sometimes diagnostically helpful, but morphology takes precedence. The annular impetigo shown in **Figure 3.8** illustrates this point. If the crust had been interpreted as scale, the annular lesions would almost certainly have been misdiagnosed as tinea corporis (ringworm). The honey-colored crust, however, should focus attention on the pustular nature of the primary process and raise the question of bacterial infection. So, for dermatologic diagnosis, the morphology of the primary lesion must be identified correctly before consideration is given to a specific configuration, if one is present. If a conflict appears to exist between the morphology and the configuration, more diagnostic weight should be given to the morphology.

Mucous membrane disorders:
1.   Erosions and ulcerations
2.   White lesions

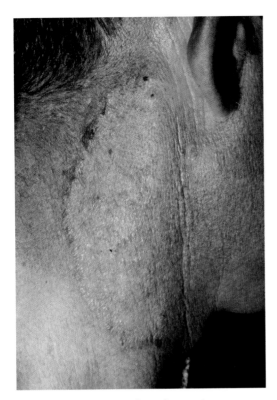

FIGURE 3.6 **Tinea corporis** – annular scaling patch.

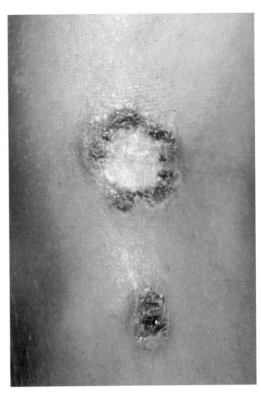

FIGURE 3.8 **Annular impetigo** – when morphology and configuration (or distribution) appear to conflict, the morphology takes precedence.

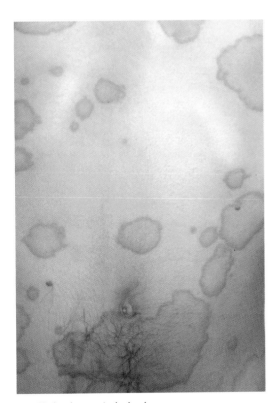

FIGURE 3.7 **Urticaria** – typical wheals.

DISTRIBUTION OF SKIN LESIONS

> **Key Points**
>
> 1. The distribution of skin lesions and the region affected can help to suggest or confirm a diagnosis

Many skin diseases have preferential areas of involvement, so the location of the eruption may help in diagnosis. A good example of this is herpes zoster, in which consideration of all three diagnostic criteria (morphology, configuration, and distribution) secures the diagnosis: vesicles in grouped configuration and dermatomal distribution are diagnostic for herpes zoster.

Many skin disorders have favored regional distributions (i.e., a propensity for a particular area of the body), such as the scalp, face, hands, groin, or feet. Sometimes, this propensity can be used as a starting point for developing a differential diagnosis. These 'regional' diagnoses are outlined in **Table 3.4**. For rashes that affect widespread areas, the distribution *pattern* may also aid in the diagnosis. This is particularly true for contact dermatitis, in which the location of the rash on the skin may be helpful, not only in leading one to suspect a contact origin but also in providing a clue about the nature of the contactant. For example, a rash on the earlobes and around the neck should lead one to suspect allergic contact dermatitis caused by the nickel present in jewelry.

TABLE 3.4 Regional diagnoses

Growths	Rashes	Growths	Rashes
Scalp		***Groin (inguinal)***	
Nevus	Seborrheic dermatitis (dandruff)	Skin tag	Intertrigo
Seborrheic keratosis	Psoriasis	Wart	Tinea cruris
Pilar cyst	Tinea capitis Folliculitis	Molluscum contagiosum	Candidiasis Pediculosis pubis Hidradenitis suppurativa Psoriasis Seborrheic dermatitis
Face		***Extremities***	
Nevus	Acne	Nevus	Atopic dermatitis
Lentigo	Acne rosacea	Dermatofibroma	Contact dermatitis
Actinic keratosis	Seborrheic dermatitis	Wart	Psoriasis
Seborrheic keratosis	Contact dermatitis (cosmetics)	Seborrheic keratosis	Insect bites
Sebaceous hyperplasia	Herpes simplex	Actinic keratosis	Erythema multiforme
Basal cell carcinoma	Impetigo	Xanthoma	Lichen planus (wrists and ankles) Actinic purpura (arms) Stasis dermatitis (legs) Vasculitis (legs) Erythema nodosum (legs)
Squamous cell carcinoma	Pityriasis alba		
Flat wart	Atopic dermatitis		
Nevus flammeus	Lupus erythematosus		
Trunk		***Hands (palmar)***	
Nevus	Acne	Wart	Nonspecific dermatitis Atopic dermatitis Psoriasis Tinea manuum Erythema multiforme Secondary syphilis
Skin tag	Tinea versicolor		
Cherry angioma	Psoriasis		
Seborrheic keratosis	Pityriasis rosea		
Epidermal inclusion cyst	Scabies	***Feet (dorsal)***	
Lipoma	Drug eruption	Wart	Contact dermatitis (shoe)
Basal cell carcinoma	Varicella	***Feet (plantar)***	
Keloid	Mycosis fungoides	Wart (plantar)	Contact dermatitis (shoe)
Neurofibroma	Secondary syphilis	Corn	Tinea pedis
Genitalia		Nevus	Nonspecific dermatitis Psoriasis Atopic dermatitis
Wart (condyloma acuminatum)	Herpes simplex Scabies		
Molluscum contagiosum	Psoriasis		
Seborrheic keratosis	Lichen planus Syphilis (chancre)		

Dermatologic Therapy and Procedures 4

Chapter Contents

ABSTRACT

Because the skin is so accessible, it can be treated with a variety of therapeutic options not available for use in diseases of internal organs. Drugs for dermatologic therapy can be administered topically, intralesionally, and systemically. In addition, physical modalities such as ultraviolet (UV) and ionizing radiation, surgery, laser, and cryotherapy can be easily administered.

At one time, dermatologic therapy was based largely on empiric approaches. However, much progress has been made in defining the scientific bases for numerous dermatologic treatments, resulting in a well-rounded rationale for choosing specific modalities.

The discussions in this chapter are limited to principles of external therapies unique to the skin. Other, more specific, topical therapies, such as those used for acne and for fungal diseases, as well as all systemic therapies, are discussed in chapters concerning the diseases in which they are used.

PRINCIPLES OF TOPICAL THERAPY

Key Points

1. Many types of drug are available in topical preparation
2. The vehicle is almost as important as the active ingredient
3. Give enough volume to treat the area of disease involvement adequately

A diverse group of medications is available in topical preparations, including antibiotics, antifungals, corticosteroids, acne preparations, sunscreens, cytotoxic agents, antipruritics, antiseptics, and pesticides. Topical therapy has the distinct advantage of delivering medications directly to the target organ. This route reduces the potential of systemic side-effects and toxicity seen with systemic therapy. The disadvantages of topical therapy are that it is time consuming, it can require large volumes of medication, it requires patient education in the technique of using topicals, and, at times, it is not esthetically pleasing because of staining or greasy preparations.

Advantages of topical medication:
1. Direct delivery to target tissue
2. Reduced systemic side-effects

For a medication to be effective topically, it must be absorbed into the skin. The main diffusion barrier of the skin is the stratum corneum, which is responsible for most of the protection offered by the skin against toxic agents, microorganisms, physical forces, and loss of body fluids.

Percutaneous absorption is influenced by: (1) physical and chemical properties of the active ingredient; (2) concentration; (3) vehicle; and (4) variations in type of skin. Cutaneous penetration of an active ingredient is enhanced when it has a low molecular weight, is lipid soluble, and is non-polar.

Percutaneous absorption depends on:
1. Active ingredient
2. Concentration
3. Vehicle
4. Skin type

Substances move across the stratum corneum by passive diffusion and follow a dose–response curve. The higher the *concentration* applied, the greater is the quantity of medication absorbed.

The *vehicle* is nearly as important as the active agent in the formulation of topical medications. This was realized when investigators found that the release of drugs varied greatly with different vehicles. The more occlusive the vehicle, the greater is the hydration of the stratum corneum and penetration of the medication. In addition, occlusive vehicles increase local skin temperature and prevent mechanical removal and evaporation of the active agent. An ointment is the most occlusive vehicle.

Percutaneous absorption is also influenced by the *location of the skin* to which it is applied. Passive diffusion is slow through the stratum corneum but rapid through the viable epidermis and papillary dermis. Therefore, absorption is generally low on the palm and sole, in which the stratum corneum is thick, and high on the scrotum, face, and ear, in which the stratum corneum is thin. Breakdown of the barrier function of the stratum corneum by disease, chemicals (soaps or detergents), and physical injury results in increased permeability.

The *selection of a topical preparation* must involve not only the active agent but also its other ingredients. The formulation of many topical medications is complex. A water-based preparation (cream), e.g., is composed of numerous ingredients, including the active agent, vehicle, and preservative, as well as an emulsifier to bring together the oil and water components of the preparation. As a general rule, it is better to select a commercially formulated preparation that is scientifically compounded than an extemporaneous preparation. The most frequently used vehicles are creams, ointments, lotions, foams, and gels.

Creams are semi-solid emulsions of oil in water that vanish when rubbed into the skin. They are white and non-greasy, and contain multiple ingredients. Preservatives are added to prevent the growth of bacteria and fungi. *Ointments* (oil-based) are emulsions of water droplets suspended in oil that do not rub in when applied to the skin. They are greasy and clear, and do not require preservatives. Ointments are selected when increased hydration, occlusion, and maximal penetration of the active ingredient are desired. *Lotions* are suspensions of

powder in water that may require shaking before application. Calamine lotion is the classic example. Itching is relieved by the cooling effect of water evaporation, and a protective layer of powder is left on the skin. Other liquids such as solutions, sprays, aerosols, and tinctures are characterized by ingredients dissolved in alcoholic vehicles that evaporate to leave the active agent on the skin. These agents are particularly useful for hairy areas. *Gels* are transparent and colorless semi-solid emulsions that liquefy when applied to the skin.

WRITING A DERMATOLOGIC PRESCRIPTION

Writing a prescription for a topical medication involves more than simply requesting the active ingredient. In addition to the medication, the vehicle, concentration, and amount must be indicated, as well as the instructions for use. Several concentrations and vehicles may be available for a given topical drug. The physician should indicate which vehicle the pharmacist is to dispense. Patient compliance is often directly related to their preference of vehicle. Greasy ointments on the face and hands can be unacceptable to the patient, and on the trunk or extremities may soak through clothing.

Elements of a topical prescription:
1. Medication
2. Vehicle
3. Concentration
4. Amount
5. How to apply

The type of error most frequently made in prescribing a topical drug probably involves the volume of medication to be dispensed. The size of the area being treated, the frequency of application, and the time between appointments or before predicted clearing of the eruption must all be taken into consideration when writing the prescription. An adequate quantity of medication is necessary to ensure the patient's compliance, successful therapy, and cost savings. Smaller volumes of medication are comparatively more expensive than larger volumes. One gram covers an area approximately 10×10 cm. A single application of a cream or ointment to the face or hands requires 2 g; for one arm or the anterior or posterior trunk, 3 g; for one leg, 4 g; and for the entire body, 30 g. Prescribing 15 g to be applied twice a day to an eruption that involves large portions of the trunk and extremities would be unreasonable; the patient would be required to return for refills twice daily.

Amount needed for one application:
- Face or hands: 2 g
- Arm: 3 g
- Leg: 4 g
- Whole body: 30 g

The physician needs to know the principles involved in writing a dermatologic prescription. For example, the patient's eruption is moderately severe and requires an intermediate-strength topical steroid such as triamcinolone acetonide. Triamcinolone acetonide is available in three concentrations: 0.025%, 0.1%, and 0.5%. A 0.1% concentration is effective for moderately severe eruptions and can generally be used without concern for local or systemic side-effects. In this example, it is dispensed in a cream vehicle because the patient prefers a non-greasy preparation that rubs into the skin. The patient is going to use the medication on extensive areas of skin, requiring approximately 10 g per application twice a day. A prescription for 454 g (1 lb) of cream will last almost 2 weeks, and two refills will allow more than enough medication until the next appointment in 4 weeks.

DRESSINGS AND BATHS

Key Points

1. Dressing may be dry, wet, or occlusive
2. Baths can be considered a form of wet dressing

Dressings are useful as protective coverings over wounds. They prevent contamination from the environment, and many absorb serum and blood.

Dry dressings are used to protect wounds and to absorb drainage. They usually consist of absorbent gauze secured with adhesive tape. Adhesive tape can cause allergic contact dermatitis, in which case hypoallergenic tapes may be used. These are made of an acrylic plastic adhesive mass with a plastic or cloth backing. After surgery, the skin is often painted with an adhesive that contains benzoin, which may also be responsible for allergic contact dermatitis. Dry dressings may be non-adherent or adherent. *Non-adherent dressings* are used for clean wounds. When changed, they should not pull off newly formed epithelium. An example of a non-adherent dressing is petrolatum-impregnated gauze. *Adherent dressings* are used for debridement of moist wounds. The dressings may be dry or wet at first. For dry dressings, gauze is applied and changed regularly. For wet-to-dry dressings, water, saline, or an antiseptic solution is added to the dressing and allowed to dry. Accumulated debris is removed, although removal may be painful. Discomfort can be reduced if adherent dressings are first moistened (i.e., remoistened) before removal.

Wet dressings are used to treat acute inflammation. They consist of gauze, pads, or towels soaked continuously with water, an *astringent* (drying agent), or an antimicrobial solution. They soothe, cool, and dry through evaporation. In addition, when changed, they remove crusts and exudate. Water is the most important ingredient of wet dressings, but astringents such as aluminum acetate (Domeboro) and antiseptics such as povidone-iodine (Betadine) are frequently added. Impermeable covers such as plastic should *not* be placed over wet dressings because of the maceration that would ensue.

Occlusive dressings made of semipermeable plastic membranes (e.g., Duoderm) promote wound healing by maintaining a moist environment. They are frequently used on chronic ulcers, e.g., stasis ulcers. The moist environment allows migration of keratinocytes over the ulcer base to proceed more rapidly. In addition, occlusive dressings allow autodigestion of necrotic tissue by accumulation of inflammatory cells. For some wounds, e.g., donor graft sites, these dressings also significantly reduce pain.

Baths may be thought of as a form of wet dressing. They are effective in soothing, in decreasing itching, and in cleansing, and they are relaxing. They are used for acute eruptions that are crusting and weeping. They hydrate dry skin, but only if a moisturizer is applied immediately after the bath. Routinely used baths include tar emulsions (Cutar), colloidal oatmeal (Aveeno), and bath oils. Baths are limited to 30 min to prevent maceration, and are performed once or twice daily.

TOPICAL STEROIDS (GLUCOCORTICOSTEROIDS)

Key Points

1. Potency depends on steroid structure, concentration, and vehicle
2. Learn to use a low (hydrocortisone 1%), moderate (triamcinolone 0.1%), and high potency steroid (clobetasol 0.05%)

Perhaps no topical therapeutic modality is used more frequently than steroids because of their anti-inflammatory effects. The use of glucocorticosteroids applied directly to diseased skin has resulted in a high therapeutic benefit with relatively little local and systemic toxicity. The mechanism of action of topical glucocorticosteroids is complex and is not thoroughly understood.

POTENCY

The potency of a topical glucocorticosteroid depends on its molecular structure. For example, triamcinolone acetonide is 100 times more potent than hydrocortisone. In addition, the vehicle carrying the steroid is important. For a steroid to be effective, it must be absorbed. Penetration of glucocorticosteroids through the stratum corneum (and, hence, increased activity) is optimized by using non-polar, lipophilic glucocorticosteroid molecules compounded in vehicles that readily release the steroid.

Dozens of different topical glucocorticosteroids (**Fig. 4.1**) have been formulated for use in skin disease, with many of these developed on the basis of potency assays. Measurement of the ability of glucocorticosteroids to induce vasoconstriction or blanching of the skin, *vasoconstrictive assay*, is the most frequently used method of estimating relative potency. The results of the vasoconstrictive assay parallel those found in clinical studies. Because this assay is much simpler to perform than

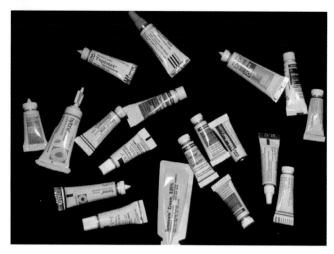

FIGURE 4.1 Multiple steroids – choose and become familiar with a low, medium, and high potency steroid.

Topical side-effects:
1. Atrophy
2. Acne
3. Enhanced fungal infection
4. Retarded wound healing
5. Contact dermatitis
6. Glaucoma, cataracts

Systemic side-effects are worrisome but rarely occur. They include adrenal suppression, iatrogenic Cushing syndrome, and growth retardation in children. These complications have been reported with long-term, extensive use of potent topical steroids, particularly when these agents are used under occlusion. The recent introduction of super-high-potency topical steroids has increased the possibility of hypothalamopituitary axis suppression. These steroids should not be used for longer than two consecutive weeks, and the total dosage should not exceed 50 g/week.

Systemic side-effects:
1. Adrenal suppression
2. Cushing syndrome
3. Growth retardation

TABLE 4.1 Topical steroids

Potency	Generic Name	(%)
Low	Hydrocortisone	1.0
Medium	Triamcinolone acetonide	0.1
High	Fluocinonide	0.05
Super-high	Clobetasol propionate	0.05

GUIDELINES FOR TOPICAL STEROID USAGE

A bewildering array of topical steroids is available in different vehicles. When prescribing a steroid preparation, one should consider several factors before making the selection of potency: vehicle, amount to be dispensed, and frequency of use. It is best to become familiar with one steroid in each class: lowest, medium, and high potency. By using only a few preparations, you will gain an enhanced appreciation of clinical efficacy, frequency of side-effects, available vehicles and volumes, and costs. Lowest-potency topical steroids are recommended for dermatoses that are mild and chronic, and involve the face and intertriginous regions. More potent steroids (medium and high) are used for dermatoses that are more severe and recalcitrant to treatment.

Once the appropriate potency has been selected, the vehicle (**Fig. 4.2**) should be chosen. Acute and subacute inflammations characterized by vesiculation and oozing are best treated with non-occlusive vehicles in a gel, lotion, or cream. Ointments, because of their occlusive properties, are better for treating chronic inflammation characterized by dryness, scaling, and lichenification. Because of their greasy nature, ointments are less acceptable esthetically. However, they have less potential for irritation and allergic reaction. Lotions and gels are best used on hairy areas such as the scalp.

complicated clinical studies, it is widely used to screen specific formulations before they are used in clinical trials.

Vasoconstrictive assay is the most common method for measuring potency.

Table 4.1 lists some topical glucocorticosteroids with different potencies. The percentage of the steroid present is relevant only when comparing percentages of the same compound. Thus, triamcinolone acetonide 0.5% is stronger than its 0.1% formulation, but hydrocortisone 1% is much weaker than triamcinolone acetonide 0.1%. In addition, potency depends on the vehicle. The same preparation tends to be more potent in an ointment base than in a cream base because of enhanced percutaneous penetration.

SIDE-EFFECTS

Numerous hazards are involved with the use of topical glucocorticosteroids. In general, the more potent the glucocorticosteroid, the greater the likelihood of an adverse reaction. However, when patients are educated on proper use, side-effects are uncommon.

Use creams on weeping eruptions, ointments on dry lichenified skin, and gels, foams, or solutions on hairy areas.

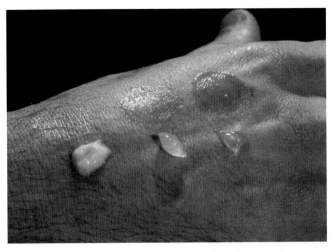

FIGURE 4.2 Steroid cream, ointment, and gel – vehicles are important.

Another consideration in topical steroid therapy is the frequency of application. The stratum corneum acts as a reservoir and continues to release topical steroid into the skin after the initial application. Applications once or twice a day are usually sufficient. Investigators have observed that chronic dermatoses, especially psoriasis, may become less responsive after prolonged use of topical steroids. This phenomenon is called *tachyphylaxis*. This diminished responsiveness after repeated applications has also been observed in vasoconstrictive assays.

Finally, the physician should instruct the patient in proper application and dispense sufficient medication to ensure adequate treatment. A good rule is to use the smallest quantity and the weakest preparation that are effective for a particular eruption. The need for continued treatment should be reviewed periodically.

PHOTOTHERAPY

Key Points

1. Positive effects are therapeutic
2. Negative effects are sunburn, photo-aging, and skin cancer

PHOTOBIOLOGY AND THERAPY

The sun emits a broad spectrum of electromagnetic radiation that is both ionizing (cosmic, gamma, and X-rays) and non-ionizing (UV, visible, infrared, and radio) (**Fig. 4.3**). The Earth's atmosphere absorbs one-third of the solar radiation. Of the radiation that reaches the Earth's surface, 60% is infrared, 37% is visible, and 3% is in the UV range. The UV spectrum is between X-ray and visible light, and composes the 200–400 nm wavelength band. It is subdivided into three groups based on physical and biologic properties: UVC (200–290 nm, germicidal spectrum); UVB (290–320 nm, sunburn spectrum); and UVA (320–400 nm). All the UVC radiation is filtered by the ozone layer, so only UVB and UVA rays reach the Earth's surface.

Because light has properties of waves and particles, two theories are used to describe its physics. The wave theory relates the speed of light to its wavelength and frequency; the light spectrum is divided according to its wavelength (nanometers, nm). The quantum theory is based on the existence of a particle of energy (photon) and relates light energy (joules, J) directly to frequency and inversely to wavelength.

The positive effects of UV radiation include vitamin D metabolism and phototherapy of cutaneous diseases. Numerous diseases are responsive to UV radiation alone or in combination with a photosensitizing drug (photochemotherapy). These diseases include psoriasis, dermatitis, pityriasis rosea, pruritus, vitiligo, and mycosis fungoides. However, these beneficial effects must be weighed against the potential adverse effects, which include sunburn, aging, and skin cancer.

For therapeutic purposes, sunlight is the least expensive source of UV radiation. However, because of its varying intensity and availability, it is often not the optimal source. To overcome these disadvantages, artificial light sources were developed. Fluorescent bulbs are placed in a light box for office use or are combined in groups of two or four for self-treatment at home. The enhancement of phototherapy using tar is sometimes used to treat psoriasis. High-intensity UVA fluorescent bulbs were developed and combined with psoralens in the photochemotherapy of psoriasis (*PUVA*, or *psoralens* plus *UVA*). PUVA is also used for selected patients with vitiligo, mycosis fungoides, and atopic dermatitis. However, close supervision, experience in use, and awareness of adverse effects are necessary for proper administration of UV radiation.

SUN PROTECTION

Excessive exposure to solar irradiation results acutely in sunburn and chronically in premature aging (**Fig. 4.4**) and carcinogenesis. These adverse effects may be prevented with the use of topical sunscreens and protective clothing, and by avoiding midday exposure when sunlight is most intense.

Sun protection includes: sunscreen with at least SPF30, protective clothing, and avoiding midday sun.

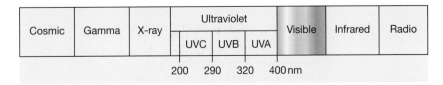

Cosmic	Gamma	X-ray	Ultraviolet			Visible	Infrared	Radio
			UVC	UVB	UVA			

200   290   320   400 nm

FIGURE 4.3 Electromagnetic spectrum.

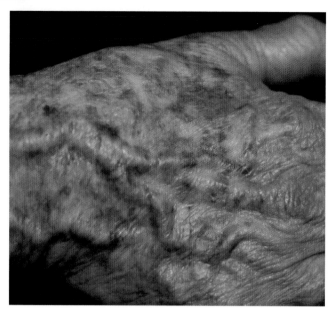

FIGURE 4.4 Photo-aged skin – note the actinic damage – brown macules, fragility, and purpura.

The amount of protection afforded by a sunscreen is measured by its sun protective factor (SPF). In general, to provide adequate protection, a sunscreen should have an SPF of 30. The SPF is calculated by comparing the amount of time required to produce erythema (minimal erythema dose, MED) in skin covered with a sunscreen divided by the time required to produce erythema in an unscreened control site. Thus, a sunscreen with a SPF of 10 would allow a person who normally burns in 20 min to be exposed for as long as 200 min before burning occurs.

The two broad categories of sunscreens are chemical and physical. The most widely used chemical sunscreens contain para-aminobenzoic acid (PABA) esters, benzophenones, salicylates, anthranilates, and cinnamates, and are available in cream, lotion, spray, or gel vehicles. Physical sunscreens contain titanium dioxide, zinc oxide, or talc in creams or pastes. Sunscreens with benzophenone combined with PABA esters are those most often used to protect against sunburn, which is primarily due to UVB radiation, and, to a lesser degree, to protect against UVA. Many moisturizers that are advertised as having 'anti-aging' properties contain sunscreens. Newer sunscreens containing avobenzone (Parsol) or ecamsule (Mexoryl) are particularly helpful for patients who have photosensitivities provoked by UVA and for those who are receiving PUVA therapy.

An additional measure of a sunscreen is its ability to remain effective when the person using it is sweating or swimming. This property is called *substantivity* and has been found to be a function of both the active sunscreen and its vehicle. At present, no universally accepted means of expressing substantivity exists, as there is with SPF. In choosing a sunscreen, phrases such as *water resistant* or *waterproof* indicate a preparation's substantivity.

Topical sunscreens are not without mild irritant cutaneous and ocular adverse reactions. However, allergic contact dermatitis or allergic photocontact dermatitis rarely occurs from sunscreen ingredients.

DIAGNOSTIC TESTS

Key Points

1. Microscopic examination is frequently diagnostic
2. Sample selection is critical in obtaining the proper diagnostic specimen

In general, laboratory tests serve as important tools that are relied on, sometimes too heavily, as diagnostic aids. Imaging studies and blood and urine tests are occasionally helpful for patients suspected of having a systemic disease. For example, an antinuclear antibody test should be ordered in a patient with skin lesions of lupus erythematosus. A serologic test for syphilis is appropriate in a patient with a skin rash in which syphilis is considered to be a possible cause. However, because most dermatologic diseases are limited to the skin, tests for systemic disease are less frequently indicated than are microscopic examinations, cultures, biopsies, and patch tests, which more specifically involve the skin.

As a highly accessible organ, the skin lends itself to direct laboratory examination. Specimen gathering is easy, minimally traumatic, and often highly rewarding diagnostically. Numerous tests can be performed in the office, with results immediately available. For other tests, specimens must be sent to the microbiology or pathology laboratory for further evaluation.

Diagnostic tests include:
- Microscopic examination
- Cultures
- Biopsy
- Patch testing

POTASSIUM HYDROXIDE MOUNT FOR DERMATOPHYTIC INFECTIONS

For undiagnosed scaling lesions of the skin, a fungal origin must be excluded. The best way to do this is with a potassium hydroxide (KOH) preparation of the scale scraping. In experienced hands, this simple test is more sensitive than fungal culture. For those just learning to perform KOH examinations, hyphae are more easily said than seen. The following steps should be followed in performing this examination:

If it scales, scrape it!

1. *Vigorously* scrape the scale from the edge of the scaling lesion onto a microscopic slide (**Fig. 4.5**). Use a no. 15 scalpel blade for scraping. Avoid

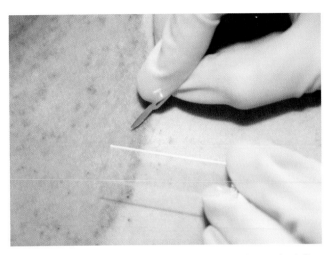

FIGURE 4.5 **Obtain scales for fungal KOH** preparation at the inflammatory margin of the patch.

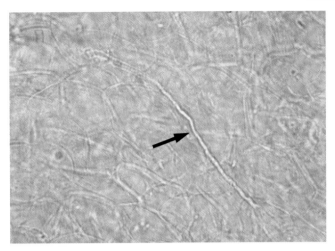

FIGURE 4.6 **Positive KOH** showing fungal hyphae (arrow).

extremely thick pieces of scale, because they are difficult to examine.

2. Place no more than 1 or 2 drops of 20% KOH with dimethylsulfoxide (DMSO) on the scale before covering with the coverslip.

3. *Blot* out the excess KOH by firmly pressing a paper towel on top of the coverslip and slide. This important step achieves two purposes. First, it spreads the cells into a thin layer on the slide. A monolayer of cells is desired for the microscopic examination; grossly, this looks like a cloudy film under the coverslip. Second, the blotting removes excess KOH on and around the coverslip; the microscope objective can be permanently etched by contact with KOH.

4. When examining the preparation under the microscope, use *low illumination*. This is most easily achieved by racking the light condenser down all the way. Bright illumination 'washes out' the preparation so that hyphae 'disappear.'

5. Scan the *entire* coverslip under low power (×10). In the cellular areas, look for the hyphae, which often appear as slightly refractile branching tubes (**Fig. 4.6**). When suspicious elements are seen, use the high dry objective (×45) for confirmation.

6. Unlike mucous membrane preparations for candidiasis, in skin scrapings, hyphae are often sparse. *Careful search*, sometimes with multiple preparations, is indicated when there is a high index of suspicion that a lesion may be fungal.

POTASSIUM HYDROXIDE PREPARATION FOR CANDIDAL INFECTION

In addition to causing scale, candidal infections may cause pustules. Sometimes, the pustules predominate and are a good source of material for KOH examination. The specimen is prepared and examined exactly as outlined above. KOH preparations are particularly useful for diagnosing candidal infections because the finding of hyphae or pseudohyphae is diagnostic of *infection* with this organism. Spores are inadequate for diagnosis of

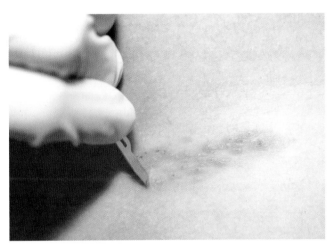

FIGURE 4.7 **Scrape the base** of the blisters for a Tzanck preparation.

infection; yeast organisms, including *Candida albicans*, can colonize skin without infecting it. For this reason, a culture growing *C. albicans* does not necessarily implicate infection, whereas finding hyphal forms on KOH examination does.

> Hyphae, not spores, are the diagnostic findings in candidal infections.

TZANCK PREPARATION

The Tzanck preparation provides an opportunity to make an immediate diagnosis of a herpes simplex or varicella-zoster infection. The preferred specimen is the scraping of the contents and base of a freshly opened vesicle (**Fig. 4.7**). This material is placed on a glass slide, air-dried, methanol fixed, and then stained for 10 s with toluidine blue. Inclusion bodies are not well seen, but the finding of multinucleate giant cells is diagnostic for infection with either herpes simplex or varicella-zoster virus (**Fig. 4.8**).

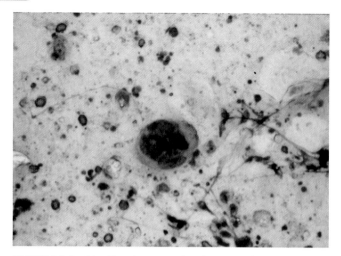

FIGURE 4.8 Positive Tzanck preparation showing multinucleated giant cell typical of a herpesvirus infection.

SCABIES SCRAPING

Finding a scabies mite under the microscope confirms the diagnosis as well as ensuring treatment compliance, should the patient be skeptical. Burrows produce the highest yield, but, because their presence alone is diagnostic, scraping a burrow serves only to dramatize the diagnosis. On close inspection of the burrow, the adult scabies mite is sometimes barely visible as a tiny black speck. Under the microscope, it appears more impressive. A scraping may be more helpful when definite burrows are not found, in which case small papules or questionable burrows are scraped. The scraping is done with a no. 15 scalpel blade moistened with oil (any oil) so that the scraped skin adheres to the blade, from which it can be easily transferred to a drop of oil on a glass slide, covered with a coverslip, and examined microscopically. In scraping, the scalpel blade is held perpendicular to the skin surface. The key to a successful test is to scrape *vigorously*. Alternatively, *KOH* can be used in place of oil on the slide.

CULTURE

The microbiology laboratory can confirm and further characterize bacterial, viral, and fungal pathogens, some of which may initially be identified in an office microscopic examination.

Organisms for both superficial and deep fungal infections can be isolated from an appropriate skin specimen. For a superficial fungal (dermatophyte) infection, this specimen is simply a collection of scales scraped or vigorously swabbed from the surface of the lesion. For deep fungal infections, skin tissue is needed and is obtained most easily with a punch biopsy from the active border of the lesion. Tissue should simultaneously be sent to the pathology laboratory for histologic examination to include special fungal stains. If the specimen is sufficiently large, it may be bisected; otherwise, two biopsy specimens should be collected.

Material for bacterial culture should be obtained from intact pustules, bullae, or abscesses. If only crusts are

present, they should first be removed so that the underlying exudate can be swabbed and cultured. More invasive procedures are required for deeper bacterial infections. For bacterial cellulitis, the responsible organisms can sometimes be retrieved from the involved site by injecting and aspirating 0.5–1 mL of non-bacteriostatic saline. Cultures of skin biopsies may also be rewarding, especially for mycobacterial infections of the skin. Some atypical mycobacteria grow only at room temperature, so to handle the skin tissue properly, the laboratory needs not only the specimen but also the clinician's diagnostic considerations.

> Intact pustules, bullae, or abscesses are the source of specimen for bacterial cultures.

Viral cultures must be transported in a viral transport medium, which can be obtained from the viral laboratory. For herpes cultures, a vesicle is opened or a crust is unroofed, and the underlying serum is swabbed. The swab is placed in the transport medium, and the container is returned to the laboratory for processing. Herpes simplex cultures have a high yield, but herpes varicella-zoster grows either slowly (7–10 days) or not at all. An immunofluorescent staining technique for herpes varicella-zoster produces a much higher yield in a much faster time (same day). The test is performed on a vesicle fluid smeared on a special slide, which is returned to the virology laboratory for testing.

SKIN BIOPSY

In no other organ-based specialty is tissue so easily available for histologic examination as in dermatology. Although a biopsy is not necessary to diagnose the majority of skin disorders, in certain circumstances its value cannot be overemphasized. The following serve only as examples. Already mentioned is the mandate that skin nodules of uncertain origin must undergo biopsy to rule out malignancy. For plaques with unusual shapes and colors, a diagnosis of mycosis fungoides, a cutaneous T-cell lymphoma, may be confirmed with a skin biopsy, but sometimes only after multiple biopsies have been taken serially over time. A skin biopsy is usually necessary to secure the exact diagnosis of a primary blistering disorder. In lupus erythematosus, the information obtained from a skin specimen may help to establish the diagnosis.

Occasionally, excisional biopsies are preferred (e.g., for melanoma), but for most skin lesions a punch or shave biopsy is more convenient to perform. For a punch biopsy, a 3 mm instrument is standard, but punches are available in sizes ranging from 2 to 8 mm. The procedure is simple. After the skin is infiltrated with a local anesthetic (**Fig. 4.9**), the punch is drilled into, and preferably through, the skin (**Fig. 4.10**). The specimen then is *gently* lifted and snipped off at the subcutaneous fat level. Hemostasis can be achieved simply with pressure or absorbable gelatin (Gelfoam) packing. Occasionally, the skin defect is closed with a suture to stop bleeding.

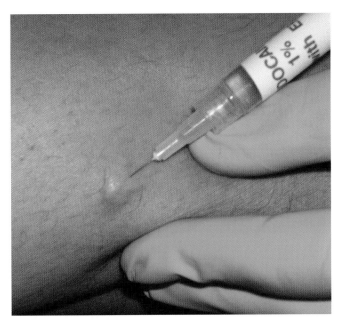

FIGURE 4.9 **Use 1% lidocaine,** usually with epinephrine (less bleeding) and a 30-gauge needle (less pain), to raise a wheal for local anesthesia.

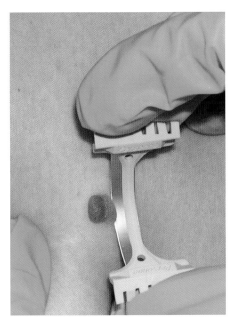

FIGURE 4.11 **Shave biopsy** is the most common technique for obtaining a superficial biopsy.

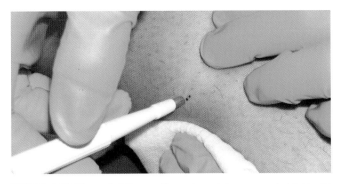

FIGURE 4.10 **Use a twisting action** when doing a punch biopsy to sample epidermal and deeper dermal tissue.

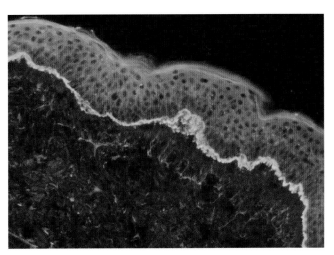

FIGURE 4.12 **Positive immunofluorescence** showing a linear deposit of immunoglobulin G at the dermal–epidermal junction, characteristic of bullous pemphigoid.

Note that, in the foregoing procedure, gentleness is emphasized. A biopsy specimen will be artifactually damaged, sometimes to the point of being histologically uninterpretable, if it is squeezed too firmly with the tissue forceps. To avoid this problem, one should either lift the specimen gently from below or grasp it by the very edge. With nodules and other dermal processes, it is particularly important that the specimen be of full thickness. For processes involving the subcutaneous fat, even deeper and larger specimens may need to be obtained.

Extremely superficial lesions can undergo biopsy or be removed with a shave technique. A wheal is raised with the anesthetic injection, after which the area is shaved with a scalpel blade maneuvered either parallel to the surface or in a slight 'scooping' fashion (**Fig. 4.11**).

For most skin lesions, adjacent normal skin is not needed, so the biopsy should be obtained from the center of the lesion. The exception is with blistering disorders, in which case the biopsy should be taken from the edge of an early lesion to include a portion of the adjacent, non-blistered skin. This is needed to identify the exact histologic origin of the blister.

For routine histologic processing and for most special stains, the specimen is placed in formalin. For electron microscopy, buffered glutaraldehyde is used. With immunofluorescence testing, the specimen must be either immediately snap-frozen or placed in a special buffered transport solution.

IMMUNOFLUORESCENCE TEST

For the diagnosis of blistering disorders such as pemphigus, bullous pemphigoid, and dermatitis herpetiformis, immunofluorescence tests on skin (direct) and, sometimes, serum (indirect) are invaluable and widely used (**Fig. 4.12**). These techniques detect autoantibodies directed against portions of skin. For example, immunoglobulin (Ig) G antibodies deposited at the basement membrane in pemphigoid are detected by direct immunofluorescence testing using the patient's skin and fluorochrome-labeled anti-IgG antibodies. The same test may also be useful in helping to diagnose lupus erythematosus, in which it is called the *lupus band test*. The presence of IgM, IgA, complement, and fibrin can also be detected with appropriate reagents.

ELECTRON MICROSCOPY

An electron microscopic examination of skin tissue is less often indicated but is helpful in diagnosing several uncommon disorders, including Langerhans cell histiocytosis and subtypes of the inherited mechanical bullous disease, epidermolysis bullosa.

PATCH TESTING

Patch testing is a valuable tool for identifying responsible allergens in patients with allergic contact dermatitis. These tests detect delayed (type IV) hypersensitivity responses to contact allergens. Patch test reactions take several days to develop and hence differ from scratch tests, which evoke immediate (type I) hypersensitivity responses (within minutes). Either specifically suspected substances may be tested, or an entire battery of allergens may be screened. For either purpose, standardized trays of common sensitizing chemicals are available, each appropriately diluted in water or petrolatum. These test materials are applied to the skin under occlusive patches that are left in place for 48 h. The patches then are removed, the sites inspected, and positive reactions noted (**Fig. 4.13**). Because these delayed hypersensitivity responses sometimes take more than 48 h, a final reading at 72–96 h is recommended. If positive tests are found, the last and most important step is to determine their clinical relevance. In itself, a positive patch test does not prove that agent to be the cause of dermatitis. Clinical correlation with an appropriate exposure history is required. Patch testing should not be done with unknown chemicals because severe irritant reactions with residual scars can result. Contact dermatitis and patch testing are discussed further in Chapter 8.

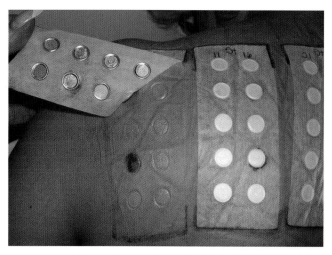

FIGURE 4.13 Removing patch tests on day 2 to detect a delayed-type hypersensitivity reaction.

> Patch tests are used to detect contact allergens and confirm allergic contact dermatitis.

DERMATOLOGIC SURGERY

> ### Key Points
>
> 1. Know the surgical options
> 2. Know how to handle complications
> 3. Obtain informed consent

Numerous techniques are available for surgery of the skin. The three most common and simplest procedures are elliptical excision, curettage and electrodesiccation, and cryosurgery. For defects that cannot be closed primarily, skin flaps or grafts may be used. A specialized form of cancer surgery, *Mohs technique*, involves serial excisions of tissue, which are systematically mapped and microscopically examined to define the extent of cancerous invasion and to ensure that surgical margins are free of tumor. This technique is the most successful means of treating basal cell and squamous cell carcinomas.

> Mohs technique is the most effective surgery for basal and squamous cell carcinoma. It is most frequently used for recurrent and facial carcinomas.

Before surgery, the patient should be informed of the procedure chosen, why it is necessary, and what to expect and do after surgery. The potential complications of the procedure, including excessive scar formation, infection, bleeding, and nerve injury, should be explained. When properly selected and technically well performed, simple excision, curettage and electrodesiccation, and cryosurgery usually have no significant complications.

> Surgery explanation includes: procedure, potential complications, and what to do after the operation.

EXCISION

The simple elliptical excision is used for obtaining tissue for biopsy and for the removal of benign and cancerous lesions. The axis of the lesion, cosmetic boundaries (e.g., the vermilion border of the lip), and skin lines should be taken into consideration when planning the excision. Most procedures require a minimal number of instruments, including a needle holder, small forceps, skin hook, small clamp, small pointed scissors, syringe, and needle (30 gauge), and a no. 15 scalpel blade plus handle. Disposable sterile gloves, eye sheet, and gauze are also necessary.

Numerous antiseptics are available for preoperative preparation of the skin, including 70% isopropyl alcohol,

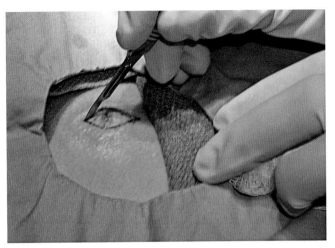

FIGURE 4.14 Excision demonstrating that the length is three times greater than the width, and the cut is perpendicular to the skin surface.

povidone-iodine (Betadine), and chlorhexidine gluconate (Hibiclens). The boundaries of the excision are marked. This is done before injection of local anesthesia because the volume of anesthetic distorts the normal skin contours. The preferred local anesthetic is 1% lidocaine because of the rarity of allergic reactions. In addition, lidocaine, an amide, does not cross-react with procaine hydrochloride (Novocain), an ester. Transdermal anesthesia with a topical anesthetic cream can be applied under an occlusive dressing 1–2 h before the procedure to reduce the pain associated with injection.

> Lidocaine (Xylocaine) does not cross-react with procaine hydrochloride (Novocain).

Normal saline or diphenhydramine hydrochloride (Benadryl) may be used for local anesthesia if lidocaine cannot be used. The addition of epinephrine to lidocaine prolongs its anesthetic effect and reduces operative bleeding. Care should be taken when using epinephrine in the earlobe and digits to avoid ischemic changes secondary to vasoconstriction.

The length of the ellipse should be three times the width to ensure easy closure. The cut should be made perpendicular to the surface and through the dermis into the subcutaneous tissue (**Fig. 4.14**). Hemostasis is achieved with pressure, electrodesiccation, or suture ligation. Repair of the wound is easy if an adequate ellipse has been formed, the edges are perpendicular, and skin lines are followed. If the defect is large, the edges may be undermined to reduce closure tension. Buried absorbable suture is used to close deeper layers. Numerous methods are used for skin closure: interrupted sutures with monofilament nylon is the simplest method. In most cases, 5-0 or 4-0 sutures are adequate for both subcuticular and skin closure. The removal of skin sutures depends on the site, wound tension, and whether buried sutures have been used. In general, facial sutures are removed in 5 days, and trunk and extremity sutures are removed in 1–2 weeks. Most wounds are dressed with

either sterile adherent bandages or gauze secured with tape. Paper tape with an acrylic adhesive mass should be used in patients with a history of tape sensitivity. Topical antibiotics are not necessary after surgery. The patient is instructed to keep the wound dry for 24 h, to change the dressings daily, and to return to the clinic if bleeding, purulent drainage, or excessive pain or swelling occurs. Postoperative pain is usually negligible, requiring only acetaminophen.

> The length of elliptical excision is three times its width.

> Suture removal:
> - Face: 5 days
> - Trunk and extremities: 1–2 weeks

CURETTAGE AND ELECTRODESICCATION

The procedure of curettage and electrodesiccation is used most often for the treatment of selected small basal cell and squamous cell carcinomas. It is a deceptively simple procedure that requires proper selection of tumor and a skilled practitioner. Otherwise, the recurrence rate is unacceptably high. The tumor is prepared and anesthetized with a local anesthetic. The *curette*, an oval instrument with a cutting edge, is used to remove the soft cancerous skin. The tumor margins are determined by 'feel,' with normal skin having a firm and gritty consistency. After curettage, the base and borders of the wound are electrodesiccated to destroy residual tumor and to provide hemostasis. The wound heals by secondary intention in 2–3 weeks.

> Curettage and electrodesiccation require experience to avoid a high recurrence rate.

CRYOSURGERY

Keratoses and warts are frequently treated with cryosurgery. Liquid nitrogen (−195.6°C) is the standard agent because it is inexpensive, rapid, and non-combustible. Tissue destruction is caused by intercellular and extracellular ice formation, by denaturing lipid–protein complexes, and by cell dehydration. This treatment usually requires no skin preparation or anesthesia. Liquid nitrogen application is accomplished with direct spray and usually requires <30 s (**Fig. 4.15**). A repeat freeze–thaw cycle results in more cellular damage than a single cycle.

During the procedure, the patient feels a stinging or burning sensation. Subsequently, burning occurs along with tissue swelling. Within 24 h, a blister often forms in the treated area. If the blister is excessively large or painful, the fluid should be removed in a sterile manner. Otherwise, it is allowed to heal spontaneously.

Treatment of skin cancers with cryotherapy requires an operator experienced with thermocouple devices to ensure adequate freezing for tissue destruction.

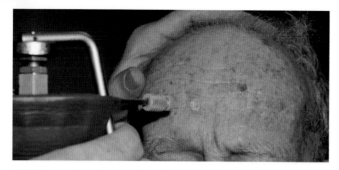

FIGURE 4.15 Cryotherapy of a seborrheic keratosis – using a spray unit, the white freeze cycle should last about 10 s.

Postoperative morbidity includes significant tissue edema and necrosis.

PATIENT EDUCATION

Key Points

1. Verbal and written communication is important
2. Education enhances understanding and compliance

A dialogue must be established between the physician and the patient. This is begun during the history and physical examination. Once a diagnosis is established, the patient should be told what the disease is, what its cause is, and what to expect from treatment. Patients are frequently hesitant to ask certain questions because they are either afraid or embarrassed. It is important that these unasked questions be answered: Is my disease contagious? Is it cancer? Do I have something wrong internally that is causing my skin problems?

Answer the unasked questions:
- Contagious?
- Cancer?
- Internal?

For therapy to be successful, patient cooperation and compliance are necessary. To ensure this goal, therapeutic options, expected outcome, and potential side-effects should be explained. Instructions on how to use topical medications must be demonstrated. All too frequently, too much medication is applied, and it is not rubbed in sufficiently. For example, when applying a white cream, patients should be instructed to apply sparingly and rub it in until it 'disappears.' If white cream remains on the surface, either too much has been applied or it has not been rubbed in sufficiently. Dressings may be either too wet or too dry, or left on too long, resulting in maceration. These pitfalls are avoided when the medication or dressing is applied to the area of dermatitis as a demonstration while the patient is in the office.

Patient instruction sheets augment the spoken word. They inform and instruct patients. Frequently, medical problems and therapies are complex, and the patient fails to understand them. Instruction sheets save time, reinforce what has been told to the patient, answer unasked questions, and provide a reference for the patient to read.

Penn State Hershey's Dermatology website (www.PennState Hershey.org/dermatology) provides a lot of patient education material and links to other trusted websites.

Epidermal Growths 5

Key Points

1. Proliferation of keratinocytes or basal cells
2. Scaling usually prominent
3. Bleeding or crusting suggests cancer

ABSTRACT

Neoplasms of the epidermis (**Table 5.1**) are derived from a proliferation of basal cells or keratinocytes. Epidermal growths are recognized clinically by a localized thickening of the epidermis that often is accompanied by thickening of the stratum corneum, which is called *hyperkeratosis* or *scale*. Large, indurated, rapidly growing, crusted, or ulcerated tumors suggest a malignant process and should undergo biopsy. Unless injured or irritated, benign growths do not bleed or become crusted or ulcerated.

ACTINIC KERATOSIS

Key Points

1. Precancerous
2. Prevent with sun protection

Definition

Actinic (solar) keratosis is a precancerous neoplasm of the epidermis caused by the ultraviolet (UV) portion of sunlight. The abnormal keratinocytes in actinic keratoses are confined to the epidermis and constitute a premalignant change. The proliferation of these abnormal cells is clinically manifest as a rough, scaling patch or papule (**Fig. 5.1**).

Incidence

The incidence of actinic keratoses varies with: (1) skin pigmentation; (2) geographic location; and (3) amount of sun exposure. Thus, the incidence of actinic keratoses is high in Caucasians who have light skin, live in the southern USA where there is an abundance of natural sunlight, and engage in frequent outdoor activity. In the authors' clinic, 1.7% of new patients were seen because of actinic keratoses, although the incidence would be higher in the 'Sunbelt.' Moreover, in many patients, actinic keratoses are an incidental finding.

> Light skin and abundant sun exposure may result in actinic keratoses.

History

Risk factors can usually be elicited in the history. The patient may have a genetic predisposition. Fair-skinned Caucasians have the least amount of protective pigment. A family history of skin cancer or an Irish or Anglo-Saxon heritage is frequently obtained. Second, the geographic location where the patient has lived directly influences the amount of UV light exposure. As one moves toward the equator, the UV light intensity increases dramatically. Last, the occupational and recreational activities of the patient with reference to sun exposure provide another clue. Farmers, sailors, and others with occupations that require working outdoors have a high amount of UV light exposure. Similarly, persons who spend many hours at the poolside or on the beach are at higher risk.

Physical Examination

Actinic keratoses are 1–10 mm, reddish, ill-marginated patches and papules that have a rough, yellowish brown, adherent scale. Their ill-defined margins make them **41**

TABLE 5.1 Epidermal growths

	Frequency (%)[a]	Etiology	Physical Examination	Differential Diagnosis	Laboratory Test (Biopsy)
Actinic keratosis	1.7	Sunlight	Ill-marginated, reddish, rough, scaling patch or papule	Squamous cell carcinoma Seborrheic keratosis Superficial basal cell carcinoma	When thick scale or indurated base
Basal cell carcinoma	1.7	Sunlight			Yes
Nodular			Pearly nodule with telangiectasia, often has central depression or ulcer	Molluscum contagiosum Squamous cell carcinoma Sebaceous hyperplasia Nevus Merkel cell carcinoma Trichoepithelioma	
Pigmented			Blue–black plaque or nodule with pearly border	Malignant melanoma Nevus Seborrheic keratosis	
Superficial			Red, scaling, crusted eczematous appearing patch	Psoriasis Eczema Bowen's disease	
Sclerosing			Whitish, slightly depressed, sometimes crusted plaque	Squamous cell carcinoma Non-healing scar	
Corn	0.4	Friction	Hyperkeratotic papule or nodule with compact clear core	Wart	No
Molluscum contagiosum	0.3	Poxvirus	Translucent papule with umbilicated center	Comedo Nodular basal cell carcinoma	No
Seborrheic keratosis	1.6	–	Tan–brown, greasy, 'pasted on' papule or plaque	Wart Actinic keratosis Nevus Malignant melanoma Pigmented basal cell carcinoma	No
Skin tag	0.5	–	Soft, skin-colored, pedunculated papule	Neurofibroma nevus	No
Squamous cell carcinoma	0.2	Sunlight Viruses Chemicals	Flesh-colored, hard, crusted or scaling nodule, often ulcerated	Keratoacanthoma Basal cell carcinoma Wart Actinic keratosis Merkel cell carcinoma Trichoepithelioma Nevus sebaceous	Yes
Wart	5.2	Papillomavirus			No
Common			Flesh-colored, scaling, vegetative papule or nodule, skin lines interrupted, studded with black puncta	Corn Squamous cell carcinoma	
Flat			Reddish, smooth, flat, well-demarcated papule	Lichen planus Comedo Corn	
Plantar			Solitary, grouped or mosaic scaling papules, skin lines interrupted, studded with black puncta	Squamous cell carcinoma	
Condyloma acuminatum			Soft, moist, cauliflower-appearing papules or nodule	Squamous cell carcinoma Secondary syphilis	No

[a]Percentage of new dermatology patients with this diagnosis seen in the Hershey Medical Center Dermatology Clinic, Hershey, PA.

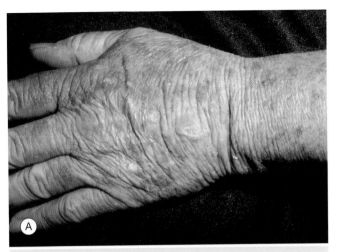

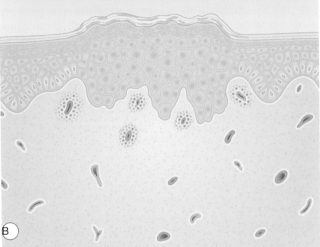

FIGURE 5.1 **Actinic keratosis. A.** Rough, scaling, ill-marginated, pinkish patches and papules on markedly sun-damaged skin. **B.** Epidermis – atypical keratinocytes in lower epidermis. Dermis – chronic inflammation.

indistinct to the casual observer. Their rough-textured surface is often easier to feel than to see. Actinic keratoses occur in sun-exposed areas: the face, dorsum of the hands and forearms, neck, upper back, and chest. They generally are found on UV-damaged skin that has a yellowish hue, wrinkles, and freckled pigmentation.

> An actinic keratosis is rough, scaling, and ill marginated; it is often easier felt than seen.

Differential Diagnosis

An actinic keratosis must be differentiated from other epidermal tumors. Most often, it is confused with a *seborrheic keratosis*. The well demarcated, 'pasted on' appearance of a seborrheic keratosis differentiates it from an actinic keratosis. *Bowen's disease* (*in situ* squamous cell carcinoma) is a larger plaque with margins that are well defined, in contrast to the margins of an actinic keratosis. Hypertrophic or indurated actinic keratosis (**Fig. 5.1**) cannot be differentiated with certainty from *squamous cell carcinoma* and should undergo biopsy. *Superficial basal cell carcinoma*, which resembles Bowen's disease clinically, is occasionally confused with actinic keratosis.

Laboratory and Biopsy

Actinic keratosis is characterized histologically by a partial-thickness dysplasia of the epidermis (**Fig. 5.1B**). A hyperkeratosis with underlying irregular hyperplasia of mildly dysplastic keratinocytes is seen. A chronic inflammatory response is present in the dermis. All thick and indurated actinic keratoses should undergo biopsy to rule out squamous cell carcinoma, as well as lesions that have not responded to previous treatment.

> Indurated and therapeutically unresponsive actinic keratoses should undergo biopsy to rule out carcinoma.

Therapy

Prevention by reducing sunlight exposure is the most effective form of therapy. Patients who are sensitive to the sun or have developed actinic keratoses should wear protective clothing such as broad-brimmed hats and long-sleeved shirts when outside. Sunscreens with a sun protective factor (SPF) of 30 should be used on exposed skin. The regular use of sunscreens prevents the development of new actinic keratoses, as well as hastening the resolution of those that already exist. Avoidance of sun exposure at midday (from 10:00 a.m. to 2:00 p.m.), when UV radiant energy is most intense, is recommended. Patient awareness and education should begin in childhood.

> Use sun protection to prevent more actinic damage.

Cryosurgery with liquid nitrogen is the most common treatment for actinic keratoses and is most useful when a few lesions are present. Thick, hypertrophic, actinic keratoses are also better treated in this way. Freezing can be accomplished in a manner similar to that described for warts. Avoid overzealous treatment of thin actinic keratoses because of possible scarring.

Topical chemotherapy with 5-fluorouracil cream 5% (Efudex) is the most common means of treating multiple actinic keratoses. 5-Fluorouracil inhibits DNA synthesis by blocking the enzyme thymidylate synthase. When 5-fluorouracil is applied to normal skin, little reaction occurs, but when it is applied to sun-damaged skin, those areas with actinic keratoses become inflamed. The medication is applied to the involved areas twice daily. Erythema develops within several days. Subsequently, within 2–4 weeks, the actinic keratoses become painful, crusted, and eroded, at which time the medication is stopped. Patients need to be warned about the discomfort and cosmetically unsightly effects of 5-fluorouracil, which are temporary and resolve after discontinuing treatment. Because of the marked amount of inflammation that can occur, small regions may be treated at a time in patients with extensive actinic keratoses. A few patients become allergic to 5-fluorouracil. Patients with severe actinic damage can be expected to require treatment every couple of years. Alternative agents include: (1) diclofenac gel 3% (Solaraze), a non-steroidal anti-inflammatory drug (NSAID), applied twice daily for 3 months, and (2) imiquimod cream 5% (Aldara), a topical immune response modifier, applied twice weekly for 4 months.

Therapy for Actinic Keratosis

Prevention
- Sunscreen ≥SPF 30
- Broad-rimmed hat, long-sleeved shirt, and pants
- Avoidance of intense midday sun (from 10:00 a.m. to 2:00 p.m.)

Initial
- Cryotherapy with liquid nitrogen

Alternative
- 5-Fluorouracil 5% cream twice daily for 2–3 weeks
- Diclofenac 3% gel twice daily for 3 months
- Imiquimod 5% cream twice weekly for 16 weeks

Course and Complications

In patients with chronically sun-damaged skin, the acquisition of more actinic keratoses can be expected. Some actinic keratoses spontaneously disappear (up to 26%), although others may develop into squamous cell carcinoma. The number that do develop into squamous cell carcinoma appears to be small, less than 1 in 1000 within 1 year. Metastases from squamous cell carcinomas arising in actinic keratoses are very uncommon.

Actinic keratosis has the potential of developing into a squamous cell carcinoma.

Pathogenesis

Actinic keratoses are produced by UV radiation-induced damage to keratinocyte DNA. This results in unrepaired or error-prone repaired DNA. Abnormal replication occurs and results in epidermal cellular hyperplasia. The cells within an actinic keratosis are arranged in a disorderly way and have increased mitoses and an abnormal chromatin pattern. Other precancerous keratinocytic neoplasms similar to actinic keratoses are caused by artificial UV light, X-irradiation, or polycyclic aromatic hydrocarbons.

BASAL CELL CARCINOMA

Key Points

1. Malignancy of the epidermal basal cell
2. Rarely metastasizes
3. Different types have different appearances

Definition

Basal cell carcinoma is a malignant neoplasm arising from the basal cells of the epidermis. Although these cancers rarely metastasize, their potential for local destruction attests to their malignant nature. UV radiation is the cause of most basal cell carcinomas in humans. Four clinically and histopathologically distinct types of basal cell carcinoma are recognized: nodular, pigmented, superficial, and scarring (sclerotic).

Incidence

Basal cell carcinoma is the most common human malignant disease; it affects more than 800 000 persons annually in the USA. In Queensland, Australia, 4.6% of adults aged 20–69 years had skin cancer, mostly basal cell carcinoma. In Tucson, Arizona, the annual incidence is 315 per 100 000 population. Two percent of the new patients in the authors' clinic are seen for basal cell carcinoma. The increased frequency in adult Caucasians is related to sun exposure.

Basal cell carcinoma is the most common skin cancer and very rarely metastasize.

History

The patient with basal cell carcinoma seeks medical attention because of a new growth, especially if it is a non-healing, easily bleeding lesion. There may be a personal or family history of skin cancer. The risk of basal cell carcinoma is higher in patients with light skin, in those who live in southern latitudes, and in those who work or play outdoors. Frequently, these patients have a history of sunburning easily and tanning poorly.

Physical Examination

The usual patient with basal cell carcinoma has fair skin, blue eyes, blonde or red hair, and actinic-damaged skin manifested by freckles, yellow wrinkling, and actinic keratoses. Basal cell carcinoma occurs in sun-exposed skin, particularly the head and neck.

A 'pearly' appearance is the most characteristic feature of a nodular basal cell carcinoma.

The *nodular type* (**Fig. 5.2**) of basal cell carcinoma is the most common. It is a 'pearly,' semi-translucent papule or nodule that often has a central depression or crater, telangiectasia, and a rolled, waxy border. Ulceration and crusting can occur. Nodular basal cell carcinoma occurs most frequently on the face, especially the nose.

Types of basal cell carcinoma:
1. Nodular
2. Pigmented
3. Superficial
4. Scarring (sclerotic)

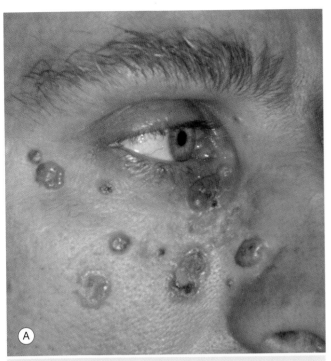

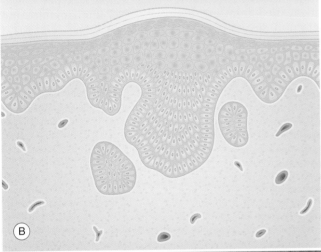

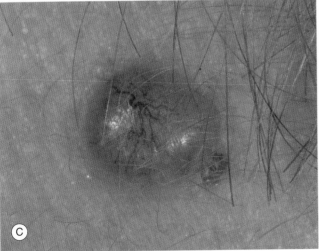

FIGURE 5.2 **A.** Nodular basal cell carcinoma. **B.** Basal cell carcinoma. Epidermis – thickened. Dermis – invasive buds and lobules of basaloid cells. **C.** Basal cell nevus syndrome – multiple pearly to flesh-colored papules and nodules with rolled border and telangiectasia and some crusting.

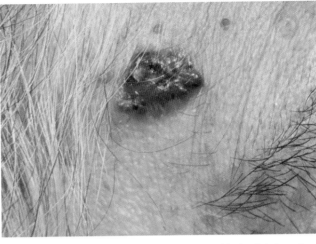

FIGURE 5.3 **Pigmented basal cell carcinoma** – black, slightly scaling, translucent plaque.

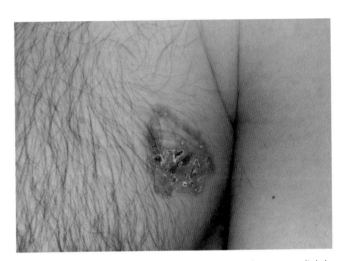

FIGURE 5.4 **Superficial basal cell carcinoma** – erythematous, slightly scaling and crusted patch.

Pigmented basal cell carcinoma (**Fig. 5.3**) is a shiny, blue–black papule, nodule, or plaque. The pigment is often speckled, and a pearly, rolled margin can be seen when the tumor is viewed from the side.

Superficial basal cell carcinoma (**Fig. 5.4**) occurs most frequently on the thorax. It is a red, slightly scaling, well demarcated, eczematous appearing patch. Centrally, it may become slightly eroded and crusted, subsequently leaving an atrophic, slightly depressed center. Its shape is oval to round, with a characteristic thread-like, pearly, rolled border. It is often referred to as multicentric superficial basal cell carcinoma because it skips islands of normal skin, similar to the way a forest fire may surround a stand of trees yet leave it unburned.

The *scarring (sclerotic or morpheaform) basal cell carcinoma* (**Fig. 5.5**) is an atrophic, white, slightly eroded, or crusted plaque that often looks like a scar. It is frequently depressed and is the least common and most aggressive type of basal cell carcinoma.

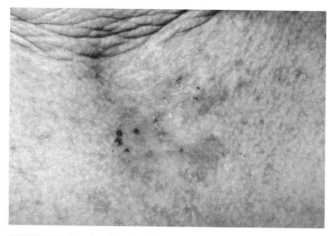

FIGURE 5.5 **Scarring basal cell carcinoma** – erythematous, atrophic white, crusted, ill-marginated patch.

Differential Diagnosis

Nodular basal cell carcinoma and *sebaceous hyperplasia* are sometimes difficult to differentiate clinically. Sebaceous hyperplasia is the proliferation of sebaceous glands surrounding a hair follicle that appears as a 1–3-mm, yellowish papule with overlying telangiectasia and a central pore. The yellowish coloration and central pore help to differentiate it from a basal cell carcinoma. Other epithelial growths that resemble a nodular basal cell carcinoma include a *non-pigmented nevus, molluscum contagiosum,* Merkel cell carcinoma, trichoepithelioma, fibrous papule of the nose, and *squamous cell carcinoma.*

Pigmented basal cell carcinoma can be confused with a *seborrheic keratosis, pigmented nevus,* and, most importantly, *malignant melanoma.* The pearly, rolled border of pigmented basal cell carcinoma helps to differentiate it from a malignant melanoma. If doubt exists, an excisional biopsy should be performed.

Superficial basal cell carcinoma resembles a patch of *dermatitis.* It can be confused with *psoriasis, nummular dermatitis,* and *Bowen's disease.* A persistent solitary lesion and lack of response to topical steroids clinically differentiate superficial basal cell carcinoma from dermatitis or psoriasis. A skin biopsy is the only way to differentiate it from squamous cell carcinoma *in situ* (Bowen's disease).

Any *non-healing scar-like lesions* should undergo biopsy to rule out a scarring basal cell carcinoma or *squamous cell carcinoma.*

> Non-healing scars should undergo biopsy to exclude carcinoma.

Laboratory and Biopsy

The diagnosis of basal cell carcinoma should be confirmed by a shave or punch biopsy. The technique of skin biopsy is reviewed in Chapter 4. The tumors are made up of uniform cells that resemble the basal layers of the epidermis (**Fig. 5.2B**). They have a uniform, large, oval, blue nucleus with indistinct cytoplasm. The tumor

extends from the epidermis into the dermis as nodular or cystic structures, bands, or strands, or as buds from the epidermis. The nodular areas have peripheral palisading with retraction from the surrounding stroma. The cells in some basal cell carcinomas have a 'squamoid' appearance, which makes them difficult to differentiate from squamous cell carcinoma. The infiltrative, morpheaform, micronodular, and mixed histologic subtypes of primary basal cell carcinoma are more aggressive and more difficult to eradicate.

> A chronic eczematous patch should be biopsied to rule out a superficial basal cell carcinoma, especially if crusted.

Therapy

Treatment of basal cell carcinoma should be individualized according to the location of the lesion, the histopathologic type, the age of the patient, the general health of the patient, the size of the basal cell carcinoma, and whether it is primary or recurrent. Recurrence of basal cell carcinoma is related particularly to location on the nose or ear, size >2 cm, and histologic pattern of micronodular, infiltrative, and morpheic types. Treatment modalities include scalpel excision, curettage and electrodesiccation, radiotherapy, cryotherapy, and topical 5-fluorouracil or imiquimod. Each treatment must be *properly* selected to achieve a high cure rate. Surgical modalities are those most frequently used and with the best cure rates. The surgical techniques are reviewed in Chapter 4.

Excision with primary suture closure is the most frequently used form of therapy and allows for histologic assessment of surgical margins. When the wound is large, grafts or tissue transposition flaps may be used to achieve closure. Excision is good for most basal cell carcinomas, but is the treatment of choice for large basal cell carcinomas, recurrent tumors, sclerosing types of basal cell carcinoma, basal cell carcinomas at sites of high recurrence such as the nose or ear, and basal cell carcinoma that extends into the subcutaneous tissue. A specialized form of excision using detailed mapping of the extent of the tumor with histologic orientation is the *Mohs micrographic surgical technique.* This meticulous procedure is most often used for recurrent basal cell carcinoma and primary tumors with a high risk of recurrence.

> Mohs micrographic surgery has the highest cure rate and preserves the most normal skin. It is indicated for most facial and for recurrent basal cell carcinomas.

Curettage and electrodesiccation is a therapeutic modality frequently used by dermatologists. The clinical margins of the tumor are defined by vigorous curettage until the firm, fibrous consistency of normal dermis is felt. This is followed by electrodesiccation. The entire procedure of curettage and electrodesiccation may be repeated to ensure removal of the tumor. The resultant wound heals by secondary intention over a 2–3-week period, with excellent cosmetic results in most cases. Experience is needed to obtain good cure rates. Curettage and electro-desiccation should not be used for basal cell carcinomas >2 cm wide, for tumors with poorly defined clinical borders, for sclerosing basal cell carcinomas, for recurrent basal cell carcinomas, or in certain anatomic locations such as the nasolabial fold, scalp, and eyelids.

Radiation therapy is reserved for elderly patients because the subsequent chronic radiodermatitis that occurs years after the therapy may be cosmetically unacceptable, and because of the potential for developing a new primary cancer in the radiotherapy site. Radiation therapy is used when the patient refuses surgical treatment or has a large tumor that would be difficult to treat surgically.

Cryosurgery with liquid nitrogen is reserved for those clinicians experienced in its use for cancer therapy. The margins and depth of the tumor must be estimated clinically. Cryoprobes are used to monitor the depth of the freeze. After surgery, marked tissue reaction occurs with edema, tissue necrosis, weeping, and crusting.

Topical chemotherapy with *5-fluorouracil* or imiquimod is, in general, inappropriate for treating skin cancer. It should not be used on deep or recurrent tumors. It is occasionally used in patients who have multiple, superficial, multicentric basal cell carcinomas that otherwise would require numerous surgical procedures. Treatment is continued for weeks until marked inflammation and erosion occur. Residual areas suspected to have tumor must undergo biopsy, and another therapeutic modality must be used if basal cell carcinoma persists.

Prevention of further sun-induced damage to the skin is mandatory. Sun protection includes the regular use of sunscreens with an SPF of 15–30, protective clothing (wide-brimmed hat and long-sleeved shirt), and avoidance of midday sun (from 10 a.m. to 2 p.m.).

> Prevention with sun protection – sunscreen, clothing, and avoid midday sun.

Therapy for Basal Cell Carcinoma

Initial
- Excision
- Curettage and electrodesiccation
- Mohs micrographic surgery

Alternative
- Radiation
- Cryotherapy
- 5-Fluorouracil or imiquimod topically for multiple superficial basal cell carcinomas

Course and Complications

Because its course is frequently indolent, a basal cell carcinoma is often ignored. It may enlarge locally and can invade underlying tissues, resulting in significant morbidity and mutilation. Vital structures such as an eye, a nose, or an ear may be totally lost.

Basal cell cancer rarely metastasizes, presumably because of stromal dependence. The metastatic rate is estimated to be <0.003% (1 in 52 000 cases in one series). The excessively large, ulcerated, locally destructive, and recurrent basal cell carcinoma is most likely to metastasize. Regional lymph nodes, lung, and bone are the most likely tissues involved. Routine follow-up every 12 months of patients with basal cell carcinoma is recommended because 35% of these patients will develop another basal cell carcinoma within 5 years.

Pathogenesis

The most common factor related to the development of basal cell carcinoma is UV radiation. Other factors to be considered are arsenic ingestion, genetic predisposition, X-irradiation, and chronic irritation. Mutations of the genes, smoothened (SMO) and patched (PTCH), in the Hedgehog pathway are implicated in over 90% of basal cell carcinomas, and the basal cell nevus syndrome. The *basal cell nevus syndrome* is a rare autosomal dominant disorder characterized by early development of multiple basal cell carcinomas (**Fig. 5.2C**), jaw cysts, macrocephaly, palmar and plantar pits, increased risk of medulloblastoma, and other congenital abnormalities. The origin of basal cell carcinoma is a pluripotential primordial epithelial cell in the basal layer of the skin or, less often, a cutaneous appendage such as the hair follicle.

CORNS

Key Points
1. Caused by pressure or friction
2. Do not interrupt skin lines

Definition

A corn is a localized thickening of epidermis secondary to chronic pressure or friction. It occurs most often on the feet. Synonyms are *clavus* and *heloma*.

Incidence

Corns are extremely common. Many patients treat themselves or see a podiatrist rather than a physician.

History

The patient seeks medical care because of painful feet when standing or walking. A history of ill-fitting footwear or foot injury may be obtained.

Physical Examination

Corns are white-gray or yellow-brown, well circumscribed, horny papules or nodules. Paring the surface with a scalpel reveals a translucent core with preservation of skin lines. Hard corns occur on the sole (**Fig. 5.6**) and

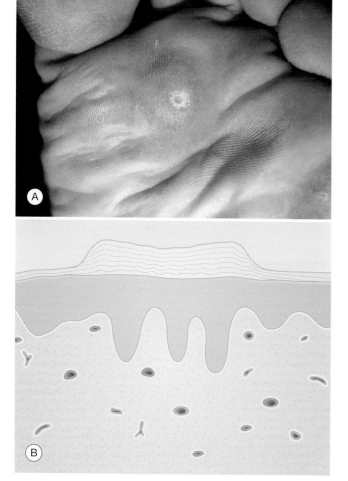

FIGURE 5.6 Corn. A. Thick, yellowish plaque with intact skin lines and compressed keratin center. **B.** Epidermis – thickened, with hyperkeratosis.

external surface of the toes, where drying occurs. Soft corns occur between the toes, where sweating results in maceration.

Corns have a clear center and intact skin lines.

Differential Diagnosis

Plantar warts and corns are commonly confused. The simple maneuver of paring the surface and identifying the presence of skin lines with a translucent core confirms that the lesion is a corn.

Laboratory and Biopsy

A biopsy is unnecessary (**Fig. 5.6B**).

Therapy

The goal of treating corns is to provide immediate relief of pain and then to reduce the friction and pressure that have caused the corn. Immediate relief is provided by paring down the hyperkeratotic surface. Softening of hard corns may be accomplished with keratolytic agents such

as salicylic acid plasters (Mediplast). Changing ill-fitting footwear and shielding the sites with pads, rings, and orthotic devices reduce mechanical trauma. When these procedures fail, surgical correction of a foot deformity or removal of a bony prominence (exostosis) should be considered.

Therapy for Corn

Initial
- Paring down with scalpel
- Softening with salicylic acid plaster
- Reduction of trauma – change of shoes, protective pads, rings, etc.

Alternative
- Surgery – correction of bony deformity

Course and Complications

Persistence of the corn can be expected unless the underlying mechanical problem is reduced or removed. Underlying bursitis from chronic inflammation and sinus formation with infection, osteomyelitis, and gangrene may occur and are particularly worrisome in patients with arteriosclerosis, diabetes mellitus, or peripheral neurologic disorders.

A corn will persist unless friction and pressure are relieved.

Pathogenesis

Repeated pressure and trauma resulting extrinsically from ill-fitting shoes and intrinsically from an exostosis or other anatomic skeletal defects result in the formation of corns.

MOLLUSCUM CONTAGIOSUM

Key Points

1. Caused by poxvirus
2. Umbilicated smooth papule
3. Destructive treatment

Definition

Molluscum contagiosum is caused by a DNA poxvirus that infects epidermal cells. Clinically, the lesions appear as smooth, dome-shaped papules that often are umbilicated (**Fig. 5.7**).

Incidence

Molluscum contagiosum is a common childhood disease. Spread among family members occurs but is uncommon.

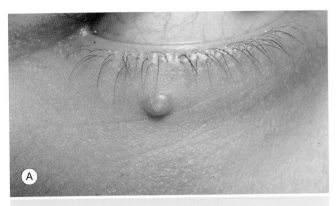

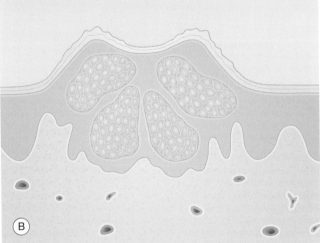

FIGURE 5.7 Molluscum contagiosum. A. Smooth, flesh-colored papule with umbilicated whitish center. **B.** Epidermis – thickened, containing molluscum bodies.

History

In adults, venereal transmission is suggested by a history of sexual exposure and the location of lesions in the genital region.

Physical Examination

The papules of molluscum contagiosum are 2–5 mm wide, hard, smooth, dome-shaped, and flesh colored or translucent. The papules have a central umbilication from which a 'cheesy' core can be expressed. They occur singly or in groups, most often on the trunk, face, and extremities of children and on the genitals of sexually active adults. Uncommonly, they become disseminated, resulting in hundreds of lesions. If inflamed, they are difficult to recognize because of secondary erythema and crusting.

Differential Diagnosis

The translucent papule of molluscum contagiosum can resemble *nodular basal cell carcinoma* or a *comedo*. Nodular basal cell carcinomas usually have telangiectasia and occur in sun-exposed skin of older patients. Comedones lack umbilication. An inflamed molluscum contagiosum may appear to be a bacterial infection of the skin.

Laboratory and Biopsy

The diagnosis usually is clinically obvious. When doubt exists, a simple office procedure is confirmatory. The molluscum papule is removed by curettage and crushed onto a slide. This unstained material readily reveals numerous oval molluscum bodies when examined with a microscope. A biopsy usually is not necessary unless the typical features are masked by secondary inflammation (Fig. 5.7B).

> When in doubt, the diagnosis may be confirmed by expressing the cheesy core and smearing it onto a glass slide for microscopic examination.

Therapy

The initial treatment is usually cryotherapy with liquid nitrogen. For children who will not tolerate the pain of curettage or cryotherapy, the careful application of the blistering chemical cantharidin (Verr-Canth) can be used in the office, or topical salicylic acid preparations can be used at home, similar to the treatment of warts. The most reliable means of eradication is by curettage. The molluscum papule, composed of many molluscum bodies, is scraped off – with some discomfort and bleeding. The topical immune response modifier, imiquimod (Aldara) cream 5% applied daily has been successful.

Therapy for Molluscum Contagiosum

Initial
- Cryotherapy with liquid nitrogen
- Salicylic acid
- Cantharidin

Alternative
- Curettage
- Imiquimod cream 5%

Course and Complications

Spontaneous remission often occurs within 6–9 months, although lesions have been known to persist for many years, and more lesions may develop by autoinoculation. Individual lesions can become secondarily inflamed and may resemble furuncles. Involvement of the eyelids is uncommon but may result in chronic conjunctivitis. The development of hundreds of lesions with little tendency for involution should alert the clinician to consider immunocompromise. Molluscum contagiosum is one of the most common cutaneous findings in acquired immune deficiency syndrome (AIDS) and AIDS-related complex, infecting 9% of these individuals. In the patient with AIDS, molluscum contagiosum is often recalcitrant to treatment and causes significant morbidity and disfigurement.

Pathogenesis

Although it is difficult to produce lesions after experimental inoculation, molluscum contagiosum is certainly contagious. Intimate physical contact such as occurs in Turkish baths, wrestling, and sexual intercourse has resulted in transmission of the disease.

The molluscum contagiosum virus replicates in the cytoplasm of the keratinocyte, with resulting large intracytoplasmic inclusion bodies (molluscum bodies) and proliferation of the epidermis. The center of the papule ultimately disintegrates, forming a crater and releasing molluscum bodies.

Spontaneous involution results from a host immune response that is presumed to be cell mediated. The stimulus that provokes this response after many months of inactivity is unknown, as with warts.

SEBORRHEIC KERATOSIS

Key Points

1. Common in older adults
2. Tan, brown, dark brown, well demarcated, 'pasted on' appearance
3. When in doubt, biopsy to rule out melanoma

Definition

A seborrheic keratosis is a benign neoplasm of epidermal cells that clinically appears as a scaling, 'pasted on' papule or plaque. It is thought to be an autosomal dominant inherited trait.

Incidence

Seborrheic keratoses usually appear in middle age, with at least a few lesions present in most elderly patients.

History

Many patients remember family members who had seborrheic keratoses. These neoplasms are gradually acquired in middle and later life, and grow slowly.

Physical Examination

Seborrheic keratoses vary in size from 2 mm to 2 cm and are slightly to markedly elevated (**Fig. 5.8**). Color ranges from flesh to tan or brown or, occasionally, black. The keratoses are oval to round, greasy-appearing, 'pasted on', sharply marginated growths. The surface is often verrucous or crumbly in appearance and may be punctuated with keratin-filled pits. The lesions occur on the head, neck, trunk, and extremities, sparing the palms and soles.

A tan/brown/dark brown well marginated, 'pasted on' appearance is distinctive.

Differential Diagnosis

Wart, *actinic keratosis*, and pigmented growths such as a *nevus*, *pigmented basal cell carcinoma*, or *malignant melanoma* may be confused with a seborrheic keratosis. The

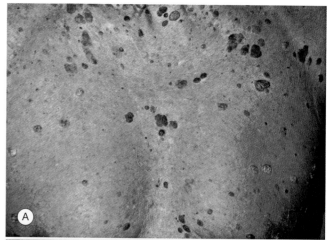

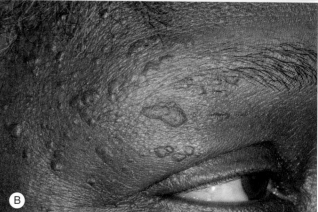

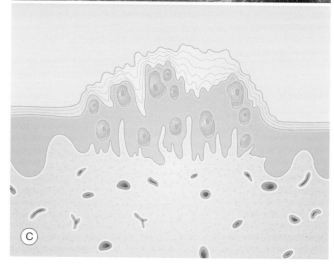

FIGURE 5.8 Seborrheic keratosis. A,B. Thick, corrugated, scaling, well marginated, 'pasted on,' brown and tan plaques. **C.** Epidermis – hyperkeratosis with thickened epidermis containing horny pseudocysts.

occurrence of multiple similar scaling growths with a greasy, well marginated, 'pasted on' appearance gives the observer the clue that these lesions are seborrheic keratoses. The superficial, exophytic, epidermal growth and keratotic surface of a seborrheic keratosis differentiate it from a nevus, a pigmented dermal growth with which it is often confused.

Laboratory and Biopsy

If there is concern for a melanoma, than an excisional or deep shave biopsy confirms the clinical impression of seborrheic keratosis. This neoplasm is characterized by a uniform, well demarcated, intraepidermal proliferation of small, benign squamous cells. Invaginations of the epidermis form small, keratin-filled pseudocysts (**Fig. 5.8C**).

> Deep shave or excisional biopsy is indicated for uncertain lesions.

Therapy

No therapy is necessary for seborrheic keratoses unless they become irritated, are cosmetically unacceptable, or require confirmation that they are benign. Cryotherapy with liquid nitrogen is an efficient and effective means of removal. As an alternative, seborrheic keratoses can be anesthetized and curetted or shaved off. Caution should be used; vigorous treatment may result in scarring. Excisional surgery is seldom needed unless concern about malignancy exists.

Therapy for Seborrheic Keratosis

Initial
- Cryotherapy with liquid nitrogen

Alternative
- Curettage
- Shave

Course and Complications

The tendency is to acquire more seborrheic keratoses with age. Sometimes, seborrheic keratoses become irritated from rubbing, clothing, or excoriations. Occasionally, their typical morphologic appearance becomes obscured by inflammation, thus making a biopsy necessary for diagnosis.

> The number of seborrheic keratoses increases with age.

Of note is the very rare *sign of Leser-Trélat*, the rapid increase in size and number of seborrheic keratoses accompanied by pruritus. This is a cutaneous sign of internal malignancy, usually adenocarcinoma involving the stomach, ovary, uterus, or breast. The extremities and shoulders are the most frequent sites of involvement.

SKIN TAG

Key Points

1. Soft pedunculated papules
2. No therapy necessary

Definition

A skin tag (acrochordon) is a benign fleshy tumor that is frequently acquired in adult life. It is characterized by a slightly hyperplastic epithelium covering a dermal connective tissue stalk. It appears as a pedunculated, flesh-colored growth.

Incidence

This benign tumor is extremely common in adulthood. The incidence of patients coming into the authors' clinic specifically for skin tags is 0.5%, but as an incidental finding 50–60% of patients older than 50 years have skin tags. A steady increase in frequency occurs from the 2nd decade (11%) to the 5th decade (59%) of life, after which the number of individuals with skin tags remains stable.

History

Most patients ignore skin tags and accept their acquisition as a sign of aging. Some patients request their removal because of irritation or cosmetic appearance.

Physical Examination

A skin tag is a soft, tan- to flesh-colored, 1–10 mm, pedunculated, fleshy papule (**Fig. 5.9A**). It has a smooth or folded surface and frequently appears boggy or filiform. It is found on any skin surface but has a predilection for the axilla, neck, inframammary region, inguinal region, and eyelids. When irritated or injured, it can appear as a necrotic, crusted papule that may not be clinically distinctive and causes concern regarding a malignancy.

Differential Diagnosis

Intradermal nevi may have a boggy, flesh-colored appearance, making them impossible to differentiate from skin tags other than by histologic examination. The acquisition of skin tags in later life would help to differentiate them historically from nevi. *Neurofibromas* can resemble skin tags, but on palpation a neurofibroma can be invaginated into what feels like a 'buttonhole' defect in the dermis. Uncommonly, *basal or squamous cell carcinoma* may have the appearance of a skin tag.

Laboratory and Biopsy

Skin tags are covered by a slightly hyperplastic epithelium consisting of hyperkeratosis, papillomatosis, and acanthosis. The underlying dermal connective tissue stalk is composed of loose collagen containing numerous capillaries (**Fig. 5.9B**). Typical multiple, 1–5 mm, flesh-colored, pedunculated skin tags need not be submitted for pathologic examination. Larger solitary and necrotic or crusted skin tags should be examined histologically.

> Large or necrotic skin tags should be sent to pathology.

Therapy

Skin tags need not be removed unless the patient requests it. The easiest means of removal of skin tags is by quickly snipping them with scissors. This usually requires no local anesthesia, and the crushing action of the scissors results in little bleeding. As an alternative, they may be frozen with liquid nitrogen.

Therapy for Skin Tags

Initial
- Snipping off with scissors

Alternative
- Cryotherapy with liquid nitrogen

Course and Complications

The number of skin tags increases with age. Tags normally are of little consequence and require no treatment. Concern has been expressed that skin tags may be a marker for the presence of colonic polyps in highly selected referral populations presenting for colonoscopy. In the primary care setting, no association exists between skin tags and colonic polyps.

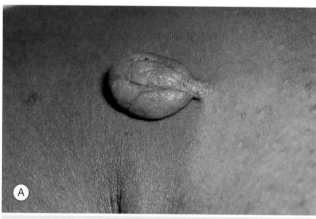

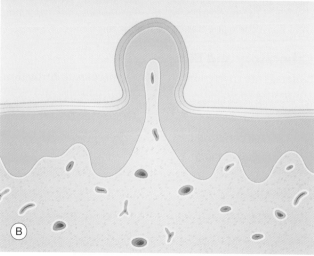

FIGURE 5.9 **Skin tag. A.** Soft, pedunculated, flesh-colored papule. **B.** Epidermis – mildly thickened. Dermis – loose connective tissue stalk.

SQUAMOUS CELL CARCINOMA

Key Points

1. Malignancy of keratinocytes
2. Potential to metastasize

Definition

Squamous cell carcinoma is a malignant neoplasm of keratinocytes. It is locally invasive and has the potential to metastasize. It appears clinically as a scaling, indurated plaque or nodule that sometimes bleeds or ulcerates (**Fig. 5.10**). The etiology of squamous cell carcinoma includes UV radiation, X-irradiation, and chemical carcinogens such as soot and arsenic.

Incidence

Squamous cell carcinoma is the second most common skin cancer, with nearly 250 000 new cases diagnosed each year in the USA. The incidence of squamous cell carcinoma varies greatly with reference to ethnic group, geographic location, and occupation. It is most common in men aged over 60 years who have light skin and abundant sunlight exposure. Closer to the equator, the incidence increases. For example, squamous cell carcinoma is five times greater in New Orleans than in Chicago. In renal transplant patients, squamous cell carcinoma is 3.5 times more frequent than basal cell carcinoma, and more than 250 times more common than in the general population. Some 9 years after renal transplantation, patients have a >40% incidence of squamous cell carcinoma.

> Squamous cell carcinoma is the second most common skin cancer.

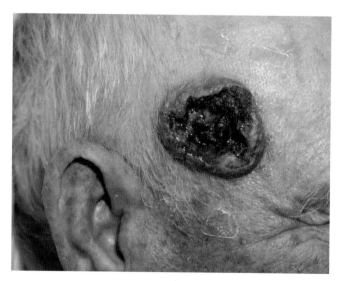

FIGURE 5.10 **Squamous cell carcinoma** – ulcerated plaque.

History

The patient's history of sunlight exposure in occupational and recreational activities is important in determining the risk of developing squamous cell carcinoma. A family history of skin cancer and a personal history of fair skin and sunburning are additional predisposing factors. The history of a chronic, non-healing, bleeding growth or ulcer should arouse suspicion of squamous cell carcinoma.

Physical Examination

Squamous cell carcinoma occurs most often in sun-exposed skin. It also develops on the mucous membranes and in sites of chronic injury such as burn scars, irradiated sites, erosive discoid lupus erythematosus, and osteomyelitis sinuses. The occurrence of squamous cell carcinoma varies with anatomic location: head and neck, 81%; upper extremities, 16%; trunk, 1.5%; legs, 1.3%. The tumor nodule is hard, is erythematous to flesh colored, and has a smooth or verrucous surface. The central portion may be hyperkeratotic, ulcerated, or crusted. Deep invasion results in fixation to underlying tissue. Squamous cell carcinoma of the lip involves the lower lip in 90% of cases and usually arises from a chronically damaged epithelium secondary to actinic exposure or smoking (**Fig. 5.11**).

> Most squamous cell carcinomas occur on the head, neck, and arms.

Differential Diagnosis

Squamous cell carcinoma can be differentiated clinically or by biopsy from a *keratoacanthoma, hypertrophic actinic keratosis, wart, basal cell carcinoma,* and *seborrheic keratosis.* All persistent ulcers or crusted lesions must undergo biopsy to rule out squamous cell carcinoma.

> Chronic ulcers should undergo biopsy to exclude malignancy.

Bowen's disease (**Fig. 5.12**) is squamous cell carcinoma *in situ* of the skin. It appears as an erythematous, scaling, crusted, well marginated patch. Squamous cell carcinoma *in situ* of the glans penis is referred to as erythroplasia of Queyrat, and appears as a red, velvety, moist patch.

Keratoacanthoma is a rapidly growing neoplasm of the epithelium that is biologically benign but histologically resembles a squamous cell carcinoma. Keratoacanthoma is a round, flesh-colored nodule that characteristically grows rapidly (within 4–6 weeks) and has a central keratin-filled crater (**Fig. 5.13**). Most keratoacanthomas spontaneously involute within 6 months. However, because some may be difficult to differentiate from squamous cell carcinoma, excision or other destructive treatment is recommended.

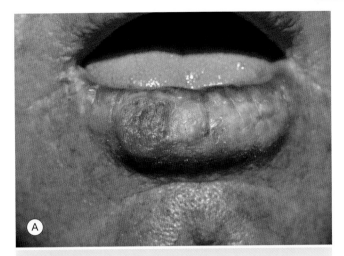

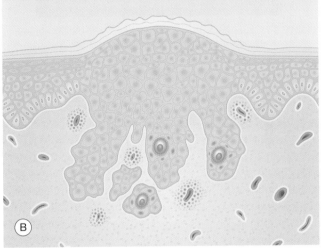

FIGURE 5.11 **Squamous cell carcinoma. A.** Slightly crusted, hyperkeratotic plaque on the lower lip, which raises concern about greater metastatic potential. **B.** Epidermis – hyperkeratosis, atypical keratinocytes. Dermis – invasive tumor, inflammation.

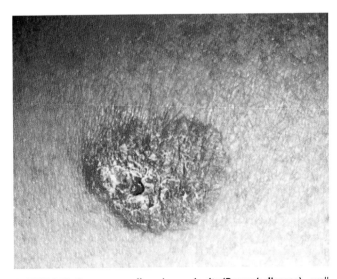

FIGURE 5.12 **Squamous cell carcinoma *in situ* (Bowen's disease)** – well demarcated erythematous, scaling, and crusted patch.

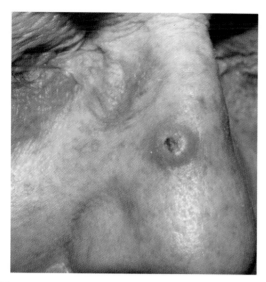

FIGURE 5.13 Keratoacanthoma. Rapidly growing erythematous nodule with a crusted, hyperkeratotic central crater.

Laboratory and Biopsy

Any lesion suspected of being squamous cell carcinoma should undergo biopsy. Squamous cell carcinoma consists of malignant epidermal cells that invade the dermis (Fig. 5.11B). It is graded according to the degree of atypicality of the tumor cells, with grade 1 predominantly mature, whereas grades 2, 3, and 4 are less well differentiated. Grade 4 tumors may be difficult to differentiate from malignant melanoma because their spindle-shape cells lack intercellular bridges.

The biopsy of squamous cell carcinoma *in situ* (*Bowen's disease*) reveals a thickened epidermis consisting of atypical, poorly oriented, dysplastic cells that lie completely within the epidermis. *Keratoacanthoma* has a large, central, keratin-filled crater surrounded by well differentiated epidermal cells that sometimes appear dysplastic, thus making it difficult to distinguish from a squamous cell carcinoma.

Therapy

Excision is the treatment of choice, although a well-differentiated small squamous cell carcinoma occurring in actinically damaged skin may be effectively treated with curettage and electrodesiccation. These surgical techniques are reviewed in Chapter 4. Large or recurrent poorly differentiated tumors, as well as those occurring on the mucous membrane and in scars, should be treated by scalpel excision with narrow margins (3–5 mm) that are checked histologically to be free of tumor or by the Mohs technique. Non-surgical therapy such as ionizing radiation is useful in selected patients. Sun protective measures such as the use of sunscreens, protective clothing, and avoiding midday UV light exposure are important for prevention of future squamous cell carcinomas.

Therapy for Squamous Cell Carcinoma

Initial
- Excision
- Curettage and electrodesiccation
- Mohs micrographic surgery

Alternative
- Radiation

Course and Complications

The course of squamous cell carcinoma is variable. Those carcinomas most likely to metastasize are relatively large, poorly differentiated, invade more deeply, and occur in damaged skin or on mucous membranes. Some 2% of all squamous cell carcinomas of the skin metastasize. Those that arise in actinic keratoses are less aggressive, with a metastasis rate of 0.5%. Much higher rates of metastasis, up to 9%, occur in squamous cell carcinoma arising in chronic leg ulcers, burn scars, radiodermatitis, osteomyelitis sinuses, and the mucous membrane of the lips, glans penis, and vulva. When metastasis occurs, it is usually through the lymphatics to the regional lymph nodes. Prophylactic lymph node dissection is not done unless the patient has lymphadenopathy.

Squamous cell carcinoma arising in actinic keratosis has a low metastatic potential.

High-risk features include: large size, >2 mm depth, perineural invasion, ear or mucous membrane, and poor differentiation.

Pathogenesis

Sir Percivall Pott in 1775 was the first to describe occupationally induced cancer and to relate cancer to an etiologic agent. He described the occurrence of squamous cell carcinoma of the scrotum in chimney sweeps and suggested that its cause was chronic soot exposure. In 1809, Lambe related squamous cell carcinoma to arsenic in drinking water. The relationship between UV radiation and squamous cell carcinoma was suggested in 1875 by Thiersch. Frieben in 1902 described the occurrence of squamous cell carcinoma after exposure to X-rays.

Experimentally, Yamagiwa and Ichikawa in 1915 were the first to produce squamous cell carcinoma in mice and rabbits after the topical application of coal tar. Several years later, in 1924, Block induced squamous cell carcinoma in rabbits after X-irradiation. Using mice repeatedly exposed to UV radiation, Findlay in 1928 was the first to produce UV radiation-induced carcinoma.

Human papillomavirus (HPV) has been implicated as the cause of cutaneous and cervical carcinoma. Patients with epidermodysplasia verruciformis, a rare genetic disorder, develop hundreds of flat warts, and those warts caused by specific types of HPV, particularly HPV-5, are prone to transform into squamous cell carcinoma. The finding of HPV-16 and -18 genomes in carcinoma of the cervix has provided strong circumstantial evidence for HPV carcinogenic potential.

All of these carcinogens – UV radiation, X-irradiation, coal tar, arsenic, and viruses – are active in the skin, initiating malignancy by altering cellular DNA, RNA, and proteins. In addition, UV radiation also alters the immune system, making the host more susceptible to these tumors. Chronic immunosuppression, as occurs in organ transplant patients, is also associated with an increased frequency of squamous cell carcinoma, especially in sun-damaged skin.

WART

> ## Key Points
>
> 1. Caused by multiple papillomavirus types
> 2. Vary in appearance
> 3. Treatments are nonspecific and destructive

Definition

Warts are benign neoplasms caused by infection of epidermal cells with papillomaviruses. The thickening of the epidermis with scaling and an upward extension of the dermal papillae containing prominent capillaries give them their 'warty' or verrucous appearance.

> Warts are caused by papillomaviruses.

Incidence

Warts generally occur in healthy children and young adults. Genital HPV infection may be the most common sexually transmitted disease. One percent of sexually active adults are estimated to have genital warts, and a further 10–20% have latent infection. For sexually active young college women, the incidence of infection is high: 43%. Some 5–7% of patients seen by dermatologists present with warts.

History

Predisposing conditions make the occurrence of multiple warts more likely. Immunosuppressed patients, such as renal transplant recipients, are prone to the development of warts. Inquiry into the patient's occupation is important because butchers and meat cutters have a significantly higher incidence of common warts. Anogenital warts (condylomata acuminata) affect sexually active individuals, and their occurrence in children should raise suspicions of sexual abuse. However, most patients with warts do not have any significant predisposing conditions.

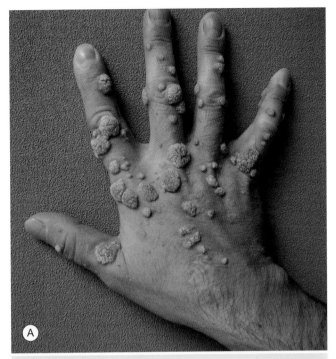

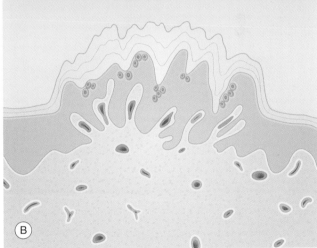

FIGURE 5.14 Wart. A. Scaling, verrucous papules with interrupted skin lines and black puncta. **B.** Thickened epidermis, with overlying hyperkeratosis. Vacuolated keratinocytes are present in the granular cell layer.

Physical Examination

The *common wart* (**Fig. 5.14**), or verruca vulgaris, is a flesh-colored firm papule or nodule that has a corrugated or hyperkeratotic surface. It interrupts the normal skin lines and is studded with black puncta. Common warts occur individually, in groups, or in a linear fashion from autoinoculation. The hands and fingers are the usual sites. Involvement around nails frequently results in extension underneath the nail plate. A filiform variant of verruca vulgaris occurs on the head and neck.

A *flat wart* has a subtle appearance (**Fig. 5.15**). It is a flesh-colored or reddish brown, slightly raised, flat-surfaced, 2–5-mm, well marginated papule. On extremely close inspection (a hand magnifying lens may be needed),

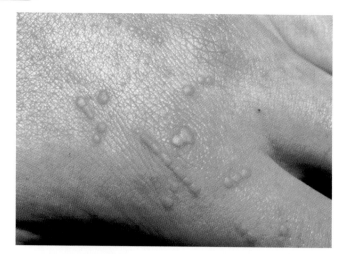

FIGURE 5.15 **Flat warts** – pinkish flat papules in a linear arrangement, suggesting autoinoculation.

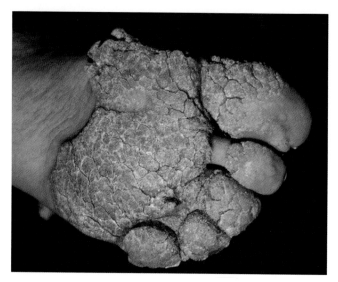

FIGURE 5.16 **Plantar warts** – confluent verrucous plaque.

the surface appears finely verrucous. Multiple lesions commonly affect the hands and face. A linear arrangement of lesions is common.

A *plantar wart* may occur as a single, painful papule on the plantar aspect of the foot. It is often covered by a thick callus. When the callus is pared down with a scalpel, the underlying wart is visualized with interruption of skin lines and black puncta. Multiple plantar warts may coalesce (**Fig. 5.16**) in a mosaic configuration or remain discrete in a mother–daughter relationship, with a central large wart surrounded by multiple smaller warts.

> Common and plantar warts interrupt skin lines and have black puncta.

Condyloma acuminatum (venereal wart) (**Fig. 5.17**) involves the rectum, perineal region, inguinal folds, external genitalia, and, occasionally, urethra and vagina. It is composed of a soft, moist papule and plaque that may be sessile or pedunculated. It has a verrucous surface that is often cauliflower-like. Soaking the genital area for

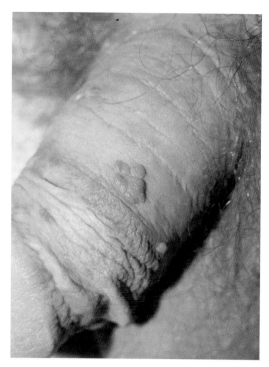

FIGURE 5.17 **Condyloma acuminatum** – verrucous, flesh-colored papules on the genitalia.

5 min with 3–5% acetic acid (white vinegar) causes warts to turn white. Subsequent use of a hand magnifying lens or colposcopy enables better visualization of small genital warts (aceto-whitening). Although aceto-whitening increases the sensitivity of detection, it is not specific for HPV lesions and is not recommended for routine screening because overdiagnosis of external genital warts may occur.

Differential Diagnosis

A common wart usually is easily recognized. When covered with thick scale, it may be confused with a *callus*, which on paring does not have interrupted skin lines. The diagnosis of *squamous cell carcinoma* should be entertained for a lesion that is resistant to treatment, is enlarging, and is crusted or ulcerated.

A flat wart on the face may be confused with a noninflammatory acne lesion, the 'whitehead' or *comedo*. The tops of comedones are smooth and dome-shaped, whereas flat warts have roughened flat tops. When flat warts occur on the hand and forearm, *lichen planus* (see Ch. 11), an idiopathic inflammatory skin disease, is in the differential diagnosis. Lichen planus papules are red to purple; warts are flesh colored.

Plantar warts and *corns* are often confused because both are painful and have a thick, scaling surface. However, paring down the surface demonstrates the interruption of skin lines and black puncta characteristic of a plantar wart.

Condyloma acuminatum may resemble the verrucous form of squamous cell carcinoma. Lesions that do not respond to treatment must undergo biopsy. *Secondary syphilis* of the anus and genitals (condyloma latum) is ruled out with a darkfield examination and serology. *Seborrheic keratoses* in the genital region also may resemble condyloma acuminatum.

Bowenoid papulosis is an uncommon disorder characterized by erythematous, sometimes pigmented, papules occurring in the genital region of sexually active young adults. Histologically, bowenoid papulosis has the appearance of squamous cell carcinoma *in situ*. Its relationship with HPV infection has been confirmed by finding HPV DNA in bowenoid papulosis, especially HPV-16. Conservative surgical modalities should be used to treat bowenoid papulosis. Radical, mutilating procedures are unwarranted.

Laboratory and Biopsy

Warts are usually not biopsied unless a suspicion of carcinoma exists. When examined by biopsy, warts demonstrate a thickened epidermis (acanthosis) with overlying hyperkeratosis (**Fig. 5.14B**). Distinctive large keratinocytes (koilocytes) with small pyknotic nuclei surrounded by clear cytoplasm are found in the upper layers of the epidermis. Typing of HPV based on DNA homology is a technique currently available in only a few laboratories.

Therapy

Prevention of warts is better than treatment. A quadrivalent vaccine (Gardasil), preventing types 6 and 11 (which cause anogenital warts), and types 16 and 18 (responsible for >70% of cervical cancers), is highly effective for young naive males and females.

> Prevention is better than treatment.

Treatment of warts is nonspecific, destructive, and usually painful. A topical local anesthetic applied under occlusion 1–2 h before painful procedures may be beneficial when treating warts in uncooperative children. The goal is destruction of the keratinocytes that are infected with HPV. This may be accomplished with a variety of physical, chemical, or biologic modalities.

> Avoid overzealous treatment, which produces scars.

The physical modalities include cryotherapy with liquid nitrogen, electrodesiccation and curettage, surgical excision, and laser therapy. Cryotherapy, the most common initial mode of treatment, uses either a cotton-tipped stick or a cryospray unit for application of the liquid nitrogen onto the verruca. A white ice ball develops at the site of freezing and should extend 1–2 mm beyond the margins of the wart. After the area has thawed, a second freezing results in greater destruction of the wart. Subsequent blister formation often occurs within 24 h. After a couple of weeks, the blister dries, and the skin containing the wart peels off. Often, follow-up treatments every 2–4 weeks are necessary to eradicate any residual wart. Eradication generally requires at least two or three visits. The advantages of cryotherapy are that it is quick, does not require local anesthesia, and the discomfort from the freezing is tolerated well by most patients, except young children. Caution must be used with all the physical modalities, especially surgical excision, because of potential scarring. The scar may be cosmetically unacceptable, or it may be painful if on the plantar surface. Although laser surgery was initially thought to be superior to other surgical procedures in removing warts, this now appears not to be true.

Numerous chemotherapeutic agents are used to treat warts either in the office or at home. The initial treatments include salicylic acid at home or trichloroacetic acid in the office. Common warts may be treated with non-prescription 17% salicylic acid preparations applied daily with or without occlusion (duct tape). The wart is softened by soaking in water for 5 min before application; any loosened tissue is gently removed. Once the acid has been applied, the wart can be covered with adhesive tape. Cantharidin, a potent blistering agent derived from the blister beetle, is an alternative office treatment that is applied to common warts and covered with tape. After 24 h, a blister forms beneath the wart. The blister roof dries and peels off, taking with it the wart. Occasionally, cantharidin or cryotherapy may result in formation of a new wart in an annular configuration (ring) at the periphery of the blister.

Tretinoin (Retin-A) is useful in the treatment of flat warts; its efficacy probably results from its irritant effect.

Therapy for Warts

Initial
- Cryotherapy with liquid nitrogen – all warts
- Salicylic acid plus occlusion with tape – common and plantar warts
- Cantharidin – especially for children
- Tretinoin 0.1% cream – flat warts
- Podophyllin 25% – genital warts
- Podofilox solution or gel – genital warts: twice daily for 3 days/week for 4 weeks
- Imiquimod cream – genital warts: once daily for 3 days/week for 16 weeks

Alternative
- Surgical excision, curettage, electrocautery
- Laser
- Interferon
- Bleomycin intralesionally
- 5-Fluorouracil
- Sinecatechins 15% ointment – genital warts: 3 times daily for 16 weeks

---

Plantar verrucae are treated with daily applications of salicylic acid plaster or 17% salicylic acid liquid under occlusion (duct tape).

Genital warts (condyloma acuminatum) are commonly treated with 25% podophyllin resin (Podocon-25), which can be very toxic and is used only in the clinician's office. Within 4–6 h after application, excess podophyllin should be washed off to prevent excessive local irritation. Caution must be used when applying podophyllin to extensive lesions because severe systemic reactions may result from absorption. The Centers for Disease Control and Prevention prefer cryotherapy over podophyllin for treatment of condyloma acuminatum. Podophyllin is a cytotoxic agent and has resulted in renal toxicity, polyneuritis, and shock. Podophyllin must never be used during pregnancy because of potential harmful effects on the fetus. Podofilox, a chemically pure ligand derived from podophyllin, is available as a 0.5% topical solution or gel (Condylox, Podofilox) for patient self-treatment of external genital warts. Application is made twice daily for 3 consecutive days followed by a 4-day rest period. This cycle may be repeated up to four times. Sinecatechins 15% ointment (Veregen) is an alternative treatment. The sexual partners of infected individuals should be examined for the presence of genital warts. Female patients with genital warts should have periodic gynecologic examinations with Papanicolaou smears. Screening for other sexually transmitted diseases should be considered.

> Podophyllin is toxic; do not apply to extensive lesions or use to treat pregnant women.

Recalcitrant warts have been treated with 5-fluorouracil topically, bleomycin intralesionally, and interferon topically, intralesionally, and systemically.

Biologic treatments have centered on the induction of immune responses. Imiquimod (Aldara) cream 5% applied topically induces the cytokines interferon α, tumor necrosis factor α, and interleukins 1, 6, and 8. It is indicated for the treatment of external genital and perianal warts, with three applications per week. Squaric acid dibutylester has been used to induce allergic contact dermatitis. Presumably, the wart is destroyed by the delayed hypersensitivity reaction that occurs at the site of application of the allergens. Currently, no wart vaccines are available.

Course and Complications

A total of 35–65% of warts resolve spontaneously within 2 years. Treatment results in cure rates of as high as 80%.

Of concern is the relationship between papillomavirus and carcinoma. Papillomavirus-associated cancers occur in humans, cattle, horses, and rabbits, and experimentally in rodents. In patients with the rare syndrome *epidermodysplasia verruciformis*, manifest by widespread refractory warts, who are infected with HPV-5 or HPV-8, sun-exposed flat warts progress into squamous cell carcinoma. Furthermore, HPV genomes have been demonstrated within the malignant squamous cells. The epidemiologic evidence for an association between papillomavirus (type 16, 18, or 33) and cervical cancer is overwhelming. HPV infection of the cervix appears to represent a necessary but not sufficient condition for developing malignancy. Other possible co-factors, such as cigarette smoking, appear to be required for carcinogenesis. HPV typing, however, has not been proven to be beneficial in the diagnosis and management of external genital warts.

> Papillomavirus is associated with some carcinomas, particularly cervical carcinoma.

Pathogenesis

The contagious nature of warts was observed in ancient times. Jadassohn in the 1800s was the first to prove conclusively the infectious nature of warts. He ground up wart material and inoculated the normal skin of volunteers. After an incubation period of 2–3 months, warts developed in the inoculation sites. In 1907 Ciuffo proved the viral nature of warts using ultrafiltration techniques.

The papillomavirus is a double-stranded DNA virus that infects and replicates in keratinizing cells in the epidermis. The HPV virion is an icosahedral particle composed of a viral genome surrounded by a proteinaceous capsid. Progeny HPV virions are assembled and become apparent in the upper layers of the epidermis, especially the stratum corneum and stratum granulosum. Viral genomes are found in lower layers of the epidermis and probably help to explain the chronicity and treatment failure of many warts. The presence of the wart virus stimulates epidermal proliferation, resulting in epidermal thickening and hyperkeratosis. Papillomaviruses have been subdivided into distinct types based on DNA homology. On this basis, >80 genotypes have been described. The

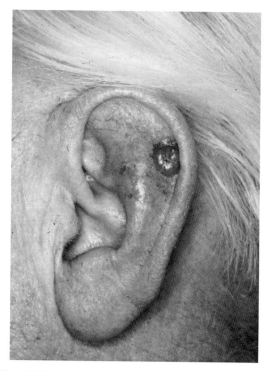

FIGURE 5.18 Merkel cell carcinoma – pearly pink nodule.

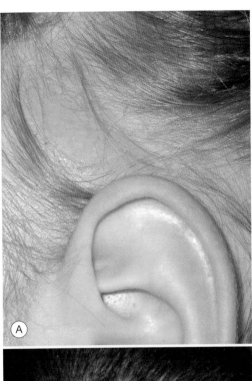

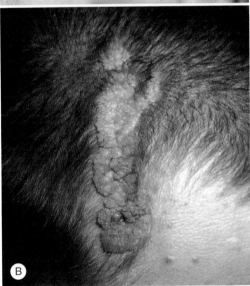

FIGURE 5.19 **Nevus sebaceous. A.** Typical smooth, yellow plaque with alopecia in a child. **B.** Yellow-brown, verrucous, linear plaque with alopecia and a pink papule (syringocystadenoma papilliferum).

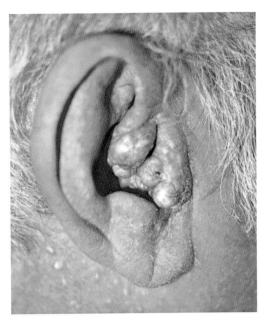

FIGURE 5.20 **Trichoepithelioma** – flesh-colored and yellowish nodular plaque.

UNCOMMON EPIDERMAL GROWTHS

MERKEL CELL CARCINOMA

Merkel cell carcinoma is a rare malignant tumor that usually occurs as an asymptomatic, solitary nodule on the head and neck of elderly, fair-skinned patients (**Fig. 5.18**). The etiology of this tumor appears to be the Merkel cell polyomavirus. Of great concern is its high rate of local recurrence, metastasis to regional lymph nodes and distant viscera, and mortality. The histologic appearance of the tumor can be confused with that of other primary and metastatic neoplasms of the skin. Treatment requires wide local excision, sentinel lymph node biopsy, and radiotherapy. Chemotherapy is administered for disseminated disease.

NEVUS SEBACEOUS

This hamartoma of the sebaceous glands and other cutaneous structures appears at birth as a thin yellowish plaque with alopecia. In adulthood, the plaque becomes verrucous, and both benign and malignant tumors may develop (**Fig. 5.19**). For this reason, excision is often recommended when the individual is a teen or young adult. Extensive nevus sebaceous may be associated with neurologic or skeletal abnormalities, as found in the epidermal nevus syndrome.

TRICHOEPITHELIOMA

Trichoepithelioma is a benign tumor of the hair follicle. It usually appears on the face as solitary or multiple, firm, smooth, flesh-colored papules or nodules (**Fig. 5.20**). Multiple trichoepitheliomas may be inherited as an autosomal dominant condition. Differentiation from basal cell carcinoma is important.

clinical type of wart had been thought to be determined by local conditions at the site of infection. However, it now appears that different HPV types are responsible for the different clinical lesions – common, flat, plantar, and condyloma acuminatum – because good correlation often exists between clinical presentation and HPV type.

The viral and host factors that influence persistence, regression, latency, and reactivation of warts are poorly understood. Serum antibodies to warts have been detected. More importantly, cell-mediated immunity appears to contribute to the regression of warts; in immunodeficient hosts (e.g., those with organ transplants or epidermodysplasia verruciformis), warts may reactivate or persist.

6   Pigmented Growths

Key Points

1. Melanocytes produce melanin, the skin pigment
2. When recognized early, malignant melanoma is curable

ABSTRACT

The skin has one pigment-forming cell: the melanocyte. Melanocytes are dendritic cells found in the basal layer of the epidermis. Nevus cells, a type of melanocyte, found in the basal layer of the epidermis as well as in the dermis, are arranged in nests, and do not have dendritic processes. Melanocytes contain tyrosinase, the enzyme necessary for pigment (melanin) synthesis, and are thought to be derived from a progenitor cell in the neural crest.

Pigmented growths (Table 6.1) are the result of an increased number of melanocytes, nevus cells, or pigment deposition. The diagnosis of malignant melanoma is important because it can be recognized early, when it is curable.

FRECKLE

Key Points

1. Sun-induced brown macules
2. Evidence of significant sun exposure and light complexion

Definition

A freckle (ephelis) is a hyperpigmented macule found in sun-exposed areas of the skin (**Fig. 6.1**). The amount of melanin in the basal area of the epidermis is increased, with no increase in the number of melanocytes.

Incidence

Freckles are a common incidental finding during a skin examination and are rarely a reason, in and of themselves, for seeking medical attention.

History

Freckles usually appear before 3 years of age and darken after ultraviolet (UV) light exposure. The patient has a history of sunburning easily.

> Sunlight darkens freckles.

Physical Examination

The freckled individual typically has a fair complexion and reddish or sandy hair. Hundreds of freckles occur on sun-exposed skin. They are 1–6 mm, irregularly shaped, discrete brown macules.

> Freckles occur only in sun-exposed areas.

Differential Diagnosis

Lentigo and *junctional nevus* can look like a freckle. *Actinic lentigo* does not darken with sun exposure and is acquired later in life. In contrast, freckles darken after sun exposure and are present from early childhood. *Lentigo simplex* is acquired in childhood, but the lentigines are not confined to sun-exposed skin. *Junctional nevi* and freckles are acquired in childhood. Darker pigmentation and lack of change after sunlight exposure favor a diagnosis of junctional nevus.

Laboratory and Biopsy

Ordinarily, freckles do not require biopsy (**Fig. 6.1B**).

TABLE 6.1 Pigmented growths

	Frequency (%)[a]	History	Physical Examination	Differential Diagnosis	Laboratory Test (Biopsy)
Freckle		Appear before age 3 years	Tan macule, sun-exposed skin	Junctional nevus Lentigo Seborrheic keratosis	No
Lentigo	0.2	Acquired at any age	Brown macule	Junctional nevus Freckle Seborrheic keratosis	If uneven color
Melanoma	0.3	Recent acquisition Itches Bleeds Growing			Excision or deep shave biopsy
Superficial spreading			Irregular surface, border, color	Nevus Seborrheic keratosis Hemangioma Pigmented basal cell carcinoma	
Lentigo maligna			Irregular surface, border, color	Actinic lentigo Seborrheic keratosis	
Acral lentiginous melanoma			Irregular surface, border, color	Nevus Tinea nigra palmaris	
Nodular			Blue–black nodule	Blue nevus Pyogenic granuloma Angioma Dermatofibroma	
Melasma	0.2	Adults	Brown macules on face	Post-inflammatory hyperpigmentation Freckle	No
Nevus	2.8	Not acquired past 3rd decade	Flesh- or brown-colored macule or papule; smooth or verrucous surface	Melanoma Seborrheic keratosis Skin tag Neurofibroma Dermatofibroma Basal cell carcinoma Lentigo Freckle	If change

[a]Percentage of new dermatology patients with this diagnosis seen in the Hershey Medical Center Dermatology Clinic, Hershey, PA.

Therapy

Freckles should be accepted as normal. Prevention by sunlight avoidance is effective but not practical.

Therapy for Freckles

- None

Pathogenesis

Ultraviolet radiation induces an increase in melanin pigment in the basal layer of the epidermis without an increase in melanocytes.

LENTIGO

Key Points

1. Lentigo simplex occurs in childhood and is idiopathic
2. Actinic lentigo occurs in adults and is sun-induced

Definition

A lentigo (plural, lentigines) is a brown macule caused by an increased number of melanocytes. Two types are recognized: lentigo simplex lesions arise in childhood and are few in number, whereas actinic (solar) lentigines

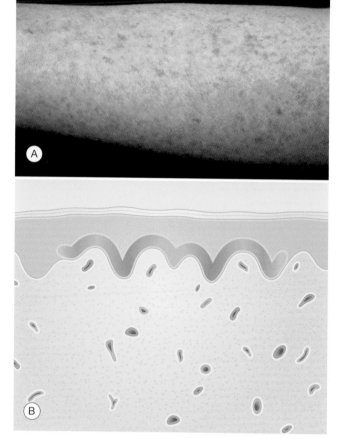

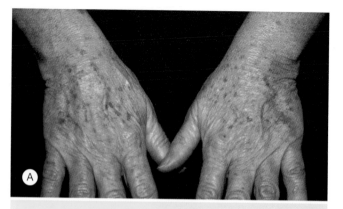

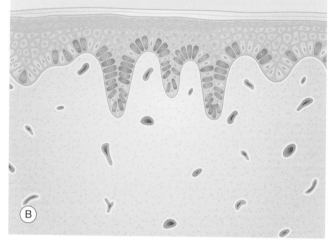

FIGURE 6.1 **Freckles. A.** Brown macules on sun-exposed skin of a youth. **B.** Epidermis – melanin pigmentation in basal layer.

FIGURE 6.2 **Actinic lentigo. A.** Small brown macules in sun-exposed skin of a middle-aged person. **B.** Epidermis – increased basal layer pigmentation resulting from increase in melanocytes and melanin; rete ridges are elongated.

(**Fig. 6.2**) arise in middle age and are numerous in sun-exposed skin.

> Types of lentigo:
> 1. Simplex – few, congenital or in childhood
> 2. Actinic – many, sun-exposed skin, in middle age

Incidence

Lentigo simplex is uncommon. Actinic lentigines are found on more than 90% of Caucasians after the age of 70 years, but seldom cause a patient to seek medical advice.

History

Lentigo simplex may be congenital or may arise in childhood. It has no relation to sun exposure. Conversely, actinic lentigo is acquired in middle age, does not fade, and occurs in sun-exposed skin. Patients often call actinic lentigo 'liver spots.'

Physical Examination

Lentigo is a uniform, tan, brown or dark brown macule. Lentigo simplex is sharply marginated and occurs anywhere on the body and mucosae. These lesions are usually few in number.

> Lentigo is a brown macule with uniform color.

Actinic or solar lentigo is a tan or brown macule, ranging in size from several millimeters to several centimeters, with distinct borders. The lesion occurs in sun-exposed areas of the body: on the dorsum of the hands, neck, head, and shoulders.

Differential Diagnosis

In childhood, the differential diagnosis of lentigo includes junctional nevus and freckle. In adults, seborrheic keratosis and lentigo maligna are included in the differential diagnosis. The most important of these is lentigo maligna, which appears as an irregularly colored (varying shades of brown and black), irregularly bordered macule on sun-exposed regions of the body. A lentigo maligna is an *in situ* malignant melanoma.

Laboratory and Biopsy

Biopsy is seldom indicated. If biopsy is performed, the histologic picture is characterized by an increased number of melanocytes within the epidermis as well as increased pigmentation within the keratinocytes. The rete ridges may be normal or elongated (**Fig. 6.2B**).

Therapy

No therapeutic intervention is required, except for cosmetic purposes. For multiple actinic lentigo, tretinoin cream 0.1% (Retin-A) applied daily is effective in lightening these photo-aging spots. Irritation, however, is common, thus requiring less frequent application (every other day or every third day) or use of a less concentrated cream (0.025% or 0.05%). Preparations containing hydroquinone are generally ineffective. A combination product, 2% mequinol plus 0.01% tretinoin solution (Solage) applied twice daily, lightens these spots. Mild freezing with liquid nitrogen or laser destruction of these pigmented lesions is effective. Sunscreens with a sun protective factor (SPF) of 30 should be used to prevent the development of more actinic lentigo.

Therapy for Lentigo

Initial
- Cryotherapy

Alternative
- Laser
- Tretinoin cream 0.1% daily or less frequently
- Mequinol 2% plus tretinoin 0.01% solution (Solage) twice daily
- Sunscreen SPF 30

Course and Complications

Lentigo has no malignant potential. The *multiple lentigines syndrome*, a rare but distinctive syndrome, is characterized by hundreds of lentigines on the trunk, head, and extremities, including the palms and soles. It is dominantly inherited and also called the *LEOPARD* syndrome (Lentigines, Electrocardiographic abnormalities, Ocular hypertelorism, Pulmonary stenosis, Abnormal genitalia, Retarded growth and development, and Deafness).

Syndromes with numerous lentigines:
1. LEOPARD
2. Peutz–Jeghers

Peutz–Jeghers syndrome is a dominantly inherited trait that is distinctive because of numerous lentigines occurring around the mouth and eyes as well as on the lips, oral mucosa, hands, and feet, in association with gastrointestinal polyps. Intussusception, hemorrhage, and malignancy are complications of these polyps.

MALIGNANT MELANOMA

Key Points

1. Thin melanoma is curable
2. Prognosis is best predicted by depth of invasion (Breslow thickness) in primary cutaneous melanoma
3. Sentinal lymph node biopsy is prognostic, not therapeutic

Definition

Malignant melanoma is a cancerous neoplasm of pigment-forming cells, melanocytes, and nevus cells. Clinically, its hallmarks are an irregularly shaped and colored papule or plaque. Four types of melanoma are recognized (**Table 6.2**): (1) superficial spreading; (2) lentigo maligna; (3) nodular; and (4) acral lentiginous.

Incidence

The occurrence of malignant melanoma is increasing faster than that of any other cancer in the USA, with increased sunlight exposure implicated as one possible factor. More than 55 000 new cases of melanoma are diagnosed yearly in the USA, with the majority occurring in the 15–50-year-old age group. The estimated lifetime risk of developing a malignant melanoma is approaching 1 in 50.

The incidence of malignant melanoma is increasing and related to UV exposure.

History

An increase in the size of the lesion or a change in its color is noted in at least 70% of patients who have melanoma. Development of a new growth, bleeding, and

TABLE 6.2 Clinical features of melanoma

Type	Location	Median Age (years)	Pre-Metastatic	Frequency (%)[a]	Ethnicity
Lentigo maligna	Sun-exposed surfaces (head, neck)	70	5–15 years	10	Caucasian
Superficial spreading	All surfaces (back, legs)	47	1–7 years	27	Caucasian
Nodular	All surfaces	50	Months to 2 years	9	Caucasian
Acral lentiginous	Palms, soles, nail beds	61	Months to 8 years	1	Black, Asian

[a]53% of melanomas are unclassified.

itching are other symptoms that may accompany a melanoma. Occasionally, patients have a family history of malignant melanoma.

Physical Examination

Lentigo maligna melanoma, superficial spreading melanoma, and acral lentiginous melanoma are characterized by a horizontal growth phase that allows for clinical identification before deeper invasion and metastasis occur. The ABCDs of identifying characteristics for these three types of melanoma are: Asymmetry, Border irregularity, Color variegation, and Diameter >6 mm. The suspicious lesion is red, white, and blue, has a notched border, and has a papule or nodule within it. However, in approximately 10% of melanomas, the ABCD rule does not apply. Therefore, any pigmented lesion or 'nevus' that looks significantly different from an individual's other nevi – the 'ugly duckling' mole – should be viewed suspiciously and biopsied.

Melanoma signs (ABCDs):
1. Asymmetry
2. Border irregularity – notched border
3. Color variegation – red, white, blue
4. Diameter >6 mm

Lentigo maligna melanoma (**Fig. 6.3**) occurs on sun-exposed skin, especially the head and neck. It is multicolored, with dark brown, black, red, white, and blue hues, and it is elevated in areas. It is preceded by lentigo maligna (*in situ* melanoma), which extends peripherally and is an unevenly pigmented, dark brown and black macule. Lentigo maligna often reaches a diameter of 5–7 cm before showing signs of invasion. The change in size and darkening are insidious, occurring over a period of years.

The most common type of melanoma is the *superficial spreading melanoma* (**Fig. 6.4**). This lesion is irregular in color (red, white, and blue), surface (papular or nodular), and border (notched), and may occur anywhere on the body. It is found most frequently on the upper back in males, and on the upper back and lower legs in females. During the horizontal growth phase, the lesion is flat, extending to approximately 2.5 cm in diameter before invasion develops.

Nodular melanoma (**Fig. 6.5**) is a rapidly growing, blue-black, smooth or eroded nodule. It occurs anywhere on the body. It begins in the vertical growth phase, so is less likely to be diagnosed in a pre-metastatic stage.

Acral lentiginous melanoma (**Fig. 6.6**) occurs on the palms, soles, and distal portion of the toes or fingers. It is an irregular, enlarging, black growth similar to a lentigo maligna melanoma. The vertical growth phase in this type of melanoma can be deceptive, showing only a small degree of papular elevation associated with a deep invasion. In contrast to the other melanomas, acral lentiginous melanoma is most frequent in the Black and Asian populations.

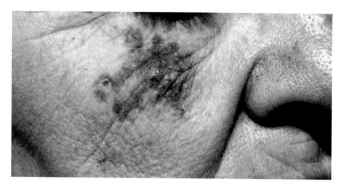

FIGURE 6.3 Lentigo maligna melanoma – large, brown, black, irregularly shaped macule that typically occurs on the face of the elderly.

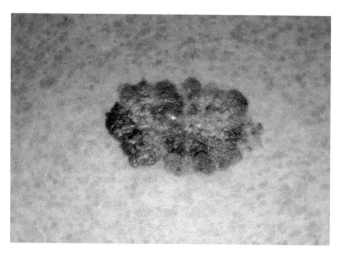

FIGURE 6.4 Superficial spreading melanoma – brown-black, irregularly surfaced and bordered plaque with a red papule.

Differential Diagnosis

Although the clinical criteria outlined above allow for the early diagnosis of malignant melanoma, other pigmented lesions must be considered before definitive therapy is undertaken. In one study, two-thirds of the pigmented lesions that were thought clinically to be malignant melanoma were not malignant by histopathologic criteria.

The differential diagnosis of lentigo maligna melanoma includes *actinic lentigo* and *seborrheic keratosis*. The brown color of these latter lesions is a reassuring sign of their benignity.

Pigmented basal cell carcinoma, seborrheic keratosis, nevus, and *angioma* can look like superficial spreading malignant melanoma.

Nodular melanoma can resemble *pyogenic granuloma, angioma, blue nevus,* and *dermatofibroma*. A pyogenic granuloma is an easily bleeding nodule composed of numerous benign blood vessels. It often occurs after minor trauma and can be viewed as excessive granulation tissue.

Tinea nigra palmaris, a rare superficial fungal infection, and nevus should be considered in the differential diagnosis of acral lentiginous melanoma. Tinea nigra palmaris can easily be diagnosed with a potassium hydroxide scraping that reveals fungal hyphae.

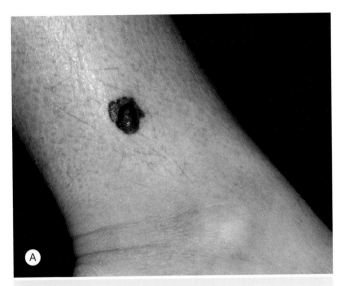

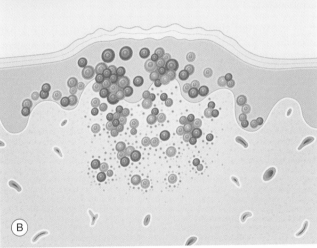

FIGURE 6.5 **A.** Nodular melanoma – blue-black nodule. **B.** Epidermis – atypical pigmented melanoma cells. Dermis – variously sized nests of atypical melanoma cells, inflammation.

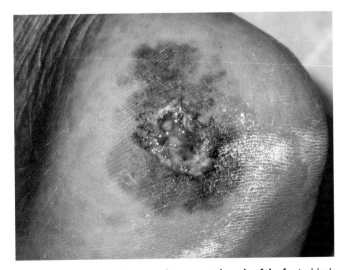

FIGURE 6.6 **Acral lentiginous melanoma on the sole of the foot** – black and whitish, irregularly shaped and bordered plaque with an erosion.

Biopsy

All suspicious pigmented lesions must undergo biopsy, by excision with narrow 2–3-mm margins of normal skin or by deep shave biopsy. Definitive treatment by wide surgical excision should not be undertaken until confirmation of malignant melanoma has been made histologically. For extensive lesions such as lentigo maligna melanoma, it is acceptable to perform an incisional biopsy before definitive therapy. The histologic features vary with the type of melanoma, and require a skilled pathologist for interpretation (**Fig. 6.5B**).

> All suspicious pigmented lesions, especially the 'ugly duckling' mole, that could be melanoma should undergo biopsy excision or deep shave.

Therapy

The survival of patients with malignant melanoma depends on early diagnosis, when surgical excision is often curative. The margin of normal skin excised around the melanoma increases with the depth of invasion, or thickness: *in situ*, 0.5 cm margin; thickness <2 mm, 1 cm margin; thickness >2 mm, 2 cm margin.

> Cure of malignant melanoma rests in the hands of the surgeon, if the lesion is treated early enough.

Radiolymphatic *sentinel node* mapping and biopsy have been used for melanomas >1 mm in thickness in patients with clinically negative lymph nodes. A radioactive tracer is injected at the site of the primary melanoma before wider excision is performed. The first draining or sentinel lymph node can be identified by lymphoscintigraphy and examined by biopsy for the presence of metastatic melanoma. In this way, the clinician can identify patients who may benefit from regional lymphadenectomy and adjuvant immunotherapy. Prognostic information is also garnered.

> Sentinal lymph node biopsy is an appropriate staging procedure. Its survival benefit is controversial.

Once a malignant melanoma has metastasized, therapy is with dacarbazine alone or in combination with other agents. Radiation therapy is used for palliation of bone and brain metastasis, and when lentigo maligna is so large that surgical removal is technically difficult.

Immunotherapeutic approaches for the treatment of disseminated melanoma include cytokines (interferons and interleukins), monoclonal antibodies, autologous lymphocytes, and specific immunization. Interferon α-2b (Intron A) and interleukin 2 (Proleukin) are approved as an adjuvant to surgical treatment in patients at high risk of systemic recurrence of the disease. These patients have melanomas >4 mm thick, or nodal involvement. Median overall survival was increased by 11 months with high-dose interferon α-2b compared with no treatment. However, high-dose interferon causes significant toxicity.

Kinase inhibitors and biologic agents have caused significant response rates. However, they are not long lasting as a solo therapy. Known mutations (BRAF, KIT, N-RAS, PTEN) provide therapeutic signaling pathway targets for inhibition of melanoma growth.

Therapy for Malignant Melanoma

Initial
- Wide excision with margins of normal skin based on thickness of melanoma: *in situ* 0.5 cm margin; thickness <2 mm, 1 cm margin; thickness >2 mm, 2 cm margin

Alternative
- Chemotherapy – DTIC (dacarbazine)
- Radiation
- Immunotherapy – interferon α-2b, interleukin, ipilimumab
- Kinase inhibitor (BRAF V600E) – vemurafenib

Course and Complications

Lentigo maligna melanoma, superficial spreading melanoma, and acral lentiginous melanoma initially have a horizontal growth phase manifested as a macular or slightly raised pigmented lesion. During the horizontal growth phase, malignant melanoma is totally curable. Nodular melanoma has only a vertical growth phase. Certain principles are important concerning malignant melanoma:

1. A horizontal growth phase makes surgical cure possible for superficial melanoma
2. The prognosis is related to tumor thickness
3. Clinical criteria allow for an early diagnosis of malignant melanoma.

Clark and Breslow correlated survival with tumor thickness. Clark and co-workers devised a system of microstaging melanoma based on level of invasion in the dermis. The difficulty with this system is variability in differentiating between level 3 and level 4 melanomas. Breslow, using an ocular micrometer, measured tumor thickness from the stratum granulosum to the depth of invasion. These measurements are reproducible and are the preferred method of calculating tumor thickness and, thus, of predicting 5-year survival (**Fig. 6.7**).

Guidelines for Recommended Follow-Up of Patients with Malignant Melanoma

- New or changing mole?
- Review of symptoms
- Examine complete skin surface + lymph nodes + liver and spleen
- Thickness >1 mm: annual chest radiography
- More extensive studies based on patient's symptoms and signs
- Follow-up visit every 6 months for 2 years, and then annually

---

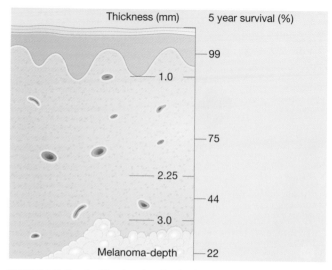

FIGURE 6.7 **Survival** is related to depth of invasion (thickness measured in millimeters).

It is estimated that patients with melanoma have a 5% chance of developing a second one. Extensive laboratory tests such as brain, bone, liver, and spleen scans, magnetic resonance imaging, or positron emission tomography are not indicated unless the history or physical examination suggests possible metastasis to these organs.

Pathogenesis

The pathogenesis of malignant melanoma is unknown. However, sunlight (sunburn) and heredity (*CDKN2A* and *CDK4* gene mutations) have been implicated as risk factors. Other risk factors for melanoma include a large number of small nevi, large nevi, and dysplastic nevi. The production of melanoma by UV radiation is suggested both epidemiologically and experimentally. The cause-and-effect relationship, however, is less well proven than with other skin cancers. Familial occurrence of malignant melanoma is rare but well established. The *familial atypical mole and melanoma syndrome* (*dysplastic nevus syndrome* or B-K mole syndrome) occurs in family members with numerous atypical-appearing, haphazardly colored and bordered nevi (*atypical moles*) and who have one or several malignant melanomas. Biopsy of these atypical moles reveals disordered melanocytic proliferation. These atypical moles are markers for an increased risk of developing malignant melanoma and, in some cases, precursors of melanoma. This syndrome occurs sporadically and in a familial pattern. Close clinical follow-up and excision of suspicious nevi are mandatory (see Nevus section, below, for guidelines). Genetic testing may be considered when: three family members have melanoma; an individual has three melanomas, or three cancer events (melanoma or pancreatic cancer) occur in a family.

MELASMA

Key Points

1. Brown macules on the face
2. Treat with 4% hydroquinone and sun protection

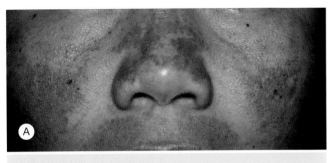
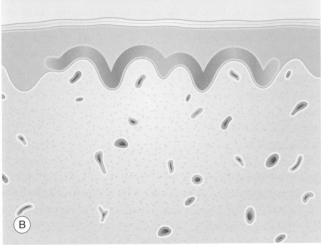

FIGURE 6.8 Melasma. A. Brown macules on the face. **B.** Epidermis – melanin pigmentation in basal layer.

Definition

Melasma (chloasma) is patchy macular hyperpigmentation of the face (**Fig. 6.8**). It usually affects women. The melanocytes in melasma produce more melanin in response to multiple factors, including UV radiation, genetic predisposition, and hormonal influences.

Incidence

Melasma is more common in women and in those from darkly pigmented ethnic groups. The frequency of new patients presenting in the authors' clinic with the chief complaint of melasma is 0.2%, but it is a common incidental finding.

History

Displeasure with their self-image causes patients to seek medical attention. Adults acquire melasma in association with sunlight exposure, pregnancy (chloasma, the 'mask of pregnancy'), and the use of birth control pills.

Sunlight, pregnancy, and birth control pills exacerbate melasma.

Physical Examination

Macular brown patches of melasma occur symmetrically on the face. They are sharply delineated and involve the malar eminences, forehead, upper lip, and mandible. The brown pigmentation is often patchy within the macule, giving it a reticulated appearance.

Differential Diagnosis

Post-inflammatory hyperpigmentation and *freckles* are pigmented macules. For the former, patients have a history of prior dermatitis. Freckles are smaller and more numerous, and involve the trunk and extremities in addition to the face.

Laboratory and Biopsy

No laboratory tests are necessary.

Therapy

Hydroquinone, a bleaching agent, is most frequently used to treat melasma. A 2% concentration is available over the counter, whereas 4% hydroquinone cream (Eldoquin-Forte) requires a prescription. It is applied twice daily to affected areas. Sunscreens with a SPF of 30 should be used prophylactically. If after several months no lightening has occurred, tretinoin cream 0.1% (Retin-A) may be cautiously applied daily in addition to the use of hydroquinone and a sunscreen. In addition, a combination product containing fluocinolone, hydroquinone, and tretinoin (Tri-Luma) is effective. Less commonly used treatments include azelaic acid cream (Azelex) and chemical peels.

Therapy for Melasma

Initial
- Hydroquinone cream 4% twice daily
- Sun protection – sunscreen SPF 30, and hat

Alternative
- Tretinoin cream 0.1% daily or less frequently
- Fluocinolone 0.01% plus hydroquinone 4% plus tretinoin 0.05% solution (Tri-Luma) twice daily
- Azelaic acid cream 20%
- Chemical peels

Course and Complications

Melasma fades postpartum, with sunlight protection, and with discontinuation of birth control pills. However, it may take months to years for normal skin color to return.

Pathogenesis

The melanocytes in the areas of involvement are increased in number as well as in activity, producing a greater number of melanosomes. Hormonal factors have been implicated because of the association with pregnancy and birth control pills, but melasma is infrequently found in menopausal women who receive estrogen replacement. Plasma measurements of β-melanocyte-stimulating hormone are normal.

NEVUS

> ## Key Points
>
> 1. Nevi generally have uniform color, surface, and border
> 2. Changing or symptomatic nevi should be viewed with suspicion
> 3. The 'ugly duckling' mole should be biopsied

> Types of nevi:
> 1. Junctional
> 2. Compound
> 3. Intradermal

Definition

A nevus (mole) is a benign neoplasm of pigment-forming cells, the nevus cell. Nevi are congenital or acquired. A junctional nevus is macular, with nevus cells confined to the base of the epidermis. Compound (**Fig. 6.9**) and intradermal nevi are papular, with nevus cells in the epidermis and dermis, and in the dermis only, respectively.

Incidence

Nevi should be considered a normal skin finding. The average number of nevi per person is 15–40 for Caucasians and 2–11 for African-Americans. In the authors' clinic, 3% of new patients are seen because of concern about nevi that have become irritated, have changed in color or size, or are cosmetically unattractive.

History

Most nevi are acquired after 6 months of age and before the age of 35 years. Thereafter, one sees a progressive decline in number, so that nevi are infrequent by age 80 years. Moles usually appear singularly, rarely in crops. It is common to have darkening in color, itching, and development of new nevi during pregnancy and adolescence. Otherwise, symptomatic nevi should be regarded suspiciously.

Physical Examination

Nevi vary greatly in appearance and coloration (**Fig. 6.10**). However, individuals tend to have similar appearing nevi that are generally uniform in color, surface, and border. The pigmented lesion that differs from other nevi – the *'ugly duckling'* – should be biopsied to rule out malignant melanoma. Nevi are flat or elevated, smooth or verrucoid, polypoid or sessile, and pigmented or flesh colored. Their coloration is orderly, with shades of brown and occasionally blue, although the latter color should be regarded with suspicion. Skin lines may or may not be present. Nevi frequently contain hair. The junctional nevus is a light to dark brown macule. Compound and

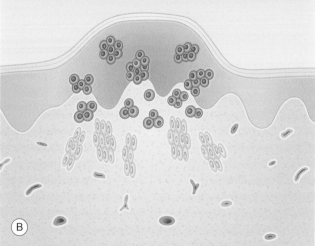
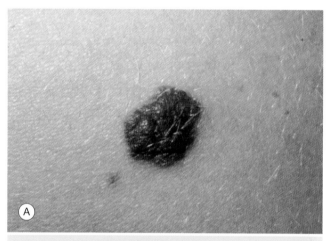

FIGURE 6.9 **Compound nevus. A.** Even bordered and surfaced, brown-colored papule. **B.** Epidermis – pigmented nevus cell nests in lower epidermis. Dermis – pigmented nests of round nevus cells in upper dermis; bundles of spindle-shaped nevus cells in lower dermis.

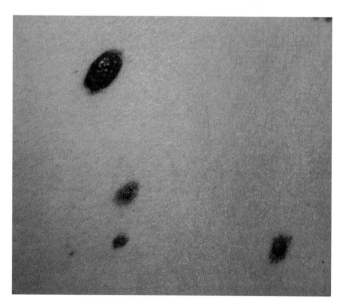

FIGURE 6.10 **Brown and tan nevi** showing variation in appearance.

intradermal nevi are flesh-colored or brown, smooth- or rough-surfaced papules that occur in older children and adults.

> Uniform color, surface, and border are characteristics of nevi. The 'ugly duckling' nevus, the one that looks different from the patient's other nevi, should be biopsied.

Differential Diagnosis

The most important task is to differentiate a nevus from a *malignant melanoma*. Regular brown color, surface, and border are characteristic features of a nevus that differentiate it from melanoma. A junctional nevus may appear similar to other pigmented macules, such as a *lentigo* or *freckle*. Compound and intradermal nevi, when flesh colored, can be confused with a *skin tag, basal cell carcinoma*, and *neurofibroma*. The presence of telangiectasia and central depression, as well as a recent acquisition, in an adult, are characteristic of a nodular basal cell carcinoma. When pigmented, these nevi can resemble *seborrheic keratoses* and *dermatofibromas*. The presence of scale and a 'pasted on' appearance is typical of seborrheic keratosis. Dermatofibromas are hard dermal papules that dimple when pinched, whereas nevi are soft.

The *Spitz nevus* (*benign juvenile melanoma*) is composed of spindle and epithelioid nevus cells. It is a smooth, round, slightly scaling, pink nodule that occurs most frequently in children. The most important aspect of dealing with this lesion is to recognize that it is a nevus and not a melanoma, and to avoid extensive surgical intervention.

> Special nevi:
> 1. Spitz
> 2. Blue
> 3. Dysplastic
> 4. Congenital

Blue nevi are small, steel-blue nodules that usually begin early in life. Their importance in diagnosis is their similar appearance to nodular melanoma. If any doubt exists, a biopsy should be performed.

The *dysplastic nevus*, or *atypical mole*, is both controversial and confusing (**Fig. 6.11**). Controversy exists regarding its propensity to develop into a malignant melanoma. The confusion stems from differing histologic criteria for diagnosis. Clinically, the atypical mole is >5 mm, is variegated in color with an erythematous background, and has an irregular, indistinct border. Atypical moles were initially recognized as markers for increased risk of melanoma in family members with inherited malignant melanoma, the *familial atypical mole and melanoma syndrome* or *dysplastic nevus syndrome*. In these families, virtually all members with atypical moles developed a melanoma in their lifetime, whereas family members without atypical moles did not. Subsequently, investigators discovered that approximately 5% of the

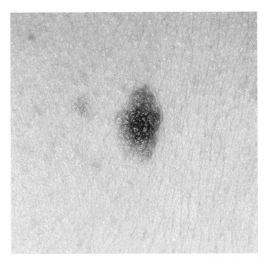

FIGURE 6.11 **Atypical mole** – pink, tan, brown, irregularly shaped papule with an indistinct border.

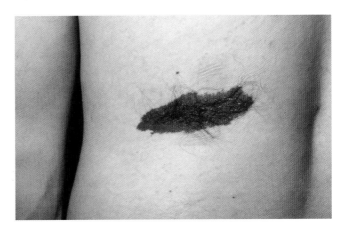

FIGURE 6.12 **Congenital nevus** – black plaque containing dark hairs.

healthy Caucasian population in the USA has atypical moles. The risk of developing a melanoma in these individuals, many of whom have only one or a few atypical moles and no personal or familial history of melanoma, is unclear, but, for most, a melanoma never develops.

Congenital nevi (**Fig. 6.12**) are present at birth or shortly thereafter, are usually elevated, and have uniform, dark brown pigmentation with discrete borders. Of newborns, 1% have congenital nevi. Large congenital nevi (>20 cm across or covering 5% of body area) have a 6–12% chance of developing into a malignant melanoma. Small congenital nevi have little to no increased risk of transformation into melanoma and therefore do not need to be removed prophylactically.

Laboratory and Biopsy

Nevus cells vary in morphology, depending on their location in the skin (**Fig. 6.9B**). They are arranged in nests in the basal layer of the epidermis and upper dermis. When they extend deeper, cord-like or sheet-like formations occur. In the upper dermis and epidermis, the individual cells are epithelioid in appearance with a cuboidal or oval shape, indistinct cytoplasm, and a round or oval nucleus, and are pigmented. In the middle dermis, nevus cells are smaller, do not contain pigment, and have a lymphoid appearance. In the lower dermis, they have a spindle cell appearance, resembling fibroblasts. Immunohistochemical markers can be used to identify melanocytic lesions. Atypical moles histologically have: (1) abnormal architecture of melanocytes within the epidermis; (2) a dermal fibrotic response; and (3) depending on the pathologist, variable cytologic atypia.

Therapy

The prophylactic removal of nevi is not required. Worrisome lesions are those that have changed in color, shape, or size; have been acquired in adulthood; bleed; or are itching. An excisional or deep shave biopsy with narrow margins (2–3 mm) is recommended for suspicious lesions. Clinically benign and cosmetically unsightly nevi may be removed by shaving off the lesion with a scalpel. However, a superficial shave biopsy leaves some residual nevus cells at the biopsy site that may become darkly pigmented.

> All nevi that are removed should be examined by a pathologist.

Therapy for Nevus

Initial
- Shave biopsy or deep shave excision for worrisome lesions.

Alternative
- Elliptical excision

The management of *congenital nevi* is difficult when these lesions are large (diameter >20 cm or covering 5% of body area), and controversial when they are small. Large congenital nevi, such as the bathing-suit nevus, cover extensive areas of the trunk in a garment-like fashion and are generally associated with many satellite lesions. They are rare but have a significant potential for developing into malignant melanoma (6–12%). The optimal treatment is excision of the lesions, although the technical difficulty of removing such wide areas of skin may preclude this therapy. At the least, patients should be followed carefully, with excision of nodules that develop within the nevus. Large congenital nevi covering the head and neck are sometimes associated with underlying meningeal melanosis, seizures, mental retardation, and development of meningeal malignant melanoma. For small congenital nevi, no excision is needed unless the lesion changes clinically.

The recommended advice to the healthy person with (multiple) atypical moles but no personal or familial history of malignant melanoma is patient education about sun exposure, self-examination, and yearly full skin examination by a physician.

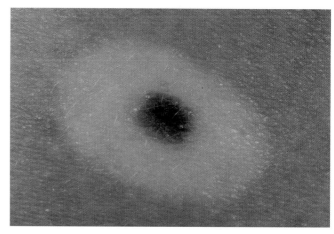

FIGURE 6.13 **Halo nevus.** Red, tan-brown papule with surrounding white halo.

Guidelines for Management and Follow-Up of Patients with Multiple Atypical Moles

- Biopsy of at least two lesions to confirm diagnosis
- Skin photographs, including close-ups of suspicious lesions
- Sun protection
- Patient self-examination periodically
- Screen blood relatives for atypical nevi and melanoma
- Frequency of follow-up:
  - Patients with no personal or family history of melanoma: yearly
  - Patients with personal or family history of melanoma: every 6 months for 2 years, then yearly

Course and Complications

Approximately 50% of malignant melanomas have associated nevi. The relative risk of melanoma increases as the number of nevi increases; that is, persons with large numbers of nevi have a greater risk of melanoma than do persons with a few nevi. No evidence indicates that mild irritation or rubbing results in transformation of a nevus into a melanoma.

Some nevi develop a surrounding depigmented zone and are referred to as *halo nevi* (**Fig. 6.13**). They occur singularly or multiply, usually on the trunk in teenagers. The development of a halo around the nevus is a harbinger of its disappearance. Both humoral and cellular immunities appear to be involved with the development of halo nevi, a process that results in destruction of nevus cells. On rare occasions, a depigmented halo develops around a malignant melanoma. If the central lesion has a uniform brown color typical of a nevus, an excisional biopsy is not necessary.

> Halo nevi are rarely a malignant melanoma.

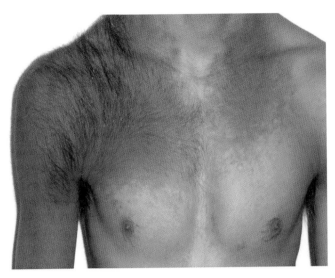

FIGURE 6.14 Becker's nevus.

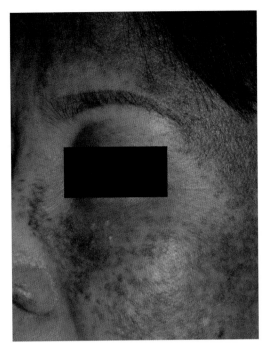

FIGURE 6.15 Nevus of Ota.

Pathogenesis

Nevus cells are derived from the neural crest. Morphologically, one can recognize the nevus cell because it has no dendritic processes and groups together in nests within the epidermis and dermis.

UNCOMMON PIGMENTED GROWTHS

BECKER'S NEVUS

Becker's nevus (melanosis) is a brown patch with dark, coarse hairs that occurs on the upper trunk and arms (**Fig. 6.14**). It usually appears in teenage and young adult males. It has no malignant potential and treatment is for cosmetic appearance.

NEVUS OF OTA

Nevus of Ota (oculodermal melanocytosis) is a mottled or confluent brown, blue, gray macule of the face that usually affects female Asians (**Fig. 6.15**). Besides the skin, the eye can be involved with associated glaucoma. Onset occurs at birth, before 1 year of age, and at puberty. Malignant melanoma is a rare complication. Laser treatment can be cosmetically successful.

7 Dermal and Subcutaneous Growths

Key Points

1. Biopsy nodules of uncertain origin
2. Suspect cancer for hard dermal nodules

ABSTRACT

This chapter deals with nodular and cystic 'lumps' in the skin (**Table 7.1**). With the exception of lipomas, the lesions are located in the dermis, often with no alteration in the overlying epidermis. For many patients, common lesions such as epidermal inclusion cysts, small angiomas, dermatofibromas, and lipomas are not troubling and are not brought to the attention of a physician. However, these lesions are often found during routine physical examinations, and it is important to be able to distinguish them from malignant dermal growths. The usual question asked by patients who present with a 'lump' in the skin is: 'Is it cancer?' This concern is appropriate and must always be addressed.

Color and consistency are helpful distinguishing clinical features. The color of the lesion sometimes reflects the nature of the proliferating elements. Vascular lesions, for example, have hues ranging from red to purple. Consistency often distinguishes a nodule from a cyst. A cyst is usually fluctuant or malleable. For nodules, a soft consistency lends reassurance that the lesion is benign, a firm consistency is of intermediate concern, and a hard consistency should lead to suspicion of a possible malignant process.

> Color and consistency are helpful distinguishing features.

Sometimes, the diagnosis can be made only with biopsy. This is particularly important for firm to hard nodules in which the clinical diagnosis is uncertain. A general and important rule, then, is that for any skin nodule of uncertain origin, a biopsy is indicated to rule out malignancy.

DERMATOFIBROMA

Key Points

1. Dermal fibrotic papule or small nodule
2. Chronic, asymptomatic, and stable

Definition

A dermatofibroma is an area of focal dermal fibrosis, often accompanied by overlying epidermal thickening and hyperpigmentation. It appears clinically as a brown papule or small nodule, often more indurated than elevated. The origin is unknown.

Incidence

Dermatofibromas are common and are often found incidentally during cutaneous examinations. Occasionally, they cause a patient to seek medical advice. They are seen most often in young adults.

History

Dermatofibromas usually are asymptomatic. The patient's concern, if any, is over the possibility of malignancy.

TABLE 7.1 Dermal and subcutaneous growths

	Frequency[a]	Physical Examination	Differential Diagnosis[b]	Laboratory Test (Biopsy)	
				Diagnostic But Usually Not Necessary	Diagnostic and Necessary
Dermatofibroma	0.2	Tan to brown, firm, flat to slightly elevated papule; 'dimples' with lateral pressure	Nevus Melanoma Dermatofibrosarcoma protuberans (rare)	✓	
Epidermal inclusion (follicular) cyst	0.5	Flesh-colored, firm, but malleable nodule	Pilar cyst Lipoma	✓[c]	
Hemangioma	0.8	Red or purple (often *blanchable*) soft-to-firm macule, papule, or nodule	Blue nevus Melanoma Kaposi's sarcoma	✓	
Kaposi's sarcoma	<0.1	*Purple* macules, plaques, or nodules	Bruise Hemangioma Bacillary angiomatosis		✓
Keloid	0.2	Pink, firm, elevated scar	Hypertrophic scar Dermatofibrosarcoma protuberans (rare)	✓	
Lipoma	0.2	Flesh-colored, rubbery, *subcutaneous* nodule	Epidermal inclusion cyst Angiolipoma Metastatic tumor	✓	
Neurofibroma	0.1	Flesh to brown, soft, and often compressible ('buttonhole' sign) papule or nodule	Skin tag Nevus	✓	
Xanthoma	<0.1	*Yellow* papules and nodules Hard subcutaneous tendon nodules	Sebaceous gland tumor Juvenile xanthogranuloma Rheumatoid nodules	✓	
Other malignant tumors	<0.1	Flesh, red, or purple, *hard* nodules	Any of the above		✓

[a]Percentage of new dermatology patients with this diagnosis seen in the Hershey Medical Center Dermatology Clinic, Hershey, PA.
[b]A malignant tumor should be in the differential diagnosis for all dermal growths.
[c]Incision and drainage reveals cheesy, foul-smelling material.

Physical Examination

Typical dermatofibromas are approximately 5 mm in size and are slightly elevated. They vary in color from light tan to dark brown. The fibrotic nature of the lesion is best appreciated by palpation, which reveals a firm consistency. A helpful diagnostic test is the 'dimple sign,' in which pinching results in central dimpling (**Fig. 7.1A**). Most dermatofibromas exhibit this sign; it is rarely seen with any other skin lesion. Dermatofibromas may occur anywhere, but the thighs and legs are the most common locations. One or several lesions may be present.

The 'dimple sign' is characteristic of dermatofibroma.

Differential Diagnosis

With its brown color, a dermatofibroma may be confused with a *nevus*. Nevi, however, are usually softer and do not exhibit the dimple sign. Darker dermatofibromas may

raise a clinical suspicion of *melanoma*. Dermatofibromas are usually purely brown (a benign color), whereas a nodular melanoma usually has shades of dark gray or blue. If any doubt exists, however, a biopsy should be performed.

Enlarging or atypically colored lesions should undergo biopsy to rule out malignancy.

Dermatofibrosarcoma protuberans is a low-grade malignant fibrous tumor that grows slowly but persistently, and rarely metastasizes. It is a rare tumor and is distinguished clinically from a dermatofibroma by its larger size, irregular shape, and continued growth.

Laboratory and Biopsy

The diagnosis is usually made clinically. If any doubt exists, a biopsy should be performed to rule out malignancy. The histologic picture is diagnostic and shows a

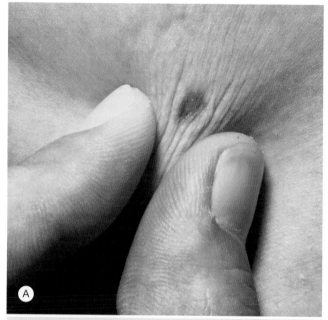

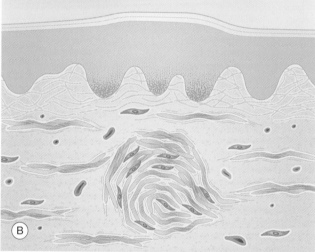

FIGURE 7.1 Dermatofibroma. A. Firm, reddish papule with 'dimple sign.' **B.** Epidermis – slightly thickened and hyperpigmented. Dermis – nodular aggregate of fibroblasts and densely packed collagen.

focal proliferation of densely packed collagen bands that are twisting and intertwining (**Fig. 7.1B**). Fibroblasts are interspersed and increased in number. Increased pigmentation of the slightly thickened overlying epidermis accounts for the frequently brown color of these lesions.

Therapy

Therapy is usually not indicated. If desired, a simple excision is sufficient for removal and histologic examination.

Therapy for Dermatofibroma

- None
- Excision if desired

Course and Complications

Dermatofibromas are chronic and usually stable in size. They are not associated with any complications.

Pathogenesis

Although the origin is unknown, trauma (e.g., an insect bite) may be an initiating factor for some of these lesions. The proliferation of fibroblasts and subsequent fibrosis may represent an exuberant healing response to injury. However, most patients do not recollect a history of trauma in the area.

Two other lesions are considered within the spectrum of a dermatofibroma. A *histiocytoma* (an aggregate of histiocytes in a focal area within the dermis) probably represents an early phase in the formation of a dermatofibroma. A *sclerosing hemangioma*, as the name suggests, shows more of a vascular component, but the end result is that of dermal fibrosis as well.

EPIDERMAL INCLUSION CYST

Key Points

1. Central pore and cheesy, foul-smelling discharge is diagnostic
2. Origin is from the hair follicle

Definition

An epidermal inclusion cyst (**Fig. 7.2**) is derived from the upper portion (infundibulum) of the epithelial lining of a hair follicle and is located in the mid and lower dermis. It is also called an epidermoid cyst. Clinically, it appears as a flesh-colored, firm, but often malleable, solitary nodule in the skin.

Incidence

These lesions are common, but usually are not brought to the attention of a physician, so the exact incidence is not known. They may occur at any age.

History

Epidermal inclusion cysts are usually asymptomatic, slow growing, and most frequently are found incidentally by either the patient or the examining physician. Occasionally, they are the primary complaint in a patient concerned about the possibility of malignancy. Another reason for medical attention is rupture of the cyst or secondary infection, either of which produces inflammation, pain, and drainage of foul-smelling material.

Physical Examination

Characteristically, the lesion is a flesh-colored, dome-shaped nodule that feels firm (but not hard). On palpation, it often feels slightly malleable, a finding that suggests the contents are semi-solid. This is a helpful diagnostic aid, as is the finding of a *central pore*, which represents the opening of the follicle from which the cyst

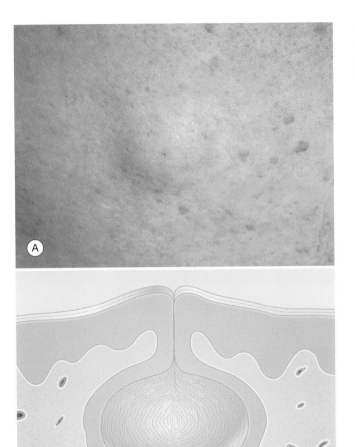

FIGURE 7.2 **Epidermal inclusion cyst. A.** Flesh-colored, firm nodule with central puncta. **B.** Epidermis – invaginates into dermis. Dermis – keratin-filled, epidermal-lined cyst.

originated. Lesions range in size from 0.5 to 5 cm. They may be located anywhere, but occur most frequently on the head and trunk. If the central pore is patent, the diagnosis is sometimes confirmed by squeezing the lesion and expressing some of the whitish, cheesy, foul-smelling material that is trapped within. This material represents macerated keratin.

> A central pore is characteristic of an epidermal inclusion cyst.

Differential Diagnosis

Pilar (trichilemmal) *cysts* arise from the middle third (isthmus) of the follicular canal. They occur most frequently on the scalp, where they are the most common type of cyst. In other locations, they are less common than epidermal inclusion cysts, but the two may be indistinguishable clinically, and histologically, some cysts may have elements of both. The difference is not critical: both are benign. A *lipoma* is usually deeper than an epidermal

inclusion cyst, and although a lipoma may feel rubbery, it is usually not malleable. When the diagnosis is uncertain, particularly if the lesion feels firm, a *malignant tumor* must be considered.

Laboratory and Biopsy

Usually, the diagnosis can be made clinically. If desired, confirmation can be obtained by incising and draining the lesion, which reveals the cheesy, foul-smelling, keratinous contents. A biopsy is equally confirmatory, but usually not necessary (**Fig. 7.2B**).

Therapy

Frequently, no therapy is requested or needed. If removal is desired, the entire cyst should be excised with its lining, to prevent recurrence. This is accomplished by incising the skin overlying the cyst without disrupting the cyst wall and then bluntly dissecting the entire cyst, along with its wall. If the cyst breaks, a curette can be used to remove the remaining contents and cyst wall. Elliptical excision is usually required for removal of cysts that have previously ruptured and scarred.

> To prevent recurrence, the entire cyst, with its lining, should be removed.

Therapy for Epidermal Cysts

- None
- Incision and drainage
- Excision

Course and Complications

Untreated, most epidermal inclusion cysts reach a stable size, often in the range of 1–3 cm, rarely larger.

Complications are rare and usually limited to occasional rupture or infection. Rupture or infection results in redness and tenderness of the cyst and, on examination, increased fluctuance. If this occurs, the lesion should be treated as an abscess with incision and drainage, and occasionally oral antibiotics.

Multiple epidermal inclusion cysts are a feature of *Gardner syndrome*, an uncommon, autosomal dominant, heritable disorder manifested by multiple epidermal cysts, fibromas, osteomas, and intestinal polyps. The intestinal polyps often undergo malignant degeneration.

Pathogenesis

Epidermal inclusion cysts arise from the upper portion (infundibulum) of a hair follicle. The epidermal lining of the cyst is identical to that of the surface epidermis and produces keratin, which, having no place to shed, accumulates and forms the cystic mass.

HEMANGIOMA

Key Points

1. Benign vascular tumor in infancy
2. Superficial and subcutaneous involvement
3. Most regress spontaneously

Definition

A hemangioma (**Fig. 7.3**) is a benign proliferation of blood vessels in the dermis and subcutis. The vascularity imparts a red, blue, or purple color to these lesions, depending on the size and depth of the proliferative vessels.

Incidence

Hemangiomas are the most common soft tissue tumor of infancy, occurring more frequently in females, premature, and white infants. They are likely to be brought to the attention of a physician because of their rapid growth or cosmetic concerns.

History

Most arise in the first few weeks of infancy. Hemangiomas are usually asymptomatic, except when they are large, ulcerate, or cause local obstruction – a fortunately rare occurrence.

Physical Examination

Superficial hemangiomas have a bright red color, whereas the deeper subcutaneous forms have a bluish hue. Mixed hemangiomas are bright red, dome-shaped nodules.

Types of hemangioma:
1. Superficial
2. Subcutaneous
3. Mixed

Differential Diagnosis

The diagnosis of childhood hemangioma is usually made clinically, without difficulty. In contrast, *vascular malformations* are generally present at birth and do not regress spontaneously.

Blanchability is a diagnostic feature found in many (but not all) hemangiomas.

Laboratory and Biopsy

A biopsy, if done, reveals a marked increase in the number of blood vessels, many of which are dilated (**Fig. 7.3B**).

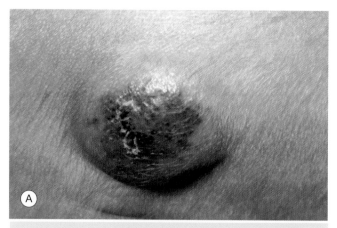

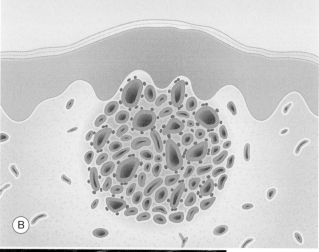

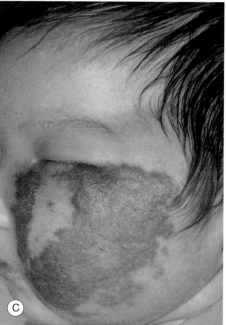

FIGURE 7.3 **Hemangioma. A.** Reddish, blue, soft nodule. **B.** Dermis – focal proliferation of blood vessels and endothelial cells. **C.** Rapidly growing hemangioma that requires systemic treatment to prevent serious complications.

Therapy

Skillful neglect is the most appropriate therapy for most childhood hemangiomas. Although these lesions grow over the first year of life (and during this time, the parents will need repeated reassurance), they usually involute spontaneously over the ensuing years with a cosmetic result that is superior to any that can be obtained by therapeutic intervention. For ulcerating, large, or head and neck hemangiomas, therapeutic intervention may be necessary as vision, respiration, or a good cosmetic result may be compromised. Therapeutic options include: systemic glucocorticosteroid therapy, 3–5 mg/kg daily, as the first line of therapy, intralesional and potent topical steroids, pulsed-dye laser, interferon α-2a, and surgical excision.

Therapy for Hemangiomas

Initial
- None
- Topical propranolol or steroids

Alternative
- Propranolol: 2 mg/kg daily
- Steroids: 3–5 mg/kg daily
- Laser
- Surgery

Course and Complications

Superficial hemangiomas often increase in size over the 1st year but then subside spontaneously, so that by the age of 5 years, 50% are involuted, and by age 9 years, 90% are involuted. Some 20% have residual changes, including scarring and fibro-fatty tissue. Depending on their location, large subcutaneous or mixed hemangiomas (**Fig. 7.3C**) may cause functional compromise of neighboring and underlying structures (e.g., the eye, ear, or oral pharynx). Hemangiomas occasionally ulcerate, become painful, and may be further complicated by infection.

> Most hemangiomas involute spontaneously during childhood.

In infants with numerous hemangiomas (*diffuse neonatal hemangiomatosis*), internal organ involvement should be suspected; this rare syndrome occasionally leads to death from high-output cardiac failure or compromise of an affected vital organ.

Pathogenesis

Although the pathomechanism of hemangiomas is unknown, a localized proliferation of endothelial cells and the supporting stroma, resulting in a cellular mass containing increased vascular channels, suggests the importance of angiogenic growth factors.

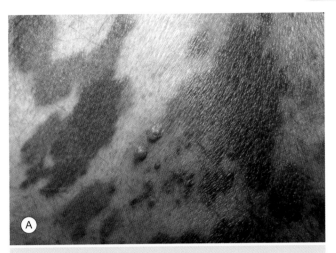
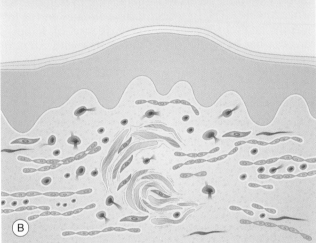

FIGURE 7.4 Kaposi's sarcoma. A. Purple macules and papules. **B.** Dermis – strands and clusters of spindle cells, hemorrhage, and blood-filled vascular slits.

KAPOSI'S SARCOMA

Key Points

1. Malignant vascular tumor
2. Human herpesvirus 8 may be pathogenetic
3. Sign of AIDS, test for HIV

Definition

Kaposi's sarcoma is a malignant tumor derived from endothelial cells. It is manifest by multiple vascular tumors that usually occur first in the skin, where they appear as purple macules, plaques, or nodules (**Fig. 7.4**).

Incidence

The disease occurs in three settings.

> Types of Kaposi's sarcoma: classic, lymphadenopathic, and AIDS-associated.

Classic Kaposi's sarcoma is a chronic cutaneous disorder that occurs primarily in elderly men, usually those of Eastern European descent. This is the type described by Moritz Kaposi in 1872. It remains an uncommon disorder with an annual incidence in the USA of approximately 0.05 per 100 000 population. It affects men 10–15 times more often than women and occurs most often in people older than 50 years.

An aggressive *lymphadenopathic* form occurs primarily in equatorial Africa, where it accounts for approximately 9% of all cancers. This type mainly affects young men and is rapidly fatal.

Acquired immune deficiency syndrome (AIDS)-associated Kaposi's sarcoma was first noted in 1979 and represents the most common neoplasm associated with AIDS. Kaposi's sarcoma occurs most frequently in homosexual patients with AIDS, in whom it disseminates and is frequently fatal. In the USA, the incidence of Kaposi's sarcoma has been decreasing in patients with AIDS in recent years because of better antiretroviral therapy and less immunosuppression.

History

The skin lesions in Kaposi's sarcoma are usually asymptomatic, so patients seek advice because of concern over appearance or uncertainty about the nature of newly appearing skin lesions. In some patients, Kaposi's sarcoma may be an incidental physical finding. In this setting, it often is the first sign of AIDS, so the physician should obtain a blood test for human immunodeficiency virus (HIV). Kaposi's sarcoma can also develop in patients receiving immunosuppressive therapy for organ transplantation and other diseases.

Test for HIV in patients newly diagnosed with Kaposi's sarcoma.

Physical Examination

Lesions of Kaposi's sarcoma may appear as macules, papules, dermal plaques, and nodules. However, in all forms, the lesions are characteristically *purple*. In the classic type of Kaposi's sarcoma, multiple lesions are usually located on the lower legs, where they may be accompanied by edema. In AIDS-associated Kaposi's sarcoma, lesions may occur anywhere on the skin, and range in number from one to innumerable. Lymphadenopathy is frequently also present in patients with AIDS. Kaposi's sarcoma may also involve the mucous membranes. When examining the mouth, one should also look for oral hairy leukoplakia (see Ch. 22) as another sign of AIDS. Additional skin manifestations of AIDS are listed in Chapter 23.

Differential Diagnosis

A solitary macule of Kaposi's sarcoma may be subtle, resembling a *bruise*. Papules and nodules may be confused with *angiomas*, although angiomas usually are redder. *Bacillary angiomatosis* is a condition that also occurs in patients with AIDS. It is manifest by red or purple papules that may resemble Kaposi's sarcoma. Biopsy of bacillary angiomatosis, however, shows a benign process, and a Warthin–Starry stain reveals clusters of *Bartonella* bacteria, the same microorganisms that cause cat scratch disease. Distinguishing bacillary angiomatous from Kaposi's sarcoma is important because bacillary angiomatosis is benign and responds to erythromycin therapy.

Laboratory and Biopsy

The diagnosis of Kaposi's sarcoma is confirmed with a biopsy that shows a proliferation in the dermis of spindle cells arranged in strands and small nodular aggregates (**Fig. 7.4B**). The spindle cells also attempt to form small blood vessels, resulting in slit-like spaces filled with red blood cells. Hemorrhage is common; lymphocytes and histiocytes may also be present. As mentioned above, patients suspected to have AIDS-associated Kaposi's sarcoma should have an HIV serologic test.

Therapy

Early classic Kaposi's sarcoma may require no therapy or only occasional excision of a papule or nodule. With more advanced cutaneous disease, local radiation therapy is highly effective. Patients with disseminated disease are treated with one or more chemotherapeutic agents.

Therapy for Kaposi's Sarcoma

Initial
- Radiation therapy
- Excision
- Cryotherapy

Alternative
- Interferon-α (intralesional or systemic)
- Chemotherapy (intralesional or systemic)

AIDS-associated Kaposi's sarcoma has been treated with local radiation therapy, cryosurgery, intralesional interferon-α, or intralesional chemotherapy (e.g., vinblastine). Disseminated disease is treated with a combination of zidovudine (AZT) and systemic interferon-α, or with systemic chemotherapy using agents such as vincristine, vinblastine, bleomycin, and etoposide, either alone or in combination.

Course and Complications

Classic Kaposi's sarcoma progresses slowly, and because it affects primarily elderly patients, many die from other causes. In the USA, the average survival time for patients with classic Kaposi's sarcoma has been reported to be 8–13 years, but much longer times have been noted, and spontaneous remissions have occurred. Patients have an increased frequency of second malignant diseases, especially lymphoma and leukemia.

Lymphadenopathic Kaposi's sarcoma disseminates rapidly to internal organs and results in early death.

AIDS-associated Kaposi's sarcoma also disseminates early in its course, but some patients respond to therapy, and many die from other causes, such as opportunistic infections.

Pathogenesis

Kaposi's sarcoma is a malignant disease in which endothelial cells proliferate to form tumors. Multiple tumors apparently result from a multifocal rather than a metastatic process. Immunosuppression may play a permissive role because, in the USA, the disease occurs most frequently in patients who are immunosuppressed by drugs or AIDS. The findings of Kaposi's sarcoma in several homosexual patients who are HIV-negative, and the epidemic occurrences of lymphadenopathic Kaposi's sarcoma in Africa, also suggest an etiologic role for an infectious, transmissible organism. In this regard, human herpesvirus type 8 has now been detected in all forms of Kaposi's sarcoma and so is strongly implicated in the pathogenetic process.

KELOID

Key Points

1. Exuberant scar tissue
2. Treat cautiously because of high recurrence rate

Definition

A keloid represents excessive proliferation of collagen (scar tissue) after trauma to the skin (**Fig. 7.5**). Clinically, a keloid appears as an elevated, firm, protuberant nodule or plaque.

Keloids occur most often in young Black people.

Incidence

Keloids are relatively common. The incidence is highest in people aged 10–30 years. Black people are particularly prone to keloids; in African populations, the prevalence is approximately 6%.

History

The trauma responsible for inducing the keloid is almost always remembered by the patient. Often, the trauma is obvious, such as ear piercing, surgical incisions, or other wounds. Keloids develop over weeks to months after the trauma. New and actively growing keloids often itch, whereas stable, long-standing ones are asymptomatic.

Physical Examination

A keloid looks like an overgrown scar – which is what it is. It is protuberant and firm, and usually conforms roughly to a pattern of the original trauma, although it is more extensive. Keloids are often pink or dark brown

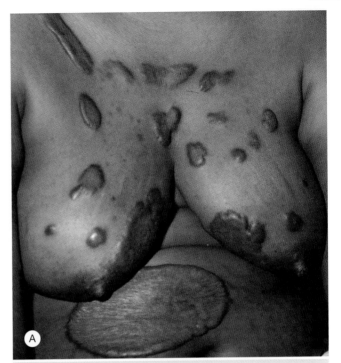
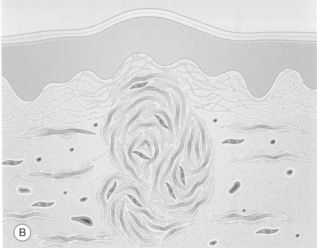

FIGURE 7.5 **Keloid. A.** Multiple hyperpigmented, smooth, firm, protuberant nodules and plaques. **B.** Dermis – highly compacted whorls of collagen.

and have an irregular border with claw-like extensions. They may occur anywhere, but they are more common on the earlobes (secondary to ear piercing), shoulders, upper chest, and back.

Differential Diagnosis

The difference between a keloid and a *hypertrophic scar* is mainly quantitative, with a keloid expanding beyond the limits of the original trauma.

A *dermatofibrosarcoma protuberans* is a rare, malignant, fibrous tumor that clinically may look like a keloid, but the patient usually has no history of prior trauma, and the lesion continues to enlarge. If malignancy is suspected, a biopsy should be performed.

Laboratory and Biopsy

The diagnosis can usually be made on clinical grounds. If doubt remains, a biopsy can be performed for confirmation. The histologic examination shows whorls and nodules of highly compacted hyalinized bands of collagen (**Fig. 7.5B**). Fibroblasts may be increased in number, but not markedly so in mature keloids. Mast cells are prominent, and release of their histamine content may be the cause of the often associated pruritus. The overlying epidermis may be atrophic.

Therapy

Surgical removal alone, although tempting, is contraindicated because it is often followed by a recurrence that is larger than the original lesion. Repeated intralesional injections of steroids (triamcinolone; Kenalog-40) at monthly intervals may cause keloids to flatten, which is a goal desired by some patients. Surgery may be used if it is combined with another modality such as intralesional steroids or low-dose radiotherapy. Pressure dressings are also helpful when applied after surgery or injections. Silicone (Silastic) gel dressings applied daily for 2 months have been shown to help flatten hypertrophic scars by mechanisms that are unknown.

Therapy for Keloids

- None
- Intralesional steroids: Kenalog-40
- Compression
- Surgery with intralesional steroids

Surgery should never be used alone in treating keloids.

Course and Complications

Untreated, the usual course of a keloid is that of gradual enlargement to a steady-state size. Keloids are much less likely to regress than are hypertrophic scars, but in either case, the time course for regression (if it occurs at all) is measured in years. The major complication is cosmetic disfigurement, which may be profound.

Pathogenesis

Increased fibroblast activity, initiated by tissue injury, results in a marked increase in collagen synthesis. Dermal ground substance (primarily the chondroitin 4-sulfate component) is also increased; investigators have suggested that this change may inhibit collagen degradation. Collagen production may also be affected by imbalance in, or altered fibroblastic responsiveness to, tissue cytokines. For example, collagen synthesis by fibroblasts is stimulated by transforming growth factor ß and is inhibited by interferon.

LIPOMA

Key Points

1. Benign subcutaneous fat tumor
2. Slow growing or stable
3. Biopsy rapidly growing tumors and if uncertain of the diagnosis

---

Definition

A lipoma represents a benign tumor of subcutaneous fat (**Fig. 7.6**). Clinically, it is a rubbery nodule that appears only slightly elevated above the skin's surface but is easily palpable deep in the skin. The origin is unknown.

Incidence

Most lipomas are never brought to a physician's attention. When they are, it is because of the patient's concern that the lesion may be malignant. They are most common in midlife.

History

Lipomas are usually asymptomatic. They may grow slowly, but most patients are not aware of any change in size.

Physical Examination

A typical lipoma is flesh colored and imparts a slight elevation to the normal-appearing overlying skin. It feels rubbery but not hard, and is usually freely movable. Lipomas range in size from 1 to 10 cm, rarely larger. They may occur anywhere but are found most often on the trunk, neck, and upper extremities.

Lipoma is a stable or slow growing, movable, rubbery, subcutaneous nodule.

Differential Diagnosis

A lipoma usually is deeper, more freely movable, and more rubbery than an *epidermal* inclusion cyst.

Angiolipomas are uncommon tumors that are often painful and sometimes locally invasive. Histologically, they have a prominent vascular component.

Metastatic *malignant tumors* of the skin can be deep, but usually are firm (if not hard) and also involve the dermis, so the skin cannot be freely moved over them. A lipoma may also be mistaken for a soft tissue sarcoma, which is harder.

Laboratory and Biopsy

The diagnosis can usually be made clinically. When any doubt exists, particularly if a malignant tumor is even remotely suspected, a biopsy should be performed. One needs to be sure to extend the biopsy deep enough to sample the tumor. A deep elliptical excision is preferred.

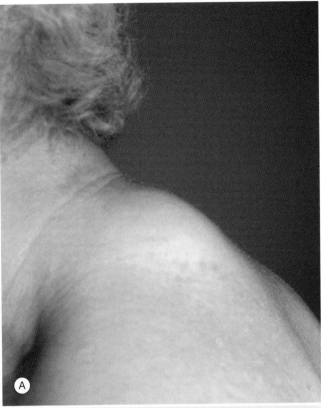

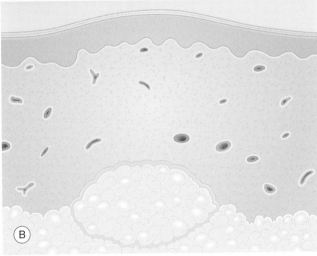

FIGURE 7.6 Lipoma. A. Deep, movable, flesh-colored, rubbery nodule. **B.** Dermis – impinged on by encapsulated tumor of normal-appearing fat cells.

Histologically, a lipoma is an encapsulated collection of normal fat cells (**Fig. 7.6B**).

Therapy

Therapy is usually not required.

Therapy for Lipoma

- None
- Excision

Course and Complications

Lipomas found incidentally by the physician are usually reported by the patient to have been present without change in size for a number of years. For lesions recently detected or those that appear to be growing, a biopsy should be considered to confirm the diagnosis. These lesions have no complications.

NEUROFIBROMA

Key Points

1. Soft, 'buttonhole,' papule or nodule
2. Think of neurofibromatosis type 1 if there is more than one neurofibroma

Definition

A neurofibroma represents a focal proliferation of neural tissue within the dermis (**Fig. 7.7**). Clinically, neurofibromas may appear in two ways: (1) most often, as soft, protruding papules and nodules; and (2) less often, as deep, firm, subcutaneous nodules. Multiple neurofibromas are a cutaneous expression of *neurofibromatosis 1* (*von Recklinghausen's disease*), a dominantly inherited neurocutaneous disorder with prominent skin, skeletal, and nervous system abnormalities. *Neurofibromatosis 2* is characterized primarily by bilateral acoustic neuromas and usually lacks the cutaneous findings of neurofibromatosis 1.

Incidence

Solitary neurofibromas are infrequent and inconsequential. Neurofibromatosis 1 is one of the more common genetic disorders, with an estimated birth incidence of 1 in 3000.

> Solitary neurofibromas are inconsequential; multiple ones are a sign of neurofibromatosis.

History

In neurofibromatosis 1, the onset of skin tumors usually occurs in late childhood, with more rapid growth occurring in adolescence and pregnancy. Inheritance is determined by an autosomal dominant mechanism, but the expressivity is variable. A family history is important and should be followed by a cutaneous examination of both parents. However, spontaneous mutations are common and account for approximately 50% of patients with neurofibromatosis 1. Patients with neurofibromatosis may have signs and symptoms relating to other organ involvement, most often the skeletal and central nervous systems.

Physical Examination

A typical neurofibroma appears as a soft, flesh-colored, protruding papule or nodule that characteristically, on

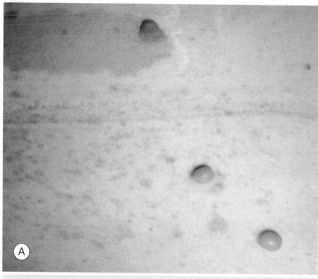

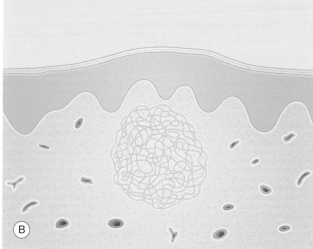

FIGURE 7.7 **Neurofibroma. A.** Multiple soft papules that invaginate into skin with pressure (buttonhole). Note the associated café-au-lait macule. **B.** Dermis – circumscribed collection of loosely packed neural fibers.

compression, can be invaginated into what feels like a defect in the skin. This is the so-called *buttonhole sign*. These soft lesions sometimes attain nodule size. Less often, neurofibromas appear as deep, firm, dermal or subcutaneous nodules, which sometimes become extremely large (plexiform neurofibromas) and are occasionally tender.

> Soft papules and nodules can often be invaginated into an apparent defect in the skin; this 'buttonhole' sign is characteristic of neurofibroma.

Neurofibromas in neurofibromatosis 1 are multiple, occasionally numbering in the thousands in a given patient. In the extreme case, particularly when combined with bony abnormalities, the condition can be remarkably disfiguring.

Diagnostic Criteria for Neurofibromatosis Type 1

Two or more of the following:
1. Six or more *café-au-lait macules* – 5 mm or larger in prepubertal individuals and 15 mm or larger in postpubertal individuals
2. Two or more *neurofibromas* of any type or one plexiform neurofibroma
3. Axillary or inguinal *freckling*
4. Optic nerve *glioma*
5. Two or more *Lisch nodules* (iris hamartomas)
6. Distinctive *osseous lesions* such as sphenoid wing dysplasia or long bone cortex thinning/dysplasia
7. A *first-degree relative* with neurofibromatosis 1

Café-au-lait spots are light brown macules and are present early in life – 99% by the age of 1 year. Six or more *café-au-lait macules* 5 mm or larger in prepubertal individuals and 15 mm or larger in post pubertal individuals are diagnostic. Axillary and inguinal freckling is another characteristic sign. Ophthalmologic evaluation is extremely helpful because iris hamartomas (*Lisch nodules*) are found in 70% of affected individuals by the age of 10 years.

> Ophthalmologic examination for Lisch nodules is useful in diagnosing neurofibromatosis 1.

Differential Diagnosis

Skin tags are also soft but more superficial, are narrower at the base (pedunculated), and lack the buttonhole sign.

A *dermal nevus* can appear as a soft, flesh-colored papule in the skin that clinically is similar to a small neurofibroma. Sometimes, only a biopsy can differentiate the two with certainty. Biopsies are more often done for solitary neurofibromas than for multiple neurofibromas, in which the diagnosis is more clinically evident.

Laboratory and Biopsy

The diagnosis of neurofibromatosis can usually be made clinically. Magnetic resonance imaging is helpful in detecting brain hamartomas in children affected with neurofibromatosis 1 and in revealing acoustic neuromas in patients with neurofibromatosis 2. For solitary neurofibromas or when histologic confirmation is needed for neurofibromatosis, a biopsy specimen provides the diagnosis. The histologic picture shows a well circumscribed collection of fine, wavy fibers loosely packed in the dermis (**Fig. 7.7B**). Special stains for nerve fibers are positive.

Therapy

Individual lesions can be removed surgically, but if excision is incomplete, recurrence is common. No known medical therapy is available to treat, prevent, or retard the progression of either the cutaneous features or the systemic disease in neurofibromatosis 1. Patients who are diagnosed with neurofibromatosis 1 should have genetic counseling.

Therapy for Neurofibroma

- None
- Excision

Course and Complications

Solitary neurofibromas are of little consequence. They are usually asymptomatic, have no complications, and are stable. In neurofibromatosis 1, the cutaneous condition is usually progressive. Lesions continue to form and grow, sometimes to the point of resulting in marked cosmetic disfigurement. With the variable expressivity of the disease, some patients are affected only mildly. Deep nodular lesions (plexiform neurofibromas) can rarely degenerate into malignant neurofibrosarcoma. Clinical clues that this is occurring include lesion enlargement and the development of tenderness. In most patients, the skin lesions remain histologically benign, although, as mentioned, they can become a source of cosmetic disfigurement and social stigmatization. Systemic complications of neurofibromatosis are potentially numerous and include the following: central nervous system involvement with tumors, mental retardation, and seizures; skeletal abnormalities, including kyphoscoliosis, pseudarthrosis, and localized gigantism; and endocrine disorders such as precocious puberty and pheochromocytoma. Patients with neurofibromatosis and hypertension should be screened for pheochromocytoma.

Pathogenesis

Neurofibromatosis 1 is caused by an abnormal gene, *NF-1*, on chromosome 17, transmitted in an autosomal dominant manner in half of the affected individuals. The other half have spontaneous mutations. The gene encodes for a protein named *neurofibromin*, which appears to possess tumor suppressing activity. Accordingly, inherited abnormalities of this gene may lead to tumor development, e.g., neurofibromas and possibly other tumors found in patients with neurofibromatosis 1. Genetic testing for NF-1 mutations is complex and a negative test does not exclude the diagnosis.

XANTHOMA

Key Points

1. Composed of lipid-laden histiocytes
2. Skin sign of hyperlipidemia

Definition

A xanthoma represents a focal collection of lipid-laden histiocytes in the dermis or tendons. Clinically, xanthomas located in the dermis appear as yellowish (*xanthous*, Greek for yellow) papules, plaques, and nodules. Tendon xanthomas are deep, flesh-colored, hard nodules located within peripheral tendons. Xanthomas usually are a manifestation of a hyperlipoproteinemic state.

Xanthomas are yellow tumors in the skin.

Incidence

Flat xanthomas on the eyelids (xanthelasmas) are the most frequently encountered xanthomas, but are still not very common. Other xanthomas are even less common, both as a presenting complaint in a dermatology clinic and as an incidental finding in the general population. Familial hypertriglyceridemia and familial hypercholesterolemia are both inherited as autosomal dominant traits, each at a frequency of 1 in 500 of the general population. Patients who are homozygous for the disease are obviously much fewer in number, but are more severely affected and more likely to have xanthomas.

History

In patients with one of the inherited hyperlipoproteinemias, a positive family history may be elicited. In addition, the patient may have systemic signs and symptoms that accompany the cutaneous xanthomas, including a history of coronary artery disease and diabetes. Patients with eruptive xanthomas have markedly raised triglyceride levels that usually result from a familial metabolic abnormality combined with a secondary factor such as alcohol, obesity, glucose intolerance, hyperinsulinemia, and drugs, including estrogens, corticosteroids, and isotretinoin. Eruptive xanthomas appear relatively quickly in several weeks, and correspondingly disappear rapidly after reduction of serum triglyceride levels.

Physical Examination

Several types of xanthoma have been characterized. In all except the tendon type, the yellow color of the lesion provides the clue to its lipid nature. The most common types are described below.

Xanthoma type	Raised plasma lipid levels
Xanthelasma	Often none
Eruptive	Triglycerides
Tendon	Cholesterol
Tuberous	Both or either of the above

Xanthelasmas are yellowish plaques on the eyelids. This is the only type that is not invariably accompanied by an increase in either plasma cholesterol or triglyceride concentration.

Eruptive xanthomas (**Fig. 7.8**) are reddish-yellowish papules and plaques that occur in patients with markedly raised triglyceride levels. They occur most frequently on extensor surfaces but may appear anywhere.

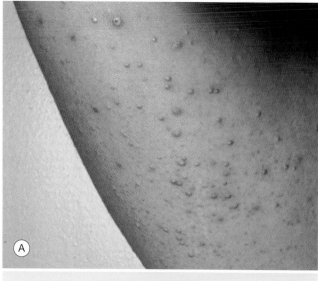

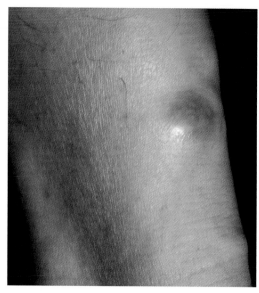

FIGURE 7.9 Tendon xanthoma – hard, pinkish, flesh-colored nodule on the Achilles tendon.

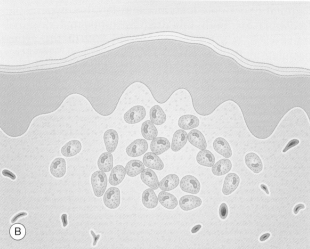

FIGURE 7.8 Eruptive xanthomas. A. Multiple yellowish-pink papules. **B.** Dermis – dense infiltrate of lipid-laden histiocytes.

Tendon xanthomas (**Fig. 7.9**) are stony hard nodules occurring on tendons, most often the Achilles tendon and the extensor tendons of the fingers. Because of their depth, the yellow color cannot be appreciated clinically. Tendon xanthomas are usually associated with severe hypercholesterolemia.

Tuberous xanthomas are 'potato-like' papules and nodules, which are yellowish and most often found on the elbows and buttocks. Tuberous xanthomas are associated with increased serum triglyceride or cholesterol levels.

Differential Diagnosis

Sebaceous glands, lipid deposits, and granulomas are the major causes of the yellow color in skin papules. The lesions of *sebaceous gland hyperplasia* usually occur on the face as small superficial papules, often with a central umbilication.

The yellowish papules and plaques of *juvenile xanthogranuloma* also contain lipid, which is responsible for their color. As the name suggests, these lesions occur in childhood and usually involute spontaneously. Histologically,

they have a distinctive appearance. They are not associated with raised plasma lipid levels.

Both *rheumatoid nodules* and *tendon xanthomas* are subcutaneous, but only tendon xanthomas are affixed to the tendon structures.

Laboratory and Biopsy

The diagnosis is usually made clinically. All patients with xanthomas should have a screening fasting lipid profile. In patients with xanthelasma, results are normal in approximately 50%. For the other types of xanthoma, lipid abnormalities are to be expected. The biopsy reveals an infiltrate of numerous lipid-laden histiocytes (**Fig. 7.8B**).

Therapy

Therapy is aimed at lowering the abnormal lipid levels with diet and, for patients with markedly increased lipid levels, drugs. Xanthelasma lesions may be removed surgically for cosmetic reasons.

Therapy for Xanthoma

Initial
- Diet
- Medications – statins, bile-acid binding resins, fibrates, nicotinic acid

Alternative
- Surgery

Course and Complications

Eruptive xanthomas involute spontaneously after lowering of the serum triglyceride concentration. The other types of xanthoma are more persistent, but may slowly regress if the lipid levels are lowered. The cutaneous lesions usually have no complications, but the lipid abnormality may be associated with significant systemic complications such as premature myocardial infarction in patients with raised cholesterol levels and pancreatitis in patients with markedly increased levels of serum triglycerides.

> Eruptive xanthomas usually resolve when triglyceride levels are lowered; other xanthomas are more persistent.

Pathogenesis

Xanthomas represent accumulations of lipid-laden histiocytes. The lipid is thought to be extracted from plasma, although some evidence suggests that intracellular lipid synthesis may also be operative in some instances.

Patients with familial hypertriglyceridemia have increased endogenous hepatic production of very low density lipoproteins (VLDLs), which are particles with a high triglyceride content. In these patients, VLDL production is further increased with high carbohydrate or alcohol ingestion, obesity, or diabetes, so triglyceride levels of more than 2000 mg/mL may be attained. Triglyceride deposits are polar and thereby more susceptible to intracellular lysosomal hydrolases; hence, eruptive xanthomas quickly resolve when the triglyceride level is lowered.

Patients with familial hypercholesterolemia have high levels of circulating low density lipoproteins (LDLs), which are particles with a high cholesterol content. In these patients, the gene affected is the one that controls the synthesis of LDL cell surface receptors. As a result, LDL cannot be adequately removed from the plasma by cellular uptake. In addition, the cells perceive an intracellular deficiency of LDL and hence are stimulated to produce more LDL, a process resulting in even higher serum levels. Individuals who are heterozygous for this disease have plasma LDL levels that are twice to three times the normal level, and develop tendon xanthomas and premature atherosclerotic cardiovascular disease in midlife. Homozygotic patients have plasma LDL levels that are six to eight times normal levels, with cholesterol levels of >800 mg/dL, and they develop symptomatic coronary artery disease before the age of 20 years. The non-polar cholesterol esters are more resistant to degradation and therefore persist in both skin (tendon xanthomas) and blood vessels (atherosclerosis).

OTHER MALIGNANT DERMAL TUMORS

Key Points

1. Rule out cancer for hard dermal nodules
2. Although uncommon, skin metastases may be the first sign of internal cancer

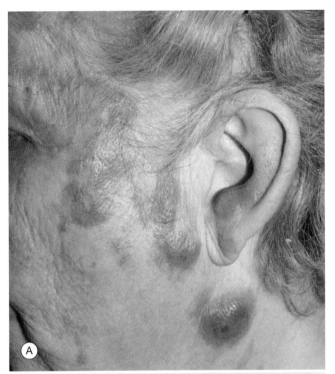

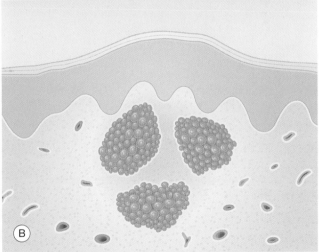

FIGURE 7.10 Metastatic lymphoma. A. Hard, plum-colored nodules. **B.** Dermis – dense aggregates of malignant cells.

Definition

These tumors result from deposition or proliferation of malignant cells in the dermis. They usually manifest clinically as hard nodules in the skin (**Fig. 7.10**).

Incidence

Malignant dermal tumors can be primary or metastatic. Kaposi's sarcoma, as discussed above, is an example of a primary (albeit multifocal) malignant tumor derived from endothelial cells in the skin. Tumors from other endogenous elements such as collagen (dermatofibrosarcoma protuberans), neural tissue (neurofibrosarcoma), vascular tissue (angiosarcoma), appendageal structures (sweat gland and sebaceous gland carcinomas), and subcutaneous fat (liposarcoma) are all extremely rare and

TABLE 7.2 Frequency of skin metastases from internal malignancies

	Frequency (%)
Malignancy	
Leukemia	
Acute myelomonocytic	10–20
Chronic lymphocytic	5–10
Acute lymphocytic	Rare
Lymphoma (not including mycosis fungoides)	
Non-Hodgkin's	3–20
Hodgkin's	0.5
Multiple myeloma	4
Metastatic carcinoma	10
Type of carcinoma responsible for skin metastases	
Women	
Breast	73
Melanoma	11
Ovary	3
Oral cavity	2
Lung	2
Men	
Melanoma	34
Lung	12
Large intestine	12
Oral cavity	10

are not discussed except with the usual admonition that, for undiagnosed nodules in the skin, a skin biopsy is necessary.

> Malignant tumors from endogenous dermal elements are rare. Metastatic tumors are more common.

The more common cause of malignant dermal tumors is metastatic disease. The authors performed a tumor registry survey of 4020 patients with metastatic carcinoma and found that 420 (10%) had cutaneous metastases. The incidence of metastatic nodules in the skin depends on the type of malignancy. For example, skin involvement is relatively common in acute myelomonocytic leukemia (occurring in 10–20% of cases) but uncommon in acute lymphocytic leukemia. Moreover, skin nodules are common in metastatic breast carcinoma but extremely rare in prostatic carcinoma. **Table 7.2** lists the tumor types that were found most likely to metastasize to skin.

Cutaneous metastases occasionally serve as the *first sign* of an internal malignancy. In a retrospective survey of 7316 patients with cancer, 59 (0.8%) presented with direct extension (22 patients), local (20) or distant (17) metastases as the first manifestation of cancer. Most had breast cancer.

History

In patients with a known history of internal malignant disease, one should be particularly suspicious of a possible malignant origin of any new skin nodule. The nodules are usually asymptomatic, but the patient may have other signs and symptoms of malignancy, including weight loss, lymphadenopathy, or symptoms related to the location of the primary tumor.

Physical Examination

Malignant tumors in the dermis are characteristically hard, or at least extremely firm. They vary in color from flesh tones to pink, red, and purple. Skin nodules of lymphoma and myeloma are frequently plum colored. Large nodules sometimes ulcerate. Lymphadenopathy or hepatosplenomegaly may also be present in patients with metastatic disease.

> Malignant tumors are hard dermal nodules.

Differential Diagnosis

A malignant tumor in the skin may be confused with any of the benign dermal growths. As is emphasized repeatedly, if any doubt exists, a biopsy is required.

Laboratory and Biopsy

The biopsy is diagnostic, showing an infiltrate of malignant cells, often in nodular aggregates (**Fig. 7.10B**). Occasionally, the histologic features are tumor specific, that is, the likely primary source is suggested by the histologic appearance of the skin involvement. Special histochemical stains for cellular components (e.g., keratin) or tumor markers (e.g., carcinoembryonic antigen) may be helpful.

Therapy

For a primary malignant process in the skin, the preferred therapy is surgical excision. Therapy of metastatic disease is that of the primary tumor. The effect of systemic therapy can often be evaluated by measuring the metastatic skin lesion, an easily assessable marker. Troublesome skin metastases are sometimes also treated with palliative radiation or surgery.

> **Therapy for Malignant Dermal Tumors**
>
> - Excision for primary tumors
> - Chemotherapy for metastases
> - Palliative surgery or radiotherapy for metastases

Course and Complications

For metastatic disease, the course is similar to that of the primary process. For many diseases, the development of skin metastasis indicates a particularly poor prognosis. Acute myelomonocytic leukemia is an example.

The skin nodules of metastatic disease may ulcerate and become secondarily infected. This condition can lead to sepsis and death. The major complications, however, do not usually result from the skin but from the systemic disease.

Pathogenesis

Spread to the skin from an internal malignant disease usually occurs by a hematogenous route. Some tumors may also reach the skin via lymphatic pathways. Once lodged in the skin, the malignant cells proliferate in a 3-dimensional fashion, clinically expressed as a nodule. Why some tumors have a greater propensity for the skin than others is not known.

UNCOMMON DERMAL AND SUBCUTANEOUS GROWTHS

GLOMUS TUMOR

Glomus tumor (glomangioma) is a benign growth of vascular smooth muscle which produces solitary or multiple flesh-colored to dusky blue nodules. Solitary glomus tumor is frequently extremely tender, occurring on the arms, fingers (subungual), and elsewhere. Multiple glomangiomas (**Fig. 7.11**) are usually non-tender and may be inherited as an autosomal dominant trait.

GRANULAR CELL TUMOR

Granular cell tumor usually presents in middle age and is benign in the great majority of cases. It is found in the skin and tongue, most frequently as a solitary, asymptomatic nodule (**Fig. 7.12**). The biopsy reveals large polyhedral cells with a characteristic granular cytoplasm.

INFANTILE DIGITAL FIBROMATOSIS

This is a rare benign tumor of myofibroblasts that occurs at birth or usually by the age of 1 year. The biopsy reveals spindle-shaped cells with characteristic eosinophilic inclusion bodies. These asymptomatic nodules affect the fingers and toes (**Fig. 7.13**). Surgical excision is usually unsuccessful because of a high recurrence rate.

LEIOMYOMA

Cutaneous leiomyoma is a benign smooth muscle tumor that is characteristically painful. It can be solitary or grouped (**Fig. 7.14**). An autosomal dominant familial form of multiple leiomyoma in women is associated with uterine leiomyomas and renal cell cancer. This is due to a germline mutation in the gene encoding fumarate hydratase.

LYMPHANGIOMA CIRCUMSCRIPTUM

This uncommon benign lymphatic tumor usually arises in infancy or early childhood. It is characterized by irregularly grouped, vesicle-like papules that are likened to frogspawn (**Fig. 7.15**). Trauma can result in weeping clear, colorless lymph. They also may be colored purple if filled with blood. These superficial lymphangiomas are frequently connected to deeper lymphatic cisterns, which makes treatment more difficult.

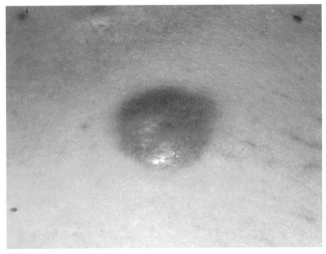

FIGURE 7.12 **Granular cell tumor** – reddish-yellow, firm nodule.

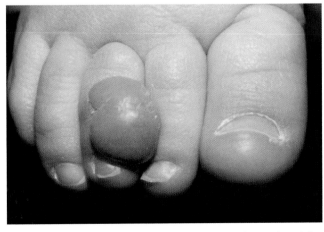

FIGURE 7.13 **Infantile digital fibromatosis** – firm, red, smooth nodule.

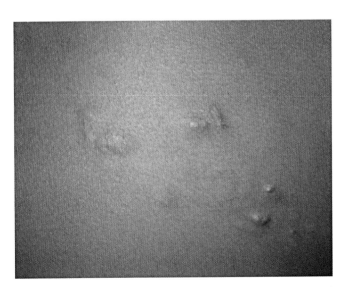

FIGURE 7.11 **Glomus tumor** – dusky blue non-tender papules and nodules.

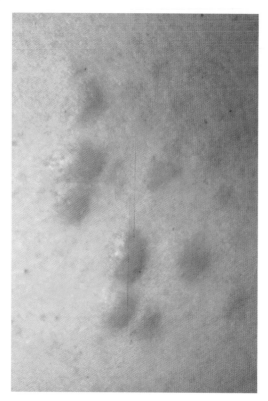

FIGURE 7.14 **Leiomyoma** – grouped, pink, tender, papules.

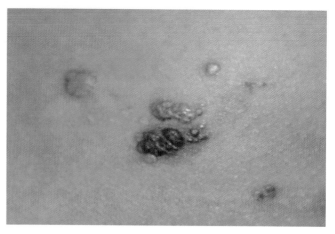

FIGURE 7.15 **Lymphangioma circumscriptum** – irregularly grouped, translucent and red papules.

MYXOID CYST

Myxoid, or digital mucous, cyst occurs as a solitary, opalescent or flesh-colored, nodule. It is found over the distal interphalangeal joint or proximal nail fold, where it can cause a characteristic nail plate groove (**Fig. 7.16**). Puncture of the cyst results in a clear, viscous, sticky drainage. Connection with the underlying joint space makes treatment disappointing, unless careful excision is accomplished.

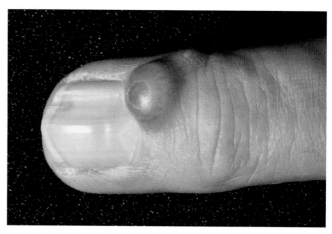

FIGURE 7.16 **Myxoid cyst** – opalescent nodule of the proximal nail fold producing a characteristic groove of the nail plate.

Eczematous Rashes 8

Chapter Contents

- Atopic Dermatitis
- Contact Dermatitis
- Essential Dermatitis
- Lichen Simplex Chronicus
- Seborrheic Dermatitis
- Stasis Dermatitis
- Uncommon Eczematous Appearing Diseases
  - Darier's Disease
  - Glucagonoma Syndrome
  - Langerhans Cell Histiocytosis
  - Lichen Sclerosus
  - Pemphigus Foliaceus
  - Wiskott–Aldrich Syndrome
  - Zinc Deficiency

Key Points

1. Appearance varies from blisters to scaling, lichenified plaques
2. Itching is prominent
3. Distribution can be localized or generalized

ABSTRACT

The term *eczema* is derived from the Greek word that means 'to boil out or over.' It is a convenient 'wastebasket' for many undiagnosed rashes but is best applied to epidermal eruptions that are characterized histologically by intercellular edema, called *spongiosis* (**Table 8.1**). *Eczema* and *dermatitis* are synonyms. Acute dermatitis has a marked amount of spongiosis causing vesiculation. Subacute dermatitis has less spongiosis, resulting in 'juicy papules.' Chronic dermatitis involves a markedly thickened epidermis (*lichenification*) with only slight spongiosis.

Types of dermatitis:
1. Acute – vesicles
2. Subacute – juicy papules
3. Chronic – lichenification

The hallmarks of dermatitis are marked pruritus, indistinct borders (except for contact dermatitis), and epidermal changes characterized by vesicles, juicy papules, or lichenification. Dermatitis may be localized or diffuse; it may be idiopathic or may have a specific cause. Contact allergy is the best understood cause of an eczematous reaction, and potentially the most correctable. For any eczematous rash, the first question to be asked is: 'Could it be contact dermatitis?'

If it does not itch, reconsider the diagnosis of dermatitis.

ATOPIC DERMATITIS

Key Points

1. Itching is prominent
2. The antecubital and popliteal fossae are typically affected
3. Chronic waxing and waning course

Definition

Atopic dermatitis is a chronic, relapsing, intensely pruritic, eczematous condition of the skin that is associated with a personal or family history of atopic disease (e.g., asthma, allergic rhinitis, or atopic dermatitis). The cause of atopic dermatitis is thought to be altered skin barrier and immune function. Patients appear to have a genetic predisposition that can be exacerbated by numerous factors, including food allergy, skin infections, irritating clothes or chemicals, change in climate, and emotions. Lichenification is the clinical hallmark of chronic atopic dermatitis (**Fig. 8.1**).

89

TABLE 8.1 Eczematous eruptions

	Frequency[a]	History	Physical Examination	Differential Diagnosis	Laboratory Test
Atopic dermatitis	2.6	Allergic rhinitis Asthma	Vesicles, juicy papules – infants Lichenified plaques – adults and older children Head, neck, antecubital and popliteal fossa	Contact dermatitis Scabies	IgE
Contact dermatitis	2.8	Irritant: contact precedes rash by hours to days Allergic: contact precedes rash by 1–4 days	Vesicles, juicy papules, lichenified plaques Sharp margins Geometric or linear configuration Conforms to area of contact	Eczematous dermatitis Fungal infection Cellulitis	Patch test
Essential dermatitis	11.4	Pruritus	Acute: vesicles, weeping, crusted patches Subacute: juicy papules Chronic: lichenified, scaling plaques	Contact dermatitis Atopic dermatitis Seborrheic dermatitis Fungal infection Psoriasis Drug rash Dermatitis herpetiformis	–
Lichen simplex chronicus	0.8	Rash subsequent to pruritus	Lichenified plaque within reach of fingers	Psoriasis	–
Seborrheic dermatitis	3.7	Dandruff	Scaling papules and patches Scalp, eyebrows, nose, sternum	Atopic dermatitis Psoriasis Fungal infection Langerhans cell histiocytosis Lupus erythematosus	–
Stasis dermatitis	0.4	Varicose veins Leg swelling Thrombophlebitis	Juicy papules Lichenified plaques Brown pigmentation Lower legs	Cellulitis Contact dermatitis Arterial disease Fungal infection	–

[a]Percentage of new dermatology patients with this diagnosis seen in the Hershey Medical Center Dermatology Clinic, Hershey, PA.

Incidence

Atopic dermatitis is predominantly a disease of childhood, with 17% of children and 6% of adults affected. It usually starts after 2 months of age, and by 5 years of age, 90% of the patients who will develop atopic dermatitis have manifested the disease. It is uncommon for adults to develop atopic dermatitis without a history of eczema in childhood.

History

A history of allergic respiratory disease is found in one-third of patients with atopic dermatitis and in two-thirds of their family members. Pruritus (**Fig. 8.1D**) is the most distressing and prominent symptom.

Diagnostic Criteria for Atopic Dermatitis

- Pruritus
- Typical morphology and distribution
- Flexural lichenification in adults and older children
- Facial and extensor papulovesicles in infancy
- Chronic – relapsing course

- Personal or family history of atopic disease
- Lichenification is the clinical hallmark of chronic atopic dermatitis

Physical Examination

The morphology and distribution of atopic dermatitis are age-dependent (**Fig. 8.2**). Infantile atopic dermatitis is characterized by acute-to-subacute eczema with papules, vesicles, oozing, and crusting. It is distributed over the head, diaper area, and extensor surfaces of the extremities. In children and adults, the eruption is a chronic dermatitis with lichenification and scaling. The distribution includes the neck, face, upper chest, and, characteristically, antecubital and popliteal fossae (see **Fig. 8.1**).

Atopic dermatitis in infants is papular or vesicular; in children and adults, it is lichenified, especially affecting the antecubital and popliteal fossae.

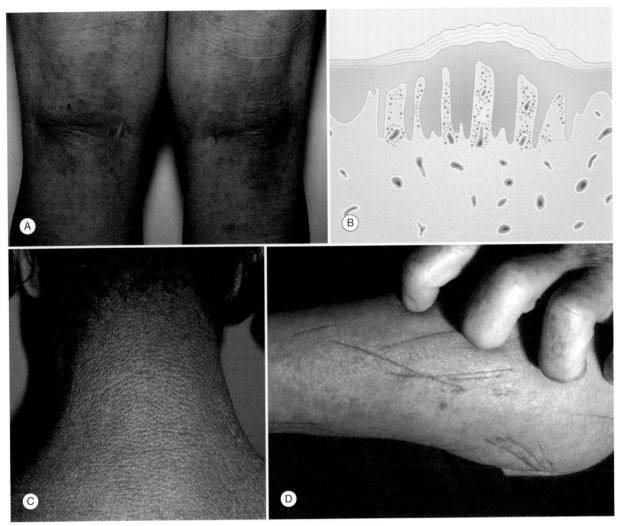

FIGURE 8.1 **Atopic dermatitis. A.** Hyperpigmented, erythematous, lichenified plaques affecting the popliteal fossae. **B.** Epidermis – thickened, hyperkeratosis. Dermis – perivascular inflammation. **C.** Hyperpigmented, lichenified plaque involving the whole neck. **D.** Severe scratching, excoriations, and erythroderma.

Atopic individuals have a characteristic expression. The face has mild to moderate erythema, perioral pallor, and infraorbital folds (Dennie–Morgan lines) associated with dermatitis and hyperpigmentation. The skin generally is dry and may have generalized fine, whitish scaling. The palms often have increased linear markings.

Differential Diagnosis

The differential diagnosis of atopic dermatitis includes other eczematous eruptions and *scabies*. The history of other family members with pruritus and a thorough skin examination that reveals burrows, particularly on the hands, are diagnostic of scabies. Infants with *histiocytosis X* and immunodeficiency syndromes such as *Wiskott–Aldrich syndrome, ataxia-telangiectasia,* and *Swiss-type agammaglobulinemia* have dermatitis that resembles atopic dermatitis, but these conditions are rare, and the infants have systemic symptoms that distinguish their conditions from atopic dermatitis.

Laboratory and Biopsy

The diagnosis of atopic dermatitis is made clinically. The skin biopsy (rarely required) reveals an eczematous change that is not specific for atopic dermatitis (see

Fig. 8.1B). Serum immunoglobulin (Ig)E concentration is frequently raised, but usually is not necessary to make the diagnosis.

Therapy

The treatment of atopic dermatitis is the same as for other eczematous eruptions and includes topical steroids, topical macrolide immunosuppressants, and systemic antihistamines. These should be given in appropriate strength and frequency to reduce inflammation and itching significantly. A common error is undertreatment. Occasionally, a short course of systemic steroids (prednisone) is necessary to bring the disease under control. Wet dressings (plain water) and baths (Aveeno) are helpful in treating acute atopic dermatitis. Avoidance of environmental factors that enhance itching, such as woolen clothes, emotional stress, and uncomfortable climatic conditions, is important. Moisturizers reduce dry skin and itching. Ultraviolet radiation B (UVB), psoralen plus ultraviolet radiation A (PUVA), or other systemic immunosuppressants – cyclosporine (Neoral), azathioprine (Imuran), and mycophenolate mofetil (CellCept) – may be considered if satisfactory control is not achieved with initial treatment.

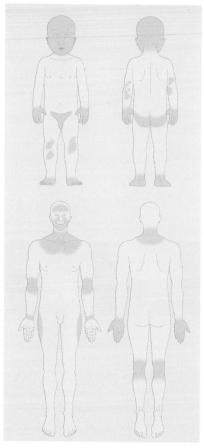

FIGURE 8.2 Distribution of atopic dermatitis.

To be successful, treatment must eliminate pruritus.

In some children, food allergy can cause atopic dermatitis. Skin testing or radioallergosorbent tests may help to identify foods that are responsible. Positive tests must be confirmed with controlled food challenges and elimination diets. Eggs, peanuts, milk, and wheat appear to be the most frequently offending foods. Investigators have suggested that atopic dermatitis can be prevented by avoiding cow's milk, wheat, and eggs for the first 6 months of life. However, this approach is controversial and not generally recommended. Patients with atopic dermatitis have a higher frequency of immediate skin test reactivity in general, but hyposensitization is rarely of value in atopic dermatitis. As a last resort, severe atopic dermatitis is treated with systemic immunomodulants.

Therapy for Atopic Dermatitis

Initial
- Moisturizers
- Avoidance of irritants – woolen clothes, harsh soaps, uncomfortable climate

- Steroids, topical macrolide immunosuppressants, antihistamines, baths, compresses, and antibiotics (see Therapy for essential dermatitis, below)
- Avoidance of food allergens (eggs, peanuts, milk, wheat) in selected patients

Alternative
- Ultraviolet light – UVB, PUVA
- Immunomodulants – azathioprine, cyclosporine, mycophenolate mofetil
- Support group – National Eczema Association for Science and Education, www.nationaleczema.org

Course and Complications

Atopic dermatitis is a chronic disease punctuated by repeated acute flare-ups followed by longer periods of slow resolution. The cause of these flare-ups is frequently unknown – a feature that adds to the frustration of this disease. Most children (90%) outgrow their disease by adolescence, although as adults some continue to have localized forms of atopic dermatitis such as chronic hand or foot dermatitis, patches of lichen simplex chronicus, or eyelid dermatitis. Longitudinal studies suggest an 'atopic march' in which over half of infants and children with atopic dermatitis will progress to develop allergic rhinitis and asthma.

Atopic dermatitis is frequently complicated by skin infections. Atopic skin has a higher rate of colonization with *Staphylococcus aureus*. The most serious cutaneous infection is *Kaposi's varicelliform eruption*. This widespread vesiculopustular eruption is caused by herpes simplex, variola, or vaccinia virus. Patients with this infection are acutely ill and may die; for this reason, smallpox immunization was contraindicated in these patients. The *hyper-IgE syndrome* refers to a syndrome of atopic dermatitis characterized by recurrent pyoderma (skin infections), raised serum IgE levels, and decreased chemotaxis of mononuclear cells.

Bacterial and viral skin infections are common in atopic dermatitis.

Pathogenesis

A disrupted skin barrier (filaggrin gene mutation) and disturbed immunologic response (Th2 + Th1 cytokines, and IgE) have been implicated in the etiology of atopic dermatitis. The epidermal barrier defect results in dry skin and penetration of irritants, microbes, and antigens. The immunologic changes are most notable and frequent in patients with severe atopic dermatitis. These changes include raised serum IgE levels, defective cell-mediated immunity, decreased chemotaxis of mononuclear cells, increased T-lymphocyte activation with production of T helper (Th)1 and Th2 cytokines, and hyperstimulatory Langerhans cells. The increased IgE concentration is thought to reflect decreased numbers of T-suppressor cells and uninhibited production of IgE. Depressed cell-mediated immunity is manifested by an increased susceptibility to cutaneous viral and bacterial infections. In addition, responses to in vitro tests of cell-mediated immunity such as lymphocyte blastogenesis to mitogens and antigens are blunted. There are also low levels of antimicrobial peptides in lesional skin resulting in increased susceptibility to pathogens such as *S. aureus*, herpes simplex virus, and vaccinia virus.

CONTACT DERMATITIS

Key Points

1. Irritant or allergic etiology
2. Distribution conforms to areas of contact
3. Avoidance of the contactant results in cure

Definition

Contact dermatitis (**Fig. 8.3**) is an inflammatory reaction of the skin precipitated by an exogenous chemical. The two types of contact dermatitis are irritant and allergic. *Irritant contact dermatitis* is produced by a substance that

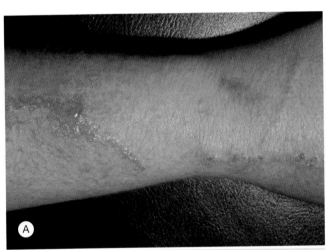

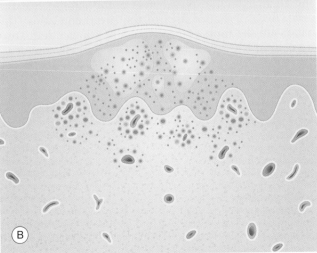

FIGURE 8.3 Allergic contact dermatitis from poison ivy. A. Linear, erythematous papules and weeping vesicles. **B.** Epidermis – vesicles, spongiosis. Dermis – perivascular inflammation.

has a direct toxic effect on the skin. *Allergic contact dermatitis* triggers an immunologic reaction that causes tissue inflammation. Examples of irritants include acids, alkalis, solvents, and detergents. Innumerable chemicals cause allergic contact dermatitis, including metals, plants, medicines, cosmetics, and rubber compounds. Clinical appearance can range from acute (vesicles) to chronic (lichenification) eczematous reactions.

Types of contact dermatitis:
1. Irritant
2. Allergic

Incidence

Contact dermatitis is a frequent problem that most people experience during their lifetime, whether it is irritant diaper dermatitis or allergic poison ivy or oak dermatitis. A significant cause of occupational illness (excluding injury) is caused by contact dermatitis, resulting in impairment and time lost from work. In occupational contact dermatitis, irritant is usually more common than an allergic etiology.

History

One should first determine whether the contact dermatitis is an allergic or an irritant phenomenon. Skin damage is usually evident within several hours of contact with a strong irritant. Weaker irritants, however, may require multiple applications days before the development of dermatitis. Allergic contact dermatitis usually appears 24–48 h after exposure, before the development of clinical disease. Occasionally, the dermatitis may develop as soon as 8–12 h after contact or may be delayed as long as 4–7 days. The history of a precipitating contactant may be either obvious or obscure. Detailed history of occupation, hygienic habits, and hobbies is frequently necessary to find the contactant.

The most common sensitizers are poison ivy or oak, cosmetics, nickel, rubber compounds, and medications.

Causes of allergic contact dermatitis:
1. Poison ivy or oak
2. Cosmetics/personal care products
3. Nickel
4. Rubber compounds
5. Topical medications

Poison ivy or *oak* is a frequent cause of allergic contact dermatitis in the summer (**Fig. 8.4**). The sensitizing allergens are pentadecylcatechol and heptadecylcatechol chemicals located in the sap (urushiol) of the plant. Another familiar member of this family of poisonous plants is poison *sumac*. Less frequently recognized family members are cashew, mango, and lacquer trees. Sensitization to poison ivy results in sensitivity to the other poisonous plants in this family. The characteristic eruption resulting from contact with poison ivy or oak is

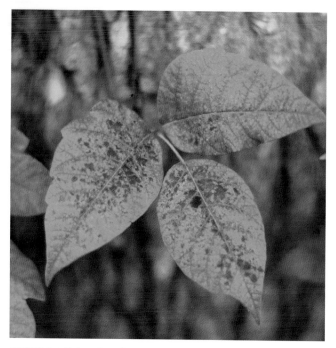

FIGURE 8.4 **Poison ivy plant** with characteristic three leaves.

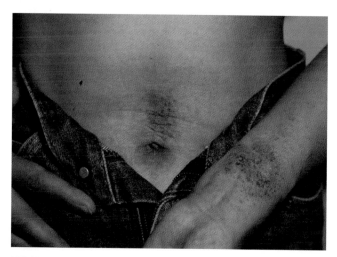

FIGURE 8.5 **Allergic contact dermatitis** from nickel-containing snap and watch band – erythematous, scaling and slightly crusted, lichenified plaques.

manifested by linear streaks of papules and vesicles along with cellulitic appearing plaques and patches. Contact with the smoke of burning plants can result in confluent severe dermatitis of the exposed skin.

> Streaks of vesicles are characteristic of contact dermatitis to poison ivy or oak.

Cosmetics (personal care products) contain fragrances and preservatives that cause allergic contact dermatitis, particularly affecting the faces of women from the use of make-up and moisturizers, for example. *Paraphenylene-diamine* is a dye found in permanent hair coloring. Sensitization to paraphenylenediamine occurs in hair-dressers and in clients who have their hair colored. When completely oxidized, as the dye on a fur coat, paraphenylenediamine is not allergenic.

Nickel sensitivity is seen most often in women as a result of wearing 'cheap' pierced earrings. It is found in many metal alloys (**Fig. 8.5**). One cannot be certain that the commonly advertised 'hypoallergenic' earrings are nickel-free. Although stainless steel contains nickel, it is bound so tightly that it usually does not allow an allergic reaction to occur.

Rubber compounds are ubiquitous. Shoes and gloves are the most common sources of allergic contact dermatitis caused by these chemicals. An eczematous reaction limited to the feet or hands is typical of shoe and glove dermatitis, respectively. The most frequent rubber allergens are *mercaptobenzothiazole* and *thiuram*.

In sleuthing the causes of contact dermatitis, one must not overlook the possibility of a *topical medication* perpetuating or exacerbating a pre-existing dermatitis. *Neomycin* and *bacitracin*, found in topical antibiotic preparations, cause allergic contact dermatitis when these agents are used to treat cuts and abrasions, chronic ulcers, and surgical wounds.

Physical Examination

Contact dermatitis may be acute or chronic. The configuration of the lesions depends on the nature of the exposure, which may result in patches or plaques with angular corners, geometric outlines, and sharp margins. Poison ivy or oak characteristically causes linear streaks of papulovesicles.

The location of the dermatitis is helpful in predicting the causative irritant or allergen. The head and neck are frequent sites of contact dermatitis from fragrances and preservatives found in cosmetics. Hair dyes, permanent wave solutions, and shampoos produce dermatitis on the scalp. Eczema of the eyelids is caused by eye cosmetics or allergens that have been transferred from the hands, such as nail polish. Photoallergic contact dermatitis from sunscreens is produced by a photoreaction between sunlight and an allergen in exposed areas of the skin, such as the head, neck, V-shaped area of the chest, and arms. The hands are the most common area of contact dermatitis from industrial chemicals, particularly an irritant reaction from detergents, petroleum products, and solvents. Dermatitis of the feet is produced by allergens in shoes, such as rubber chemicals and leather tanning agents. The groin and buttocks in infants are frequently affected by *diaper dermatitis* (**Fig. 8.6**). This condition is an irritant contact dermatitis from moisture and feces. Diaper dermatitis is often complicated by secondary infection with bacteria and yeast.

> The location of the dermatitis often provides a clue to the nature of the contactant.

Differential Diagnosis

Morphologically, contact dermatitis is identical to other *eczematous eruptions* and may complicate atopic or stasis

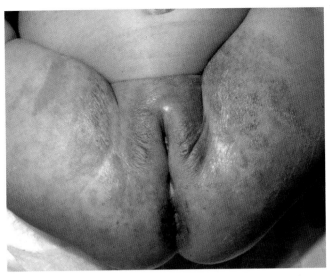

FIGURE 8.6 **Irritant contact dermatitis** (diaper dermatitis) – erythematous patches.

dermatitis if the patient becomes sensitized to the topical preparation used to treat these dermatoses. Other causes of eczematous appearing dermatoses that may need to be ruled out include superficial *fungal infections* and *bacterial cellulitis*. In bacterial cellulitis, the skin is painful (rather than pruritic), and the patient is often febrile.

> For any dermatitis, ask: 'Could it be contact dermatitis?'

Laboratory and Biopsy

No standard testing method is available for diagnosing irritant contact dermatitis. For allergic contact dermatitis, the causative agent can be identified by patch tests, but these tests must be properly performed and interpreted (see Ch. 3). Patch testing is done with a screening patch test series. This series is composed of medications, fragrances, preservatives, metals, rubber compounds, and miscellaneous chemicals. Individual chemicals and special trays (e.g., allergens found in plants) supplement the screening series. The chemicals are applied to patches that are taped on the back of the test subject. After 48 h, the patches are removed and the test site is examined for an eczematous reaction that is graded according to a standard interpretation key: a +1 reaction indicates palpable erythema; a +2 reaction indicates papules and vesicles; and a +3 reaction indicates bullae. A further delayed reading 1–2 days after patch removal is mandatory. Although the patch-testing procedure is simple, its interpretation is often difficult. A positive patch test must be relevant to the eruption to be meaningful. Unknown chemicals and potential irritants must be patch tested cautiously and are best left to trained personnel who have experience in patch testing.

> Patch tests help in identifying the responsible allergen or allergens.

Biopsy (see **Fig. 8.3B**) of contact dermatitis cannot differentiate between irritant and allergic causes. Contact dermatitis also cannot be differentiated histologically from other causes of eczematous eruptions such as atopic or seborrheic dermatitis.

Therapy

Prevention of contact dermatitis is the most logical, but often most difficult, solution. Avoidance of an irritant or allergen may require a change in lifestyle or occupation. Sometimes, protective clothing is curative. Allergens that have high sensitizing potential are best used in closed systems in which workers have virtually no contact with the offending chemicals. Protective or barrier creams are of benefit when matched to the contactant they block. Application of IvyBlock before exposure reduces the development of poison ivy or oak dermatitis. Sometimes, the offending material can be substituted with another, less toxic or allergenic, chemical. Predictive testing for contact irritancy or sensitivity is standard procedure before introducing new cosmetics or chemicals.

Acute, severe, generalized contact dermatitis is treated with a short course of systemic steroids: 40–60 mg prednisone daily for a *minimum* of 5 days and then tapered over the next 5 days or 1 mL triamcinolone suspension (Kenalog-40) intramuscularly. Astringent dressings (Domeboro) or soothing baths (Aveeno) reduce weeping and itching. Milder dermatitis responds to topical steroids (see **Table 4.1**) or to macrolide immunosuppressants (Protopic or Elidel). Systemic antihistamines such as 10–25 mg hydroxyzine (Atarax) or 25–50 mg diphenhydramine (Benadryl) four times daily are helpful for pruritus.

Therapy for Contact Dermatitis

Initial
- Avoidance of irritant or allergen
- Protective clothing – gloves, etc.
- Barrier creams – IvyBlock – poison ivy and oak

Alternative
- Steroids, antihistamines, baths, and compresses (see Therapy for essential dermatitis, below)

Course and Complications

Acute allergic contact dermatitis subsides within 3–4 weeks. If the patient has repeated exposure to the contactant, chronic dermatitis will develop. With the breakdown of the epidermal barrier, secondary bacterial infection may complicate contact dermatitis. Although contact dermatitis may start locally, generalized hypersensitivity of the skin can occur, with resultant generalized dermatitis autosensitization.

Pathogenesis

Irritant contact dermatitis is a nonspecific inflammatory reaction resulting from toxic injury of the skin. Allergic contact dermatitis is a cell-mediated, delayed type IV immunologic reaction. It is divided into a sensitization phase and an elicitation phase. The sensitization phase occurs when a chemical (hapten) is applied to the skin of a non-sensitized individual. This chemical in itself is unable to induce an allergic reaction because of its small molecular size, which is usually less than 500 Daltons (Da). It must combine with an epidermal protein thought to be on the surface of the Langerhans cell (epidermal macrophage). After the formation of the hapten–protein complex, the Langerhans cell presents the allergen to T lymphocytes in the lymph node, where effector, memory, and suppressor lymphocytes are produced. The period of sensitization requires approximately 7–10 days. The elicitation phase occurs in sensitized individuals 1–2 days after re-exposure to the antigen. After presentation of the antigen by Langerhans cells to memory T cells in the skin, effector T cells produce lymphokines, which recruit other inflammatory cells and produce allergic contact dermatitis. The dermatitis usually appears clinically 1–2 days after the elicitation exposure. The reaction is thought ultimately to be extinguished by suppressor T cells.

> Allergic contact dermatitis is a cell-mediated, delayed type IV immunologic reaction.

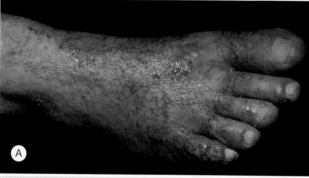

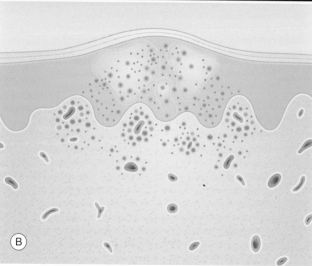

FIGURE 8.7 **Acute essential dermatitis. A.** Erythematous, weeping, vesicles. **B.** Epidermis – vesicles, spongiosis. Dermis – perivascular inflammation.

ESSENTIAL DERMATITIS

Key Points

1. Idiopathic etiology
2. Diagnosis of exclusion
3. Treatment is symptomatic: suppress inflammation and itching

Definition

Essential (nonspecific) dermatitis is an epidermal eruption that may be acute (**Fig. 8.7**) or chronic (**Fig. 8.8**), and localized or generalized. It is a diagnosis that is made by exclusion when an underlying cause such as an allergen or irritant cannot be found, and its distribution is not typical of defined eczematous eruptions such as atopic or seborrheic dermatitis.

Incidence

Essential dermatitis is one of the eruptions most frequently seen by the clinician. Some 11% of the authors' patients had this diagnosis.

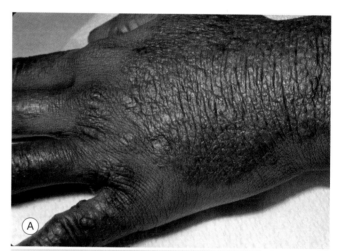

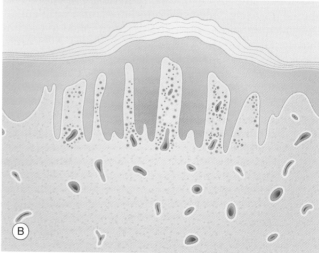

FIGURE 8.8 **Chronic essential dermatitis. A.** Hyperpigmented, lichenified plaque. **B.** Epidermis – thickened, hyperkeratosis. Dermis – perivascular inflammation.

History

Itching is the chief complaint prompting patients to seek medical attention. It is often severe enough to interfere with normal daily activities and to interrupt sleep. The itching may be episodic or constant. The patient frequently has a history of 'sensitive skin' that is intolerant to topical preparations such as moisturizers, soaps, and detergents and to irritating fabrics such wool.

Physical Examination

The varied appearance of essential dermatitis occurs because of its evolution from an acute to a chronic process. Acutely, intercellular edema leads to vesiculation. Chronically, lichenification occurs. The polymorphism is manifest by vesicles, juicy papules, patches, and plaques. Secondary changes include oozing, crusting, scaling, and fissuring. Characteristic of essential dermatitis is the indistinct border between normal and abnormal skin.

Depending on the morphology and location, various types of dermatitis have been classified. *Dyshidrotic eczema* is characterized by deep-seated vesicles (which resemble the pearls in tapioca pudding) involving the hands (palms), feet (soles), and sides of the digits. It occurs bilaterally and symmetrically. *Autosensitization* or *id eruption* is a generalized subacute dermatitis that follows a localized acute dermatitis, usually of the feet or hands. It is thought to be a hypersensitivity reaction to a substance produced by the acute dermatitis. *Xerotic eczema* (**Fig. 8.9**) is the result of low humidity and dry skin. It occurs in the winter and is manifest by dry fissured skin of the trunk and extremities. It particularly affects the elderly and the lower legs of all age groups. *Nummular eczema* is characterized by oval, weeping patches with crusted papulovesicles. It occurs on the trunk and extremities.

Types of idiopathic eczema:
1. Dyshidrotic – hands and feet
2. Autosensitization – generalized
3. Xerotic – dry skin
4. Nummular – oval patches

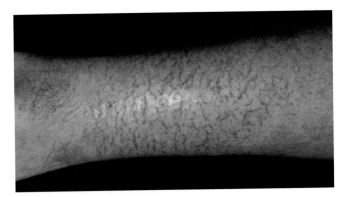

FIGURE 8.9 Xerotic (dry skin) eczema – erythematous, scaling, fissured, reticulated patch.

Differential Diagnosis

The differential diagnosis of an acute vesiculopapular essential dermatitis includes, first, *contact dermatitis*. Also to be considered are infectious processes by a *dermatophyte, herpes simplex virus, varicella-zoster virus,* or *bacterium,* as in impetigo. The appearance of rectangular or linear areas of dermatitis would lead one to suspect contact dermatitis. Removal of the top of the vesicle or scales from the edge of the patch for potassium hydroxide (KOH) examination reveals the typical hyphae of a fungal infection. Scraping the base of the vesicle for a Tzanck preparation reveals the multinucleated giant cells of herpesvirus, which clinically appear as grouped vesicles on an erythematous base. Impetigo can be ruled out by Gram-staining or culture of the yellow crusts typical of this infectious process.

The differential diagnosis of chronic essential dermatitis includes: chronic *contact dermatitis, psoriasis, drug eruption, fungal infection,* and *dermatitis herpetiformis.* The history and patch tests differentiate chronic nonspecific dermatitis from contact dermatitis. Clinically, psoriasis is usually easy to distinguish by its sharply demarcated, silvery, scaling plaques that affect but are not limited to the scalp, elbows, and knees. In any nonspecific dermatitis, one should consider drugs as the cause. Discontinuation of medication with subsequent clearing is the only reliable way to rule out a drug eruption. Fungal infections of the skin can mimic dermatitis, especially if lesions are treated with topical steroids. Any scaling patch, particularly if it has an annular inflammatory border, should be scraped and the scale examined for fungal hyphae (KOH preparation). Dermatitis herpetiformis (see Ch. 10) should be considered for any eczematous-appearing eruption involving the extensor elbows, knees, and low back (**Fig. 8.10**). A biopsy for routine and immunofluorescent staining will be diagnostic.

Biopsy

The histologic hallmark of dermatitis is intercellular edema of the epidermis leading to widening of intercellular spaces with a sponge-like appearance of the epidermis (spongiosis). When the process is acute and severe, it results in intraepidermal vesicle formation (see **Fig. 8.7B**). When it is chronic, the epidermis becomes hyperkeratotic and thickened (acanthotic) (see **Fig. 8.8B**). The dermis is characterized by a lymphocytic infiltrate.

Spongiosis is the histologic hallmark of eczema.

Therapy

Corticosteroids are the cornerstone of dermatitis treatment. They may be applied topically, injected intralesionally, or administered systemically. Steroid creams are used for acute papulovesicular eczema, whereas ointments are better for chronic lichenified dermatitis. Therapy with topical steroids such as hydrocortisone 1% (Cortaid), triamcinolone 0.1% (Kenalog), fluocinonide 0.05% (Lidex), and clobetasol 0.05% (Temovate) is discussed in

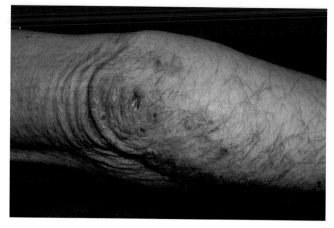

FIGURE 8.10 Dermatitis herpetiformis – erythematous, slightly scaling, and excoriated patch.

detail in Chapter 4. An alternative to topical steroids are the macrolide immunosuppressants, tacrolimus (Protopic) and pimecrolimus (Elidel). These non-steroidal topicals have the advantage of not causing skin atrophy and, when used near the eyes, glaucoma or cataracts. Thick, hyperkeratotic plaques that are unresponsive to topical steroids may be injected with intralesional steroids (Kenalog-10). This should be done cautiously because skin atrophy may occur. Severe, widespread acute or subacute dermatitis is treated most effectively with prednisone, but long-term use must be avoided if possible. In adults, prednisone, starting at a dosage of 40–60 mg daily and tapered over 2–4 weeks, is usually effective. Topical steroids may be added during the tapering period for recurrence of small areas of dermatitis. An alternative to prednisone is triamcinolone at a dose of 40 mg intramuscularly (Kenalog-40), which has an effect for 2–4 weeks. Again, long-term administration should be avoided.

> Avoid the use of long-term systemic steroids because of systemic side-effects.

Astringent dressings (Domeboro) applied for 15 min twice daily are helpful in treating acute weeping dermatitis. For widespread dermatitis, baths have a soothing effect on the skin by reducing inflammation and oozing, and by removing crust and scaling. Colloidal oatmeal (Aveeno) or tar (Cutar) may be added to the bath water. Patients should soak in the bath for 15–20 min once or twice daily, and should apply a steroid to the dermatitis *immediately* after towel drying.

Itching is a prominent component of dermatitis and must be reduced to prevent scratching. Antihistamines such as hydroxyzine (Atarax) or diphenhydramine (Benadryl) can be used three or four times daily, particularly at bedtime. The non-sedating antihistamines, unfortunately, are not effective in reducing pruritus. An alternative antipruritic is gabapentin (Neurontin).

Secondary bacterial infections with *Staphylococcus aureus* often complicate dermatitis, in which case a course

of dicloxacillin or cephalexin for 7 days is indicated. Penicillin is *not* prescribed because *S. aureus* is usually resistant to this antibiotic For methicillin-resistant *Staphylococcus aureus* (MRSA), trimethoprim-sulfamethoxazole or doxycycline are the preferred choices. Nasal and skin disinfection with Polysporin ointment and bleach baths, respectively, can be implemented. Impetiginized eczema has yellow crusting, purulent weeping, and pustules.

Therapy for Essential Dermatitis

Initial
Topical Steroids – Cream, Ointment, Solution
- Hydrocortisone 1% (lowest potency)
- Triamcinolone 0.1% (medium potency)
- Fluocinonide 0.05% (high potency)
- Clobetasol 0.05% (super potent)

Antihistamines
- Hydroxyzine: 10–25 mg q.i.d.; syrup, 10 mg/5 mL – 2 mg/kg daily in four divided doses
- Diphenhydramine: 25–50 mg q.i.d.; elixir, 12.5 mg/5 mL – 5 mg/kg daily in four divided doses

Alternative
Intralesional Steroid
- Triamcinolone suspension (Kenalog-10)

Systemic Steroid
- Prednisone: 1 mg/kg or 40–60 mg daily in adults
- Triamcinolone suspension (Kenalog-40): 1 mL IM.

Macrolide Immunosuppressants
- Tacrolimus ointment 0.03% and 0.1%
- Pimecrolimus cream 1%

Baths and Compresses
- Oatmeal
- Tar
- Aluminum acetate
- Bleach: ¼–½ cup of bleach in ½ tub of water

Antibiotics If Secondary Infection
- Dicloxacillin: 500 mg b.i.d.
- Erythromycin: 500 mg b.i.d.
- Cephalexin: 500 mg b.i.d.; suspension, 250 mg/5 mL – 25–50 mg/kg daily in divided doses
- Trimethoprim-sulfamethoxazole DS b.i.d., suspension, 1 mL/kg per day b.i.d.
- Doxycycline 100 mg b.i.d.
- Polysporin ointment

Antipruritic
- Gabapentin: 100–300 mg q.i.d.

Pathogenesis

The cause of essential dermatitis is unknown. Scratching results in histamine release, which causes more itching, more dermatitis, and a chronic, self-perpetuating eruption.

LICHEN SIMPLEX CHRONICUS

Key Points

1. Localized chronic dermatitis from scratching
2. Goal is to break itch–scratch–itch cycle
3. Occluded steroids may help

Definition

Lichen simplex chronicus (also called 'neurodermatitis') is a chronic eczematous eruption of the skin that is the result of scratching (**Fig. 8.11**). Pruritus precedes the scratching and may be precipitated by frustration, depression, and stress. The scratching then causes the lichenification and further itching, resulting in an 'itch–scratch–itch' cycle that perpetuates the process.

Incidence

Of all new patients seen in the authors' clinic, 0.8% have presented with lichen simplex chronicus.

History

Some patients with lichen simplex chronicus have a history of emotional or psychiatric problems. However, for most, it is simply a nervous habit. Preceding the eruption, the patient has a pruritic area of skin that is scratched, producing a plaque of chronic dermatitis.

Itching typically precedes the rash of lichen simplex chronicus.

Physical Examination

The patient may appear anxious and may talk with pressured speech. There may be little insight into the cause of the eruption. The lichenified plaque always occurs within reach of scratching fingers.

Differential Diagnosis

The diagnosis of lichen simplex chronicus is usually obvious in patients who have a localized itching plaque of chronic dermatitis. Several more serious 'psychodermatoses' are habitual (neurotic) excoriations, factitious dermatitis, and delusions of parasitosis.

Types of 'psychodermatoses':
1. Lichen simplex chronicus
2. Habitual (neurotic) excoriations
3. Factitious dermatitis
4. Delusions of parasitosis

Habitual (neurotic) excoriations (**Fig. 8.12**) are characterized by linear, 'dug-out' lesions that typically spare the upper mid-back, where scratching fingers cannot reach. Patients are usually neurotic women.

Factitious dermatitis is a self-inflicted injury of the skin that presents as a bizarre eruption (often ulcerated) with

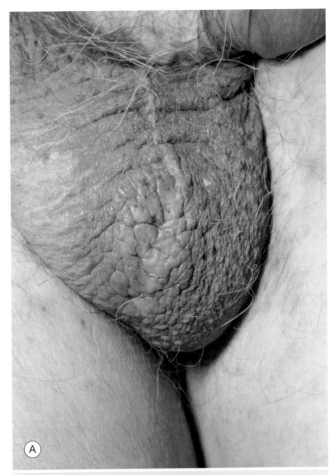

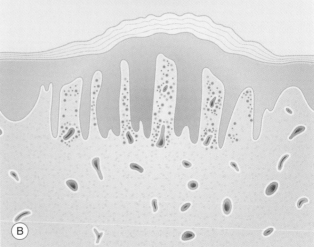

FIGURE 8.11 Lichen simplex chronicus. A. Lichenified, erythematous plaque. **B.** Epidermis – thickened. Dermis – perivascular inflammation.

linear and geometric outlines. The patient's history is vague and unclear. The diagnosis is made when the clinician has a high index of suspicion in a patient who has apparent secondary gain from perpetuating the condition.

Delusions of parasitosis occur in disturbed or anxious eccentric individuals. This disorder begins as intractable pruritus with a crawling sensation in the skin. The patients are convinced that they are harboring parasites and

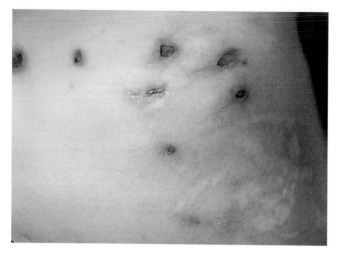

FIGURE 8.12 **Habitual (neurotic) excoriations** – linear white scars and dug-out excoriations.

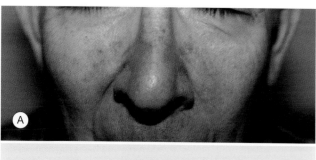

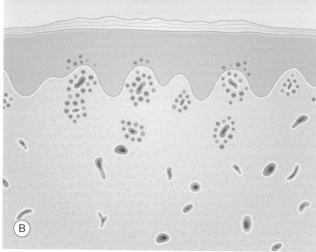

FIGURE 8.13 **Seborrheic dermatitis. A.** Erythematous, slightly scaling patches. **B.** Epidermis – hyperkeratosis. Dermis – perivascular inflammation.

usually bring 'specimens' to prove infestation. These bits of material or skin must be examined to rule out a true infestation and to assure the patient of your interest in the problem. More than half of these patients have no visible skin lesions. Those with active lesions have excoriated, crusted papules secondary to picking. Illicit drug addiction should also be ruled out.

Laboratory and Biopsy

The biopsy in lichen simplex chronicus is nonspecific, showing only chronic dermatitis (see **Fig. 8.11B**).

Therapy

Treatment may be difficult, particularly if the patient has poor insight concerning the nature and cause of the eruption. Topical steroids under occlusion, which protect the area from scratching fingers, and intralesional steroids (Kenalog-10) are helpful. Tranquilizers and antidepressants have a role in treating underlying emotional difficulties if such conditions are present.

Therapy for Lichen Simplex Chronicus

Initial
- Steroids
  - Topical under occlusion
  - Intralesional – triamcinolone suspension: 10 mg/mL
- Emotional support

Alternative
- Tranquilizers and antidepressants

Course and Complications

Lichen simplex chronicus is a chronic, waxing and waning problem that accompanies the mood changes of the patient.

SEBORRHEIC DERMATITIS

Key Points

1. Face and scalp most commonly involved
2. Treat with anti-yeast and anti-inflammatory agents
3. Check HIV status in severe cases

Definition

Seborrheic dermatitis is a chronic, superficial, inflammatory process affecting the hairy regions of the body, especially the scalp, eyebrows, and face (**Fig. 8.13**). Its cause is thought to be an inflammatory reaction to the *Malassezia* yeast (formerly *Pityrosporum ovale*). Dandruff is scaling of the scalp without inflammation.

Malassezia yeast may contribute to the cause of seborrheic dermatitis.

Incidence

Seborrheic dermatitis is a common problem affecting 3–5% of the healthy population.

History

The occurrence of seborrheic dermatitis parallels the increased sebaceous gland activity occurring in infancy and after puberty. It has a waxing and waning course with

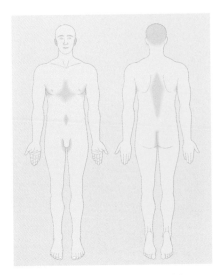

FIGURE 8.14 Distribution of seborrheic dermatitis.

a variable amount of pruritus. It has been associated with Parkinson's disease and acquired immune deficiency syndrome (AIDS). Approximately one-third of patients with AIDS and AIDS-related complex have seborrheic dermatitis.

Physical Examination

Seborrheic dermatitis has a predilection for the hairy regions of the skin, where sebaceous glands are numerous (**Fig. 8.14**). These regions are the scalp, eyebrows, eyelids, nasolabial creases, ears, chest, intertriginous areas, axilla, groin, buttocks, and inframammary folds. The rash is bilateral and symmetrically distributed. In its mildest form, dandruff, one sees fine, white scale without erythema. The patches and plaques of seborrheic dermatitis are characterized by indistinct margins, mild to moderate erythema, and yellowish, greasy scaling. It is uncommon for hair loss to result from seborrheic dermatitis.

Differential Diagnosis

The differential diagnosis of seborrheic dermatitis includes atopic dermatitis, psoriasis, tinea capitis, histiocytosis X, lupus erythematosus, and rosacea. The distinction between *seborrheic dermatitis* and *atopic dermatitis* in infancy is often difficult, so many clinicians use the term 'infantile eczema.' When the dermatitis involves solely the diaper area and axillae, a diagnosis of seborrheic dermatitis is favored. Lesions on the forearms and shins favor the diagnosis of atopic dermatitis. *Psoriasis* may also enter into the differential diagnosis. Psoriasis limited to the scalp may be impossible to differentiate from seborrheic dermatitis. Involvement of nails, knees, and elbows favors the diagnosis of psoriasis. *Tinea capitis* should be considered in the differential diagnosis of seborrheic dermatitis, especially when the usual antiseborrheic agents have failed, when the patient has hair loss, and when the patient is a Black person living in an urban area. *Otitis externa* is not usually due to a fungal infection, but rather is a manifestation of seborrheic dermatitis. *Histiocytosis X*, an uncommon Langerhans cell neoplasm, may appear as a seborrheic dermatitis-like eruption. The occurrence of

petechiae and the failure of standard therapy should make one suspect this cancer and obtain a skin biopsy. Facial involvement with seborrheic dermatitis may mimic lupus erythematosus or rosacea. *Lupus erythematosus* lacks yellowish, greasy scales and generally does not involve the eyebrows, as does seborrheic dermatitis. If in doubt, the history, physical examination, laboratory tests, and skin biopsy will rule out lupus. *Rosacea* has inflammatory papules and pustules not seen in seborrheic dermatitis. *Perioral dermatitis* is a hybrid of acneiform papules and pustules plus eczematous patches surrounding the mouth and nares. When the dermatitis predominates, topical steroids are often prescribed, which cause steroid addiction to suppress the acneform eruption that will flare badly when the steroid is discontinued.

> Seborrheic dermatitis is the most common cause of a 'butterfly' rash.

Laboratory and Biopsy

Seborrheic dermatitis usually is not examined by biopsy unless concern exists about the possibility of another disease such as histiocytosis X. The histopathologic changes in seborrheic dermatitis are those of dermatitis and therefore are non-diagnostic with reference to other eczematous conditions (see **Fig. 8.13B**).

Therapy

Non-prescription antiseborrheic shampoos containing zinc pyrithione (Head & Shoulders), selenium sulfide (Head & Shoulders Intensive Treatment), or ketoconazole (Nizoral) are the mainstay of treatment. The shampoo must be rubbed into the wet scalp, rinsed, and then reapplied for 3–5 min before the final rinse. Patients with inflammatory seborrheic dermatitis that has not responded to shampoos benefit from a topical steroid lotion or gel. High-potency steroids should be used sparingly, particularly on the face. Tacrolimus ointment 0.1% or pimecrolimus cream can be used as steroid sparing agents.

> High-potency topical steroids should be avoided in prolonged treatment of seborrheic dermatitis, especially the face and intertriginous skin.

Therapy for seborrheic dermatitis

Initial
- Shampoos – two or three times per week
  - Zinc pyrithione 1%
  - Selenium sulfide 1% or 2.5%
  - Ketoconazole 1% or 2%
- Hydrocortisone cream 1% or 2.5% b.i.d. as needed

Alternative
- Tacrolimus ointment 0.1% or pimecrolimus cream

Course and Complications

In infants, seborrheic dermatitis can be expected to remit after 6–8 months. In adults, the course is chronic and unpredictable. However, it is usually easily controlled with shampoos and topical hydrocortisone preparations. Rarely, it can cause widespread exfoliative dermatitis. In infants, the association of a seborrhea-like dermatitis with failure to thrive and diarrhea is called *Leiner's disease*.

Pathogenesis

The pathogenesis of seborrheic dermatitis is thought to be an inflammatory reaction to the resident skin yeast *P. ovale*. This lipophilic yeast is normally found on the seborrheic regions of skin, and proliferation is believed to play a role in this disease. The most effective antiseborrheic shampoos have antifungal activity against these yeast organisms.

STASIS DERMATITIS

Key Points

1. Eczematous patches or plaques overlying lower leg edema
2. Chronic and itchy
3. Treat venous hypertension with compression stockings

Definition

Stasis dermatitis is an eczematous eruption of the lower legs secondary to peripheral venous disease (**Fig. 8.15**). Venous incompetence causes increased hydrostatic pressure and capillary damage with extravasation of red blood cells and serum. In some patients, this condition causes an inflammatory eczematous process.

Incidence

Stasis dermatitis is a disease of adults, predominantly of middle and old age.

History

Patients have a history of a chronic, pruritic eruption of the lower legs preceded by edema and swelling. Patients with stasis dermatitis have often had thrombophlebitis.

Physical Examination

Varicose veins are often prominent, as is pitting edema of the lower leg. The peripheral pulses are intact. The involved skin has brownish hyperpigmentation, dull erythema, petechiae, thickened skin, scaling, or weeping. Any portion of the lower leg may be affected, but the predominant site is above the medial malleolus.

Characteristics of stasis dermatitis:
1. Edema
2. Brown pigmentation
3. Petechiae
4. Subacute and chronic dermatitis

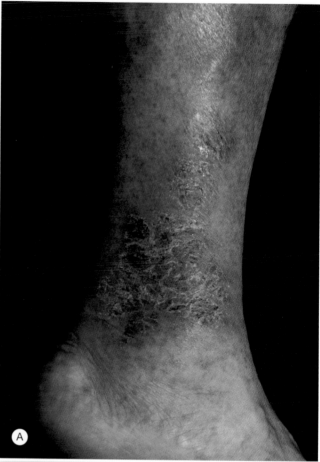

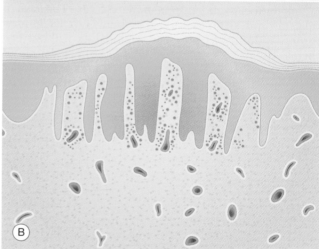

FIGURE 8.15 **Stasis dermatitis. A.** Erythematous, scaling, crusted, plaque. **B.** Epidermis – hyperkeratosis, thickened. Dermis – perivascular inflammation.

Differential Diagnosis

Contact dermatitis, superficial fungal infection, and *bacterial cellulitis* must be considered in the differential diagnosis of stasis dermatitis. The history of application of a topical preparation to the skin and KOH testing will help to differentiate the first two conditions from stasis dermatitis. Gram-staining and bacterial culture from bacterial cellulitis may be helpful, but often are negative. An acute onset with fever particularly favors bacterial cellulitis.

Laboratory and Biopsy

The diagnosis of stasis dermatitis is usually made clinically. The biopsy shows a subacute or chronic dermatitis with hemosiderin, fibrosis, and dilated capillaries in the dermis (**Fig. 8.15B**). Vascular laboratory studies may be used to assess for peripheral vascular disease (see Ch. 19).

Therapy

The cornerstone of stasis dermatitis management is the prevention of venous stasis and edema. This is done by the use of supportive hose (Futuro), while the patient is ambulatory. Standing should be restricted, and patients who are obese should be placed on a weight reduction program. If this approach fails, bed rest with elevation of the legs is required. The dermatitic skin is treated with topical steroids (Kenalog, Lidex) and wet compresses (Domeboro), if oozing or crusting is present.

Therapy for Stasis Dermatitis

Initial
- Support stocking (knee high, 20–30 mmHg pressure)
- Leg elevation
- Topical steroids
- Compresses if weeping

Alternative
- Unna boot
- Surgery

Course and Complications

Stasis dermatitis is a chronic and slowly progressive disease unless treated. Dusky erythema in areas of stasis dermatitis is the harbinger of leg ulceration.

Allergy to topical preparations may occur in 60% of patients with stasis dermatitis. The compromised epidermal barrier from stasis allows sensitization to occur more easily than in normal skin. Contact dermatitis can easily be misdiagnosed as a flare-up of stasis dermatitis. Topical antibiotics are particularly prone to cause allergic contact dermatitis.

Avoid the prolonged use of topical antibiotics since allergic contact dermatitis is frequent.

Pathogenesis

Venous incompetence results in increased venous pressure of the lower legs. This increased hydrostatic pressure results in swelling and edema. Capillary proliferation and leakage of red blood cells and vascular fluids result in inflammation. If the condition is unchecked, fibrin deposition will occur around the capillaries, resulting in tissue hypoxia, sclerosis, and necrosis with ulceration.

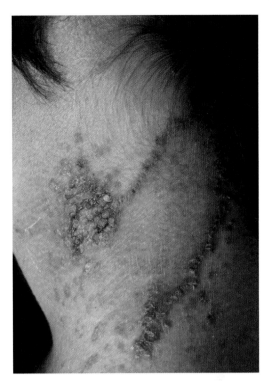

FIGURE 8.16 **Darier's disease** – erythematous patch with annular crusted border.

UNCOMMON ECZEMATOUS APPEARING DISEASES

DARIER'S DISEASE

Darier's disease, also known as keratosis follicularis, is a rare, autosomal dominantly inherited genodermatosis. It is characterized by a chronic, waxing and waning course beginning in childhood and lasting a lifetime. The eruption (**Fig. 8.16**) involves the scalp, face, neck, trunk, and extremities with accentuation in the seborrheic areas. It has tan, pink, brown, rough-feeling papules that coalesce into large plaques that can become secondarily infected, resulting in crusting and weeping. The skin biopsy is diagnostic, demonstrating epidermal suprabasilar clefts with acantholytic keratinocytes. Mutations in the ATP2A2 gene result in markedly reduced calcium dependent epidermal adhesion molecules.

GLUCAGONOMA SYNDROME

Glucagonoma syndrome is a multisystem disorder characterized by migrating erythematous, scaling, and crusted papules, patches, and plaques along with the occasional vesicle and pustule (**Fig. 8.17**). Skin biopsy demonstrates characteristic superficial epidermal necrosis. Hence, this condition is also known by the descriptive name, *necrolytic migratory erythema*. The eruption is periorificial, flexural, and acral, with associated glossitis. It is caused by a pancreatic tumor of the islet alpha cell, which secretes raised plasma glucagon levels. Besides the skin findings, patients with this syndrome also have weight loss, anemia, diarrhea, and diabetes.

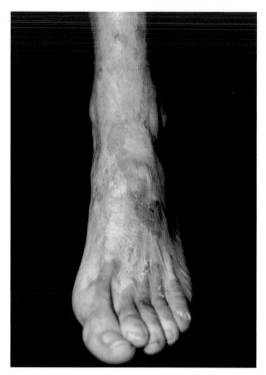

FIGURE 8.17 **Glucagonoma syndrome** – erythematous, scaling, slightly crusted patches.

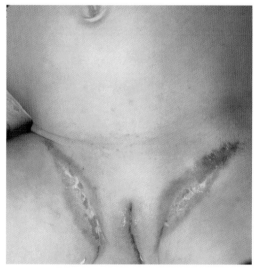

FIGURE 8.18 **Langerhans cell histiocytosis** – erythematous, slightly eroded patches.

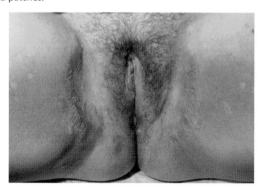

FIGURE 8.19 **Lichen sclerosus** – erythematous, slightly whitish, confluent macules and plaques.

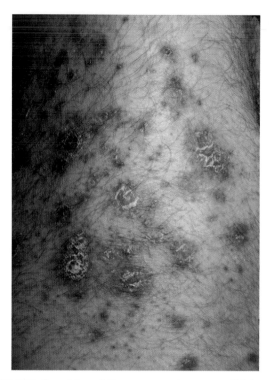

FIGURE 8.20 **Pemphigus foliaceus** – erythematous, slightly scaling papules and small plaques.

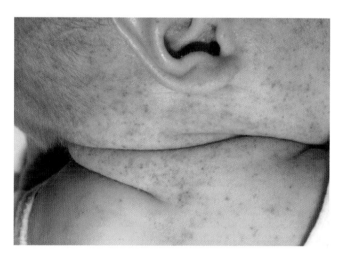

FIGURE 8.21 **Wiskott–Aldrich syndrome** – diffuse erythematous and petechial papule and macules.

LANGERHANS CELL HISTIOCYTOSIS

Langerhans cell histiocytosis, formerly known as histiocytosis X, is a neoplasm of Langerhans cells that affects the skin and extracutaneous organs, particularly bone, bone marrow, spleen, liver, lungs, and lymph nodes. It can be acute and disseminated (Letterer–Siwe disease), chronic and multifocal (Hand–Schüller–Christian disease), and localized (eosinophilic granuloma). The acute, disseminated form (**Fig. 8.18**) typically presents in infancy and involves the scalp, trunk, and intertriginous areas (recalcitrant diaper dermatitis). There are tan, pink, sometimes hemorrhagic, papules, and scaling, slightly eroded, patches. The skin biopsy demonstrates a proliferation of Langerhans cells in the epidermis and dermis that stain with S-100 antibody, and are seen on electron microscopy to contain Birbeck granules.

LICHEN SCLEROSUS

Lichen sclerosus can initially be confused with a pruritic eczematous patch, especially in the anogenital region of females (**Fig. 8.19**). On close inspection, or with time, the typical ivory white papules and atrophic patches are seen (see Ch. 13).

PEMPHIGUS FOLIACEUS

This rare, milder form of pemphigus affects the superficial epidermis, causing erythematous scaling with some crusting (**Fig. 8.20**), and a few flaccid bullae and erosions. Like pemphigus vulgaris (see Ch. 10), a skin biopsy with immunofluorescence is diagnostic.

WISKOTT–ALDRICH SYNDROME

Wiskott–Aldrich syndrome is a rare X-linked recessive disorder that may appear like atopic dermatitis. Recurrent, severe infections suggest an immunodeficiency that is characterized by increased IgA and IgE levels, decreased IgM concentration, and impaired cell-mediated immunity. Petechiae (**Fig. 8.21**) and bleeding episodes are a manifestation of thrombocytopenia, as well as platelet dysfunction. Infection, bleeding, and lymphoreticular malignancy are causes of childhood death in these patients.

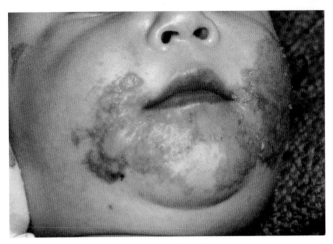

FIGURE 8.22 **Zinc deficiency** – perioral erosion.

ZINC DEFICIENCY

Zinc deficiency is an inherited (acrodermatitis enteropathica) or acquired (parenteral nutrition) malady characterized by perioral (**Fig. 8.22**), genital, and acral dermatitis plus diarrhea. It usually begins in infancy, with the diagnosis confirmed by low serum zinc levels. Essential fatty acid and biotin deficiencies have a similar dermatitic appearance.

Scaling Papules, Plaques, and Patches

Chapter Contents

Key Points

1. Scaling disorders have multiple causes – immunologic, infectious, and neoplastic
2. Borders are usually distinct, in contrast to eczema
3. Scaling (stratum corneum) is not crusting (dried fluids and blood)

ABSTRACT

Scale is the common characteristic of the diseases discussed in this chapter. Scaling disorders have also been called the papulosquamous (squamous means scaly) diseases. As previously emphasized, *scale* represents thickened stratum corneum and is to be distinguished from *crust*, which represents dried surface fluid, as found in the vesicular and pustular disorders. The elevation of scaling papules and plaques results from thickening of the epidermis (acanthosis) or underlying dermal inflammation. A *patch* is a scaling macule. It is flat because it has no

epidermal thickening (the epidermis may even be atrophic) and little dermal inflammation.

The papulosquamous disorders have diverse causes, as seen in **Table 9.1**. The lesions, in addition to being scaly, are sharply demarcated. The latter feature helps to distinguish them from scaling lesions of eczematous dermatitis, in which the borders usually are indistinct. Exceptions are *nummular (coin-shaped) eczema*, which can resemble tinea corporis, and *seborrheic dermatitis*, which in the scalp can be confused with psoriasis and on the chest can be confused with tinea corporis. *Lichen planus* often is also included in the papulosquamous disorders, but usually, the scale is not readily evident, so we have designated this disease as a papular disorder (see Ch. 11). *Tinea versicolor* can appear as finely scaling patches, but patients more often present because the lesions appear as white spots; hence, this disease is discussed in Chapter 13.

> In papulosquamous lesions, the borders are sharply demarcated; in eczematous lesions, they are not.

The diagnostic approach to scaling diseases should include consideration of the distribution of the lesions, and sometimes also the presence or absence of nail and mucous membrane involvement. Of the laboratory tests that are listed, the one that should be done most frequently is a potassium hydroxide (KOH) preparation of the scale to look for fungal elements. The general rule for scaling rashes of uncertain etiology is: 'If it scales, scrape it!'

> For scaling rashes of uncertain etiology, 'If it scales, scrape it!'

DISCOID LUPUS ERYTHEMATOSUS

Key Points

1. Whitish, scaling, scarring plaques in sun-exposed areas
2. A small proportion have systemic lupus erythematosus
3. Skin biopsy is diagnostic

TABLE 9.1 Scaling papules, plaques, and patches[a]

	Frequency (%)[b]	Etiology	Physical Examination		Differential Diagnosis	Laboratory Tests
			Appearance of Lesions	Characteristic Distribution		
Lupus, discoid	0.2	'Autoimmune'	Red to *purplish* papules and plaques with adherent scale and *follicular plugging*; older lesions atrophic	Sun-exposed areas favored	Psoriasis	Biopsy with immunofluorescence; antinuclear antibodies
Fungus	2.5	Infection (dermatophyte)	*Annular* patches with elevated borders surmounted by scale	Anywhere	(See **Table 9.2**)	Potassium hydroxide preparation; fungal culture
Mycosis fungoides	0.2	Neoplastic (lymphoma)	*Yellowish-red* or *violaceous*, irregularly shaped patches and plaques with only slight scale	*Asymmetric*; girdle area is often the first area involved	Psoriasis Eczematous dermatitis	Biopsy
Pityriasis rosea	1.1	Human herpesvirus 6 and 7	Tannish-pink *oval* papules and patches with delicate *collarette of scale*; rash preceded by *herald patch*	'Christmas tree' pattern on trunk; spares face and distal extremities	Secondary syphilis Tinea corporis	
Psoriasis	5.2	Unknown	Erythematous plaques with *silvery scales*	Anywhere; scalp, elbows, knees, and *intergluteal cleft* are favored locations; nails often involved	Seborrheic dermatitis (scalp) Fungal infection (nails)	
Secondary syphilis	<0.1	Infection (spirochete)	*Red–brown* or *copper-colored* scaling papules and plaques, sometimes annular in shape	Generalized; *palms* and *soles* often included; mucous membranes sometimes involved	Pityriasis rosea Lichen planus Drug eruption	Serologic test for syphilis

[a]See also discussions of seborrheic dermatitis (Ch. 8), lichen planus (Ch. 11), and tinea versicolor (Ch. 13).
[b]Percentage of new dermatology patients with this diagnosis seen in the Hershey Medical Center Dermatology Clinic, Hershey, PA.

Definition

Discoid lupus erythematosus (DLE) is one of several rashes that can occur in lupus. DLE is the rash that scales and scars. Immunoglobulins are found in the skin in this autoimmune disease. Clinically, the lesions appear as disk-shaped plaques surmounted by a white adherent scale that also involves the hair follicles. DLE may be limited to the skin, or it may be one of the manifestations of systemic lupus erythematosus (SLE).

> Discoid lupus erythematosus (DLE) may be limited to the skin or may be a manifestation of systemic lupus erythematosus (SLE).

Incidence

The disease affects primarily young and middle-aged adults. It is uncommon, but the exact incidence in the general population is not known. Of all new patients seen in the authors' dermatology clinic, 2 per 1000 were seen for DLE.

History

The eruption may be slightly pruritic but is more often asymptomatic. Patients may give a history of exacerbation after exposure to sunlight. In patients with DLE, a history should be taken for symptoms of possible SLE, including photosensitivity, hair loss, nasal and oral ulcerations, Raynaud's phenomenon, arthritis, and other systemic systems.

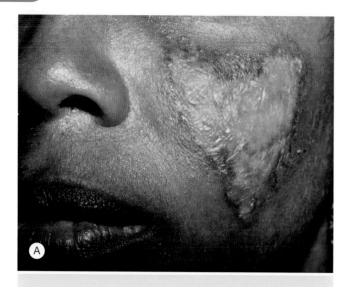

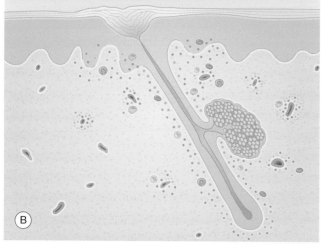

FIGURE 9.1 **Discoid lupus erythematosus. A.** Erythematous, scaling, atrophic plaque with hyperpigmented border. **B.** Epidermis – hyperkeratosis with follicular plugging; vacuolar degeneration of basal cell layer. Dermis – perivascular and periappendageal inflammatory cell infiltration.

Physical Examination

The earliest lesion is a purplish-red plaque, which accumulates scale as it matures. The scale is white and usually cohesive, so it can often be removed in one piece. When this is done, the underside of the scale may show small, spiny projections. These have been called 'carpet tacks,' and they represent the keratinous plugs that had been present in dilated hair follicles. The oldest lesions appear as *depressed*, atrophic plaques, often with pigmentary change, usually hypopigmentation in the center with a hyperpigmented rim (**Fig. 9.1**).

The distribution of the lesion of DLE favors sun-exposed areas (i.e., the face, neck, upper trunk, and dorsal arms). An occasional patient has widespread cutaneous involvement. Erosions in the oral cavity, particularly of the palate, are occasionally found in patients with DLE. The scalp is frequently involved with scarring alopecia (see Ch. 20).

Differential Diagnosis

Psoriasis may be the most common misdiagnosis. The finding of atrophy helps to differentiate the two. *Lichen planus* lesions are also purplish, but they are usually small (papular), have scant scale, and do not result in depressed scars. The scaling patches and plaques that occur in *subacute cutaneous lupus erythematosus* (SCLE) also do not scar, are frequently annular, and are often accompanied by circulating anticytoplasmic antibodies-anti-Ro (SSA) and anti-La (SSB).

Laboratory and Biopsy

Skin biopsy establishes the diagnosis (**Fig. 9.1B**). With routine processing, the diagnosis is strongly supported by the findings of: (1) hyperkeratosis with follicular plugging; (2) vacuolar degeneration of the basal cell layer; and (3) a dermal inflammatory cell infiltrate that is both perivascular and periappendageal. Epidermal atrophy is also seen in older lesions. Diagnosis can be further confirmed with direct immunofluorescent techniques (the lupus band test). In more than 90% of patients with DLE, immunoglobulins (usually IgG or IgM) are deposited as a 'band' at the dermal–epidermal junction in lesional skin. However, direct immunofluorescent staining is usually not necessary. Caution must be exercised when the biopsy is taken from facial skin, as false-positive immunofluorescent results may occur.

In addition to the history and physical examination, a laboratory screen for SLE should be done on all patients with DLE. This includes a complete blood cell count, a urinalysis, and an antinuclear antibody (ANA) test. If the latter is positive, an anti-DNA antibody test should be ordered. Patients with DLE who have positive ANA tests or persistent complete blood cell count abnormalities are more likely to develop SLE subsequently.

Patients with DLE should be screened for SLE with:
1. Complete blood cell count
2. Urinalysis
3. Antinuclear antibody test

Therapy

Topical therapy is usually adequate. Steroids, applied topically or injected intralesionally, are used most often. Sun protection is important, and sunscreens that protect against both short UV (UVB) and long UV (UVA) light should be strongly recommended to all patients. Patients with extensive or recalcitrant disease sometimes require systemic therapy; antimalarials, such as chloroquine (Aralen) 250 mg daily or hydroxychloroquine (Plaquenil) 200–400 mg daily are used most often. Patients receiving these antimalarial drugs should undergo ophthalmologic examination every 6–12 months to monitor for the retinal toxicity that rarely is encountered with the dosages used in DLE. For patients with DLE not responding to the above measures, alternative systemic therapies, including retinoids (isotretinoin or acitretin), dapsone, thalidomide, azathioprine, methotrexate, and oral gold may be used.

Therapy for Cutaneous Lupus

Initial
- Topical steroids (e.g., clobetasol cream 0.05% b.i.d.)
- Sunscreens (Anthelios) and sun protective clothing

Alternative
- Antimalarials (e.g., hydroxychloroquine 200 mg b.i.d., chloroquine 250 mg daily)
- Retinoids (e.g., isotretinoin, acitretin)
- Thalidomide
- Azathioprine
- Methotrexate
- Dapsone
- Gold

Course and Complications

The course of the disease is chronic but, with therapy, usually controllable. New lesions may continue to appear over a course of years as old ones become inactive. Eventual remission occurs spontaneously in approximately 50% of patients. Scarring and post-inflammatory hypopigmentation and hyperpigmentation are common and may result in disfigurement, particularly in African-Americans. In the scalp, the scarring leads to permanent alopecia; if extensive, this can be a cosmetic problem. In patients presenting with only DLE lesions, the risk of subsequently developing SLE is 5–10%.

> Some 5–10% of patients presenting with DLE subsequently develop SLE.

Pathogenesis

Lupus erythematosus has been classified as an autoimmune disease because of the autoantibodies found in the disease. In DLE, these are in the form of IgG and IgM deposited at the dermal–epidermal junction. The cause of this deposition and the role that these immunoglobulins play in the pathogenesis of the skin lesions are not clear. UV light has been implicated as a pathogenic factor. Circumstantial evidence for this includes the localization of lesions mainly in sun-exposed areas, the finding that many patients note that sun exposure exacerbates their skin disease, and experimental induction of skin lesions with UV light. A sequence of pathogenic events has been proposed as follows. UV light damages epidermal cells, releasing their nuclear antigens. These diffuse to the dermal–epidermal junction, where they combine with antibodies from the circulation, initiating an inflammatory reaction resulting ultimately in the clinical lesion.

T-cell dysregulation has also been implicated in the pathogenesis of cutaneous lupus. For example, increased activity of the Th2 subset of helper T cells has been found in lesional skin. The main function of these cells is to augment humoral immunity. Genetic predisposition to

DLE is possible, but familial disease and association with specific HLA phenotypes have been reported more frequently with SLE than with DLE. Current evidence suggests that most patients with DLE have a genetically different disease from that in patients with SLE, a concept that accounts for the observation that most patients with DLE never develop SLE.

FUNGAL INFECTIONS

Key Points

1. If it scales, consider scraping it for a KOH preparation
2. Superficial fungi, dermatophytes, cause tinea infections

Definition

These disorders result from infection of the skin by fungal organisms collectively called dermatophytes (*phyte* is the Greek word for plant). Various clinical lesions can result, but the most common are scaling, erythematous papules, plaques, and patches, which often have a serpiginous or worm-like border. The word *tinea* (Latin for worm) is used for these superficial fungal infections. It is followed by a qualifying term that denotes the location of the infection on the body. For example, *tinea capitis* is a fungal infection of the scalp, and *tinea pedis* is a dermatophyte infection of the feet. *Tinea versicolor* is the only exception; its name derives from the several shades of color that lesions may have in this disease.

> Synonyms for fungal infection of the skin:
> 1. Dermatophytosis
> 2. Tinea
> 3. 'Ringworm'

Incidence

Dermatophytic infections are common, in aggregate representing 2.5% of the authors' new patients. The incidence is higher in warmer, more humid climates. **Table 9.2** gives the prevalence of four of the more common skin infections in the general US population.

History

In most dermatophytic infections, the patient presents with a scaling rash. Pruritus is common, and often the chief complaint. A history of exposure to infected persons or other mammals (e.g., dogs, cats, cattle) may be elicited.

Physical Examination

The physical findings and differential diagnosis vary with the different tineas. The findings in *tinea capitis* are discussed in Chapter 20, and those in *tinea unguium* in Chapter 21. Because *tinea versicolor* most often presents as white spots, it is discussed in Chapter 13. The physical findings and differential diagnosis of the remaining dermatophyte infections are considered below.

TABLE 9.2 Fungal infections

	Prevalence in General Population (rate per 1000)[a]	Location	Clinical Appearance	Differential Diagnosis
Tinea capitis[b]		Scalp	Round, scaling area of alopecia Diffuse scaling Red, boggy, swollen area with pustules (kerion)	Alopecia areata Seborrheic dermatitis Bacterial infection
Tinea corporis		Body	Annular, 'ringworm'	Nummular eczema Pityriasis rosea (herald patch)
Tinea cruris	7	Groin	Sharply demarcated area with elevated, scaling, serpiginous borders	Psoriasis Impetigo Intertrigo Candidiasis
Tinea faciale		Face	Slightly scaling, erythematous patches and plaques; border may not be well demarcated in all areas	Photodermatitis Lupus erythematosus Seborrheic dermatitis
Tinea manuum		Hand	Diffuse dry scaling, usually on only one palm	Contact dermatitis Psoriasis
Tinea pedis	39	Feet	Interdigital maceration Diffuse scaling on soles and sides of feet ('moccasin') Vesicles and pustules on instep	Hyperhidrosis Dry skin Contact dermatitis Dyshidrotic eczema
Tinea unguium (onychomycosis)[c]	22	Nails	Subungual debris with separation from the nail bed	Psoriasis Trauma
Tinea versicolor[d]	8	Trunk	White, tan, or pink patches with fine desquamating scale	Vitiligo (white) Seborrheic dermatitis (tan or pink)

[a]Data from the United States National Health Survey, 1978.
[b]See Ch. 20.
[c]See Ch. 21.
[d]See Ch. 13.

TINEA CORPORIS

Key Points

1. Round (annular) patch with clear center and scaling border
2. Scrape the border scales for the KOH preparation

Tinea corporis is the classic 'ringworm.' Often, patients have a history of exposure to an infected animal such as a pet dog or cat.

Physical Examination

The typical lesion is annular, with an elevated, scaling border and tendency for central clearing. One or several lesions may be present. In patients predisposed to chronic infection, the eruption may be widespread, and not all the lesions may be annular. In these instances, the finding of elevated serpiginous borders in some of the lesions is a helpful clue (**Fig. 9.2**).

Differential Diagnosis

The coin-shaped lesions of *nummular eczema* are usually multiple and are located on the extremities. They are often mistaken by the patient, and sometimes by the physician, as ringworm. In nummular eczema, one usually sees no central clearing, and the KOH preparation is negative.

Pityriasis rosea starts with a single herald patch, which is frequently mistaken for tinea. The correct diagnosis usually becomes evident when the generalized eruption develops within a few weeks. Although occasionally annular, lesions of psoriasis are usually thicker and more scaling than those of fungal infections. More typical lesions of psoriasis usually are also found, and, of course, the KOH examination is negative.

Uncommonly, *impetigo* presents in an annular configuration (see **Fig. 3.8**). The finding of vesicles, pustules, and crusts in annular lesions should lead one to suspect a bacterial, rather than fungal, cause.

Erythema annulare centrifugum and *granuloma annulare* are two uncommon diseases that may be confused with

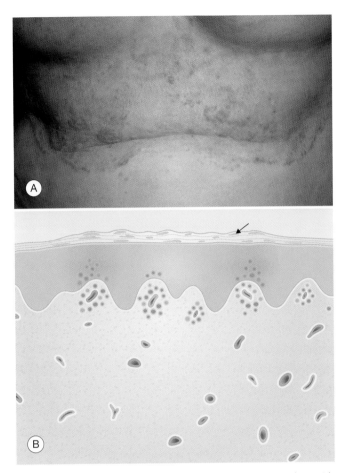

FIGURE 9.2 **A.** Tinea corporis – erythematous, scaling patches with serpiginous borders. **B.** Tinea. Epidermis – thickened stratum corneum infiltrated with fungal hyphae (arrow). Dermis – inflammation.

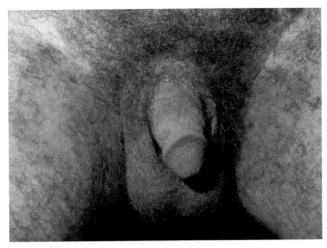

FIGURE 9.3 **Tinea cruris** – sharply marginated oval groin patches. Note typical sparing of penis and scrotum.

Physical Examination

Dermatophytic infection in the groin may not appear as an annular lesion, but the border is elevated, serpiginous, and scaling. Often, lesions have a tendency for central clearing. The scrotum and penis are seldom involved.

Differential Diagnosis

In addition to dermatophytic infection, there are two other common causes of a groin rash. *Candidiasis* appears as a bright, intensely erythematous ('beefy red') eruption with poorly defined borders and satellite papules and pustules. The scrotum is often affected. *Intertrigo* represents simple irritant dermatitis, most often found in obese patients in whom moisture accumulates between skin folds in the inguinal area and, along with friction, causes skin irritation. The eruption is not as erythematous as that of candidiasis, and not as sharply demarcated as tinea cruris. The KOH preparation is positive in tinea cruris and candidiasis but negative in intertrigo. On occasion intertrigo can be complicated by a candidal infection.

Three major causes of a groin rash:
1. Tinea cruris
2. Candidiasis
3. Intertrigo

Less often, *psoriasis* and *seborrheic dermatitis* selectively affect the groin. *Erythrasma* is an uncommon disease of intertriginous skin caused by *Corynebacterium minutissimum*. Clinically, it appears as a velvety patch with fine scale that, under Wood's light examination, fluoresces a diagnostic coral pink.

TINEA FACIALE

Key Points

1. Look for a sharp serpiginous border
2. When in doubt, do a KOH preparation

ringworm. Clinically, the differences are that in erythema annulare centrifugum the scale is inside the elevated border and the KOH preparation is negative. In granuloma annulare, the border is more indurated and is *not* scaling. A skin biopsy is helpful in confirming the diagnosis of these two disorders. Both conditions are idiopathic and are usually localized, but occasionally generalized. The generalized form of erythema annulare centrifugum is called *erythema gyratum repens*, a rare condition that is almost always associated with an internal malignant disease. Generalized granuloma annulare is sometimes associated with diabetes mellitus.

TINEA CRURIS

Key Points

1. Erythematous patch with a serpiginous scaling border
2. Scrotum and penis are not involved

A groin rash has several common causes (**Fig. 9.3**); dermatophytic infection is one. Patients with tinea cruris ('jock itch') frequently also have tinea pedis ('athlete's foot'). The perspiration that occurs with exercise is probably the common predisposing denominator in these 'athletic' rashes.

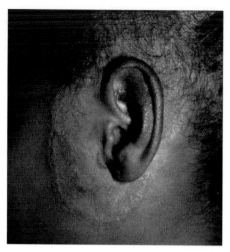

FIGURE 9.4 **Tinea faciale** – oval, sharply demarcated, erythematous patch with slightly scaling inflammatory border and cleared center.

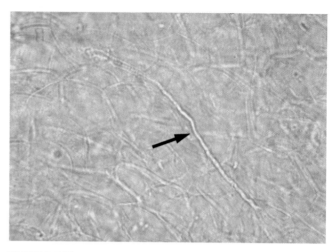

FIGURE 9.6 **Tinea** – positive potassium hydroxide examination showing hyphae (arrow).

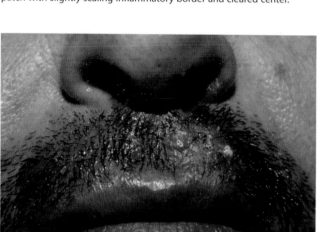

FIGURE 9.5 **Tinea barbae** – erythematous plaque with alopecia and pustule.

This is an uncommon but often missed fungal infection of the skin (**Fig. 9.4**).

Physical Examination

Tinea faciale appears as an erythematous, usually asymmetric, eruption on the face. An annular pattern is frequently not evident, but usually at least some of the borders are well demarcated and are often serpiginous, providing the clue to the fungal origin. Pustules may be present and may further obscure the clinical diagnosis (**Fig. 9.5**).

Differential Diagnosis

The lesions in *seborrheic dermatitis* are usually symmetric and are not well demarcated.

Rashes resulting from sunlight (*photodermatitis*) are distinguished by their distribution, which usually is symmetric, sparing areas that are relatively protected from the sun, such as the eyelids and under the chin. *Contact dermatitis* may also be confused with tinea faciale.

Occasionally, tinea faciale can appear as a butterfly rash, resembling that of *lupus erythematosus*. The finding of sharp serpiginous borders should heighten the suspicion of a fungal origin. However, for any of these conditions, if there is scale and any doubt, scrape it!

Laboratory Tests

The single most important laboratory test for all of these fungal infections is the KOH preparation (**Fig. 9.6**). The details of this procedure are outlined in Chapter 3. The finding of hyphae on a KOH preparation is diagnostic of a dermatophytic infection, whereas a candidal infection will have hyphae and oval yeast on microscopic exam. Usually, the clinical presentation distinguishes between the two, with candida having satellite pustules around a beefy red patch and tinea having an annulare scaling patch with a clear center.

If desired, one can also obtain scales for fungal culture. Cultures distinguish between candidal and dermatophytic infections, and are sometimes helpful in patients in whom dermatophytic infections are suspected but the KOH examination is negative.

A skin biopsy is not indicated. If a biopsy is done to rule out other disorders, the dermatopathologist may miss the fungal elements in the stratum corneum (see **Fig. 9.2B**). Contrary to some misconceptions, a Wood's light (black light) is of no help in diagnosing dermatophytic infection of the skin. A Wood's light fluoresces infected scalp hairs in one type of tinea capitis, but infected skin does not show fluorescence.

Therapy

For dermatophyte infections involving limited areas, the authors recommend one of the over-the-counter creams, which include clotrimazole (Lotrimin), miconazole (Micatin), and terbinafine (Lamisil). The patient is instructed to apply the topical antifungal to the infected area until the skin is clinically clear and then to apply it for 1–2 weeks longer in the hope of preventing recurrence.

Dermatophytes are unresponsive to nystatin.

Chronic *tinea pedis* is notoriously refractory to curative therapy, particularly when the patient has nail involvement. For suppressive therapy, an antifungal powder, such as miconazole powder, should be used daily on an indefinite basis after the skin has been clinically cleared.

For patients with disease that is either widespread or resistant to topical measures, systemic therapy is indicated. Systemic treatment is also most effective for treating scalp and nail infection. The five available oral systemic agents are griseofulvin, ketoconazole (Nizoral), itraconazole (Sporanox), fluconazole (Diflucan), and terbinafine (Lamisil). For dermatophytic infection, griseofulvin was the standard treatment. Adult patients are treated with either microsized griseofulvin (e.g., Fulvicin U/F), 500 mg twice daily, or ultramicrosized griseofulvin (e.g., Gris-PEG), 250 mg twice daily for 4–6 weeks. The newer systemic antifungals, however, can achieve better results with shorter courses of treatment (and fewer side-effects). For example, most dermatophyte infections of the skin can be treated with a 1–2-week course of terbinafine (250 mg daily). Doses for children are adjusted downward according to bodyweight.

Initial therapy:
1. Limited skin involvement – topical antifungals
2. Hair, nails, and extensive skin involvement – systemic therapy

Treatment of *tinea capitis* requires 4–8 weeks of therapy. Adjunctive twice-weekly use of a dandruff shampoo containing selenium sulfide (Selsun) can shorten the time course of this infection.

Therapy for Dermatophyte Infections

Initial (for Limited Skin Disease)
*   Azoles – miconazole 2% or clotrimazole 1% cream, gel, spray, or powder b.i.d.)
*   Allylamines – terbinafine 1% cream or gel daily

Alternative (for Scalp, Nails, or Extensive Skin Involvement)
*   Griseofulvin – microsize: 20 mg/kg daily
*   Terbinafine:
    *   <20 kg: 62.5 mg daily
    *   20–40 kg: 125 mg daily
    *   >40 kg: 250 mg daily

Course and Complications

Some acute dermatophytic infections resolve spontaneously. Even in these patients, however, the time course can be shortened by use of the therapy mentioned above.

Complications are rare. Secondary bacterial infections are uncommon. Recognizing that fungal infections can produce pustules (particularly when hair follicles are affected), one must be cautious about misdiagnosing such pustules as being bacterial in origin. KOH examinations and cultures clarify the matter if one is in doubt. Intertriginous tinea pedis can allow bacteria to gain access to deeper tissues. This is a common portal of entry in patients with recurrent cellulitis of the lower extremities, so treatment of the dermatophyte infection can prevent subsequent episodes of cellulitis.

Pathogenesis

The three genera of dermatophytes are *Trichophyton*, *Microsporum*, and *Epidermophyton*. Some of these organisms grow only on human hosts (anthropophilic), whereas others can also exist in soil (geophilic) or on animals (zoophilic). All the dermatophytes are keratinophilic, i.e., they feed on keratin. They all produce keratinases, a necessary requirement for their keratinophilia. Stratum corneum, hair, and nails are attractive substrates for these fungi, not only because of their keratin composition but perhaps also because of their low density of bacterial inhibitors and competitors. Dermatophytes form hyphae through which nourishment is obtained from the keratin-rich host environment.

The clinical appearance and behavior of a fungal infection of the skin depend partly on the host response. Slow-growing dermatophytes infecting only the outermost layers of the stratum corneum may not elicit an inflammatory response. The diffuse plantar scaling type of tinea pedis is an example. The clinical reaction may also be influenced by the type of dermatophyte; some are more likely than others to elicit an inflammatory reaction. In general, zoophilic dermatophytes provoke more inflammation than anthropophilic ones. Tinea corporis from *Microsporum canis* (*canis*, Latin for canine, or relating to the dog) is an example of an infection from a zoophilic dermatophyte that produces an inflammatory erythematous, scaling annular lesion.

Human dermatophytic infections may resolve spontaneously, probably as a result of cellular immune responses provoked by antigenic material from the organisms. Persistent infections occur in patients who do not mount this immune reaction, either because the fungus has failed to provoke it (e.g., in chronic tinea pedis, in which the fungus growth remains superficial in the thick stratum corneum and does not gain access to the circulation) or because of dermatophyte-specific host immune deficiency. Dermatophytic infections do not invade beyond the epidermis because of their dependence on keratin for nutrition and the fungistatic properties of transferrin and β-globulin in human serum.

TINEA MANUUM

Key Points

1. One hand, two feet are typically involved
2. For the hand with the 'dry' scaling unilateral palm, do a KOH preparation

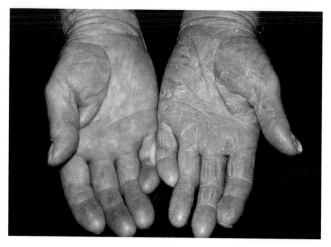

FIGURE 9.7 **Tinea manuum** – diffuse scaling patch of only one hand in a patient with tinea pedis – the 'one hand, two feet' syndrome.

Dermatophytic infection of the palm is uncommon but not rare. It virtually always occurs in a patient who has coexisting tinea pedis.

Physical Examination

Typically, tinea manuum involves only one hand, resulting in the 'one hand, two feet' syndrome (**Fig. 9.7**). It appears as diffuse scaling of the palmar surface, much like the plantar scaling type of tinea pedis. The border on the wrist side is often sharply demarcated.

Differential Diagnosis

Chronic irritant contact dermatitis and dry skin, *xerosis*, can also appear as chronic scaling of the palms. However, these conditions usually involve both palms, and the border is generally not well demarcated.

Psoriasis can affect the palms with sharply demarcated scaling plaques. Usually, these plaques are bilateral, and are more elevated and erythematous than in tinea manuum; often, lesions of psoriasis elsewhere on the body support the diagnosis. KOH preparation is necessary in case of doubt.

TINEA PEDIS

Key Points

1. Interdigital, diffuse, plantar scaling, and vesiculopustular forms
2. Onychomycosis (nail tinea) occurs frequently with tinea pedis

As noted in **Table 9.2**, the feet are most often involved with dermatophytic infection. Tinea pedis affects approximately 4% of the general population and occurs in three forms, each of which has a different appearance.

Physical Examination

Interdigital tinea pedis appears as a macerated scaling process between the toes. It is most common in patients with sweaty feet.

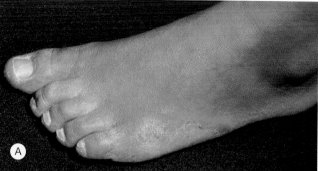
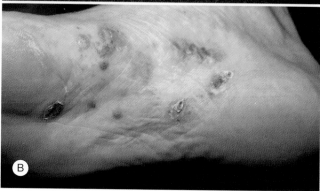

FIGURE 9.8 **Tinea pedis. A.** Diffuse plantar scaling patch, which extends onto the side of the foot and is usually associated with onychomycosis. **B.** Acute vesiculopustular form.

Diffuse plantar scaling is extremely common in older patients. It is usually asymptomatic. The skin of the feet appears dry, with diffuse scaling on the soles extending onto the sides of the feet (**Fig. 9.8A**). The border may or may not be sharply demarcated. The distribution of this process on the feet has been likened to a 'moccasin.' Often, patients have accompanying nail involvement.

The *vesiculopustular* form (**Fig. 9.8B**) is the least common type of tinea pedis and the one that is most often misdiagnosed. Vesicles and pustules on the instep of the feet should lead to a suspicion of this type of tinea pedis. A KOH preparation of the roof of the vesicle or pustule reveals fungal hyphae.

Differential Diagnosis

Patients with sweaty feet (hyperhidrosis) may develop *maceration* between the toes, simply as a result of retained moisture in these occluded areas. This then provides a good culture medium for fungus to become secondarily involved. Clinically, simple maceration may be indistinguishable from interdigital tinea pedis. A KOH preparation enables one to diagnose fungus infection, but in both situations measures to decrease sweating are also important.

Diffuse plantar scaling is most often passed off as *dry skin*. *Contact dermatitis* and *dyshidrotic eczema* are the two diseases most often confused with the vesiculopustular type of tinea pedis. In contact dermatitis and dyshidrotic eczema, however, the vesicles are usually smaller and rarely progress to pustules. *Pustular psoriasis* of the palms and soles is an uncommon disease that can also be confused with vesiculopustular tinea pedis. If doubt exists, a KOH preparation should be performed.

MYCOSIS FUNGOIDES

Key Points

1. T-cell cutaneous lymphoma
2. Survival decreases with progression of skin involvement from patches to plaques to tumors
3. Treatment is usually palliative, not curative

Definition

Mycosis fungoides is not a fungal infection; rather, it is a cutaneous T-cell lymphoma with a misleading label. Cutaneous T-cell lymphoma is a more appropriate name. The skin lesions result from proliferation in the dermis of malignant T lymphocytes, which have a propensity to migrate into the epidermis. The clinical appearance of the lesion depends on the stage of the disease, which may evolve from patch through plaque to noduloulcerative lesions, reflecting the progressive increase of the cellular infiltrate in the skin.

> Mycosis fungoides is a cutaneous T-cell lymphoma, not a fungal infection.

Incidence

Mycosis fungoides is uncommon. A survey in Rochester, Minnesota, discovered an annual incidence of 0.5 per 100 000 population. In the USA, mycosis fungoides accounts for less than 1% of all lymphomas and fewer than 200 deaths per year. The disease affects adults, most often those in the older age groups.

History

In the usual case, the eruption slowly evolves over a period of years. It often starts as a nonspecific rash, which may be diagnosed as 'atypical' psoriasis or eczema. *Parapsoriasis*, an uncommon idiopathic disorder characterized by salmon-colored, slightly scaling patches, may be a precursor. With evolution, the lesions become more elevated and indurated. Most patients with mycosis fungoides have pruritus, ranging from mild to severe.

Physical Examination

The key to the diagnosis rests with the following features. The lesions are irregular in shape, peculiar in color (often reddish brown, violaceous, or orange), and asymmetric in distribution (**Fig. 9.9**). The degree of elevation of the lesions depends on the stage of the disease. In the patch stage, the lesions are flat, surmounted by a slight scale, and sometimes accompanied by epidermal atrophy, which clinically appears as 'cigarette paper' wrinkling of the surface. Other lesions may show *poikiloderma*, a term used to describe a reticulate pattern of hyperpigmentation, hypopigmentation, and erythema with telangiectasia. In

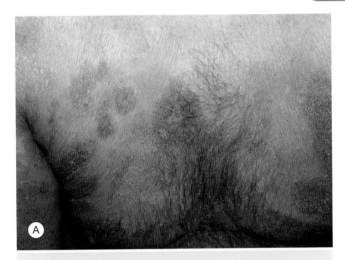

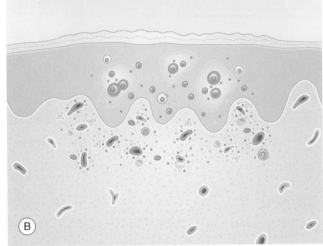

FIGURE 9.9 **Mycosis fungoides. A.** Erythematous to violaceous and brownish, slightly scaling and wrinkled, irregularly shaped patches. **B.** Epidermis – hyperkeratosis; epidermal atrophy (especially in patch stage); exocytosis of malignant lymphocytes, sometimes in focal collections (Pautrier's microabscesses). Dermis – mild to marked infiltrate of mixed inflammation cells, including cerebriform lymphocytes.

poikiloderma, the epidermis also shows atrophy. As the disease progresses, increased cellular infiltration of the skin occurs, expressed clinically as elevated, indurated plaques. These plaques are generally more widespread (**Fig. 9.10**). In advanced disease, nodules appear and frequently ulcerate. Lymphadenopathy is also often found in more advanced disease.

> Mycosis fungoides should be suspected in rashes with lesions that are:
> 1. Irregular in shape
> 2. Peculiar in color
> 3. Asymmetric in distribution

Sézary syndrome represents a leukemic variant of mycosis fungoides; this syndrome is characterized by total body erythema (erythroderma), lymphadenopathy, and a high number of mycosis (or Sézary) cells in the peripheral circulation.

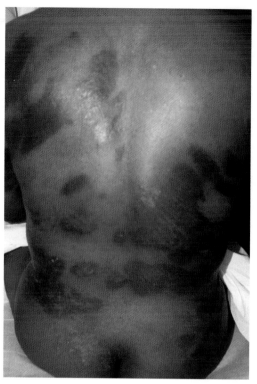

FIGURE 9.10 **Mycosis fungoides** – irregularly shaped, asymmetric, indurated plaques.

Differential Diagnosis

Mycosis fungoides may appear as *parapsoriasis*, *atypical eczema*, or *psoriasis*. In patients with nodular disease, other malignant tumors may be considered. In patients with Sézary syndrome, the differential diagnosis includes other causes of generalized erythema (see Ch. 14).

> Mycosis fungoides should be considered in patients with 'atypical' eczema or psoriasis.

Laboratory and Biopsy

The most important laboratory test is the skin biopsy. Frequently, multiple biopsies must be performed before a histologic diagnosis can be secured, particularly in patients with early, patch stage disease.

> Multiple skin biopsies, often over time, may be needed to establish the diagnosis.

The most important histologic feature is the presence of *Pautrier's microabscesses* within the epidermis (**Fig. 9.9B**). These represent collections of lymphocytes, many of which are atypical. Atypical lymphocytes are also found in varying numbers in the dermal infiltrate. With high-power examination, the nuclei of these lymphocytes are characteristically highly convoluted or cerebriform. In the early stages of the disease, they may be present only in small numbers; in the nodular stage, a dense infiltrate of malignant cells is seen.

The malignant cells in mycosis fungoides are derived from a monoclonal proliferation of helper T cells and, less commonly, suppressor T cells. The *T-cell receptor gene rearrangement test* may be used to determine monoclonality in T-cell infiltrates in skin and other tissues. Differentiated helper T cells have specific cell surface receptors that possess specificity that is determined by rearrangement of the receptor gene. The T-cell receptor gene rearrangement test detects a population of cells with the same rearrangement, thereby determining monoclonality, a finding that is supportive of malignancy. This test has been used as an aid in diagnosing mycosis fungoides in skin, blood, and lymph nodes. False-positive results occasionally occur.

A complete blood cell count, with careful examination of peripheral smear, should also be performed when looking for circulating mycosis fungoides cells. If lymph nodes are enlarged, a lymph node biopsy should be performed.

Therapy

For disease localized to the skin, external therapy is preferred. Four modalities have been used: (1) for extremely early skin involvement, topical steroids are sometimes employed successfully; the other 'external' modalities are (2) UV light, either UVB or UVA in combination with psoralens (PUVA); (3) topical nitrogen mustard, which is applied as a liquid or ointment to the total cutaneous surface; and (4) electron beam therapy. Orally administered low-dose methotrexate, retinoid or rexinoid, and intramuscular inteferon α have been used in patients with recalcitrant skin disease.

In patients with systemic disease, chemotherapy is usually used, sometimes in combination with one of the topical modalities. Some patients with Sézary syndrome have also been successfully treated with extracorporeal photochemotherapy. In this treatment, white blood cells are removed from the patient several hours after psoralen ingestion, are externally exposed to UVA, and reinfused into the circulation. Treatments are given monthly.

Therapy for Mycosis Fungoides

Initial
- Steroids (e.g., clobetasol cream 0.05% b.i.d.)
- Ultraviolet B light (UVB)
- Nitrogen mustard
- Radiotherapy (electron beam)

Alternative
- Psoralens with ultraviolet A light (PUVA)
- Methotrexate
- Retinoids (e.g., isotretinoin) or rexinoid (e.g., bexarotene)
- Interferon α-2b
- Extracorporeal photochemotherapy
- Combination chemotherapy
- Vorinostat

Course and Complications

In most patients, mycosis fungoides is a chronic, smoldering disease with slow progression over many years. Treatment in the early stages often results in complete clearance of the skin lesions, although relapses are common after therapy is discontinued. Systemic involvement develops in advanced disease, usually affecting the lymph nodes first and the internal organs later. Mean survival in patients with systemic involvement is approximately 2 years.

Pathogenesis

Mycosis fungoides is a neoplastic disease of helper (CD4+) T cells and, less commonly, suppressor (CD8+) T cells. Its first manifestation usually appears in the skin. A debate is ongoing about whether the process is malignant from the start, or whether it begins as a chronic inflammatory condition in which activated T cells eventually undergo malignant transformation. Either way, the end result is a monoclonal proliferation of helper or suppressor T cells in the skin.

> In mycosis fungoides, there is a monoclonal proliferation of helper (CD4+) or suppressor (CD8+) T cells in the skin.

The initiating events in this disease are not well established. Langerhans cells in the epidermis have been implicated as participating in the initial phases, perhaps themselves stimulated by external factors and, in turn, interacting with T cells, which are subsequently activated. Environmental chemicals have been implicated as a causative factor in some patients, but this has not been well proven. A T-cell lymphotrophic virus (HTLV-I) has been recovered from a subset of patients with aggressive cutaneous T-cell lymphomas. However, for most patients with mycosis fungoides, the underlying origin remains unknown, and the pathogenetic pathway is a matter of debate.

PITYRIASIS ROSEA

Key Points

1. Herald patch is the harbinger of a more generalized eruption
2. Oval, slightly scaling patches on the neck, trunk, and proximal extremities
3. Reconsider the diagnosis if the condition lasts for more than 2–3 months

Definition

Pityriasis rosea (*pityriasis* means 'bran-like scale,' and *rosea* means 'rose colored') is an acute, self-limiting, inflammatory dermatosis which appears to be caused by human herpesviruses 6 and 7. It is characterized clinically by oval, minimally elevated, scaling patches, papules, and plaques that are located mainly on the trunk (**Fig. 9.11**).

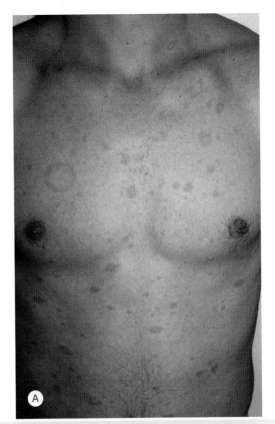

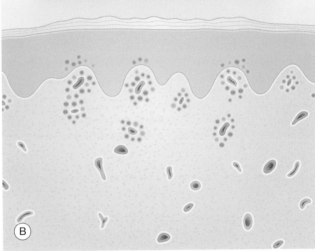

FIGURE 9.11 **Pityriasis rosea. A.** Oval erythematous patches with delicate scaling near border. **B.** Epidermis – slight hyperkeratosis and acanthosis with focal spongiosis and scattered lymphocytes. Dermis – moderate perivascular lymphocytic infiltrate.

Incidence

The exact incidence is not known, but the disease is relatively common. It is the third most common papulosquamous disease, affecting 1% of the new patients seen in the authors' dermatology clinic. The disease affects mainly older children and young adults, and occurs with some seasonal variation, being least common during the summer months.

History

Characteristically, the generalized eruption is preceded by a single lesion, called the 'herald patch.' This is frequently misdiagnosed as ringworm. The herald patch is followed after several days to weeks by the generalized rash. The patient usually feels well. Itching is often present and ranges in severity from mild to moderate.

A 'herald patch' precedes the generalized eruption.

Physical Examination

The herald patch is the largest of the lesions and ranges from 2 to 5 cm (**Fig. 9.12B**). The multiple lesions that follow resemble the herald patch but are smaller. They are typically tannish pink or salmon colored, round to oval, and surmounted by a delicate scale that in the mature lesion is located near the border. Typically, oval lesions on the neck and trunk follow the skin cleavage lines in a pattern that, with imagination, has been likened to that of a 'Christmas tree.' The rash is distributed mainly on the trunk and neck, and sometimes on the proximal extremities. In children, the face may also be affected. In addition, in children, papular or vesicular variants of the disease can occur. Oral lesions, although not prominent, have been described, and range from erythematous macules to hemorrhagic puncta to small ulcerations.

Differential Diagnosis

Although the diagnosis of pityriasis rosea is usually straightforward, sometimes other disorders must be considered in the differential diagnosis. In *tinea corporis*, patients usually have only a few lesions. If doubt exists, however, a KOH preparation should be done. The explosive onset of the small lesions of *guttate psoriasis*, distributed mainly on the trunk, can be confused with pityriasis rosea. However, the scale in psoriasis is thicker and more silvery, and the course is more prolonged. Uncommonly, generalized *lichen planus* can resemble pityriasis rosea. The purple color of the lesions in lichen planus helps to distinguish the two. *Pityriasis lichenoides chronica* is an uncommon disorder in which the lesions may resemble those of pityriasis rosea but (as the name implies) are chronic rather than transient. *Drug eruptions* should be considered in any patient with acute generalized dermatosis. Usually, however, a drug eruption is more brightly erythematous, more confluent, less scaling, and itchier than pityriasis rosea.

The most important diagnosis to consider in the differential is *secondary syphilis*, particularly if the eruption is atypical; e.g., if the patient has no herald patch, if the distal extremities (particularly the palms and soles) are involved, or if the patient is systemically ill. In all cases of 'atypical' pityriasis rosea, a serologic test for syphilis should be ordered.

For patients with 'atypical' pityriasis rosea, a serologic test for syphilis must be performed to rule out secondary syphilis.

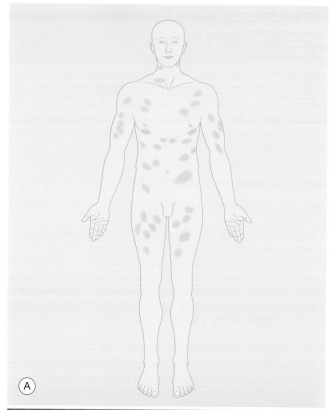

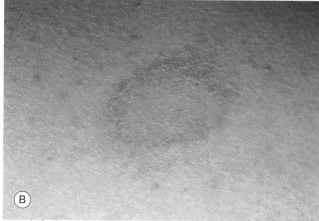

FIGURE 9.12 **Pityriasis rosea. A.** Distribution has been likened to that of a Christmas tree. **B.** Herald patch.

Laboratory and Biopsy

The diagnosis is made with the characteristic history and physical findings. Skin biopsy is nonspecific and rarely indicated. If it is performed, the findings will include mild hyperkeratosis with focal parakeratosis, minimal acanthosis with focal spongiosis, and a moderate dermal inflammatory infiltrate, with a few of the cells migrating into the epidermis (**Fig. 9.11B**).

Therapy

Treatment is usually not necessary for this self-limiting disease. Occasionally, antihistamines are needed for pruritus, and moisturizing creams for the dry scaling that occurs as the lesions evolve. UV light therapy (UVB) or erythromycin appears to accelerate resolution, but these are usually not needed.

> **Therapy for Pityriasis Rosea**
>
> **Initial**
> - None unless symptomatic
>
> **Alternative**
> - UV light
> - Erythromycin 500 mg b.i.d. for 2 weeks

Course and Complications

The disease involutes spontaneously in a time course ranging from 2 weeks to 2 months, with an average time of approximately 6 weeks. It recurs in only approximately 2% of patients. No complications occur, except for occasional postinflammatory hypopigmentation or hyperpigmentation, which resolves slowly over time, often months.

> Pityriasis rosea clears spontaneously within 2 months.

Pathogenesis

The rash appears to be mediated by a cellular (type IV) immune reaction. A possible viral trigger, human herpesviruses 6 and 7, has been implicated. However, the disease does not occur endemically, and occurrence in household contacts is uncommon.

PSORIASIS

> **Key Points**
>
> 1. Well demarcated erythematous, silvery, scaling plaques
> 2. Elbows, knees, and scalp are typically involved, as well as other sites
> 3. Inflammation and epidermal proliferation provides opportunities for therapeutic intervention

Definition

Psoriasis is an inflammatory rash with increased epidermal proliferation (acanthosis) resulting in an accumulation of stratum corneum (scale). The etiology is unknown. The clinical appearance is that of sharply demarcated, erythematous papules, patches, and plaques, surmounted by silvery scales (**Fig. 9.13**).

Incidence

Some 2–5% of Caucasian and 0.1–0.3% of the Asian populations are affected by psoriasis. Onset may occur at any age but is most common in adults, with an average age of 35 years.

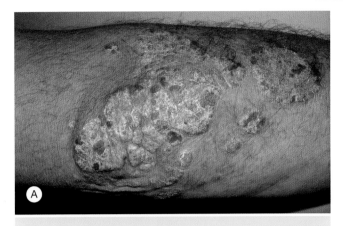

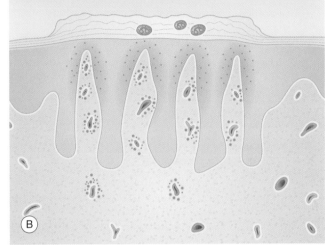

FIGURE 9.13 **Psoriasis. A.** Well demarcated, erythematous plaque with silvery scales involving the elbow. **B.** Epidermis – hyperkeratosis, acanthosis with elongated rete pegs, and infiltration by neutrophils, forming microabscesses in the stratum corneum. Dermis – capillary proliferation with perivascular inflammation.

History

The disease usually starts gradually, although occasionally it is explosive in onset or exacerbation. The sudden appearance of multiple small (guttate) lesions of psoriasis in a generalized distribution is often preceded by a streptococcal throat infection. In patients with severe sudden onset or rapidly worsening large-plaque psoriasis, a predisposing human immunodeficiency virus (HIV) infection should be considered: 1% of patients with acquired immune deficiency syndrome (AIDS) develop severe psoriasis, and sometimes the psoriasis is the presenting manifestation of AIDS. Other aggravating factors that have been implicated in psoriasis include trauma to the skin that precipitates a psoriatic lesion (Koebner phenomenon) and emotional stress, which, although difficult to document scientifically, is believed by many patients to be a contributing factor. A few drugs have been found to aggravate psoriasis. Lithium is the best proven culprit, but beta-blockers and nonsteroidal anti-inflammatory drugs have also been implicated. Itching (*psoriasis* is derived from the Greek word for 'itching') ranges from mild to severe. A family history of psoriasis can be elicited from approximately one-third of patients.

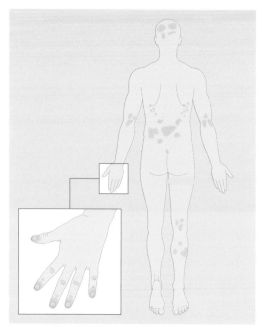

FIGURE 9.14 **Typical distribution of psoriasis** – elbows, knees, scalp, and intergluteal cleft.

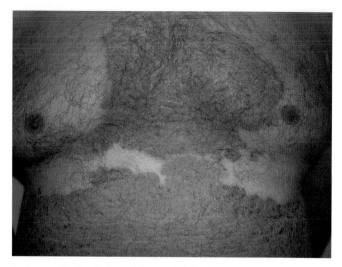

FIGURE 9.15 **Psoriasis** – widespread pink plaques.

Physical Examination

The lesions are sharply demarcated, erythematous papules, patches, and plaques surmounted by scale, which is characteristically silvery. In intertriginous areas, maceration prevents scales from accumulating, but the lesions remain red and sharply defined. Psoriasis is classically distributed on the scalp, elbows, and knees (**Fig. 9.14**). The intergluteal cleft is also a common site, and is frequently overlooked. Although these are typical sites, psoriatic lesions can occur anywhere and may cover the entire skin surface (**Fig. 9.15**).

Nail involvement (see Ch. 21) is present in as many as 50% of patients with psoriasis and can be associated with involvement of the hands (**Fig. 9.16**). The nails may be pitted with small, ice pick-like depressions in the nail plate. Onycholysis (separation of nail plate from nail bed) can also occur. This condition is caused by a plaque of psoriasis in the distal nail bed with accumulation of scale, which lifts the plate from the nail bed. The nails may be thick, irregular, and discolored.

Pustular psoriasis is an uncommon variant. In this form of the disease, superficial pustules occur in one of three presentations: (1) pustules studding more typical plaques; (2) pustules confined to the palms and soles; and (3) a rare generalized eruption in which the pustules erupt abruptly on large areas of erythematous skin and are accompanied by fever and leukocytosis (**Fig. 9.17**).

Differential Diagnosis

Diagnosis usually is not difficult, especially when the lesions have the characteristic silvery scale and involve the typical locations. It may be more difficult when scale is not present, as in extremely early lesions or in intertriginous areas. Intertriginous lesions may be confused

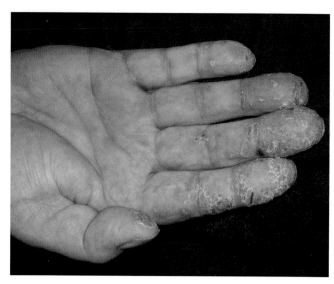

FIGURE 9.16 **Psoriasis** – erythematous, scaling, patches on the hand, often associated with nail involvement.

with *tinea cruris*, *candidiasis*, and *intertrigo* (see Tinea cruris, above). Psoriasis of the scalp is most often confused with *seborrheic dermatitis*, in which the scaling is usually finer, yellower, and more diffuse with indistinct borders. Guttate psoriasis on the trunk is sometimes confused with *pityriasis rosea* or *tinea corporis*. Nail involvement may be clinically indistinguishable from a *fungal infection*; a positive KOH preparation or fungal culture enables diagnosis of the latter.

Laboratory and Biopsy

A biopsy usually is not necessary; in fact, the clinical picture often is more characteristic than the histologic findings. If a biopsy is performed, the pathologic examination shows hyperkeratosis, parakeratosis, decreased granular layer with an acanthotic epidermis, and inflammatory infiltrate in the dermis that includes neutrophils, some of which may migrate into and through the epidermis, forming small collections within the stratum corneum (Munro's abscesses) (see **Fig. 9.13B**).

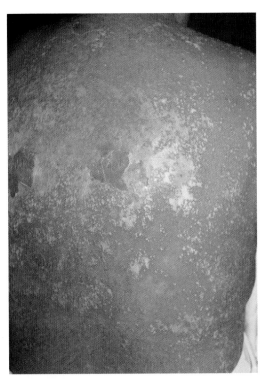

FIGURE 9.17 **Pustular psoriasis** – erythroderma studded with pustules.

Therapy

The goal of therapy is to decrease the epidermal proliferation and the underlying dermal inflammation. Five types of topical agents are used: steroids; tar and anthralin preparations; calcipotriene (a vitamin D derivative); tazarotene (a vitamin A derivative); and UV light.

Topical steroids are both antimitotic and anti-inflammatory. Over-the-counter hydrocortisone preparations are usually ineffective, requiring the stronger prescription steroids (see Ch. 4). These agents are expensive but are useful in patients with limited areas of involvement. A good response is usually noted within several weeks, but tachyphylaxis (loss of effect with continued use of a drug) may develop. Therefore, for long-term use of topical steroids, we instruct patients to use an intermittent regimen; e.g., use the agent for only 2 of every 3 weeks. This practice may also reduce the potential for developing steroid atrophy of the skin. Psoriasis also responds to systemic steroids, but these should be avoided because of their well known long-term side-effects and because psoriasis may rebound badly after the drug is discontinued.

Topical tars and *anthralin* are hydrocarbons with antimitotic activity; tars can also be anti-inflammatory. These products can stain skin (temporarily) and fabrics (permanently), and are slow to produce a response, although the responses that are achieved tend to last longer and tachyphylaxis is less likely to develop than with topical steroids. Tar oil (Cutar) added to a bath is a convenient way to apply tar to the total skin surface. The patient should be advised, however, that these tar oils stain plastic (but not porcelain) bathtubs. Tar preparations applied directly to the skin may be more effective than tar baths but are messier to use. Hence, we instruct patients to apply tar at bedtime. Commercial tar preparations are available, but we more often prescribe a compounded preparation containing a tar liquid – 5% liquor carbonis detergens (LCD) – contained in Aquaphor. To this, 3% salicylic acid may be added as a keratolytic to help remove thick scales if they are present. Anthralin is commercially available in a cream preparation (Drithocreme), ranging in concentration from 0.1% to 1.0%. Because of potential irritancy, this therapy is initiated with low concentrations and advanced as tolerated. A 30-min short-contact regimen can be used, but we usually suggest an overnight application. Skin irritation and staining are the main disadvantages of anthralin therapy.

Calcipotriene (Dovonex ointment, cream, and lotion) is a vitamin D derivative with antimitotic activity. It is applied twice daily and requires several months of use for full effect. Some patients respond well, but many do not. It is expensive and may cause irritation, but is otherwise safe for long-term use in limited plaque disease. We often alternate weekly treatments with topical steroids and calcipotriene to reduce the side effects of steroids and maintain disease control.

Tazarotene (Tazorac gel 0.05% and 0.1%) is a retinoid (vitamin A derivative). In general, retinoids promote differentiation and inhibit proliferation – desirable effects for an antipsoriatic drug. Topical tazarotene is applied at bedtime, often in conjunction with a topical steroid applied in the morning. It is effective for many patients, but it is expensive and may cause irritation (which is ameliorated by the morning steroid). Tazorac gel is also rated as category X for pregnancy, so it should not be used in women with childbearing potential.

UV light therapy can be used alone or in combination with other therapies. The least expensive source of UV light is the sun. However, this is often impractical. Tanning saloons are another source of UV light, which the patient can use three or four times weekly. Intensive UV light therapy can be provided in the offices of many dermatologists. Some patients find it convenient to purchase an expensive commercial UV light unit for their use at home, although home UV light should be used only with a physician's guidance.

Systemic agents are reserved for patients with severe or widespread disease that is poorly responsive to topical measures.

> Systemic agents for psoriasis are reserved for patients with severe disease.

PUVA is the least toxic systemic approach, but requires frequent clinic visits. The psoralen drug intercalates between the DNA strands and binds to them during irradiation with UVA. Therefore, although when the drug is taken by mouth it reaches all the body's tissues, only those tissues that receive the UVA radiation (i.e., the skin and the eyes, unless shielded) are affected. This treatment could result in cataracts, so the eyes must be protected with special glasses. The major long-term concerns involve premature aging of the skin and the development of skin cancer, including melanoma.

Methotrexate, a folate antagonist, inhibits cellular proliferation and is highly effective in many patients with psoriasis. It is administered on a weekly schedule. Complete blood cell counts need to be monitored at frequent intervals. The major long-term concern is liver toxicity, so regular liver function blood tests and intermittent liver biopsies are required. Familiarity with methotrexate and careful follow-up of patients are necessary to avoid serious side-effects of this drug.

Acitretin (Soriatane) is a retinoid with profound effects on keratinization. It is administered orally on a daily basis and is particularly effective for pustular psoriasis. Acitretin often improves but seldom clears the more common plaque-type psoriasis. It can be used in conjunction with UV light for additive effect. Acitretin is a *teratogen*, and is not safe for use in women with childbearing potential. Additional common side-effects include drying of skin and mucous membranes, hair loss, peeling of palms and soles, and numerous other less common problems, including effects on bones, eyes, liver, and blood lipids.

Systemic *cyclosporine* (Neoral) is also approved for treating psoriasis and is very effective in this role. It is, however, potentially nephrotoxic and requires careful monitoring.

Biologic agents that suppress the inflammatory response are quite effective in treating psoriasis without some of the serious sideeffects of other systemic treatments. These agents include etanercept (Enbrel), alefacept (Amevive), adalimumab (Humira), and infliximab (Remicade), and ustekinumab (Stelara). They are administered subcutaneously, intramuscularly, or intravenously.

Therapy for Psoriasis

Initial
- Steroids – mid-potency to strong potency (e.g., triamcinolone 0.1% or clobetasol 0.05% b.i.d.)
- Tars and anthralin
- Calcipotriene ointment, cream, or solution b.i.d.
- Tazarotene gel 0.05% or 0.1% daily
- Ultraviolet light

Alternative
- UV light – tanning or UVB, PUVA
- Methotrexate
- Acitretin
- Cyclosporine
- Biologics (etanercept, adalimumab, infliximab, ustekinumab, and alefacept)

Course and Complications

Psoriasis is a chronic condition that waxes and wanes, frequently without obvious cause. Perhaps because of the favorable influence of sunlight, many patients note that their psoriasis is better in summer and worse in winter. With use of the above therapies, the disease can usually be controlled, although not cured. This skin disease, like many others, can be socially stigmatizing and, in some individuals, physically disabling. The impact on quality of life can be enormous, with disruption of activities of daily life, impaired interpersonal relationships, and diminished self-esteem.

Psoriatic skin may be colonized with *Staphylococcus aureus*. With scratching, secondary infection occasionally occurs. Uncommonly, psoriasis affects the total body surface, resulting in erythroderma with its associated complications, which include loss of heat, fluid, and protein; hospitalization may be required.

Arthritis accompanies psoriasis in approximately 5% of patients. It classically affects the distal interphalangeal joints, but more often occurs as asymmetric arthritis involving small and medium-sized joints. Ankylosing spondylitis can also occur in psoriatic arthritis. Psoriatic arthritis is usually treated with non-steroidal anti-inflammatory drugs, although these sometimes aggravate the skin lesions. Methotrexate and etanercept are often useful for psoriatic arthritis, and are indicated particularly in the rapidly destructive type – arthritis mutilans (**Fig. 9.18**). Moderate to severe cutaneous psoriasis appears to be a risk factor for cardiac disease.

Arthritis accompanies psoriasis in approximately 5% of patients. Five clinical types are recognized:
1. Asymmetric small and medium-sized joint involvement
2. Distal interphalangeal joint disease
3. Rheumatoid arthritis-like
4. Ankylosing spondylitis
5. Mutilating

Pathogenesis

Many patients with psoriasis are genetically predisposed. Some 35% have a family history of psoriasis, and in

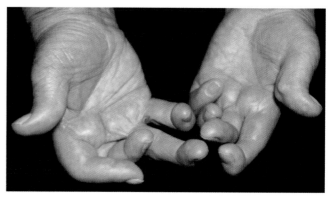

FIGURE 9.18 **Psoriatic arthritis mutilans.**

identical twins, the disease occurs concurrently in 80%. The precipitating factors responsible for unmasking this genetic predisposition include streptococcal infection, stress, smoking, drugs, and physical trauma.

Others have implicated the dermal inflammatory process as being primary in the evolution of a psoriatic lesion and epidermal hyperplasia. Clinical observations, laboratory studies, and targeted therapies support the immunologic basis of psoriasis. T-cell mechanisms have been strongly implicated. Many experimental data now suggest that psoriasis may be a T-cell-mediated autoimmune disease driven by T helper cell (Th1) and 17 cytokines. The therapeutic effectiveness of cyclosporine and biologic agents, which are T-cell-targeted drugs, supports this theory. The understanding of the immunopathogenesis of psoriasis has translated into the development of therapeutic biologic agents, which reduce the number of pathogenic T cells, inhibit T-cell activation and migration, or block the activity of inflammatory cytokines. Investigators have noted that neutrophils extravasated from the superficial dermal capillaries invade the epidermis. Raised levels of leukotrienes (one of the products of arachidonic acid metabolism) have been found in psoriatic skin, where, as mediators of inflammation (tumor necrosis factor-α, interleukins12 and 23), they may attract neutrophils and may provoke epidermal proliferation.

> Psoriasis is an inflammatory disease that provides opportunities for therapeutic intervention.

Whatever the provocation, the end result for the epidermis is an accelerated cell cycle or an increased number of cycling cells recruited from the normal resting cell population. This leads to an increased number of dividing cells, culminating in an orgy of epidermal proliferation. Cellular turnover is increased seven-fold, and the transit time from the basal layer to the top of the stratum corneum is decreased from the normal 28 days to 3 or 4 days. This process is too fast for the cells to be shed, so they accumulate, resulting in the characteristic scale.

> In a psoriatic plaque, epidermal cell production is increased seven-fold.

SECONDARY SYPHILIS

Key Points

1. *Treponema pallidum* is causative
2. Involvement of the palms and soles is typical
3. Serologic test for syphilis (RPR or VDRL) is sensitive. Confirm with FTA-ABS test

Definition

The rash of secondary syphilis represents an inflammatory response in the skin and mucous membranes to the hematogenously disseminated *Treponema pallidum* spirochete. Clinically, the rash may appear in various ways, but the most common is scaling papules and plaques.

Incidence

Despite the availability of penicillin, secondary syphilis is still present in our society, and its incidence has been increasing in recent years, both in the general population and in patients infected with HIV.

History

The secondary phase of syphilis starts 6–12 weeks after the appearance of the primary chancre. The chancre has usually (but not always) healed by the time the secondary phase develops, but it may be remembered by the patient. Systemic symptoms are usually present and include fever, headache, myalgia, arthralgia, sore throat, and malaise. Pruritus, once thought not to occur in secondary syphilis, is noted occasionally.

Physical Examination

The rash of secondary syphilis is a great imitator. It may appear as macules, non-scaling papules and annular plaques, scaling papules, patches, and plaques, and, occasionally, pustules or nodules. Vesicles or bullae are not present, however, except in newborns with congenital disease and occasionally in patients with HIV infection. The most common lesions are scaling papules and small plaques in which the color is a clue. Lesions are most frequently not just red but rather reddish brown (ham colored) or yellowish (copper colored). The eruption is often generalized, but palmar and plantar involvement with lesions of these colors is particularly noteworthy (**Fig. 9.19**). Other possible mucocutaneous features include: (1) white mucous patches in the mouth; (2) condylomata lata, which are flat-topped, moist, warty-appearing lesions in the genital areas; and (3) spotty alopecia of the scalp, which has been described as 'moth-eaten' in appearance. The general physical examination usually reveals the presence of lymphadenopathy.

> The rash of secondary syphilis is a great imitator. Involvement of the palms and soles suggests this diagnosis.

Differential Diagnosis

As mentioned, the rash of secondary syphilis can mimic many other skin disorders, the most common of which are: *pityriasis rosea*, as has been discussed; *drug eruption*; *viral exanthem*; and (for the annular lesions seen especially in African-American patients) *sarcoidosis*. A general guideline to remember is that, for patients with a generalized rash of unknown origin and systemic complaints, secondary syphilis should be considered and the patient should be tested for it.

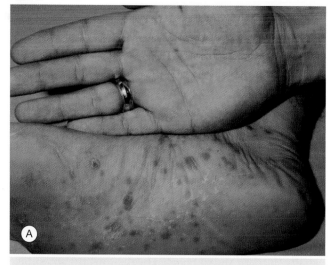

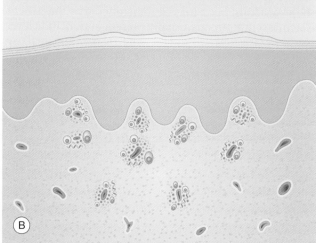

FIGURE 9.19 **Secondary syphilis. A.** Characteristic plantar and palmar, 'ham'-colored, slight scaling patches and macules. **B.** Epidermis – slight hyperkeratosis. Dermis – perivascular infiltrate with lymphocytes, plasma cells, and spirochetes (with silver stain).

In patients with fever and rash of unknown origin, a serologic test for syphilis should be done.

Laboratory and Biopsy

In secondary syphilis, the serologic test for syphilis (STS), rapid plasma reagin (RPR) or Venereal Disease Research Laboratory (VDRL), is always positive in immunocompetent hosts and is usually present in high titer. A positive STS should be followed by a fluorescent treponemal antibody-absorption (FTA-ABS) test, which is a more specific test for syphilis. Positivity of these two blood tests confirms the diagnosis. False-positive tests, usually in low titer, occur in some patients with SLE.

The STS may be negative in a patient with coexisting HIV infection and secondary syphilis. If syphilis is suspected in this setting, a darkfield examination or biopsy of a skin lesion can confirm the diagnosis. These procedures visualize the spirochetes in serous fluid obtained from the lesion or in special stains of biopsy material. The histologic findings otherwise are frequently nonspecific, showing simply an inflammatory infiltrate and, in lesions with scale, hyperkeratosis and mild acanthosis. Plasma cells are often present in the inflammatory infiltrate and may suggest the diagnosis (**Fig. 9.19B**). Patients diagnosed with syphilis should also be tested for HIV infection because the presence of the former indicates a risk factor for acquiring the latter.

Therapy

Penicillin remains the treatment of choice for syphilis. For primary and secondary syphilis in immunocompetent hosts, a single intramuscular injection of 2.4 million units of benzathine penicillin G is adequate therapy. HIV-infected patients require more intensive therapy, either with benzathine penicillin injections weekly for 3 weeks or with a course of intravenous aqueous penicillin or intramuscular ceftriaxone. Immunocompetent patients who are allergic to penicillin may be treated with a 14-day course of either tetracycline 500 mg q.i.d. or doxycycline 100 mg b.i.d. With therapy, many patients experience a febrile reaction (Jarisch–Herxheimer reaction) beginning within 12 h and resolving within 1 day.

In patients with HIV infection, syphilis progresses rapidly and requires more intensive therapy.

Therapy for Secondary Syphilis

Initial
- Benzathine penicillin G 2.4 million units IM.

Alternative
- Doxycycline 100 mg b.i.d. or tetracycline 500 mg q.i.d. for 2 weeks

Course and Complications

Without therapy, the lesions of secondary syphilis resolve spontaneously in 1–3 months in the immunocompetent host. With therapy, the lesions resolve promptly, and the titer of the STS is reduced markedly by 12 months. The FTA-ABS test often remains positive indefinitely.

In the secondary phase, the treponemal organism spreads not only to the skin but also to other organs. Hepatitis occurs in approximately 10% of the patients, bone and joint disease in approximately 4%, and nephritis even less often. Central nervous system involvement, as reflected by abnormal cerebrospinal fluid findings, occurs in approximately 10% of immunocompetent patients but is much more frequent in HIV-infected patients, in whom rapid progression to symptomatic neurosyphilis may occur.

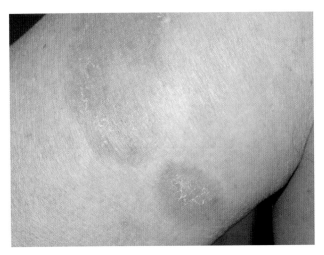

FIGURE 9.20 **Erythema annulare centrifugum** – polycyclic pink patches with a 'trailing' scale.

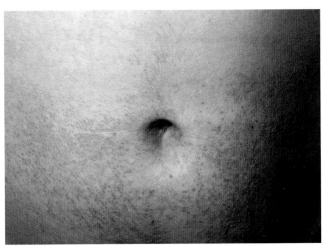

FIGURE 9.21 **X-linked ichthyosis** – 'dirty' brown scaling, more prominent on lower abdomen.

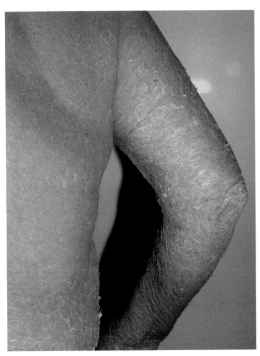

FIGURE 9.22 **Acquired ichthyosis** – diffuse, fine, whitish scaling in a generalized distribution. Look for a systemic association with lymphoma, metabolic disorder, or medications.

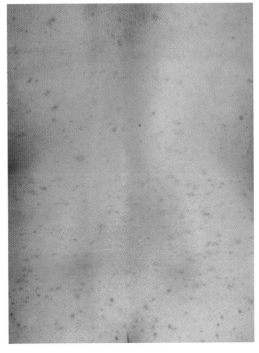

FIGURE 9.23 **Parapsoriasis** – diffuse, slightly scaling, mildly erythematous, small plaques.

Approximately one-third of untreated immunocompetent patients develop late (years later) complications of syphilis (tertiary), of which the most important are the cardiovascular and central nervous system manifestations. In patients with HIV infection, progression to tertiary syphilis is more frequent and can occur within months after primary infection.

Pathogenesis

The disease is caused by the spirochete *T. pallidum*. The organism is traumatically inoculated into mucous membranes or skin, most often during sexual intercourse. After a 10–90-day incubation period, the *primary* lesion appears as an ulcer (chancre). After another brief latent period, during which the organism continues to multiply, hematogenous dissemination occurs (*secondary* syphilis). Organisms infecting the skin provoke an immunologic response, which is clinically manifested by a variety of inflammatory lesions.

UNCOMMON SCALING DISORDERS

ERYTHEMA ANNULARE CENTRIFUGUM

This annular or polycyclic eruption is characterized by waxing and waning patches with a 'trailing' scale that is

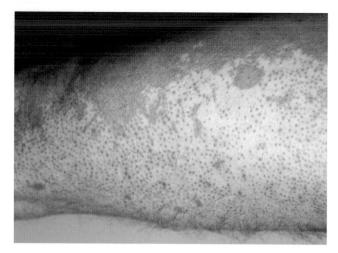

FIGURE 9.24 **Pityriasis rubra pilaris** – erythematous, slightly scaling, follicular papules and plaques.

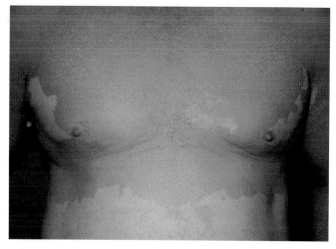

FIGURE 9.25 **Pityriasis rubra pilaris** – bright pink, slightly scaling, confluent plaques with islands of normal skin.

chronic and recurrent over months and years (**Fig. 9.20**). For most, it is idiopathic. However, on occasion it has been associated with dermatophyte infections, foods, medications, and, rarely, malignancy. Treatment is symptomatic with topical steroids.

ICHTHYOSIS

The ichthyoses are a heterogeneous group of distinct genodermatoses characterized by generalized scaling seen at birth or shortly thereafter. Genetic mutations resulting in abnormal epidermal cornification cause the dry scaling of the skin. Severity ranges from mild 'dry' skin involvement (*ichthyosis vulgaris*) to severe, 'thick' scaling (*lamellar ichthyosis*). X-linked ichthyosis is characterized by 'dirty' appearing, large brown scales, most prominent on the extensor extremities and trunk of males (**Fig. 9.21**). It is caused by a deletion of the *steroid sulfatase* gene on the X-chromosome and inherited as a recessive trait. Mothers carrying the gene often have a history of failure of labor to begin or progress. Corneal opacities and cryptorchidism are frequent findings. *Acquired ichthyosis* (**Fig. 9.22**) begins in adults and is associated with malignancy (e.g., lymphomas), metabolic disease (e.g., hypothyroidism), and drugs (e.g., retinoids).

PARAPSORIASIS

Parapsoriasis is a group of confusing scaling disorders that is most easily divided into small and large plaque parapsoriasis. Both groups have fairly well demarcated, slightly scaling, erythematous to tan patches, and thin plaques, which are asymptomatic and chronic. Small plaque parapsoriasis (**Fig. 9.23**) appears very similar to pityriasis rosea but lasts longer than 2–3 months and has a benign course. Large plaque parapsoriasis has an irregularly shaped, well demarcated, and sometimes wrinkled

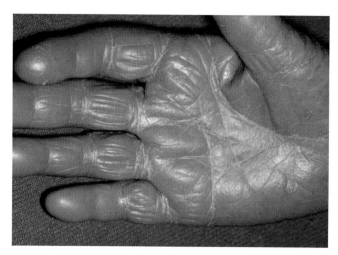

FIGURE 9.26 **Pityriasis rubra pilaris** – thickened, erythematous, shiny palms.

appearance, which in about 10% of cases evolves into mycosis fungoides. Skin biopsies are non-diagnostic and treatment with UV light is usually successful.

PITYRIASIS RUBRA PILARIS

Pityriasis rubra pilaris is a chronic idiopathic disorder characterized by scaling follicular papules (**Fig. 9.24**), diffuse and confluent, yellowish-pink, well demarcated plaques with islands of normal appearing skin (**Fig. 9.25**), and thick scaling palms and soles (**Fig. 9.26**). It affects all ages and is generally mildly pruritic. Painful fissuring of the palms and soles can cause significant disability. The skin biopsy is characteristic and treatment with oral retinoids or methotrexate is often disappointing.

Vesicles and Bullae 10

Key Points

1. Blistering is an easily recognized primary lesion
2. Weeping and crusting suggest a blistering process
3. There are multiple causes of blistering

ABSTRACT

Vesicles and bullae, when intact, are easily recognized primary lesions (**Table 10.1**). Crusts (dried serum and blood) are secondary lesions that should lead one to suspect a preceding vesicle/bulla or pustule. The etiology of vesicular and bullous diseases includes viral and bacterial infections, allergic and irritant contact dermatitis, and autoimmune, genetic, and metabolic diseases. Pathogenesis of the blister formation is helpful in understanding the location of the lesion within the skin. The blister may occur within the epidermis (intraepidermal) or beneath it (subepidermal).

Where blisters occur:
1. Intraepidermally
2. Subepidermally, help in making the diagnosis

The following diseases illustrate the pathogenetic mechanisms involved in blister formation at the different levels of the skin. Detachment of the horny layer by an epidermolytic toxin produced by *Staphylococcus aureus* causes a subcorneal blister. Invasion of epidermal cells by herpesvirus causes degenerative changes and intraepidermal vesicles. Intercellular edema caused by contact dermatitis results in stretching of the intercellular bridges (spongiosis) until they disappear, forming intraepidermal vesicles. Dissolution of the intercellular adhesion molecules secondary to autoantibodies in pemphigus vulgaris causes loss of epidermal cohesion (acantholysis) and blisters within the epidermis.

Damage to the structures within the basement membrane zone causes loss of coherence between basal cells and dermis. These subepidermal bullae are characteristic of bullous pemphigoid, dermatitis herpetiformis, and porphyria cutanea tarda.

Blisters usually rupture, producing crusting and weeping. If they become filled with purulent material, they are called *pustules*.

BULLOUS IMPETIGO

Key Points

1. Fragile, clear or cloudy bullae
2. *S. aureus* toxin causes blister
3. Treat with penicillinase-resistant antibiotic

Definition and Etiology

Bullous impetigo is an intraepidermal (subcorneal) bacterial infection of the skin caused by certain strains of *S. aureus* (**Fig. 10.1**). Impetigo is also discussed in Chapter 12.

Incidence

Bullous impetigo occurs most frequently in preschool-age children.

History

Crowding, poor hygiene, chronic dermatitis, and neglected injury of the skin are predisposing factors in the **127**

TABLE 10.1 Common blistering diseases

Disease	Frequency[a]	Etiology	History	Physical Examination	Differential Diagnosis	Laboratory Test
Bullous impetigo	0.1	*Staphylococcus aureus*	Pruritus	Circular yellow crusts, purulent bullae Head, neck, extremities	Contact dermatitis Herpes simplex Fungus	Gram-stain Culture
Contact dermatitis	2.8	Allergen Irritant	Irritant: exposure occurs hours to days before rash Allergic: exposure occurs 1–4 days before rash	Papulovesicles Conforms to area of contact with sharp margins Often has a geometric or linear configuration	Atopic dermatitis Cellulitis Fungus	Patch test
Herpes simplex	1.5	Herpes simplex virus	Itching or pain prodrome	Grouped vesicles Perioral and perineal location most frequent	Impetigo Fungus Contact dermatitis	Tzanck smear Culture Immunofluorescent staining
Herpes zoster	0.4	Varicella-zoster virus	Itching or pain prodrome	Grouped vesicles Dermatomal distribution	–	Tzanck smear Culture Immunofluorescent staining
Varicella	<0.1	Varicella-zoster virus	Marked pruritus	Macules, papules, vesicles, pustules Generalized	Rickettsialpox Smallpox	Tzanck smear Culture Immunofluorescent staining

[a]Percentage of new dermatology patients with this diagnosis seen in the Hershey Medical Center Dermatology Clinic, Hershey, PA.

development of impetigo. An initial site of involvement is followed by multiple sites that may be pruritic.

Physical Examination

Fragile, clear or cloudy bullae (**Fig. 10.1A**) are characteristic of bullous impetigo. A thin, varnish-like crust occurs after rupture of the bulla. A delicate, collarette-like remnant of the blister roof is often present at the rim of the crust. Gyrate lesions may be formed with clear centers and active margins of 0.5–2 cm. Autoinoculation results in satellite lesions. The face, neck, and extremities are most often affected. Regional adenopathy may be present, but patients have no systemic symptoms.

Differential Diagnosis

Contact dermatitis, herpes simplex virus (HSV) infection, and occasionally *superficial fungal infections* may produce vesiculobullous or crusted lesions similar to those of impetigo. The history, patch tests, Tzanck and potassium hydroxide (KOH) preparations, and appropriate cultures differentiate these entities. *Pemphigus vulgaris* may also produce crusted lesions and should be suspected in patients with chronic, apparently impetiginized, plaques that have not responded to appropriate antibiotics.

Staphylococcal scalded skin syndrome (**Fig. 10.1B**) is an uncommon disorder affecting primarily infants and young children. It is characterized by the sudden onset of fever, skin tenderness, and erythema, followed by the formation of large, flaccid bullae and shedding of large sheets of skin, leaving a denuded, scalded-appearing surface. In contrast to bullous impetigo, in which *S. aureus* may be recovered, the bullae of staphylococcal scalded skin syndrome are sterile. The usual source of infection is in the conjunctiva, nose, or pharynx. In the newborn, an infected umbilical stump may be the source.

Laboratory and Biopsy

Gram-staining of the clear or cloudy fluid from a bulla reveals Gram-positive cocci. *S. aureus* grows out in more than 95% of the cultures. Biopsy of impetigo, which is usually not done because the diagnosis is obvious, reveals a subcorneal pustule or blister (**Fig. 10.1C**).

Therapy

Most *S. aureus* cultured from impetigo lesions is penicillin resistant. Therefore, a cephalosporin such as cephalexin (Keflex), erythromycin (Ilosone), or penicillinase-resistant semisynthetic penicillin such as dicloxacillin (Dynapen) should be chosen. Mupirocin (Bactroban) ointment 2% applied three times daily is as effective as oral antibiotics in treating impetigo that is limited to a small area. For community acquired methicillin-resistant *S. aureus* (MRSA), trimethoprim-sulfamethoxazole or doxycycline can be used as alternative treatments.

General hygiene should also be implemented to prevent spread. Cleansing with antibacterial soaps and gentle removal of crust hasten healing. Daily changing of items that contact the area of impetigo such as towels, washcloths, and shavers is recommended. For widespread or recurrent impetigo, bleach baths can be helpful.

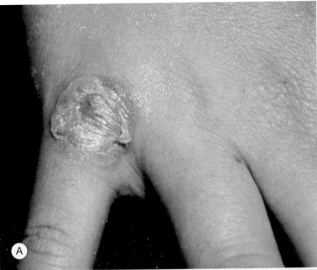

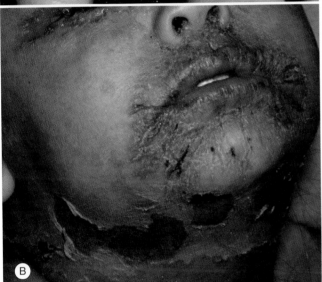

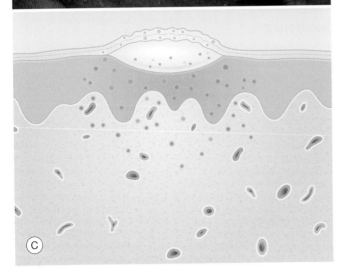

FIGURE 10.1 **Bullous impetigo. A.** Erythematous fragile bullae. **B.** Staphylococcal scalded skin syndrome – denuded and crusted, erythematous, scalded-appearing patches involving the typical distribution: periorbital, perioral, and neck. **C.** Subcorneal bulla, inflammation.

Therapy for Bullous Impetigo

Initial

Antibiotics

- Cephalexin: 25–50 mg/kg daily in oral suspension, 500 mg b.i.d.
- Erythromycin: 30–50 mg/kg daily in oral suspension, 500 mg b.i.d.
- Dicloxacillin: 500 mg b.i.d.
- Mupirocin ointment or Polysporin: applied t.i.d.

General Hygiene

- Antibacterial soap: Hibiclens
- Changing of towel, washcloth, shaver, etc., daily
- Bleach baths: ¼–½ cup of bleach in ½ tub of water daily

Alternative – for Methicillin-Resistant *S. Aureus* (MRSA)

- Trimethoprim-sulfamethoxazole (TMP) one double strength table b.i.d. or 4–6 mg/kg b.i.d.
- Doxycycline 100 mg b.i.d.

Course and Complications

Even without treatment, impetigo heals spontaneously in 3–6 weeks. Antibiotics hasten healing (within 1 week of starting therapy) and reduce contagiousness.

Pathogenesis

An epidermolytic toxin targeting desmoglein 1, a desmosomal adhesion molecule, causes the subcorneal cleavage characteristic of bullous impetigo and staphylococcal scalded skin syndrome. This toxin is from pathogenic phage group II *S. aureus.* In bullous impetigo, the toxin is produced at the site of the lesion. In staphylococcal scalded skin syndrome, it is produced remotely and then carried hematogenously to the skin.

> Epidermolytic toxin causes bullae.

CONTACT DERMATITIS (ACUTE)

Because acute contact dermatitis is characterized by a vesicular eruption (**Fig. 10.2A**), it is mentioned briefly here. In Chapter 8, it is discussed in more detail, along with other eczematous eruptions.

Contact dermatitis is an inflammatory reaction of the skin caused by an irritant or allergenic chemical. It may be an acute or chronic process. Intraepidermal vesicles are the hallmark of acute contact dermatitis. Additional characteristics are weeping, crusting, edema, and erythema. The areas involved frequently have sharp margins with geometric and linear configurations. Poison ivy and other plants characteristically cause linear streaks of papulovesicles. Treatment is with steroids (topical or systemic), antihistamines, and wet dressings or soaks. The biopsy of acute contact dermatitis reveals spongiosis and

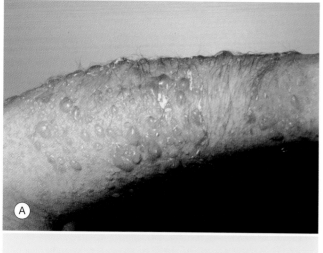

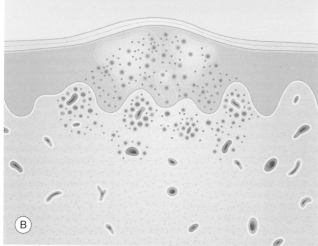

FIGURE 10.2 **Acute contact dermatitis. A.** Multiple bullae in area of contactant – poison ivy. Note sparing of area covered by watch band. **B.** Epidermis – bulla, spongiosis. Dermis – perivascular infiltrate. Intercellular staining for immunoglobulin G or complement.

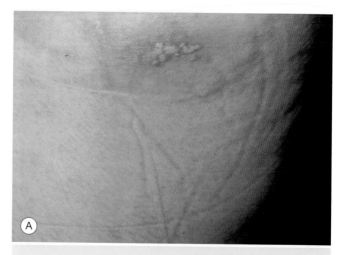

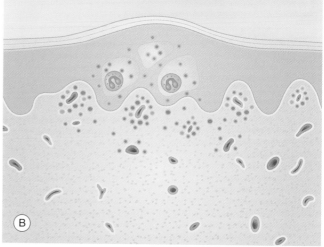

FIGURE 10.3 **Herpes simplex. A.** Grouped vesicles on an erythematous base. **B.** Epidermis – bullae, multinucleated giant cells. Dermis – perivascular inflammation.

intraepidermal vesicle formation with inflammation (**Fig. 10.2B**).

HERPES SIMPLEX

Key Points

1. Recurrent grouped vesicles in the same location
2. Tzanck smear is diagnostic
3. Treatment is suppressive, not curative

Definition

Herpes simplex is an acute, self-limiting, intraepidermal vesicular eruption caused by infection with HSV (**Fig. 10.3**). HSV is a medium-sized DNA virus that replicates within the nucleus. Based on culture and immunologic characteristics, it is divided into two types: HSV-1 and HSV-2. Usually, HSV-1 causes oral infection and HSV-2 causes genital infection. Primary infections with these viruses are characteristically followed by recurrent attacks.

Incidence

Infection with HSV is common worldwide. It is estimated in the USA that more than 50% of adults are seropositive for HSV-1 and more than 20% for HSV-2.

History

Primary infection with HSV-1 usually occurs in children, in whom it is subclinical in 90% of cases. The remaining 10% of infected children have acute gingivostomatitis. In contrast, HSV-2 primary infection usually occurs after sexual contact in postpubertal individuals, and it produces acute vulvovaginitis or progenitalis. Primary infections are frequently accompanied by systemic symptoms that include fever, malaise, myalgia, headache, and regional adenopathy. Localized pain and burning may be so severe that drinking and eating, or urinating, may be compromised.

Infection of the lips (herpes labialis) is usually caused by HSV-1, whereas the genitals and buttocks are more often infected with HSV-2. The risk of a woman developing genital herpes on exposure to an infected man is estimated to be 80–90%. The risk of recurrence after primary genital infections is less with HSV-1 (14%) than with HSV-2 (60%). Recurrent attacks are preceded by localized itching or burning and are characterized by occurrence in the same location. This prodrome usually begins within 24 h before the appearance of the eruption and occurs in approximately two-thirds of patients.

> Herpes should be suspected if a vesicular eruption is:
> 1. Recurrent in same location
> 2. Preceded by a prodrome

HSV infections are not limited to the lips and genital area; either type can infect any area of skin. Therefore, a history of a vesicular eruption recurring in the *same* location should lead to a suspicion of HSV infection.

Physical Examination

Indurated erythema followed by grouped vesicles on an erythematous base is typical of herpes infections. The vesicles quickly become pustules, which rupture, weep, and crust. Affected skin sometimes becomes necrotic, resulting in punched-out ulceration.

> Grouped vesicles on an erythematous base are characteristic of HSV infection.

Primary infections – gingivostomatitis or vulvovaginitis – are characterized by extensive vesiculation of the mucous membranes. This results in erosions, necrosis, and a marked purulent discharge. Herpes infection can develop in any area where inoculation has occurred. *Recurrent herpes* infections are characterized by localized grouped vesicles in the same location. *Herpetic whitlow* is infection of the fingers. This is an occupational hazard of medical and dental personnel that can be prevented by wearing gloves. Traumatic herpes simplex has been reported in epidemics among wrestlers (herpes gladiatorum). *Eczema herpeticum* is a generalized cutaneous infection with HSV in individuals with predisposing skin diseases such as atopic dermatitis. It is accompanied by severe toxic symptoms and may be fatal.

Differential Diagnosis

Impetigo, contact dermatitis, and, less often, *superficial fungal infections* may be confused with herpes simplex and can be ruled out by the history, Gram-staining and culture of the blister fluid, patch testing with suspected allergens, and KOH preparation test of the blister roof.

Laboratory and Biopsy

The occurrence of grouped vesicles on an erythematous base is characteristic of HSV infection. It can be confirmed with a Tzanck smear, which reveals multinucleated giant cells (**Fig. 10.4**). The Tzanck smear is a simple yet reliable method of confirming a herpetic infection. Smears from the base of the lesion stained with Giemsa, Wright, or toluidine blue demonstrate multinucleated giant cells diagnostic of HSV infection. A detailed

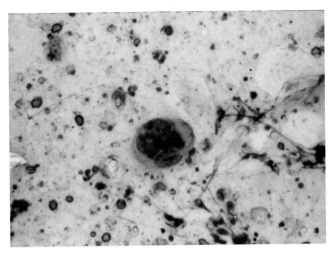

FIGURE 10.4 **Tzanck smear** – multinucleated giant cell.

description of preparing a Tzanck preparation is presented in Chapter 3. The positivity of the Tzanck preparation varies with the lesion sampled: vesicle, 67%; pustule, 55%; and crust-ulcer, 16.7%. A high correlation exists between the Tzanck preparation and viral culture. However, when performed properly, the culture has a greater positivity: vesicle, 100%; pustule, 73%; and crust-ulcer, 33%. Direct immunofluorescent staining of vesicle smears compares favorably with viral cultures. Although usually not necessary, the biopsy (see **Fig. 10.3B**) reveals an intraepidermal blister with multinucleated epidermal giant cells and an acute inflammatory process. Patients with genital herpes should be screened for other sexually transmitted diseases.

> Tzanck smear revealing multinucleated giant cells confirms a herpetic infection.

Therapy

Acyclovir (Zovirax), valacyclovir (Valtrex), famciclovir (Famvir), penciclovir (Denavir), and docosanol (Abreva) are the drugs of choice for HSV infections. Their low toxicity and specificity for HSV have resulted in widespread acceptance. Their unique mechanism of action accounts for their selectivity against HSV. Acyclovir is a synthetic acyclic purine nucleoside analog. Phosphorylation of acyclovir depends on HSV-specific thymidine kinase. This enzyme converts acyclovir to acyclovir monophosphate, which is further converted into acyclovir triphosphate by cellular enzymes. Acyclovir triphosphate inhibits viral DNA polymerase and replication of viral DNA. It is effective against replicating virus but does not eliminate latent virus. Valacyclovir is a prodrug that is better absorbed than its metabolite acyclovir. Famciclovir, also a prodrug, is metabolized to penciclovir, a synthetic acyclic guanosine derivative. Penciclovir shares similar activation pathways with acyclovir that depend on viral thymidine kinase to form penciclovir triphosphate, which halts DNA synthesis. In active infections, these antiviral drugs decrease the duration of viral shedding, accelerate healing of the lesions, and may reduce local and systemic symptoms. For genital herpes infection, condom use can prevent transmission of HSV-2 by 50% and should be encouraged for individuals with active and asymptomatic shedding of the virus.

> Treatment does not prevent recurrent infection. However, condom use prevents transmission of HSV-2.

Intravenous acyclovir is indicated in the treatment of severe primary HSV, and in initial and recurrent infections in severely immunocompromised patients. The most important adverse reactions are deposition of drug crystals in the renal tubules of patients with inadequate hydration or impaired renal function. Resistant strains of HSV have emerged in immunocompromised patients and have posed a significant clinical problem. Foscarnet is an alternative drug if acyclovir fails because of acyclovir-resistant thymidine kinase-deficient HSV.

Therapy for Herpes Simplex

Initial

First Episode – Primary
- Acyclovir: 400 mg t.i.d. for 7 days, 5–10 mg/kg IV every 8 h for 5–7 days
- Valacyclovir: 1000 mg b.i.d. for 7 days
- Famciclovir: 250 mg t.i.d. for 7 days

Recurrent
- Acyclovir: 800 mg t.i.d. for 2 days, 5% ointment every 2 h for 7 days
- Valacyclovir: 2000 mg b.i.d. for 1 day
- Famciclovir: 1 g b.i.d. for 1 day.
- Acyclovir 5% ointment: six times daily for 7 days
- Penciclovir 1% cream: every 2 h while awake for 4 days
- Docosanol 10% cream: five times daily until healed

Chronic Suppressive
- Acyclovir: 400 mg b.i.d.
- Valacyclovir:1000 mg daily
- Famciclovir: 250 mg b.i.d.

Alternative
- Foscarnet 40 mg/kg every 8–12 h for 1–2 weeks

Course and Complications

The incubation period after contact with HSV is approximately 1 week. The clinical course of the primary herpes infection lasts approximately 3 weeks. A prodrome of 1–2 days is followed by a vesiculopustular eruption that continues for about 10 days. This phase is followed by crusting, ulceration, and healing after a further 10 days. For most patients, HSV is an asymptomatic chronic infection of sensory ganglia. Overt eruptions recur in a minority of infected persons after varying periods of latency, during which the virus remains dormant within the dorsal nerve root ganglion corresponding to the site of infection. Recurrences have a shorter course of 1–2 weeks.

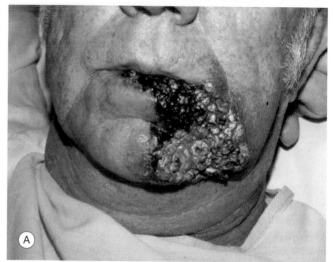

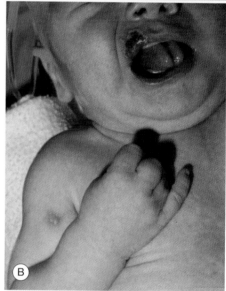

FIGURE 10.5 **A.** Chronic cutaneous herpes simplex – erythematous crusted patch. **B.** Neonatal herpes simplex – grouped vesicles on an erythematous base on the lip and arm.

Several factors, including fever, ultraviolet light, physical trauma, menstruation, and emotional stress, are attributed to initiating recurrence. Asymptomatic, subclinical shedding of the HSV is common, and is instrumental in transmitting HSV to others.

The immunocompromised host is most at risk for developing complications from HSV infections. These complications include chronic ulcerative herpes simplex (**Fig. 10.5A**), which lasts for weeks to months; generalized acute mucocutaneous herpes simplex; and systemic infection involving the liver, lung, adrenal glands, and central nervous system.

HSV infection of the neonate, *neonatal herpes* (**Fig. 10.5B**), is a devastating but fortunately uncommon disease. The fatality rate without treatment is more than 50%, and at least 50% of the survivors have significant neurologic sequelae. Significant reduction of mortality and morbidity occurs with acyclovir treatment. For women who have evidence of active HSV infection at delivery, cesarean section is recommended. Complicating neonatal HSV infection, however, are the findings that: (1) cultures to screen women immediately before delivery do not predict infection for the fetus; (2) more than 70% of mothers of babies with neonatal HSV have no history of genital HSV infection; and (3) symptomatic disease may not occur for as long as 1 month after delivery. Two-thirds of affected infants have mucocutaneous manifestations of HSV infection.

> Untreated neonatal herpes is frequently fatal and has severe morbidity.

> In most cases of neonatal herpes, the mother has no history of genital disease and it may take up to 1 month after delivery for symptoms to develop.

A relatively uncommon complication of HSV infection is *erythema multiforme*. Immune complexes composed of antibody and HSV antigen have been found in the serum of patients with erythema multiforme after HSV infection. These immune complexes may be the pathogenesis of the vascular changes seen in erythema multiforme. In addition, HSV DNA has been found in the lesions of erythema multiforme associated with HSV infection.

> Erythema multiforme may occur after HSV infection.

Pathogenesis

HSV is a highly contagious virion spread by direct contact with infected individuals who are often asymptomatically shedding the virus. Studies of shedding and survival of HSV from patients with herpes labialis have detected herpesvirus in their saliva (78%) and on their hands (67%), with virus viability on skin, cloth, and plastic for 2–4 h.

The virus penetrates the epidermal cell, in which a complex series of steps occurs. The virus undergoes a replicative cycle and induces protein and DNA synthesis with the assembling of intact virions and eventual lysis of the host cell membrane. New copies of viral DNA are packaged into capsids, which are then covered with an amorphous tegument. The viral envelope, which contains virus-specific glycoproteins, is formed by budding through the host nuclear membrane. This process requires an intact host cellular metabolism for substrate synthesis and replication. The destructive effect on epidermal cells results clinically in intraepidermal vesicles.

Latent HSV, undetectable by tissue culture, electron microscopy, and immunofluorescence, presumably resides in the dorsal nerve root sensory or autonomic ganglia in a non-replicative state. Outbreaks recur with reactivation of the replicative cycle, production of new virus, and spreading back down the nerve. Latency within the ganglion cells is possible, apparently because the HSV genomes

within these cells are relatively well protected from immunologic attacks.

HERPES ZOSTER

> ### Key Points
>
> 1. Grouped vesicles in a dermatome
> 2. Vaccinate
> 3. Treat early in the middle-aged and elderly to prevent severe post-herpetic neuralgia

Definition

Herpes zoster ('shingles') is an intraepidermal vesicular eruption occurring in a dermatomal distribution (**Fig. 10.6**). It is caused by the recrudescence of latent varicella-zoster virus in persons who have had varicella.

> Vesicular dermatomal eruption is distinctive for herpes zoster.

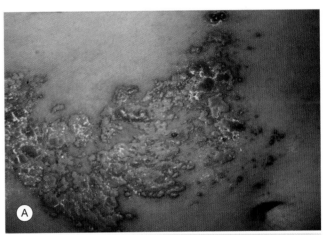

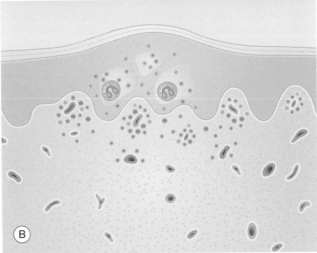

FIGURE 10.6 Herpes zoster. A. Grouped, cloudy and hemorrhagic vesicles on an erythematous base in a dermatomal distribution. **B.** Epidermis – bullae, multinucleated giant cells. Dermis – perivascular inflammation.

Incidence

Some 10–20% of individuals develop herpes zoster during their lifetime. Two-thirds of these individuals are older than 50. The attack rate is age-dependent, with a rate of: 1 case per 1000 among healthy people less than 20 years old; three cases per 1000 in patients between 20 and 49 years old; and a peak of 11 per 1000 at age 80–89 years. Patients with cancer and acquired immune deficiency syndrome (AIDS) have a higher incidence than the general population (e.g., 8–25% of patients with Hodgkin's disease develop herpes zoster). The frequency of second attacks may be 5%. However, what is thought to be recurrent zoster may be HSV in a dermatomal distribution

History

A prodrome of radicular pain and itching precedes the eruption. It can stimulate migraine, pleurisy, myocardial infarction, or appendicitis.

> The prodrome may mimic migraine, pleurisy, myocardial infarction, or appendicitis.

Physical Examination

The eruption is characterized by groups of vesicles on an erythematous base situated unilaterally along the distribution of a cranial or spinal nerve. Bilateral involvement is rare. Frequently, the eruption involves the immediately adjacent dermatomes.

Differential Diagnosis

The dermatomal distribution of herpes zoster is diagnostic. However, *herpes simplex* may occur in a dermatomal fashion.

Laboratory and Biopsy

Usually, no laboratory tests are necessary. The Tzanck preparation, direct immunofluorescent staining of vesicle smears (most sensitive test), biopsy (**Fig 10.6B**), and culture are confirmatory in unusual cases. Although herpes zoster has a higher incidence in patients with established malignant disease, patients presenting with herpes zoster who are otherwise healthy do not have a higher incidence of occult cancer and therefore do not need a screening laboratory examination for malignancy. In patients at risk for HIV infection, herpes zoster may be the presenting sign, and serologic testing for HIV is indicated.

> Herpes zoster is not a marker for occult malignant disease. It may be the presenting sign of HIV infection.

Therapy

Prevention with zoster vaccine live OKA/Merck (Zostavax), is very effective and indicated in individuals aged over 60. When the vesiculopustules of herpes zoster rupture, crusting and weeping are reduced with astringent (Domeboro) compresses. Analgesics commensurate with the amount of pain experienced by the patient are indicated. Acyclovir (Zovirax), at a dosage of 10 mg/kg every 8 h intravenously or 800 mg five times daily orally for 7–10 days, halts the progression of herpes zoster in *immunocompromised* patients and is most effective when started within 3 days of the beginning of the eruption. Effects are less cutaneous and visceral dissemination, cessation of new vesicle formation, and reduced pain. The modest benefit of acyclovir, valacyclovir (Valtrex), and famciclovir (Famvir) for the *otherwise healthy* patients may not justify the expense, except in severe infections and in patients more than 50 years old, to reduce post-herpetic neuralgia. The use of corticosteroids in otherwise healthy patients to prevent post-herpetic neuralgia has been advocated, but has not been convincingly proven to be worthwhile. Amitriptyline (Elavil) at a dosage of 50–100 mg daily, or gabapentin (Neurontin) 100–300 mg three times daily, may be helpful in managing post-herpetic neuralgia once it occurs. Capsaicin analgesic cream 0.075% (Zostrix-HP), used topically three or four times daily on affected skin, can also provide pain relief. Caution must be maintained to avoid inadvertent contact with the eyes or unaffected skin, because capsaicin normally produces transient burning. Foscarnet is indicated for resistant herpes zoster

Therapy for Herpes Zoster

Prevention
- Zoster vaccine live OKA/Merck

Initial
Antivirals[a]
- Acyclovir: 800 mg five times daily for 7 days, 10 mg/kg IV every 8 h for 5–7 days
- Valacyclovir: 1 g t.i.d. for 7 days
- Famciclovir: 500 mg t.i.d. for 7 days

Compresses
- Aluminum acetate

Pain Medication
- Analgesics
- Amitriptyline: 25–100 mg at bedtime
- Gabapentin: 100–300 mg t.i.d.

Alternative
- Foscarnet 40 mg/kg every 8 h for 10 days

[a]Treatment is optional in individuals with: (1) mild rash and pain; (2) eruption >72 h; (3) less than 50 years of age.

Course and Complications

The succession of lesions begins with macules, which develop into vesicles. Over the next several days, pustules develop and are followed by crusting and eventual healing in 2–3 weeks. Hemorrhagic bullae and gangrenous changes may occur, and may result in scarring.

Cutaneous dissemination of herpes zoster from the original dermatome develops in some patients, particularly immunocompromised patients in whom the condition is more likely to be severe and prolonged. It occurs within 5–7 days of the initial eruption and may be accompanied by fever, malaise, and prostration. The immunocompromised patient is susceptible to visceral involvement of the liver, lung, and central nervous system.

Post-herpetic neuralgia is uncommon in patients less than 40 years old, but 27%, 47%, and 73% of untreated adults older than 55, 60, and 70 years of age, respectively, develop this complication, which frequently is difficult to control and very troubling to the patient. Besides older age, the risk for developing post-herpetic neuralgia increases if you are female, have a prodrome, and have more severe acute pain and eruption. However, 80% of patients with post-herpetic neuralgia become asymptomatic within 12 months.

The nasociliary branch of the ophthalmic division of the trigeminal nerve innervates the eye and the tip of the nose. Therefore, herpes ophthalmicus should be suspected when herpes zoster involves the tip of the nose. Scarring of the cornea and conjunctiva may occur. Other occasional complications of herpes zoster are full-thickness skin necrosis and Bell's palsy.

> When herpes zoster involves the tip of the nose, suspect eye involvement.

Pathogenesis

After primary varicella infection (which the patient often does not recall), the virus becomes latent within the sensory nerve ganglia. With reactivation, replication again occurs with migration of the virus along the nerve to the skin. Viremia frequently occurs, sometimes resulting in disseminated lesions.

VARICELLA

Key Points

1. Generalized pruritic vesicles
2. Lesions in all stages
3. Treatment is usually symptomatic

Definition

Varicella (chickenpox) is an acute, highly contagious, intraepidermal vesicular eruption caused by varicella-zoster virus. Clinically, it appears as a generalized vesicular eruption (**Fig. 10.7A**).

Incidence

Varicella is predominantly a childhood disease, with 90% of cases occurring before the age of 10 years. Investigators estimated that 3.5–4.0 million cases occurred annually in the USA prior to the advent of vaccination. Chickenpox occurs throughout the year, but the incidence peaks sharply in March, April, and May. Varicella vaccine has

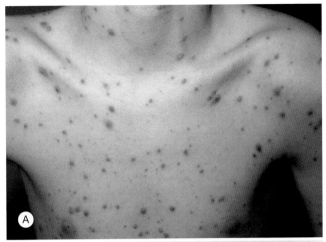
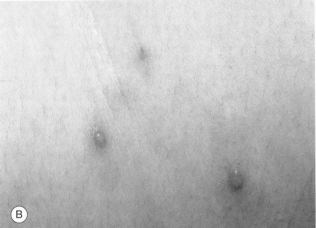
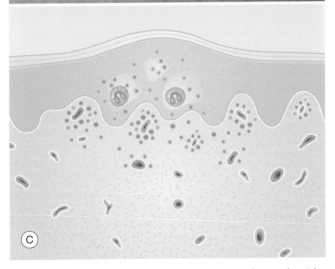

FIGURE 10.7 Varicella. A. Individual erythematous and crusted vesicles in a generalized distribution. **B.** 'Dewdrop' vesicle on a 'rose petal' erythematous base. **C.** Epidermis – bullae, multinucleated cells. Dermis – perivascular inflammation.

reduced the incidence of hospitalization greatly since its introduction.

History

After a 2–3-week incubation period, a 2–3-day prodrome of chills, fever, malaise, headache, sore throat, anorexia, and dry cough precedes the onset of the markedly pruritic vesicular eruption. The patient is infectious for approximately 1 week (1–2 days before the rash and a further 4–5 days until the vesicles have become crusted).

Physical Examination

Varicella is a generalized pruritic eruption that is most prominent on the trunk but also involves the head; the extremities including palms and soles; and the mucous membranes of the mouth and conjunctiva. It is characterized by successive crops of rapidly progressive lesions over an 8–12 h period. The lesions begin as macules, which quickly develop into papules, vesicles, and pustules. Crusting and, sometimes, necrosis precede healing. Characteristically, all types of lesions are present at the same time. The vesicles are 2–3 mm in diameter, occur on an erythematous base, and have a 'dewdrop on a rose petal' appearance (**Fig. 10.7B**). They are often umbilicated and hemorrhagic.

Differential Diagnosis

Before its eradication, *smallpox*, which is characterized by a febrile prodrome, lesions in the same stage of development, and centrifugal distribution, was the most important disease to exclude. The presence of lesions in all stages in varicella helped to differentiate it from *smallpox*, in which all lesions are in the *same stage* of development. *Disseminated herpes simplex, coxsackievirus,* and *echovirus,* as well as *rickettsialpox,* can produce vesicular eruptions similar to those of varicella. Diagnosing varicella usually is not difficult, but if there is any doubt, cultures can rule out these other infections.

> Chickenpox has all types of lesions: macules, papules, vesicles, pustules, and crusts.

Laboratory and Biopsy

The diagnosis of varicella is usually obvious. A Tzanck preparation reveals multinucleated giant cells typical of herpesvirus infection. Viral cultures, direct fluorescent antibody stain of vesicle smears, biopsy (**Fig. 10.7C**), and serologic studies may also be done to confirm the diagnosis, although usually these are not necessary. Culture of the varicella-zoster virus is difficult; therefore, direct identification of the virus in vesicle smears by immunofluorescent staining is the preferred test. The biopsy, which is rarely done, reveals an intraepidermal blister with multinucleated giant cells (**Fig. 10.7C**).

Therapy

The treatment of chickenpox is largely symptomatic. Antihistamines and topical agents such as calamine lotion are used to reduce itching. Baths (Aveeno) are used for their cleansing and anti-inflammatory actions. Aspirin should be avoided in children because of its association with Reye syndrome. Acyclovir (Zovirax) reduces complications in adults and immunosuppressed children. The use of acyclovir in immunologically normal children generally is not indicated unless rare visceral involvement is present, such as varicella pneumonia.

Varicella vaccination (Varivax) is safe and effective in healthy children and adults, especially in preventing moderately severe and severe cases. Passive immunization with varicella-zoster immune globulin (VZIG-VariZIG) is used in high-risk patients. VZIG is prepared from plasma containing high titers of varicella-zoster antibody. It is effective in preventing or modifying varicella infection in immunodeficient patients if it is administered shortly after exposure. VZIG is not given to patients with active disease. Patients with leukemia or lymphoma, those with congenital or acquired immune deficiency, those receiving immunosuppressive medication, and newborns of mothers who have varicella are candidates for treatment.

Therapy for Varicella

Prevention
- Varicella virus vaccine
- Varicella-zoster immune globulin

Initially for Symptomatic Infection
- Antihistamines:
  - Diphenhydramine: 25–50 mg q.i.d.; elixir – 12.5 mg/5 mL, 5 mg/kg daily in four divided doses
  - Hydroxyzine: 10–25 mg q.i.d.; syrup – 10 mg/5 mL, 2 mg/kg daily in four divided doses
- Oatmeal bath
- Calamine lotion

Alternative for Adults, Severe Infection, Immunosuppression
- Acyclovir: 20 mg/kg (800 mg max) orally q.i.d. for 5 days or 10 mg/kg intravenously every 8 h

---

Course and Complications

Approximately 100 deaths occurred each year in the USA as the result of varicella before vaccination was instituted. The major complications (pneumonia, encephalitis, and hepatitis) are disproportionately high in adults and in extremely young children. The estimated complication rate in children between the ages of 1 and 14 years includes encephalitis in 17 per 100 000 cases, Reye syndrome in 3.2 per 100 000 cases, and death in 2 per 100 000 cases. Approximately 200 per 100 000 patients with varicella require hospitalization. In adults, death occurs in 50 per 100 000 cases. The immunocompromised patient has a complication rate of 32%, with a 7% death rate.

> Morbidity and mortality rates are greatly increased in immunocompromised patients.

Varicella during pregnancy poses an approximately 10% risk of intrauterine infection of the fetus, resulting in congenital varicella syndrome or neonatal varicella, with devastating effects on the child.

Pathogenesis

Varicella primary infection begins in the nasopharynx. After local replication, viremia seeds the reticuloendothelial tissue. Secondary viremias cause dissemination to the skin and viscera. Varicella-zoster virus then enters a latent phase in the sensory ganglia.

UNCOMMON BLISTERING DISEASES

Bullous pemphigoid, dermatitis herpetiformis, epidermolysis bullosa, pemphigus vulgaris, and porphyria cutanea tarda are rare, blistering disorders that are important because of their significant mortality or morbidity (**Table 10.2**). They should be considered when the more common causes of blistering disease have been ruled out and appropriate laboratory data have been collected. Three of the five diseases – pemphigus vulgaris, bullous pemphigoid, and dermatitis herpetiformis – are examples of immunologically mediated disorders. Porphyria cutanea tarda is a metabolic disorder characterized by defective heme synthesis and excessive porphyrin production. Epidermolysis bullosa is a group of genetic disorders with mutations that produce structural defects in the epidermis or dermis.

BULLOUS PEMPHIGOID

Bullous pemphigoid is an autoimmune disorder characterized by large and tense blisters that occur on normal or erythematous/urticarial appearing skin (**Fig. 10.8A**). Subepidermal bullae (**Fig. 10.8B**) are characteristic

pathologic findings. The condition occurs in elderly patients (6th, 7th, and 8th decades). The preferred sites of involvement are the groin, axillae, and flexural areas. Approximately one-third of patients have oral involvement. The bullae do not extend laterally (negative Nikolsky's sign) like those of pemphigus vulgaris. Healing usually occurs without scarring.

Direct and indirect immunofluorescence studies reveal a linear band of IgG and complement C3 deposited along the basement membrane zone, where blister formation occurs (**Fig. 10.9**). The IgG autoantibodies are directed against two hemidesmosome-associated proteins (the bullous pemphigoid antigens, BP230 and BP180) in the basement membrane zone. These antigens are found intracellularly in association with the hemidesmosome and extracellularly in the lamina lucida, which is the uppermost portion of the basement membrane zone between the epidermis and dermis.

The prognosis is excellent, and the disease usually subsides after months or years. The tendency for the blistered skin to heal results in a low mortality rate. However, the morbidity caused by widespread blistering requires treatment with systemic steroids and immunosuppressive agents.

DERMATITIS HERPETIFORMIS

Dermatitis herpetiformis is a chronic, intensely pruritic, vesicular disease characterized by grouped (herpetiform) papules, vesicles, and urticarial plaques, which are distributed symmetrically on the elbows, knees, buttocks, low back, and shoulders (**Fig. 10.10A**). The vesicles are often not intact, secondary to scratching as a result of

TABLE 10.2 Uncommon blistering diseases

Disease	Pathogenesis	Physical Examination	Blister Location	Laboratory Test	Therapy
Bullous pemphigoid	Autoimmune	Tense bullae on inflamed or non-inflamed skin Flexor surfaces	Subepidermal	DIF (+) IgG and C3 basement membrane zone IIF (+)	Prednisone Azathioprine Methotrexate
Dermatitis herpetiformis	Immune complex?	Excoriated, crusted papules, vesicles, and urticarial plaques Elbows, knees, back, buttocks	Subepidermal	DIF (+) IgA dermal papillae IIF (+)	Dapsone Sulfapyridine Gluten-free diet
Epidermolysis bullosa simplex	Gene mutation	Tense bullae on hands and feet	Intraepidermal	Biopsy	Prevent trauma, wound care
Pemphigus vulgaris	Autoimmune	Flaccid bullae, erosions, and crusts Generalized	Intraepidermal	DIF (+) IgG and C3 intercellular in epidermis IIF (+)	Prednisone Azathioprine Methotrexate, mycophenolate mofetil, rituximab Gold
Porphyria cutanea tarda	Metabolic	Tense bullae, crusted erosions, milia Dorsum of hands	Subepidermal	Raised urinary uroporphyrin DIF (+) IIF (−)	Phlebotomy Antimalarials

DIF, direct immunofluorescence; Ig, immunoglobulin; C3, complement; IIF, indirect immunofluorescence; +, positive; −, negative.

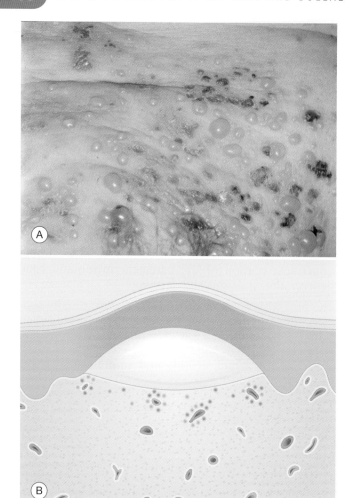

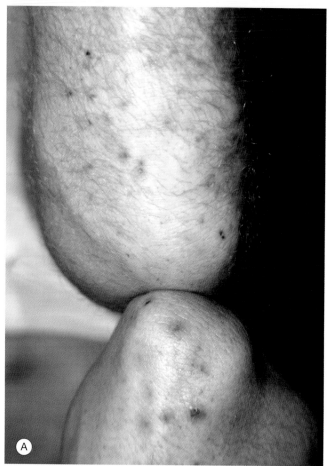

FIGURE 10.8 **Bullous pemphigoid. A.** Tense bullae on non-inflammatory skin and crusted residual bullae. **B.** Dermis – subepidermal bulla.

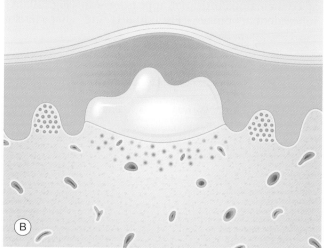

FIGURE 10.10 **Dermatitis herpetiformis. A.** Crusted vesicles on the elbow and knee – typical distribution. **B.** Dermis – subepidermal bulla, neutrophils in dermal papillae.

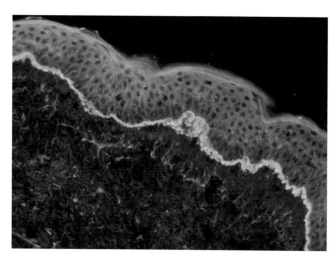

FIGURE 10.9 **Bullous pemphigoid** – direct and indirect immuno-fluorescent staining shows linear deposit of immunoglobulin G or complement at the dermal–epidermal junction.

intense pruritus. The disease usually begins in early adult life, and the general health of the patient is otherwise excellent.

Because of scratching, excoriations, rather than vesicles, may be all that is seen.

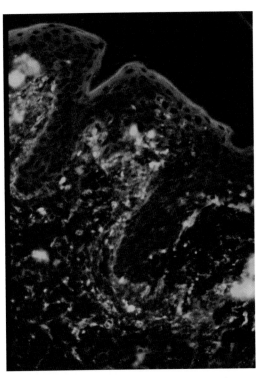

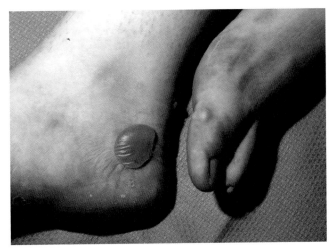

FIGURE 10.12 **Epidermolysis bullosa simplex** – tense bullae in areas of friction on the feet.

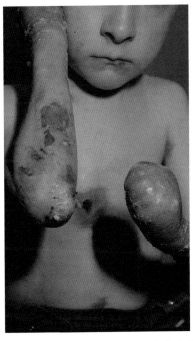

FIGURE 10.11 **Dermatitis herpetiformis** – direct and indirect immuno-fluorescent staining shows granular deposits of immunoglobulin A in the tips of dermal papillae.

The typical histologic change of dermatitis herpetiformis is a subepidermal blister (**Fig. 10.10B**) with neutrophilic abscesses in the dermal papillae. Direct immunofluorescence testing demonstrates granular deposits of IgA at the tips of the dermal papillae (**Fig. 10.11**). Indirect immunofluorescence testing for IgA antiendomysial antibodies is also sensitive and specific.

Dermatitis herpetiformis characteristically clears rapidly after treatment with dapsone or sulfapyridine, although the disease recurs promptly when therapy is stopped. Approximately 75% of patients have associated (but usually asymptomatic) gluten-sensitive enteropathy. In these patients, a strict gluten-free diet causes remission or allows a significant reduction of the medication dose.

EPIDERMOLYSIS BULLOSA: SIMPLEX AND RECESSIVE DYSTROPHIC TYPES

Epidermolysis bullosa is a group of disorders characterized by mutations in genes that encode for the structural proteins of the epidermis and dermis. This results in epidermal, junctional, and subepidermal blisters produced by minor friction or trauma. These genodermatoses range in severity from being relatively minor to being severely disabling and fatal. Epidermolysis bullosa simplex (**Fig. 10.12**) has blistering limited to the hands and feet, and is caused by dominant keratin 5 and 14 gene mutations. This defect produces keratinocyte fragility and intraepidermal cleavage. Recessive dystrophic epidermolysis bullosa (**Fig. 10.13**) results from mutations in the gene encoding type VII collagen, *COL7A1*. The severe form is characterized by 'mitten-like' deformity of

FIGURE 10.13 **Recessive dystrophic epidermolysis bullosa** – 'mitten' deformity.

the hands and feet, contractures, blistering and scarring of the mouth and eyes, esophageal strictures, growth retardation, anemia, and nutritional deficiency. Treatment of epidermolysis bullosa is symptomatic and supportive including protection from trauma, good wound care, treatment of infections, and nutritional supplements.

PEMPHIGUS VULGARIS

Pemphigus vulgaris is an autoimmune disease characterized by blistering of the skin and mucous membranes. It occurs predominantly in middle and old age, with an estimated incidence of 1 per 100 000. The bullae are flaccid and superficial, and range from 1 to 10 cm in size. They

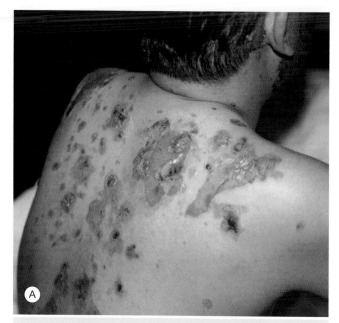

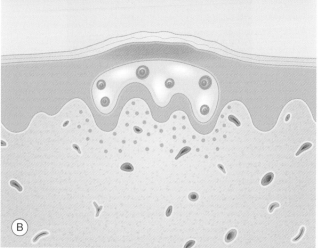

FIGURE 10.14 **Pemphigus vulgaris. A.** Flaccid bullae and erosions. **B.** Epidermis – suprabasal bulla, acantholytic epidermal cells.

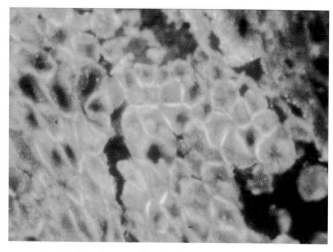

FIGURE 10.15 **Pemphigus vulgaris** – direct and indirect immunofluorescent staining shows.

autoantibodies and epidermal cell surface antigens (adhesion molecule desmoglein 3) contained in intercellular adhering junctions (desmosomes) leads to blister formation. In addition, the production of proteolytic enzymes that hydrolyze the cell surface proteins causes loss of adhesion between keratinocytes.

Before the introduction of systemic steroids, pemphigus vulgaris was associated with an extremely high mortality rate. Systemic steroids and immunosuppressive agents such as methotrexate, cyclophosphamide, azathioprine, mycophenolate mofetil, gold, and rituximab are used. The overall mortality rate is 8–10%, and death now occurs more frequently as a result of steroid-induced complications than from the disease. Two other major types of pemphigus are pemphigus foliaceus and paraneoplastic pemphigus.

> Untreated pemphigus vulgaris has a high mortality rate.

rupture easily, leaving large denuded, bleeding, weeping, and crusted erosions (**Fig. 10.14**). Pressure applied laterally to the bulla results in extension (Nikolsky's sign). The oral mucosa (erosions of the mouth) is almost always involved, and is frequently the presenting site.

> The bullae break easily, leaving erosions and crusts.

The bulla of pemphigus vulgaris occurs intraepidermally, just above the basal layer (**Fig. 10.14B**). It is formed by the loss of cohesion between epidermal cells (acantholysis). Direct (with patient skin) and indirect (with patient serum) immunofluorescence studies are positive, showing deposits of immunoglobulins (Ig) (predominantly IgG) or complement C3 between epidermal cells (intercellular space) (**Fig. 10.15**). Experimental evidence suggests that the interaction between the circulating IgG

PORPHYRIA CUTANEA TARDA

The porphyrias are a group of disorders characterized by abnormalities in the heme biosynthetic pathway resulting in abnormal porphyrin metabolism and excessive accumulation of various porphyrins. Porphyria cutanea tarda is the most common form of porphyria. It is characterized by subepidermal blisters on the hands and excessive uroporphyrin excretion in the urine. Bullae, vesicles, erosions, crusts, milia, and mild scarring occur on sun-exposed skin, especially the dorsum of the hands (**Fig. 10.16A**). Facial hair, predominantly on the temples and cheeks, and mottled facial pigmentation resembling melasma also occur.

The bullae of porphyria cutanea tarda occur subepidermally (**Fig. 10.16B**). Direct immunofluorescence reveals immunoglobulin and complement around the dermal blood vessels and at the dermal–epidermal junction. The metabolic changes in porphyria cutanea tarda are

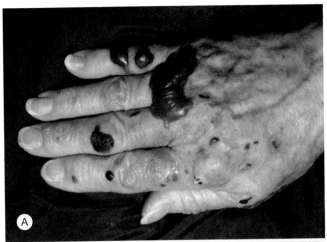

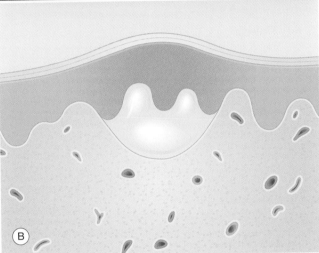

FIGURE 10.16 **Porphyria cutanea tarda. A.** Tense hemorrhagic bullae on the dorsal hand, the classic location. **B.** Dermis – subepidermal bulla.

diagnostic, so immunofluorescence testing is not warranted. Characteristically, urinary levels of uroporphyrins and coproporphyrins are markedly raised, with a ratio of uroporphyrin to coproporphyrin of at least 3:1. Liver function test results and serum iron levels are usually increased. The urine is dark brown and fluoresces orange-red under Wood's light. *Variegate porphyria* and hereditary coproporphyria have neurologic and abdominal symptoms as well as the same cutaneous findings as porphyria cutanea tarda. The ratio of urinary uroporphyrin to coproporphyrin is 1:1 in variegate porphyria and further serum or fecal porphyrin measurements are necessary to diagnose hereditary coproporphyria.

Variegate porphyria, hereditary coproporphyria, and porphyria cutanea tarda have identical skin findings.

Porphyria cutanea tarda is familial or sporadic. It is often precipitated by alcohol, hepatitis C, or hormones (contraceptive pills). It is also strongly associated with hereditary hemochromatosis. The biosynthetic pathway for heme requires the conversion of uroporphyrinogen to coproporphyrinogen by the enzyme uroporphyrinogen decarboxylase. When this enzyme is absent, uroporphyrins accumulate and produce porphyria cutanea tarda. The treatment of choice is phlebotomy or antimalarials when these drugs are used cautiously in low dosage.

11 Inflammatory Papules

Chapter Contents

Key Points

1. Itching is usually prominent
2. Primary lesion is usually a papule
3. Skin biopsy when needed confirms clinical suspicion

ABSTRACT

The common diseases discussed in this chapter are characterized by discrete, small, erythematous papules that do *not* become confluent. Most of these disorders are pruritic, some markedly so. As a result, the papules are often crusted secondary to excoriation. Papules are common primary lesions found in numerous skin diseases, including acne, eczematous diseases, and the scaling disorders. However, in these diseases, other features are present that allow for their characterization. For example, comedones and pustules accompany papules in acne, eczematous papules coalesce into plaques in atopic dermatitis, and plaques as well as papules are present in psoriasis. The diseases in this chapter feature individual papules as the predominant finding or primary lesion (**Table 11.1**). History and physical exam often establish the diagnosis but a biopsy, when needed, confirms the clinical suspicion.

INSECT BITE REACTIONS

Key Points

1. Immediate hives after insult suggest the diagnosis
2. Develop only in people who are allergic
3. Insect stings, not insect bites, are a common cause of anaphylaxis

Definition

Insect bites, stings, and infestations produce local inflammatory reactions (**Fig. 11.1**) in response to injected foreign chemicals and protein. Acute skin reactions appear as hives, and more chronic reactions appear as inflammatory papules. Insects that sting (usually when threatened) include bees, wasps, and fire ants. Insects that bite (usually out of hunger) include mosquitoes, fleas, flies, bedbugs, and lice. Spiders, ticks, and chiggers are other arthropods that sometimes attack human skin.

Incidence

Most insect bites are recognized as such and are not brought to a physician's attention. Anaphylactic reactions occur in 0.5–1.5% of stings. In the USA, yellow jackets are the leading cause of allergic insect sting reactions. In southern USA, fire ants are the leading cause of these reactions.

History

When someone is stung by an insect, the insult is usually remembered because the sting induces immediate pain. This is not always the case for biting insects; some delay may occur between the actual bite and the itching that follows. If the physical examination suggests insect bites (even when the patient is unaware of having been bitten), the history should be pursued carefully for possible exposures. For indoor exposure, fleas are common offenders. We inquire not only about pets currently living in the dwelling but also about whether pets recently occupied the premises. If a house had been occupied previously by flea-infested pets, the abandoned hungry fleas may form a welcoming party for the newly arrived human guests. We also ask about pets in homes visited by the patient. Spiders are sometimes responsible for indoor bites; their

TABLE 11.1 Papules

	Frequency (%)[a]	Etiology	History	Physical Examination	Differential Diagnosis	Laboratory Test
Insect bite reactions	0.7	Stinging and biting arthropods	Insect often not seen by patient	Papules with central puncta, and often *grouped* *Asymmetric* distribution	Urticaria Impetigo Mucha–Habermann disease	–
Keratosis pilaris	Not known	Unknown	Bothersome rough bumps	Follicular, monomorphic papules Extensor arms and thighs and facial checks	Acne Lichen nitidus Lichen spinulosus	–
Lichen planus	0.6	Unknown	–	Purple, polygonal flat-topped papules with Wickham's striae Can be generalized: wrists, ankles, and *mucous membranes* favored	Lupus erythematosus Lichen planus-like drug eruption Graft-versus-host disease	Biopsy
Miliaria	0.1	Sweat duct occlusion	Fever or occlusion of affected skin	Numerous small papules Trunk, especially back, usually affected	Contact dermatitis Folliculitis Candidiasis	Biopsy (not usually necessary)
Scabies	1.5	Mite	Other close contacts often affected	*Burrows* (when found) diagnostic Generalized distribution sparing head Genitalia often affected	Essential dermatitis	Scraping

[a]Percentage of new dermatology patients with this diagnosis seen in the Hershey Medical Center Dermatology Clinic, Hershey, PA.

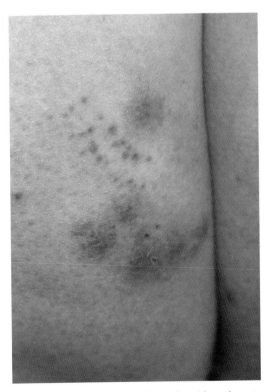

FIGURE 11.1 **Insect bites.** Grouped red papules with erythematous flare.

presence requires a careful search of the home. Bedbugs are becoming an increasingly recognized household insect that likes to bite in groups of three, commonly referred to as 'breakfast, lunch, and dinner' (**Fig. 11.2**). Bedbugs often infest bats and birds and then hide in cracks and crevices, attacking the sleeping victim. Infestations with head lice often occur epidemically in school children, so a history of affected playmates should be sought and the school nurse consulted.

'Indoor' insects:
1. Fleas
2. Spiders
3. Bedbugs
4. Lice

Contrary to some misconceptions, it is not necessary for other persons dwelling in the same household to be affected. For insect bite reactions, two factors are required: a biting insect and a host who is allergic to the bite. Not all people are sensitive, and not all people attract insects equally.

Papules occur only in people who are allergic and who attract the insects.

Physical Examination

The reaction to a sting is usually an immediate hive, often with a central punctum, that resolves within a few hours. Large local reactions, manifesting as extensive erythema

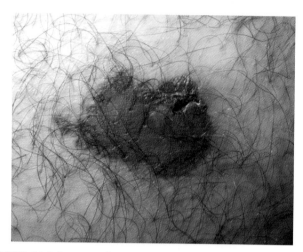

FIGURE 11.3 **Brown recluse spider bite** – impending necrotic skin reaction.

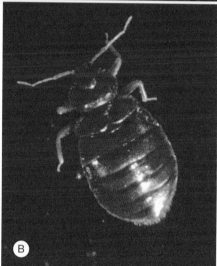

FIGURE 11.2 **A.** Bedbug insect bites – characteristic 'breakfast, lunch, and dinner.' **B.** Recovered bedbug – *Cimex lenticularis*.

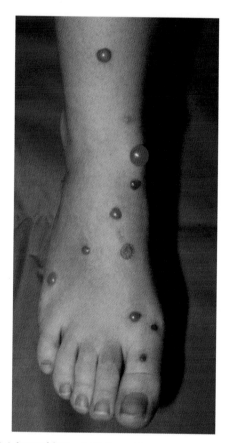

FIGURE 11.4 **Insect bites** – multiple vesicles.

and swelling at the bite site, resolve after several days. Of the stinging insects, only the honey bee leaves behind its stinger, which on close inspection appears as a sharp barb projecting from the skin. If found, this stinger should be removed gently to prevent release of additional venom from the attached venom sack. Fire ants produce multiple itching hives, which quickly progress to painful papulovesicles and pustules. The bite of a recluse spider is unique in that it produces a severe local necrotic reaction with ulceration (**Fig. 11.3**). Although the bite may be 'quiet,' the reaction that ensues over the following days is not. Chiggers favor the legs and areas of tight-fitting clothing where they produce inflammatory papules and vesicles, and occasionally even bullae (**Fig. 11.4**). Ticks painlessly burrow their heads in the skin, and pubic lice (pediculosis pubis) attach to hair; both can be visualized macroscopically. Head lice (pediculosis capitis) may be difficult to find but should be suspected in the presence of itching of the scalp, particularly the occiput or peripheral scalp (**Fig. 11.5**). The eggs (nits) are most often found and appear as small, 2–3-mm, oval, translucent concretions affixed to hair shafts. Similar findings occur in body lice (pediculosis corporis) and pubic lice (crabs, pediculosis pubis).

Physicians are most often consulted for insect bites that produce itching papules. These typically are grouped and asymmetric. Flea bites frequently occur in streaks of three: 'breakfast, lunch, and dinner.' Sometimes, a central punctum can be identified in the papule; this is diagnostic. If the offending insects remain in the environment, new lesions will continue to appear. Occasionally, only excoriations are found.

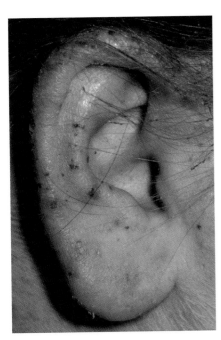

FIGURE 11.5 **Lice** – multiple vesicles; excoriated papules and white nits in hair.

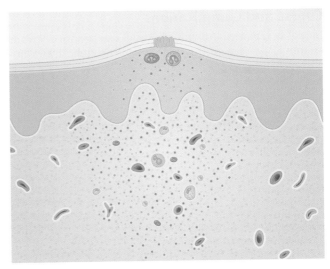

FIGURE 11.6 **Insect bite reaction.** Epidermis – crust; spongiosis; inflammation cell infiltrate. Dermis – dense infiltrate of mixed inflammatory cells, often including eosinophils.

Differential Diagnosis

For patients with urticarial reactions, other causes of urticaria (see Ch. 16) may be considered. When the hive has a central punctum, however, its cause is an insect bite. *Other foreign bodies* can induce pruritic papules in the skin. Fiberglass is an example. This diagnosis can be suggested by the history, and confirmed by the presence of refractile material in the epidermis on biopsy or skin scraping. *Dermatitis herpetiformis* (see Ch. 10) is in the differential diagnosis, particularly when only excoriations are found. Excoriation may also lead to secondary infection and a diagnosis of impetigo (see Ch. 12). An uncommon idiopathic disorder, *Mucha–Habermann disease*, presents with scattered necrotic papules and vesicles that can resemble insect bites but are usually more generalized and symmetric. A skin biopsy helps to distinguish Mucha–Habermann disease from an insect bite reaction (see later in this chapter).

Laboratory and Biopsy

The diagnosis is usually made clinically. Skin testing with commercial venom kits can be performed by an allergist. A biopsy, if performed, shows a wedge-shaped superficial and deep cellular infiltrate, so dense that it may be mistaken for malignant lymphoma. An insect bite is suggested by virtue of a mixed inflammatory cell infiltrate, which includes numerous eosinophils (**Fig. 11.6**).

Therapy

The primary therapy is to remove the offending insect from the environment of the patient, or vice versa. Insects that are attached to the skin can be gently removed with tweezers (e.g., ticks) or killed chemically (e.g., lice) with agents such as permethrin creme rinse (Nix). For lice, fomite transmission is proven as adult lice can live away

from human host for 3 days and nits can live for 10 days. Most lice treatments are pediculicidal, but not ovicidal, and require a retreatment in 7–10 days. For fleas, not only must the pet be treated, but also the house must be professionally fumigated. Insect repellent containing diethyltoluamide (DEET) remains a safe and effective deterrent to insect bites, especially ticks, with lowest effective dose of approximately 30%. Permethrin application to clothing also repels ticks, agents responsible for Lyme disease (see Ch. 16) and Rocky Mountain spotted fever. Colognes, perfumes, and scented hair sprays can attract insects and should be avoided in sensitive individuals.

> Successful treatment of flea bites includes fumigation of the home.

Treatment of the inflammatory reaction of the skin is symptomatic. Topical steroids, systemic antihistamines, and occasionally systemic steroids may be helpful in relieving the itching.

Therapy for Insect Bite Reactions

Initial
- Separation of host from insect
  - Lice: topical permethrin
  - Fleas: house fumigation
  - Bedbugs: house fumigation
  - Ticks: DEET repellent and permethrin on clothing
- Symptomatic therapy for itching:
  - Topical steroids
  - Antihistamines

Alternative
- Lice: topical benzyl alcohol and malathion
- Symptomatic therapy for itching:
  - Systemic steroids

Course and Complications

In highly sensitive individuals, stings can produce serious anaphylactic reactions, mediated through immunoglobulin E, that occasionally result in death. Patients with anaphylactic reactions require prompt therapy with epinephrine, antihistamines, and, often, systemic steroids. Patients with severe reactions are likely to have severe reactions to future stings. Subsequent 'desensitization' immunotherapy is frequently indicated for future prophylaxis. Immunotherapy is not necessary, however, in most children with urticarial reactions, even when these reactions are severe and generalized, as long as symptoms are confined to the skin. It is advisable, however, for such patients to have injectable epinephrine (Ana-Kit, EpiPen) readily available, especially when picnicking, hiking, or camping.

Most insect bite reactions resolve spontaneously and uneventfully. Secondary infection may occur, particularly when the patient has been scratching excessively. Scratching and infection can lead to scarring. A persistent local reaction to the bite of an infected deer tick is a characteristic finding in Lyme disease and is called *erythema migrans* (see Ch. 16).

Pathogenesis

Most insect bite reactions are the result of host allergy to injected secretions, including venoms (from stinging insects) and enzymes. Histamine, acetylcholine, and other vasoactive chemicals have also been isolated from the venom of stinging insects, and these, too, may play a role in the immediate reaction. However, the primary mechanism for insect bite reactions is allergic. The degree of host allergy determines the intensity of the reaction, which ranges from none to severe. As exemplified by *erythema migrans*, cutaneous reactions to insect bites may also be caused by microorganisms transmitted by the bite.

KERATOSIS PILARIS

Key Points

1. Involves extensor arms and thighs and face
2. Follicular papules
3. Appearance is bothersome

Definition

Keratosis pilaris is a disorder characterized by keratinized hair follicles. Monomorphic, follicle-based papules with a central horny spine are located predominantly on the extensor upper arms and thighs, with the face less commonly affected (**Fig. 11.7**).

Incidence

Almost one-half of the population is affected by keratosis pilaris. It is most common in adolescents, especially

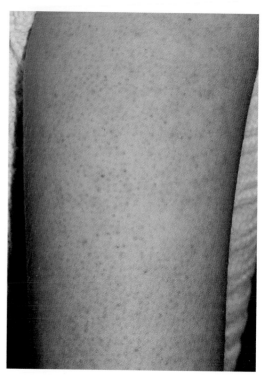

FIGURE 11.7 **Keratosis pilaris** – minute, rough, slightly inflamed papules on upper outer arm.

those with a history of dry skin. A positive family history is often present.

History

Patients often report 'rough bumps' that do not go away with washing, especially scrubbing. The condition is often mistaken for acne. Keratosis pilaris is not pruritic or painful. However, patients do not like their 'bumpy' appearance. Signs and symptoms worsen in the winter and improve with age.

Physical Examination

Keratosis pilaris is characterized by individual, small, follicular papules with a central horny spine. The lesions can be non-inflamed or inflamed. Keratosis pilaris is monomorphic. Common areas of involvement include the extensor upper arms and thighs, and, less commonly, the facial cheeks. With facial involvement, background erythema is commonly seen (**Fig. 11.8**).

Differential Diagnosis

Clinical recognition makes the diagnosis straightforward. To distinguish acne from keratosis pilaris involving the cheeks, look for pustules and comedones that are diagnostic of acne. Lichen spinulosus, which can appear clinically similar to keratosis pilaris, has a sudden onset, is located most commonly on the abdomen, extensor arms, knees, and neck, and may remit spontaneously after 1–2 years. The papules of lichen nitidus are flat-topped and not as rough as keratosis pilaris. In addition, koebnerization (linear streaks of papules) is seen in lichen nitidus, not keratosis pilaris.

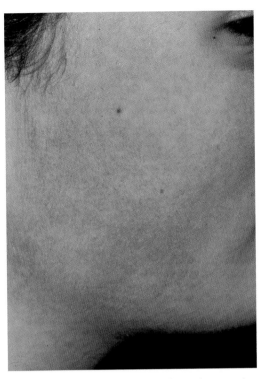

FIGURE 11.8 Keratosis pilaris – minute rough papules, sometimes better felt than seen, with background erythema on a child's face.

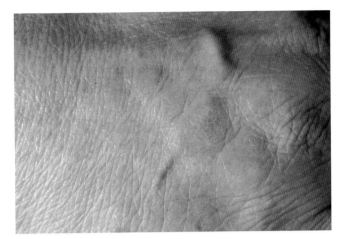

FIGURE 11.9 Lichen planus – flat-topped (planar) purple papules with Wickham's striae.

Laboratory and Biopsy

Keratosis pilaris is a straightforward clinical diagnosis. Laboratory work-up and biopsy are not necessary.

Therapy

Education and reassurance are the mainstays of treatment. An emollient cream can soften the rough papules. Therapeutic emollients containing 20% urea (Carmol 20), salicylic acid 6% (Keralyt), and ammonium lactate 12% (Lac-Hydrin, prescription only or AmLactin, available over the counter) have keratolytic properties, thereby decreasing corneocyte adhesion. Tretinoin cream 0.05% (Retin-A) can also be used successfully.

Therapy for Keratosis Pilaris

Initial
- Reassurance and education
- Therapeutic emollients
  - Urea 20%
  - Salicylic acid 6%
  - Ammonium lactate 12%

Alternative
- Tretinoin cream 0.05%

Course and Complications

Keratosis pilaris can improve with age but tends to be persistent, especially in individuals with a history of dry skin (e.g., ichthyosis vulgaris). Complications are uncommon.

Pathogenesis

Although the etiology of keratosis pilaris is unknown, abnormal keratinocyte desquamation most likely leads to keratin plugging of the hair follicle.

LICHEN PLANUS

Key Points

1. Purplish papules favor flexor wrists and distal lower extremities
2. Can affect hair, skin, nails, and mucous membranes
3. Biopsy confirms clinical suspicion

Definition

Lichen planus is an idiopathic inflammatory disorder of the skin. Clinically, the papules are flat (planus) and are surmounted by subtle, fine, white dots and lines that, with imagination, resemble the appearance of lichen (**Fig. 11.9**).

Lichen planus is characterized by five Ps:
1. Purplish
2. Planar
3. Pruritus
4. Polygonal
5. Papule

Incidence

The disorder is uncommon but not rare. It is the presenting problem in 6 per 1000 of the authors' new dermatology patients. The prevalence of lichen planus in the USA is estimated at 4.4 per 1000. Lichen planus occurs in children and adults.

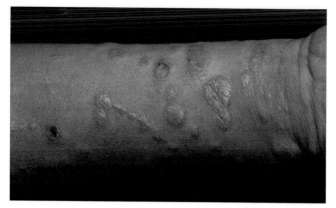

FIGURE 11.10 **Lichen planus** – papules in streaks (Koebner's phenomenon).

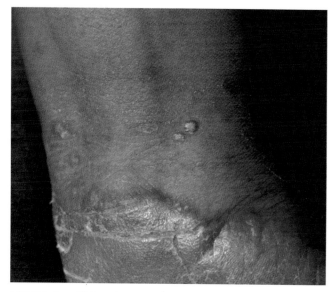

FIGURE 11.11 **Lichen planus** – palmar plaque with characteristic papule involving flexor wrist.

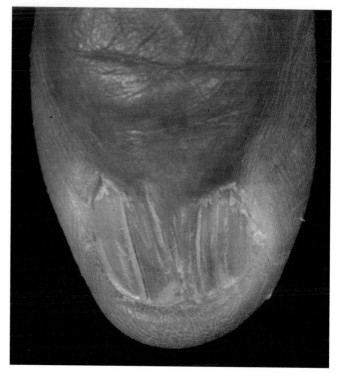

FIGURE 11.12 **Lichen planus** – nail matrix involvement leads to dystrophic nail.

generalized distribution. Uncommonly, individual lesions may attain plaque size. Residual hyperpigmented macules, more often appreciated in dark-skinned individuals, typically result from the inflammatory process. The nails and hair follicles are occasionally involved with dystrophic changes and even scarring (**Fig. 11.12**).

Mucous membrane involvement is common and, in some patients, is the sole manifestation of the disease. Most often, this condition appears as white streaks in a reticulate pattern (see Ch. 22). Blisters and erosions also sometimes occur. The buccal mucosa is affected most often, but the tongue, lips, and gums also may be involved (**Fig. 11.13**)

Differential Diagnosis

The white lines on the surface of violet lichen planus papules are often subtle, so the disease usually does not appear as a scaling disorder. Occasionally, however, more scale can be present, in which case, the papulosquamous disorders (see Ch. 9) must be considered, including *psoriasis*, *pityriasis rosea*, and *discoid lupus erythematosus*. Of these, *discoid lupus* is the most commonly confused, and in some patients, the two diseases may overlap. Lichen planus presenting with only a few scattered papules can be confused with *insect bites*. *Drug eruptions* can mimic lichen planus. Drugs that most often cause lichenoid eruptions are thiazides, phenothiazines, gold, quinidine, and the antimalarials quinacrine and chloroquine. When the palms and soles are involved, a serologic test for syphilis should be performed to rule out *secondary syphilis*. Some patients with *graft-versus-host disease* also develop a skin eruption that closely resembles lichen planus both

History

The major complaint is itching, which is often severe. Mucous membrane involvement sometimes results in painful erosions. Lichen planus-like eruptions can be induced by drugs, so a careful drug history should be elicited.

Physical Examination

The primary lesion is a purple, polygonal, flat-topped papule. Its surface has a fine reticulate pattern of white dots and lines (Wickham's striae) that can be visualized on *close* inspection. Wickham's striae are more readily visible through a hand-held lens after the application of a drop of oil on the surface of the papule. The papules are sometimes arranged in streaks, presumably resulting from the trauma of scratching (Koebner's phenomenon; **Fig. 11.10**). The wrists and ankles are favored locations for lichen planus, but any area may be affected, including the palms, soles, and genitalia (**Fig. 11.11**). Patients may have only a few papules, or innumerable ones in a

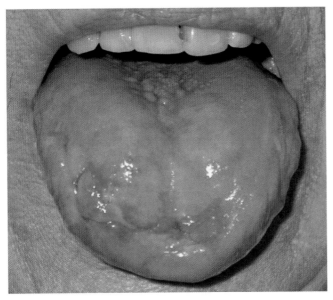

FIGURE 11.13 **Oral lichen planus** – ulcers on tongue require biopsy to exclude malignancy.

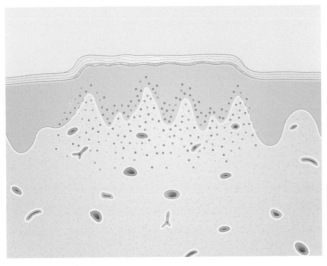

FIGURE 11.14 **Lichen planus.** Epidermis – hyperkeratosis; degeneration of the basal cell layer; 'saw-tooth' pattern of rete pegs. Dermis – dense, band-like, lymphocytic infiltrate in the upper dermis.

clinically and histopathologically. The differential diagnosis for mucous membrane involvement with lichen planus includes 'leukoplakia,' candidiasis, and secondary syphilis (see Ch. 22).

Drugs that can cause lichen planus-like eruptions:
1. Thiazides
2. Phenothiazines
3. Gold
4. Quinidine
5. Quinacrine
6. Chloroquine

Laboratory and Biopsy

If the clinical diagnosis is in doubt, a biopsy may be performed. In lichen planus, the histologic features are characteristic. The typical constellation of findings includes hyperkeratosis, thickened granular layer, degeneration of the basal cell layer, colloid bodies (necrotic basal cells), and a dense, 'band-like' inflammatory infiltrate in the papillary dermis that obscures and disrupts the dermal–epidermal junction (**Fig. 11.14**).

Therapy

The treatment is nonspecific and often not totally successful. The inflammatory reaction is suppressed with steroids. Localized disease is treated with strong topical steroids such as fluocinonide 0.05% cream, especially in children. For severe widespread disease, a course of systemic steroids is sometimes required, but caution is advised when administering these agents on a long-term basis because of the well known side-effects. Acitretin (Soriatane 25–50 mg daily) can clear cutaneous and oral lichen planus in more severe cases. Topical retinoids (e.g., tretinoin gel) and topical steroids (e.g., clobetasol gel) have been successful in some patients with mucous membrane lesions. Topical tacrolimus (Protopic) has also been used effectively for oral and cutaneous lichen planus. Cyclosporine has been used as a treatment of last resort in selected patients with severe disease.

Therapy for Lichen Planus

Initial
- Topical steroids (e.g., fluocinonide cream 0.1% b.i.d.)

Alternative
- Topical tacrolimus
- Systemic steroids
- Retinoids (acitretin)
- Cyclosporine

Course and complications

The course may be chronic, ranging from months to years. Almost two-thirds of patients experience spontaneous resolution within 1 year. Patients with mucous membrane involvement usually have a more prolonged course, often lasting years. Recurrences are uncommon, occurring in less than 20% of patients.

Serious complications are uncommon. Post-inflammatory hyperpigmentation may be cosmetically unpleasing but usually fades with time. Complications of mucous membrane lichen planus include candidiasis and squamous cell carcinoma.

Pathogenesis

The cause of lichen planus remains unknown. Evidence that immune factors play a role includes: (1) the finding of immunoglobulins at the dermal–epidermal junction in 95% of lichen planus lesions; (2) the observation that certain drug reactions can mimic lichen planus; and

(3) the occurrence of lichen planus-like eruptions in patients who have undergone bone marrow transplantation and who are experiencing a graft-versus-host reaction.

MILIARIA

> ### Key Points
>
> 1. Miliaria rubra and miliaria crystallina seen commonly in infants
> 2. Caused by occlusion of sweat ducts
> 3. Resolves with cooling and avoiding occlusion

Definition

Miliaria, or heat rash, represents an inflammatory reaction around a sweat duct. The reaction is caused by occlusion of the duct with extravasation of its contents into the surrounding tissue. Clinically, miliaria most often appears as multiple small papules (**Fig. 11.15**).

Incidence

Miliaria is an uncommon presenting complaint in the authors' outpatients. In the infant, heat rash is recognized by the parents and seldom causes them to seek a dermatologic consultation. However, it is seen frequently in hospitalized patients, in whom it is responsible for approximately 1% of the authors' inpatient consultations. It is more common in warm, humid environments, particularly in skin that has been occluded.

History

In the ambulatory patient, miliaria results from exposure to a hot, humid environment. In the bedridden patient, fever, sweating, and occlusion of the skin are predisposing factors. Pruritus is often the presenting complaint.

Physical Examination

Miliaria rubra is the most common form of miliaria and appears as multiple discrete, small, red papules. It occurs most often on the trunk, particularly the back. Although sweat ducts are not visible, miliaria is suspected when a patient has multiple small, discrete, uniform-size papules not associated with hair follicles. Less common variants are *miliaria crystallina*, with superficial non-inflamed vesicles containing crystal-clear fluid ('dewdrops'), commonly seen in infants (**Fig. 11.16**), and *miliaria pustulosa*, with erythematous pustules.

Differential Diagnosis

Miliaria rubra may be confused with *contact dermatitis*, but in contact dermatitis the papules tend to be confluent rather than discrete, and itching is often more pronounced. Miliaria pustulosa may be confused with *folliculitis*. In miliaria, the pustules are usually smaller and more numerous, and do not have a centrally placed hair. Sometimes, however, the two conditions coexist because they may share the same predisposing factor of occlusion. Candidiasis also occurs in moist occluded skin, but

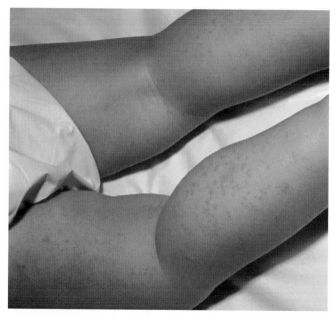

FIGURE 11.15 **Miliaria** – multiple red papules in an infant.

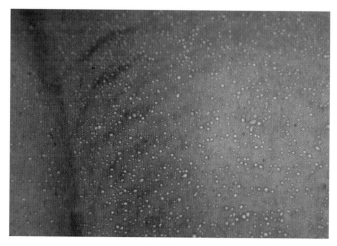

FIGURE 11.16 **Miliaria crystallina** – superficial, non-inflamed vesicles ('dewdrops').

the eruption is usually 'beefy red,' confluent, scaling, and surrounded by satellite papules and pustules. The word *milia* sounds similar to miliaria, but the condition it denotes is different. Milia are small, non-inflamed, superficial, epidermal keratin cysts often found on the face of young infants and adults.

> Miliaria is heat rash – milia are small, keratin-filled cysts.

Laboratory and Biopsy

The diagnosis is usually made clinically. For pustules, Gram-staining and culture rule out bacterial folliculitis. A potassium hydroxide preparation enables *Candida* to be identified. If a biopsy is performed, serial sections must be done to reveal the intraepidermal portion of the sweat duct, which is surrounded by spongiosis and a chronic inflammatory cell infiltrate in the epidermis and superficial dermis (**Fig. 11.17**).

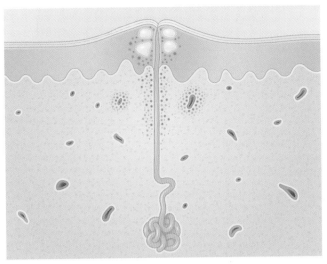

FIGURE 11.17 **Miliaria.** Epidermis – occluded sweat duct with underlying intraepidermal edema and inflammation. Dermis – superficial inflammatory cell infiltrate.

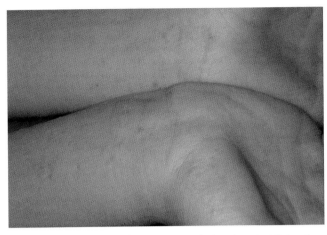

FIGURE 11.18 **Scabies** – inflammatory papules in a characteristic location.

Therapy

Therapy is directed at removing the predisposing conditions. Most important are cooling measures and air exposure for occluded skin. For ambulatory patients, this is easily accomplished. For bedridden patients, this means ensuring that the bed is dry and the patient turned frequently. Hydrocortisone lotion 1% can be applied to help relieve the itching, but this must be done sparingly to avoid any further contribution to the occlusive process.

Therapy for Miliaria

Initial
- Cooling measures
- Air exposure
- Topical steroid

Course and Complications

With decreasing heat and increasing air exposure, the condition resolves spontaneously within days. Complications are uncommon. Conditions that predispose to miliaria, however, can also contribute to coexisting infection with bacterial and candidal organisms.

Pathogenesis

Occlusion of the sweat duct is the primary event in the pathogenesis of miliaria. In miliaria rubra, this occurs within the epidermis at the level of the granular cell layer. Increased hydration appears to play the major role, resulting in swelling of the stratum corneum and compromise of the ductal lumina. After occlusion, sweat extravasates into the epidermis, where it produces an irritant reaction. In miliaria crystallina, sweat duct obstruction occurs in the stratum corneum. Experimentally, stripping of the stratum corneum with adhesive tape restores sweat flow, providing evidence that the occlusive process occurs in the stratum corneum. Bacteria and increased sweat

tonicity have also been implicated pathogenetically in miliaria, but their pathogenetic roles have not been proved conclusively.

SCABIES

Key Points

1. This is the worst itch of the patient's life
2. Burrows in characteristic locations are diagnostic
3. Treat entire body of patient and close contacts with topical agent

Definition

Scabies is an infestation of the epidermis with the 'itch' mite, *Sarcoptes scabiei* var. *hominis*. Clinically, a few burrows are usually found and are diagnostic. Inflammatory papules resulting from host hypersensitivity, however, constitute the more frequent and obvious findings (**Fig. 11.18**).

Incidence

Scabies is a common disease. It can occur endemically among school-age children, and may be hyperendemic among rural populations of less developed countries. Immobilized geriatric patients in nursing homes, patients with HIV/AIDS, and medically compromised patients (e.g., Down syndrome) are predisposed to infestation with high mite counts.

History

Generalized pruritus is the major complaint. Scabies causes the worst itch of the patient's life – often severe enough to interrupt sleep. Frequently, a history of itching can be elicited in family members and other close personal contacts. The incubation time from inoculation to the onset of pruritus is usually approximately 1 month, so in early cases, other contacts may not yet be symptomatic. Because scabies also occurs in pets (canine scabies), a pet history should be elicited, particularly in patients with recurrent disease.

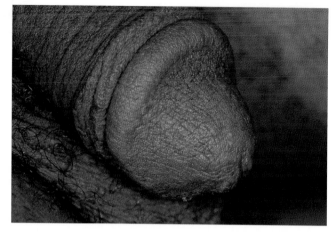

FIGURE 11.19 **Scabies** – papules on head of penis. This is scabies until proven otherwise!

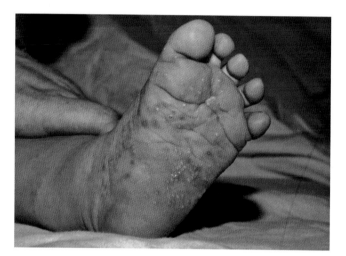

FIGURE 11.20 **Scabies** – vesicles on soles in infant.

Itching is often severe enough to interrupt sleep.

Family members and friends often also itch.

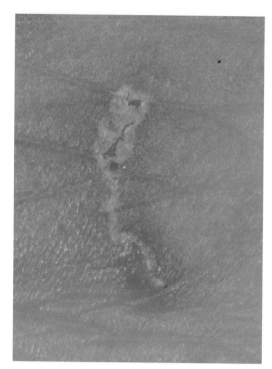

FIGURE 11.21 **Diagnostic burrow.**

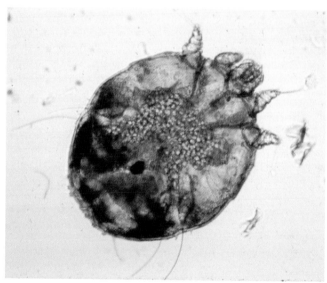

FIGURE 11.22 **Scabies mite** (×400).

Physical Examination

Small inflammatory papules predominate. They are often excoriated. The distribution is generalized, but favored locations include the finger webs, wrists, elbows, axillae, girdle area, and feet. In addition, the male genitalia are usually involved (**Fig. 11.19**). Itching papules and small nodules on the penis should be considered the result of scabies unless proved otherwise. In temperate climates, the head is almost always spared in adults but may be involved in children. In infants, vesicles may also be present, particularly on the palms and soles (**Fig. 11.20**).

The diagnostic finding is a burrow, which appears as a 2–5-mm, delicate, white, serpiginous, superficial, thread-like line (**Fig. 11.21**). The most common location for burrows is on the hands. With close inspection, a tiny black speck can often be seen at the end of the burrow.

This black dot represents the adult mite, which is best visualized under the microscope. In some patients with scabies, particularly when the condition has been long-standing, scattered nodules may also be found.

Differential Diagnosis

Because of the intense pruritus, in some patients, only excoriations are seen. In these patients, a misdiagnosis of neurotic excoriations could be made. Widespread disease may be misdiagnosed as *essential dermatitis*.

Laboratory and Biopsy

The presence of mites or eggs is diagnostic (**Fig. 11.22**). This is accomplished by a skin scraping with a no. 15

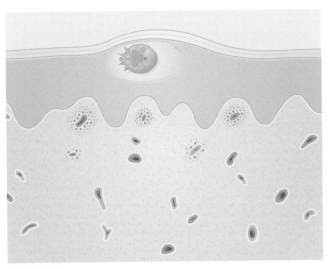

FIGURE 11.23 **Epidermis** – mite burrowed in superficial epidermis. Dermis – inflammation.

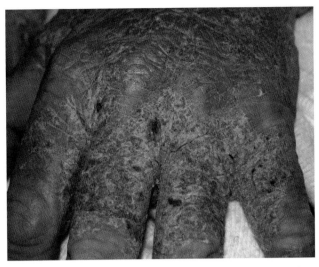

FIGURE 11.24 **Crusted scabies.** Crusted plaque with high mite load.

blade, as described in Chapter 3. The highest yield is from a black dot at the burrow, but mites and eggs also can be recovered from papules and nodules.

A biopsy is usually not necessary but may provide the diagnosis when it previously had not been suspected. Microscopically, one sees edema in the epidermis, which may be sufficient to result in a microvesicle. An inflammatory reaction occurs in the superficial dermis with lymphocytes and eosinophils. A fortuitous but diagnostic finding is the presence of a mite in the stratum corneum (**Fig. 11.23**).

Therapy

Permethrin cream (Elimite) is considered the drug of choice. The topical agent must be applied to the *entire body surface*, including under fingernails. A *single application* of 5% permethrin cream is applied at bedtime from the head to the toes and is washed off in the morning. Some physicians recommend a single reapplication after 1 week, but no controlled studies have documented that two applications are better than one. Permethrin cream is preferred for infants older than 2 months of age and for pregnant females. Treatment at the same time is recommended for household contacts; those who are asymptomatic require only one application. Clothes and bed linens can be decontaminated by machine washing at a hot temperature.

> The entire body is treated.

Most recently, systemic ivermectin has been used successfully for treating scabies. A single oral dose of 0.1–0.2 mg/kg is sufficient for cure in most patients, although residual itching may persist for up to 1 month after this systemic treatment. Ivermectin may require repeated treatment in 1 week. Ivermectin is often used in outbreaks in institutions such as a nursing home.

Therapy for Scabies

Initial
- Permethrin cream 5%

Alternative
- Ivermectin: 0.1–0.2 mg/kg

Course and Complications

When untreated, itching progresses and may become unbearable. After treatment, many patients continue to itch for 1–2 weeks. This possibility must be explained so that the patient avoids overuse of the medication. Residual itching can be treated symptomatically with topical steroids and oral antihistamines. Nodules, if present, may last for 1 month or longer.

> Itching may persist for 1–2 weeks after treatment.

Complications are uncommon. Secondary bacterial infection may occur in excoriated skin. In immunocompromised patients (particularly patients with AIDS), patients with Down syndrome, and debilitated patients with neurologic disorders, scabies may appear as a widespread, crusted eruption that often *does not* itch. This uncommon variant is called crusted scabies (Norwegian scabies) and is easily misdiagnosed as eczema or psoriasis (**Fig. 11.24**). On close inspection, however, burrows and mites are usually numerous, and their presence confirms the diagnosis.

> Crusted scabies occurs in immunosuppressed and debilitated patients.

Pathogenesis

The discovery in 1687 of the 'itch mite' made this parasite one of the first causes of human disease to be identified.

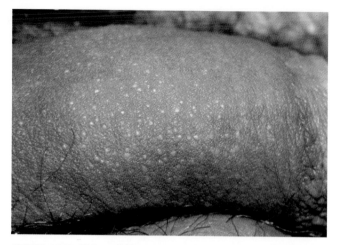

FIGURE 11.25 **Lichen nitidus** – minute, flat-topped papules with shiny appearance.

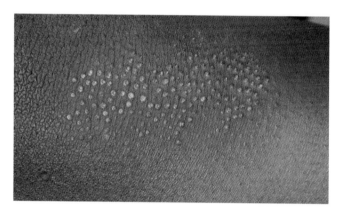

FIGURE 11.26 **Lichen spinulosus** – grouped follicular papules with central keratosis spine located on the knee.

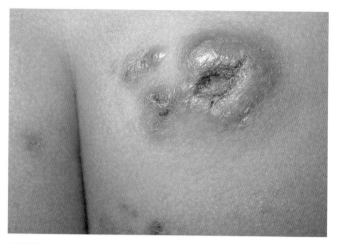

FIGURE 11.27 **Lymphomatoid papulosis** – papules and nodules with necrotic centers on the buttocks.

The *S. scabiei* mite lives in and on human skin, where it completes its life cycle in approximately 2 weeks. The impregnated female burrows into the stratum corneum, where she lays two or three eggs daily for as long as 30 days. Each egg produces a larva, which leaves the burrow and molts to produce a nymph. Several further moltings result in a mature mite, which then mates. After mating, the male dies, and the female completes the life cycle by burrowing back into the stratum corneum. Secretions from the burrowing female mite cause intraepidermal edema fluid, on which she feeds.

The itching and inflammation are thought to be a result of a hypersensitivity reaction by the host to the foreign material (i.e., mites, eggs, and feces) in the skin. This may account for the persistence of the itching for 1–2 weeks after successful treatment; it may take that long for the stratum corneum to turn over and to shed the foreign material, and for the hypersensitivity reaction to subside.

During the Second World War, studies were performed on the natural history and the contagious nature of scabies. From these studies, the following were found:

1. It is difficult to transmit scabies through fomites such as bedding and clothing (human-to-human transmission is most common).

2. The incubation time from inoculation to itching usually is approximately 1 month.
3. Untreated, the course is one of progressive itching.
4. Previously infested individuals are more difficult to reinfest, possibly because the hypersensitivity reaction is partially protective.

UNCOMMON INFLAMMATORY PAPULES

LICHEN NITIDUS

Lichen nitidus is an uncommon eruption of minute, flat-topped papules with a shiny appearance (**Fig. 11.25**). Common areas of involvement include the upper extremities, dorsal hands, genitalia, and trunk. Unlike lichen planus, oral involvement is rarely appreciated and the lesions rarely itch. Skin biopsy shows the characteristic finding of the 'ball and claw' configuration: inflammatory cells (the ball) held between elongated rete ridges of the epidermis (the claw). Treatment is directed at the symptoms, with spontaneous resolution occurring within several years.

LICHEN SPINULOSUS

Lichen spinulosus is characterized by the sudden onset of symmetrically distributed, often grouped patches of follicular papules that are topped by a centrally located keratotic spine (**Fig. 11.26**). It affects mainly children and young adults. Lichen spinulosus can occur on the abdomen, extensor arms, knees, and neck. No cure exists, but most cases remit spontaneously in 1–2 years.

LYMPHOMATOID PAPULOSIS

This uncommon, chronic disorder occurs mostly in adults but can affect children. It is similar to PLEVA (see below), but the lesions tend to be larger and fewer in number. The primary lesion is an inflammatory papule that commonly develops with a necrotic center (**Fig. 11.27**). Spontaneous healing often occurs with a

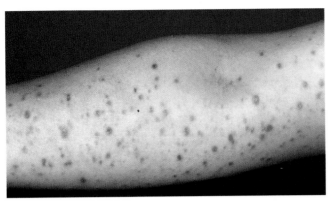

FIGURE 11.28 Pityriasis lichenoides et varioliformis acuta (PLEVA).
– papules with hemorrhagic crust.

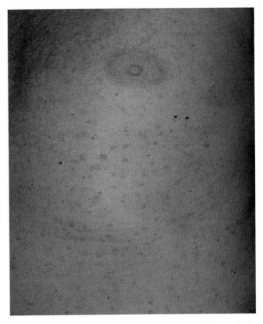

FIGURE 11.29 Transient acantholytic dermatosis (Grover's disease) – reddish brown, crusted papules with characteristic truncal location

relapsing course of crops of lesions. Histologic examination confirms the diagnosis, revealing a typical 'wedge shaped' dermal infiltrate with CD30+ cells. Approximately 10–20% of patients develop lymphoma, most commonly cutaneous T-cell lymphoma.

PITYRIASIS LICHENOIDES ET VARIOLIFORMIS ACUTA (PLEVA) (MUCHA–HABERMANN DISEASE)

This rare condition is characterized by recurrent crops of crusted, reddish papules (**Fig. 11.28**) that regress spontaneously within weeks. PLEVA is seen most commonly in children and is rarely associated with fever and malaise. The skin lesions can be in various stages: vesicular, pustular, and crusted. Skin biopsy can confirm the diagnosis. When the lesions persist for months and appear as reddish brown papules with scale, the condition is referred to as pityriasis lichenoides chronica. Rare cases eventuate into cutaneous T-cell lymphoma. Treatment includes topical steroids and oral antibiotics for their anti-inflammatory effect (e.g., tetracycline or erythromycin).

TRANSIENT ACANTHOLYTIC DERMATOSIS (GROVER'S DISEASE)

Grover's disease is a pruritic eruption of truncal, reddish brown, keratotic papules (**Fig. 11.29**), most commonly affecting middle-aged to elderly Caucasian males. Pruritus is the hallmark of this disease. Heat tends to exacerbate the condition. Biopsy shows the characteristic finding of focal separation of keratinocytes (e.g., acantholysis) in the epidermis. Potent topical steroids can diminish the pruritus but the disease is hardly 'transient.' Consider Grover's disease in a middle-aged male who presents with pruritic, keratotic papules limited to the trunk.

12 Pustules

Chapter Contents

Key Points

1. Pustules represent collections of neutrophils
2. Rule out infection when you see pustules
3. Pustules can be sterile

ABSTRACT

Pustules are collections of neutrophils that are situated superficially, usually in a hair follicle (e.g., acne and folliculitis) or just below the stratum corneum (e.g., impetigo and candidiasis). Although pustules represent the unifying clinical feature of these disorders, they may not always be the predominant finding; sometimes, they are not even present. For example, in some patients with acne, only comedones or papules are found. In impetigo, often only crusts are found because the pustules have been broken and dried. Pus often indicates infection. For pustules (and crusts) in the skin, infection is an appropriate diagnostic consideration, but, as can be seen from **Table 12.1**, not all pustular dermatoses are caused by pathogenic microorganisms. However, if infection is suspected, simple laboratory tests can be performed for confirmation.

The most common pustular diseases are listed in **Table 12.1**. Other rare causes of pustules are mentioned briefly at the end of the chapter.

ACNE

Key Points

1. Acne is the most common dermatologic disease with negative psychosocial ramifications
2. Comedones are the hallmark of the disease
3. Treatment targets multifactorial causes of acne: androgens, follicular obstruction, and *Propionibacterium acnes*

Definition

Acne vulgaris (common acne) is a disorder affecting pilosebaceous units in the skin (**Fig. 12.1**). The cause is multifactorial. Clinical lesions range from non-inflamed *comedones* to *inflammatory papules, pustules,* and *nodules.*

Incidence

Acne is the most common disease seen by a dermatologist. It begins at a surprisingly young age; comedones can be found on examination in 50% of boys aged 9–11 years. The incidence and severity of the disease increase during the teenage years and early adulthood, affecting approximately 85% of young people between the ages of 12 and 24 years. Contrary to popular belief, acne is not confined to teenagers. It may continue into the 3rd and 4th decades of life, especially in women; in some patients, it does not begin until then.

History

The patient usually makes the diagnosis and often has attempted therapy with over-the-counter medication. A history of hirsutism or irregular menses in a woman with acne should lead to the consideration of possible androgen excess. Adult women often complain of acne along the jawline that worsens around the time of their period (**Fig. 12.2**). Topical or systemic corticosteroids can also cause an acneiform eruption.

Physical Examination

The non-inflamed lesions in acne are called comedones and are of two types: (1) the *open comedone* or 'blackhead,' which appears as a dilated pore filled with black

TABLE 12.1 Common pustular diseases

	Frequency (%)[a]	Etiology	Physical Examination			Differential Diagnosis	Laboratory Test
			Appearance of Lesions	Distribution			
Acne	13	Multifactorial	Pustules, papules, nodules, and *comedones*	Face and upper trunk		Folliculitis Rosacea	None
Candidiasis	0.3	Infection (*C. albicans*)	Satellite pustules around a '*beefy red*' erythematous area	Moist areas, particularly the groin		Tinea cruris Intertrigo Miliaria Folliculitis Contact dermatitis	Potassium hydroxide preparation
Folliculitis	1.1	Infection (*S. aureus*)	Scattered pustules, many with *centrally placed hairs*	Buttocks and thighs, beard area, scalp		Acne Fungal infection	Gram-stain Culture
Impetigo	0.6	Infection (*S. aureus*)	Crusts (often honey-colored) predominant	Anywhere, most common on face		Ecthyma Herpes simplex	Gram-stain Culture
Rosacea	1.3	Unknown	Papules and pustules on a background of *erythema* and *telangiectasia*	Central portion of face		Acne Lupus erythematosus Seborrheic dermatitis	None

[a]Percentage of new dermatology patients with this diagnosis seen in the Hershey Medical Center Dermatology Clinic, Hershey, PA.

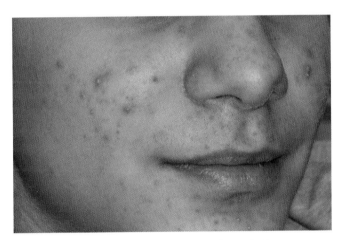

FIGURE 12.1 Acne – characteristic papules and pustules in a teenager.

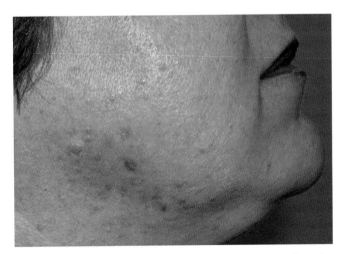

FIGURE 12.2 Adult female acne – papules and comedones along the jawline.

keratinous material (not dirt); and (2) the *closed comedone* or 'whitehead,' which is a small, flesh-colored, dome-shaped papule that often is difficult to see (**Fig. 12.3**). Inflammatory acne lesions are seen more easily by both patient and physician. They appear as papules, pustules, or nodules, depending on the magnitude of the inflammatory response. Acne is found in areas with numerous sebaceous glands, usually the face and upper trunk. The lower trunk is much less often involved, and the distal extremities are always spared.

Non-inflammatory lesions:
1. Open comedones
2. Closed comedones

Inflammatory lesions:
1. Papules
2. Pustules
3. Nodules

Differential Diagnosis

The diagnosis of acne is rarely difficult, particularly in teenagers. Occasionally, acne comedones may be confused with *flat warts*, which are small, flesh-colored, flat-topped papules usually located on the face. On close inspection, the flat wart is seen to have a sharp right-angled edge and a finely textured surface, whereas a closed comedone has a dome-shaped, smooth surface (**Fig. 12.4**)

Steroid acne is caused by use of corticosteroids and is distinguished from acne vulgaris by its sudden onset (usually within 2 weeks of starting high-dose systemic or potent topical corticosteroid therapy) and appearance

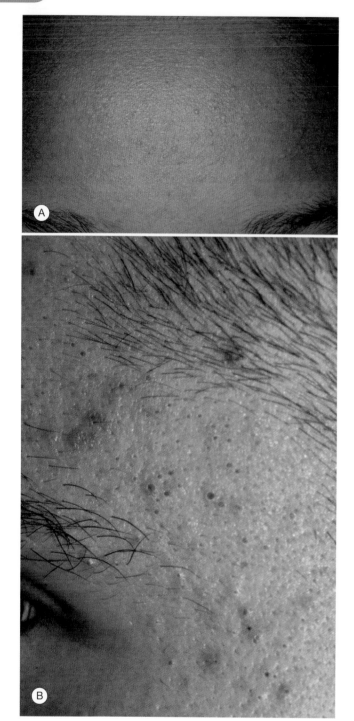

FIGURE 12.3 **A.** Closed comedones or 'whiteheads.' **B.** Open comedones or 'blackheads.'

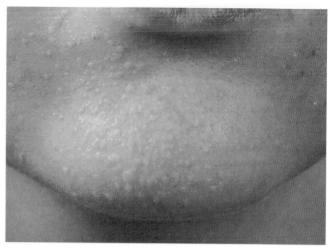

FIGURE 12.4 **Flat warts** – flesh colored papules often mistaken for acne (*Courtesy of O. Fred Miller, MD*).

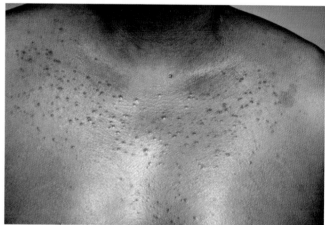

FIGURE 12.5 **Steroid acne** – uniform, red papules in a kidney transplant patient on high doses of systemic steroids.

(uniform, 2–3–mm, red, firm papules and pustules) (**Fig. 12.5**). Steroid acne caused by topically applied agents occurs most often on the face. With systemic corticosteroids, the eruption is most prominent on the upper trunk.

Pustular acne vulgaris can be confused with bacterial folliculitis or rosacea. In *bacterial folliculitis*, hairs are visible in some of the pustules and a bacterial culture is positive, usually for *Staphylococcus aureus* or, less often, a Gram-negative organism. *Rosacea* is distinguished from acne vulgaris by the presence of a background blush of erythema and telangiectasia, and the absence of comedones. Rosacea also usually occurs later in life.

Papular acne is occasionally confused with angiofibromas. Angiofibromas are a skin manifestation of tuberous sclerosis and are often incorrectly diagnosed as acne. Clinically, the lesions appear as firm, pink papules that are clustered primarily in the center of the face, are persistent, and are, of course, resistant to acne therapy.

Laboratory and Biopsy

The diagnosis is almost always made clinically. Occasionally, a bacterial culture is indicated to rule out infection. A biopsy is not indicated but would show an occluded pilosebaceous unit along with inflammation (**Fig. 12.6**).

Therapy

Four categories of medication have proved efficacious in the treatment of acne: topical agents, systemic antibiotics, systemic retinoids, and hormonal agents. The type of acne guides the choice of treatment. For the majority of

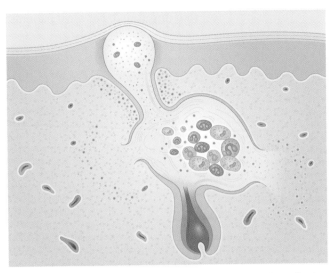

FIGURE 12.6 Acne. Epidermis – intraepidermal, intrafollicular collection of neutrophils. Dermis – occluded pilosebaceous unit with accumulation of keratin, sebum, and inflammatory cells. Extravasation of material through the ruptured wall leads to further dermal inflammation.

patients, systemic retinoids and hormonal therapy are not required.

Therapy for Acne

Initial
Comedonal
- Topical retinoids

Papules and Pustules
- Topical: retinoid in PM and benzoyl peroxide (alone or in combination with topical clindamycin)
- Systemic: tetracyclines (add if topicals fail)

Nodules
- Topical and systemic therapy in combination as outlined for papules and pustules

Alternative
Comedonal
- Topical adapalene (for sensitive skin)
- Topical tazarotene (for resistant comedones)

Papules and Pustules
- Oral isotretinoin if severe and fails initial treatment

Nodules
- Oral isotretinoin

Hormonal Treatment for Females
- Oral contraceptives
- Spironolactone

Topical Agents. Topical agents are most effective for superficial lesions. For comedones, the mainstay of treatment remains topical retinoids: tretinoin (Retin-A Micro cream), adapalene (Differin gel), and tazarotene (Tazorac). Benzoyl peroxide has mild comedolytic activity and also exerts an antibacterial effect. Topical antibiotics (erythromycin, clindamycin) should be used in combination with topical benzoyl peroxide in order to prevent bacterial resistance.

The authors usually start treatment with a topical retinoid at bedtime and a benzoyl peroxide wash (available over the counter) in the morning. The patient should apply these medications to the *entire affected area* (e.g., the entire face) rather than just to the individual lesions. In addition, patients must be advised that retinoids and benzoyl peroxide preparations can cause skin irritation, which usually is worst during the first 1–2 weeks of use and afterwards diminishes. In part because of the irritation, the patient may notice that the condition appears worse rather than better after the first several weeks of use.

Systemic Antibiotics. Systemic antibiotics are indicated in patients with inflammatory papules or pustules, especially if there is truncal involvement. Tetracycline (500 mg twice daily) and doxycycline (50–100 mg twice daily) are the two most commonly prescribed oral antibiotics because of low cost, efficacy, and relative safety, even when administered for a prolonged period. Because foods, particularly dairy products, interfere with the absorption of tetracyclines, this drug should be taken on an empty stomach. Minocycline (100 mg twice daily) is used mostly in persons who cannot tolerate the other tetracyclines.

Systemic Retinoids. The oral retinoid isotretinoin became available commercially in September 1982 for use in the treatment of patients with severe acne (**Fig. 12.7**). This potent vitamin A analog decreases follicular keratinization, sebum production, and intrafollicular bacterial counts. Side-effects are common. Almost all patients experience chapped lips and dry skin, and extracutaneous complications also occur, for example increased levels of liver enzymes and plasma lipids. Most importantly, systemic retinoids are *teratogenic*. It is mandatory that female patients not be pregnant when taking isotretinoin. Special consent forms, strict birth control measures, and monthly pregnancy tests are required for women taking isotretinoin. A consent form acknowledging the risk of depression and suicide while on isotretinoin is required for both men and women. Because of these restrictions, the drug is recommended mainly for the treatment of selected patients with severe, therapy-resistant popular/pustular acne or scarring nodular acne. The drug should be prescribed only by physicians who are familiar with its use and participate in a national risk management program (www.ipledgeprogram.com).

Isotretinoin is teratogenic.

Hormonal Therapy. This class of treatment can help females who have acne that fails to responds to initial treatment outlined above and that flares with their menstrual cycle. Birth control pills with low androgenicity improve acne in many patients. Several products are available, including Ortho Tri-Cyclen and Estrostep, for

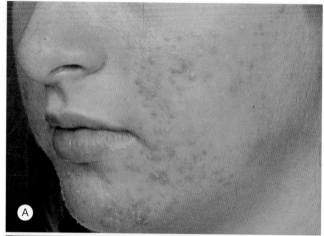

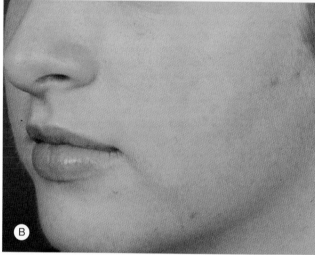

FIGURE 12.7 Acne. A. Pre-isotretinoin. Severe nodular 'cystic' acne with scarring. **B.** Post-isotretinoin.

which the US Food and Drug Administration has approved acne as an indicated use.

Antiandrogens have also been used for treating therapy-resistant acne in women. Cyproterone acetate is available in Europe, whereas spironolactone has been used in the USA. Again, these agents should be prescribed only by physicians who are fully aware of their potential side-effects.

Patient Education. The most important aspect of a successful acne treatment program is patient compliance. Instructions should be given both verbally at the time of the patient's initial visit and on a written take-home sheet that reinforces what was said. Patients are best able to comply if medications are used only twice daily, so that the medication schedule can be centered on an already established daily habit such as teeth brushing. At the time of the initial visit, answers can also be given to several common questions (often unasked) that patients with acne or their parents frequently have regarding the following:

1. *Diet.* Some evidence indicates that a 'Western' diet may have an adverse effect on acne, but specific foods have not been implicated. For most patients, a sensible diet is all that is suggested.
2. *Cleanliness.* Acne is not a function of poor hygiene. In general, acne cleansing agents are also not recommended because they cause irritation that unnecessarily compounds the irritation from the recommended topical comedolytics. Instruct patients to wash their face with their hands and not with a washcloth.
3. *Cosmetics.* If cosmetics are used, they should be water-based and used sparingly.
4. *Picking.* In many patients with acne, much of the skin damage is self-inflicted. Although the temptation to squeeze a fresh pustule is often overwhelming, it should be vigorously discouraged because it can produce more tissue damage, sometimes resulting in scars.

Course and Complications

With therapy, the prognosis for acne is good, if not excellent. The patient should understand that most therapies provide control of the disease rather than cure, and that improvement does not occur overnight. If improvement has not been noted after 2 months, more intensive therapy can be prescribed, including increased concentrations of the topical agents, increased dosage of the oral antibiotic, or change in the antibiotic therapy. Continued improvement in the disease is expected with continued therapy. Many patients can discontinue systemic antibiotics after a number of months, but most require prolonged (often lasting for years) maintenance therapy with topical agents, and some also require continued antibiotics. However, bacterial resistance to antibiotics is becoming more frequent, thereby limiting the usefulness of long-term antibiotic therapy for acne. Isotretinoin induces prolonged remissions, if not 'cures,' in many patients.

Acne remits spontaneously with time, to a degree that varies widely. For individual patients, there is no way to predict in advance when they will 'outgrow' their acne. The goal of therapy is to keep the condition under control as long as it is active.

The major complication of acne is its psychosocial ramifications, which can be devastating for some patients. Patients with severe cystic acne may even be socially ostracized. In an ironic quirk of timing, acne occurs at a time of life when personal appearance is a prime concern and self-consciousness is at its peak. Regardless of the severity of the acne, for patients seeking help (even those with apparently mild disease), the disease is important and deserves serious attention. Patients are not impressed with soothing advice that trivializes their disease and reassures them that they will eventually 'outgrow' it.

In addition to the cosmetic liability of active lesions, scars further compound and perpetuate a poor self-image in some patients long after the acne has remitted. Scars are difficult to treat. Dermabrasion, laser 'resurfacing,' chemical peels, and surgery have all been employed, with varying results. Because scars are more easily prevented than treated, the emphasis in acne is on early and aggressive medical therapy.

Pathogenesis

Multiple factors are involved in the pathogenesis of acne. The three most significant are:

Factors involved in acne pathogenesis:
1. Androgens
2. Follicular obstruction
3. *Propionibacterium acnes*

1. *Androgenic hormones.* Under androgen stimulation, sebaceous glands enlarge and increase their sebum production. Before puberty, the responsible androgens are secreted by the adrenal gland. During puberty, the addition of gonadal androgens provides further sebaceous gland stimulation.
2. *Follicular obstruction.* For acne to occur, outlet obstruction of the follicular canal is required. All acne lesions begin with a microcomedone. This obstruction occurs because of accumulation of adherent keratinized cells within the canal, forming an impaction. The cause of follicular obstruction is not known, but may also be influenced by androgens.
3. *Bacteria.* Proximal to the follicular outlet obstruction, sebum and keratinous debris accumulate. This provides an attractive environment for the growth of anaerobic bacteria, specifically *Propionibacterium acnes*. These bacteria produce lipase enzymes that hydrolyze the sebaceous lipids, resulting in the release of free fatty acids, which are presumed to cause inflammation. *P. acnes* play other roles in the pathogenesis of acne; e.g., these bacteria are chemotactic for neutrophils. Regardless of the mechanism, the therapeutic benefit of antibiotics supports the notion that bacteria play a pathogenetic role in acne.

CANDIDIASIS

Key Points

1. 'Beefy red' erythema with satellite papules and pustules
2. Common in setting of diaper dermatitis
3. Moisture is the major predisposing factor

Definition

Candidiasis represents an inflammatory reaction in the skin resulting from infection of the epidermis with *Candida albicans*. Clinically, the infection appears as a 'beefy red' erythematous area with surrounding satellite papules and pustules (**Fig. 12.8**). The pustules, when present, help in the diagnosis. In this section, candidiasis of the skin is discussed. Mucous membrane infection is discussed in Chapter 22.

Incidence

Candidiasis can affect people of all ages. Although only 0.3% of the authors' new patient visits are for candidiasis; in some situations this disease is much more common.

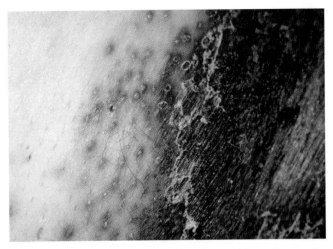

FIGURE 12.8 **Candidiasis** – 'beefy red' erythema with satellite papules and pustules.

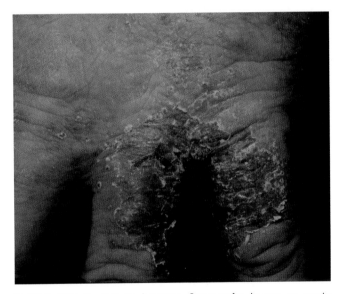

FIGURE 12.9 **Candidiasis between finger-webs** known as erosio interdigitalis blastomycetica.

It is particularly common in diaper-clad infants and in hospitalized patients. Some 2% of the authors' in-hospital consultations are for candidiasis.

History

Patients usually complain of itching and burning of the skin. A moist environment is the most important local predisposing factor for the development of this disease. For infections in the perineal area, diapers and excessive skin folds help to provide this moist environment. Wet surgical dressings can do the same in other locations. On the hands, *C. albicans* infection between the fingers occurs in patients who frequently have their hands in water, such as bartenders and dishwashers (**Fig. 12.9**). In women with recurrent candidal vulvovaginitis, a history should be taken for predisposing factors, such as pregnancy, diabetes mellitus, birth control pills, and antibiotics.

Moisture predisposes to candidiasis.

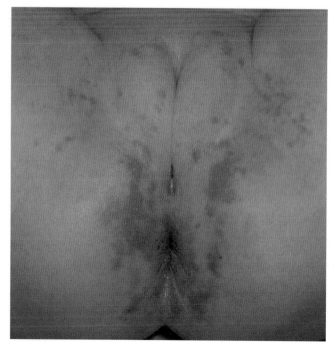

FIGURE 12.10 **Candidiasis** – Perineal location with satellite papules in a diapered infant.

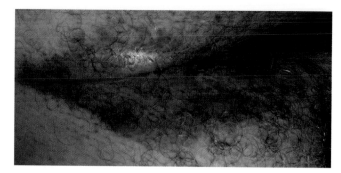

FIGURE 12.11 **Intertrigo.**

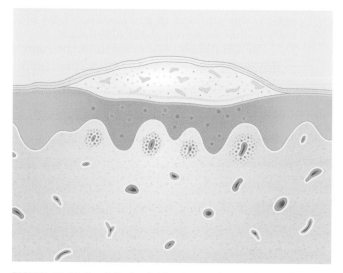

FIGURE 12.12 **Candidiasis.** Epidermis – subcorneal pustules; note associated hyphae and spores. Dermis – perivascular inflammation.

Physical Examination

The most consistent finding in cutaneous candidiasis is bright red erythema of the affected skin, characteristically surrounded by satellite pustules and papules. Pustules are not always present, but often their residua are noted. These appear as small, 2–3 mm, erythematous macules rimmed with a collarette of scale that represents the remnant of the pustule roof. As noted, the distribution of candidiasis favors moist areas. Perineal infection is most common in diapered infants (**Fig. 12.10**) and in women, in whom it is often accompanied by candidal vaginitis. In bedridden patients, especially those taking antibiotics, perianal involvement occurs and often extends up the back with multiple papules and pustules. Other favored locations are the intertriginous areas under the breasts, in the axillae, between the fingers, and under wet dressings.

> Cutaneous candidiasis is 'beefy red' with satellite papules and pustules.

Differential Diagnosis

The differential diagnosis depends in part on the location of the infection. In the groin area, candidiasis may be confused with *tinea cruris* or *intertrigo*, an irritant dermatitis caused by maceration and rubbing in intertriginous folds, usually the inguinal folds in obese patients (**Fig. 12.11**). Compared with candidiasis, tinea cruris is much more sharply demarcated, and intertrigo is less likely to be so brightly erythematous. Neither exhibits the satellite papules and pustules of candidiasis.

On the back of a bedridden patient, candidal infection may be confused with *miliaria* (heat rash) or *folliculitis*.

In candidiasis, however, the papular and pustular lesions are usually accompanied by confluent erythematous involvement in the perianal and, often, perineal areas from which the infection spread. A potassium hydroxide (KOH) preparation is negative in miliaria and folliculitis. Candidiasis developing under wet dressings can be confused with contact dermatitis. The finding of pustules favors candidiasis. The KOH preparation confirms the diagnosis.

Laboratory and Biopsy

The important laboratory test is the KOH examination of scrapings from pustules or peripheral scale. If a pustule is present, a scraping of its roof and contents has a high positive yield. The finding of hyphae and pseudohyphae is diagnostic for infection (**Fig. 12.12**). Spores alone are not diagnostic, because *C. albicans* and other yeast organisms can colonize skin without causing infection. For this reason, a skin culture for *C. albicans* is less helpful than a positive KOH scraping; a positive culture from skin does not distinguish between colonization and infection, whereas the KOH preparation does, because the KOH examination detects the infectious filamentous form of the organism. It can be difficult, if not impossible, to distinguish between the hyphae and pseudohyphae of candidiasis and the hyphae of dermatophytic infections. Usually, however, the clinical picture is sufficient to distinguish between the two. A biopsy is not needed.

Hyphae and pseudohyphae are found on KOH examination.

Therapy

Candidiasis is best treated with one of the topical imidazole creams. Over-the-counter creams include clotrimazole (Lotrimin) and miconazole (Micatin). Creams containing econazole (Spectazole) and ketoconazole (Nizoral) require a prescription. The imidazole cream should be applied twice daily. The clinician should instruct the patient to apply the medication *sparingly*, because excessive application of creams to already moist areas can contribute to maceration and may cause further irritation.

Topical medication should be applied sparingly.

Widespread candidiasis is treated with systemic therapy. Ketoconazole (Nizoral; 200 mg daily) and fluconazole (Diflucan; 100 mg daily) are effective oral agents, but are seldom needed for local cutaneous infection. These oral agents are more often indicated for severe, persistent, or recurrent mucous membrane candidiasis.

Widespread candidiasis is treated systemically.

Attention should also be given to predisposing factors, especially moisture. Drying measures depend on the situation. For example, an infant with candidal diaper dermatitis should have more frequent diaper changes, and a bedridden patient should be turned more frequently to increase air exposure to the back and buttocks.

Therapy for Candidiasis

Initial
- Topical creams b.i.d.
  - Clotrimazole
  - Miconazole
  - Ketoconazole

Alternative
- Systemic
  - Ketoconazole 200 mg daily
  - Fluconazole 100 mg daily

Course and Complications

In most instances, response to topical therapy is prompt and, if the predisposing factors have been corrected, recurrence is unlikely. In patients with recurrent disease, both local (e.g., occlusion, moisture) and systemic (e.g., diabetes, acquired immune deficiency syndrome (AIDS), systemic corticosteroids), predisposing factors should be considered. Most patients with local candidiasis are not immunologically deficient, and the disease resolves with

treatment of the infection and correction of the predisposing factors. *Systemic candidiasis* occurs exclusively in severely immunocompromised patients, particularly those with hematologic malignant diseases. In such patients, mucous membrane or cutaneous candidal infection may serve as the portal of entry for the systemic infection. *Chronic mucocutaneous candidiasis* is another rare disorder, and represents chronic infection of the skin and mucous membranes in patients who are deficient in cellular immunity against *C. albicans*.

Pathogenesis

No special pathogenic strains of *C. albicans* exist. The organism commonly colonizes skin and bowel, particularly the colon. Pathogenicity in tissue is associated with conversion of the organism from its yeast to its filamentous form. The most important local factor that encourages this conversion is moisture. Accordingly, skin folds are most commonly involved, as are areas occluded with wet dressings, including diapers. After penetration of the stratum corneum barrier, the organism elicits a complement-mediated acute inflammatory response that produces the dermatitis, as well as preventing deeper tissue invasion.

FOLLICULITIS

Key Points

1. Bacterial infection of hair follicle
2. *S. aureus* is the most common cause
3. Colonization of *S. aureus* can occur in the nose, axillae, and groin

Definition

Folliculitis is an inflammatory reaction in the hair follicle caused by bacteria, usually *S. aureus*. Clinically, the lesion appears as a pustule, often with a central hair (**Fig. 12.13**).

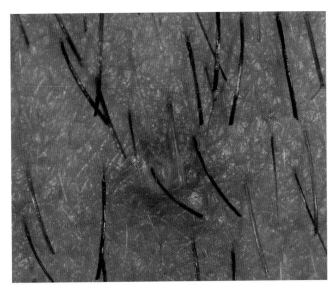

FIGURE 12.13 Folliculitis – pustule with centrally placed hair.

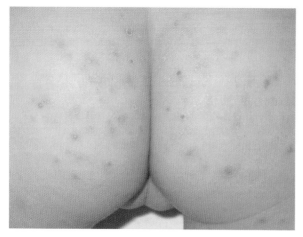

FIGURE 12.14 **Folliculitis** – Pustules and crusted papules on buttocks of infant that cultured positive for *S. aureus*.

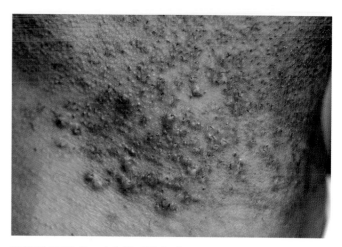

FIGURE 12.16 **Pseudofolliculitis barbae.**

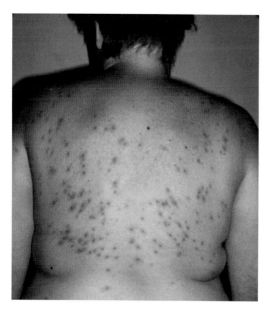

FIGURE 12.15 **Hot-tub folliculitis** – originally pustules that became hemorrhagic centrally with characteristic red flare; often appear under area of bathing suit occlusion.

Incidence

Folliculitis is relatively common, representing approximately 1% of the authors' new patients. The disorder affects primarily young adults but can occur at any age.

History

Folliculitis is usually asymptomatic; occasionally, patients complain of mild discomfort associated with the lesions. The process may be chronic or recurrent.

Physical Examination

A pustule is the predominant lesion, although papules may be found. The lesions are individual and do not become confluent. They are usually distributed on the buttocks and thighs (**Fig. 12.14**), but may also occur in the beard area and sometimes on the scalp. The key to the diagnosis is appreciated only on close inspection,

whereby hairs can be seen in the exact center of many of the lesions.

Differential Diagnosis

The distribution, absence of comedones, and presence of a hair growing from the pustules help to differentiate folliculitis from *acne*. Gram-negative organisms can cause *Gram-negative folliculitis*, mainly in two settings: patients with acne who are receiving antibiotic therapy in whom Gram-negative pathogens are selected out, and individuals exposed to hot-tubs and swimming pools contaminated with *Pseudomonas aeruginosa* (**Fig. 12.15**). Both types are uncommon. *Pseudofolliculitis barbae* is a disorder of the neck and jaw of men whose beard hairs are sharply curved. This configuration causes the hairs to re-enter the skin, where they induce an inflammatory reaction, resulting in papules and pustules (**Fig. 12.16**). The ingrowing hairs can often be visualized. *Keratosis pilaris* is a common follicular disorder that presents as tiny, rough, scaling, follicular papules (*no* pustules) on the backs of the upper arms, buttocks, thighs, and facial cheeks. Rarely, *fungal infections* can result in follicular pustules. These are usually associated with scaling plaques and therefore are not usually confused with the individual pustules of bacterial folliculitis. *Eosinophilic folliculitis* is manifested by pruritic papules on the face and trunk. It is most frequently found in human immunodeficiency virus (HIV)-infected patients (**Fig. 12.17**).

Laboratory and Biopsy

In staphylococcal folliculitis, Gram-staining of the pus reveals Gram-positive cocci, and bacterial culture confirms the diagnosis. A biopsy is not necessary but, if done, would reveal a collection of neutrophils in the superficial portion of the hair follicle (**Fig. 12.18**). It is important to send a culture and sensitivity to check for methicillin-resistant *S. aureus* (MRSA), a growing hospital and community problem.

Therapy

Most cases of staphylococcal folliculitis are mild and can be managed with an antiseptic cleanser such as povidone-iodine (Betadine), chlorhexidine (Hibiclens), benzoyl

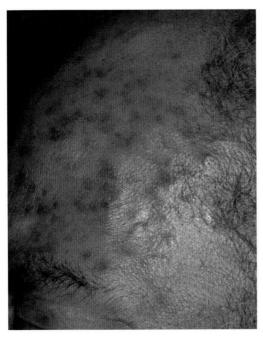

FIGURE 12.17 **Eosinophilic folliculitis.** Red papules with post-inflammatory hyperpigmentation in an HIV+ individual.

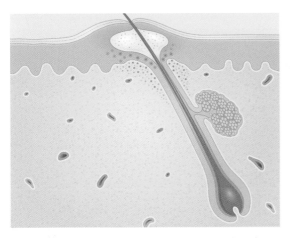

FIGURE 12.18 **Folliculitis.** Epidermis – subcorneal pustule at the opening of a hair follicle. Dermis – inflammation in the upper dermis.

peroxide used daily or every other day for at least several weeks. Antibiotic ointments may be used for localized disease (bacitracin or mupirocin 2%). For more extensive involvement, a 10-day course of a systemic antibiotic such as dicloxacillin (250 mg four times daily) is suggested in addition to the cleansers. If a bacterial culture reveals MRSA, then therapy should be directed by antibiotic sensitivities. The authors use doxycycline or trimethoprim-sulfamethoxazole most frequently for MRSA.

Course and Complications

Response to therapy usually is good, but recurrences are common. Such patients may be carriers of *S. aureus*, and more prolonged use of antiseptic cleansers is recommended. In addition, the authors often ask these patients to apply an antibiotic ointment (e.g., mupirocin) twice daily in their nares, because this is a common site for *S. aureus*. Other sites of colonization include the axillae

Therapy for Folliculitis

Initial
Topical
- Antiseptic cleansers:
  - Betadine
  - Hibiclens
  - Benzoyl peroxide
- Topical antibiotics
  - Mupirocin
  - Bacitracin

Oral
- Dicloxacillin 250 mg q.i.d.

Alternative
- Doxycycline or minocycline (MRSA)
- Trimethoprim/sulfamethoxazole (MRSA)
- Mupirocin to nares for chronic carriers

and groin. Complications are uncommon and local. Occasionally, the follicular infection can extend more deeply, resulting in a furuncle that requires incision and drainage.

> Patients with recurrent folliculitis may be chronic 'carriers' of *S. aureus*.

Pathogenesis

In folliculitis, the bacteria gain entry into the skin through the follicular orifice and establish low-grade infection within the epidermis surrounding the follicular canal. Patients who carry *S. aureus* on their skin are more susceptible to this disorder. Occlusion and maceration sometimes are also predisposing factors.

IMPETIGO

Key Points

1. Characterized by honey-colored crust
2. *S. aureus* is the most common cause
3. Treat with oral or topical antibiotics

Definition

Impetigo represents a superficial skin infection caused by Gram-positive bacteria, usually *S. aureus*, and less commonly *Streptococcus pyogenes*. The early lesions are pustules, which quickly break to form crusts (**Fig. 12.19**). Crusts are the most commonly encountered clinical lesions. Some strains of *Staphylococcus aureus* can also cause blisters (bullous impetigo), as discussed in Chapter 10.

> Most impetigo is caused by *S. aureus*.

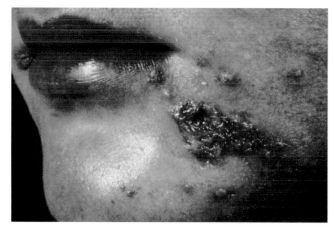

FIGURE 12.19 **Impetigo** – pustules and crusted plaque with surrounding erythema. *(Courtesy of O. Fred Miller, MD)*

Incidence

Impetigo occurs most often in children and is the most common bacterial infection in children. Although less than 1% of the authors' new patients present with impetigo, this rate would be higher in a general medical practice, particularly a pediatric practice. Nasal carriage of *S. aureus* leads to higher risk of occurrence in children.

History

The eruption often starts as a single lesion, but patients and parents often do not seek medical help until multiple new lesions develop. Other family members are sometimes affected. Staphylococcal bacterial infection also occurs secondarily (impetiginization) in association with certain skin diseases, especially atopic dermatitis.

Physical Examination

The most commonly encountered clinical finding is a honey-colored crust. Intact pustules usually are not found. When the crust is removed, a superficial glistening base is revealed. Impetigo does not extend deeply, so ulcerations are not present. Lesions can be found anywhere, but are most often located on the face around the nose and mouth. Brown or honey-colored crusts are also the hallmark of secondary bacterial infection.

Differential Diagnosis

Different from the staphylococcal impetigo described above, *ecthyma* is caused by group A streptococci, but much confusion exists regarding these two types of bacterial skin infection. In both, the presenting lesion usually is a crust, but the more important clinical difference is the depth of the infection. With staphylococcal impetigo, the process is superficial (just below the stratum corneum), so when the crust is removed only a shallow, glistening erosion is seen (**Fig. 12.20**). In streptococcal pyoderma, the infection is usually deeper, extending through the epidermis, so when the crust is removed a deeper defect (i.e., an ulcer) is noted (**Fig. 12.21**). In addition, with staphylococcal impetigo, there is usually little or no surrounding erythema, whereas with

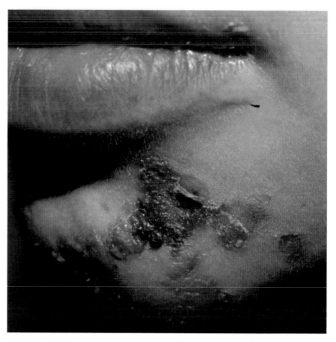

FIGURE 12.20 **Impetigo on the chin** – 'honey-colored' crusts are characteristic; culture taken from the glistening base beneath the crust grew *Staphylococcus aureus*. *(Courtesy of O. Fred Miller, MD)*

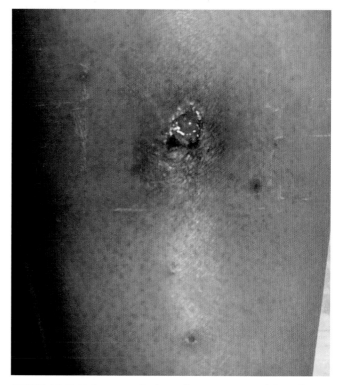

FIGURE 12.21 **Ecthyma on the lower leg** – streptococcal skin infection extends more deeply, often forming an ulcer (ecthyma).

streptococcal infection erythema is moderate to marked. Finally, staphylococcal impetigo is most common on the face, whereas ecthyma is usually found on the lower extremities, occurring after a scratch or insect bite.

When the vesicles in *herpes simplex* age, they become cloudy and eventually form crusts. At this stage, herpes is

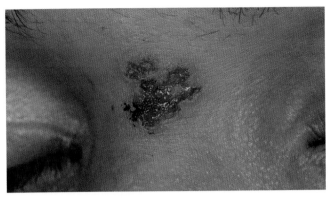

FIGURE 12.22 **Herpes simplex.** Note erosions with scalloped borders. Honey-colored crusts represent secondary impetiginization.

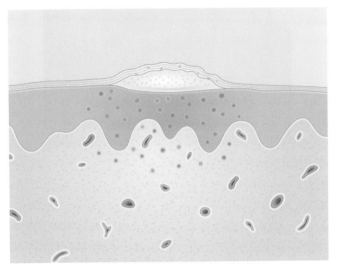

FIGURE 12.23 **Impetigo.** Epidermis – subcorneal pustules. Dermis – mild inflammatory reaction in upper dermis.

often misdiagnosed as impetigo. Features favoring herpes include the recognition (by patient or physician) of clear vesicles present at the start; a history of recurrence in the same location; and the presence of erosions with scalloped borders (**Fig. 12.22**). Inflammatory *fungal infections* can cause pustules and are in the differential diagnosis for 'sterile' pustular processes. KOH examination and fungal cultures are indicated in patients with negative Gram-stains and bacterial cultures or poor response to antibiotic therapy.

Laboratory

A Gram-stain reveals Gram-positive cocci. Bacterial culture typically grows *S. aureus*. In obtaining material for Gram-staining and culture, the clinician should first remove the crust so that the specimen can be obtained from the weeping, glistening erosion. Biopsy is rarely performed, but would show a subcorneal pustule (**Fig. 12.23**).

Therapy

Both topical and systemic antibiotics have been advocated for treating impetigo. Uncomplicated impetigo resolves on its own after approximately 2 weeks. Topical preparations such as bacitracin and mupirocin (Bactroban) have long been used, especially for small lesions. Nevertheless, for more extensive lesions, systemic antibiotic therapy is preferred. Most *S. aureus* strains, including those encountered in outpatients, produce penicillinase, so penicillin is not appropriate treatment. The preferred antibiotics are oral cephalexin or penicillinase-resistant penicillins such as dicloxacillin used over a 7–10-day course. The increasing resistance of *S. aureus* to erythromycin may limit the usefulness of this agent in impetigo. MRSA has also been encountered, and requires a tailored antibiotic regimen based on sensitivities.

> Resistance patterns of causative bacteria guide treatment decisions.

Therapy for Impetigo

Initial
- General hygiene
  - Antibacterial soaps – Lever 2000, Dial, Hibiclens
  - Changing of towel, washcloth, shaver, etc. daily
- Topical antibiotics
  - Mupirocin ointment – applied t.i.d.

Alternative
- Systemic antibiotics
  - Dicloxacillin
  - Cephalexin
- Other – based on bacterial resistant patterns

Course and Complications

With appropriate antibiotic therapy, prompt healing is to be expected, with marked improvement within several days in most patients. Bacteriologic cure is achieved in 7–10 days in nearly all cases. If a rapid response to therapy does not occur, the physician should consider the possibility that the infection is caused by an antibiotic-resistant strain. In such instances, the result of the initial culture, if obtained, serves as a guide in selecting an alternative antibiotic.

The bacteria can colonize skin without causing actual infection. This is particularly true in patients with chronic dermatoses such as atopic dermatitis or psoriasis. More than 10% of patients with atopic dermatitis have *S. aureus* colonizing their eczematous skin. Impetiginization, characterized by honey-colored crusts, occurs more often in these patients than in those with psoriasis. Naturally occurring antimicrobial peptides in the skin are deficient in patients with atopic dermatitis, and present in normal quantities in patients with psoriasis.

> Honey-colored crusts indicate that the skin is secondarily infected.

Complications are rare. Acute glomerulonephritis may occur as a sequela to skin infection from streptococcal but not from staphylococcal infections. This emphasizes the importance of discriminating between these two types of skin infection.

Pathogenesis

S. aureus is ubiquitous in the environment. With staphylococcal infection, 'trauma' to the skin is often subclinical, and most patients cannot recall obvious trauma to their skin. Once bacteria have gained entry, they establish infection in the uppermost layer of the viable epidermis just below the stratum corneum. Inflammatory cells, primarily neutrophils, respond and are responsible for the pus that is clinically evident and eventuates into the characteristic crusts.

Infection with group A streptococci is more difficult to establish. These organisms do not colonize normal skin but must be inoculated through a damaged surface such as a scratch or insect bite. Once established, the organism produces proteolytic enzymes, which are in part responsible for the surrounding inflammation.

ROSACEA

Key Points

1. Papules and pustules with a background of erythema affect the central third of the face
2. Eye involvement is common
3. Treat with topical and oral antibiotics
4. Disease of adults

Definition

Rosacea is a chronic inflammatory disorder affecting the blood vessels and pilosebaceous units of the face (**Fig. 12.24**). The etiology is unknown. Clinically, papules and pustules are superimposed on a background of erythema and telangiectasia.

Incidence

Rosacea is a relatively common disorder that affects primarily middle-aged adults. Approximately 1% of the authors' new patients are seen for this disease.

History

The disorder often has a gradual onset. Usually, the patient first notices erythema; with time, telangiectasia appears. The development of papules and pustules is usually sufficient for the patient to bring the problem to a physician's attention. Trigger factors, such as exercise and alcohol, cause a flare of the redness. Most patients have a fair complexion and light colored irises.

Physical Examination

There are four major clinical subtypes of rosacea: (1) vascular; (2) papulopustular; (3) rhinophyma; and (4)

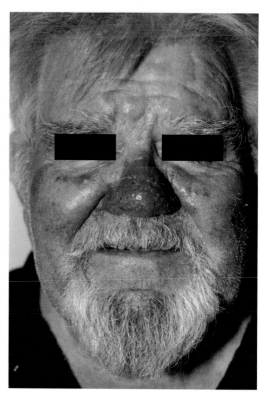

FIGURE 12.24 Rosacea – papules and pustules superimposed on background of erythema.

ocular. Each type may occur independently and there is no typical progression from one to the other. Usually a patient with rosacea presents with a combination of vascular, papulopustular, and ocular findings. Typically, papules and pustules are superimposed on a background of erythema and telangiectasia. Sometimes, only the erythema and telangiectasia are present. Characteristically, comedones are not found. The disease affects the central third of the face and spares the lateral aspects of the forehead and cheeks. Blepharitis and conjunctivitis are common. Bulbous thickening of the nose is rare and occurs most commonly in men (**Fig. 12.25**).

Papules and pustules are superimposed on a background of erythema and telangiectasia.

Differential Diagnosis

Rosacea is distinguished from *acne vulgaris* by the absence of comedones, the background of erythema and telangiectasia, the onset in middle life, and the distribution in the central third of the face. Rashes that may be confused with the vascular element in rosacea occur in lupus erythematosus, photodermatitis, and seborrheic dermatitis (**Fig. 12.26**), but none of these exhibit pustules. Interestingly, seborrheic dermatitis is often seen in conjunction with rosacea. Seborrheic dermatitis affects the convex surfaces (nasolabial fold) while rosacea affects the convex surfaces. In patients with rosacea with a prominent flushing component, the *carcinoid syndrome* sometimes enters the differential diagnosis.

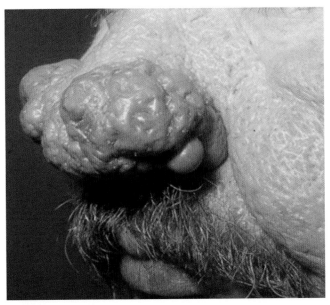

FIGURE 12.25 **Rosacea.** Extreme phymatous change leading to bulbous thickening.

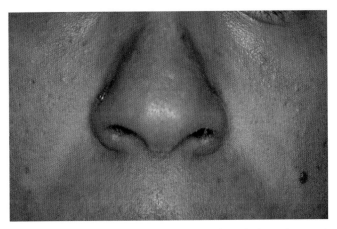

FIGURE 12.26 **Seborrheic dermatitis** – scaly red, hypopigmented patches affecting nasolabial (convex surface) folds.

Laboratory and Biopsy

The diagnosis is almost always made clinically. A biopsy is rarely needed, but if performed, shows vascular dilatation, often with degenerative changes in the collagen and elastic fibers in the upper dermis (**Fig. 12.27**). The papules and pustules in rosacea are similar histologically to those found in acne vulgaris, but in rosacea, the inflammatory infiltrate is more likely to have a granulomatous component. This represents a foreign body reaction in the dermis to the extravasated contents of affected pilosebaceous units. The granulomatous response can be impressive and has been confused occasionally with granulomatous disorders such as sarcoidosis and tuberculosis.

> Histologically, a granulomatous reaction is often present and may be confused with sarcoidosis or tuberculosis.

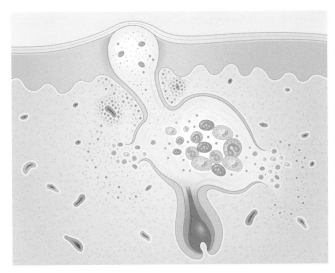

FIGURE 12.27 **Rosacea.** Epidermis – intrafollicular inflammation; granulomatous reaction to the contents of a ruptured pilosebaceous unit.

Therapy

Topical metronidazole 0.75% (MetroGel, MetroCream) or topical azelaic acid 15% (Finacea) applied twice daily is also effective in treating the papules, pustules, and erythema of rosacea. The mechanism of action is unknown. Systemic antibiotics are used frequently for the papular and pustular components and are especially beneficial in treating ocular rosacea (do not forget to ask each patient with rosacea if they have eye symptoms!). Sometimes, the erythema is also improved. Low-dose doxycycline (20 mg twice daily) exerts an anti-inflammatory effect and is the usual treatment. Most patients respond within 1 month, after which the drug often can be tapered but some patients require long-term maintenance treatment. Systemic isotretinoin (formerly Accutane), usually in low doses, is reserved for the rare patient with severe disease that has resisted all other therapy but it does not lead to a lasting response as seen in acne. Laser treatment (e.g., pulse-dye laser) is the only effective and definitive therapy for the erythema of rosacea.

Topical steroids should not be used because they are well known to aggravate the disease. Sun exposure can also be an aggravating factor, and sun protective measures should be recommended.

> Strong topical steroids are contraindicated.

Therapy for Rosacea

Initial
- Metronidazole gel or cream b.i.d.
- Azelaic acid gel b.i.d.
- Daily moisturizer containing sunscreen

Alternative
- Doxycycline 20 mg twice daily
- Pulse dye laser (vascular rosacea)

Course and Complications

The disease is usually chronic, but most patients respond well to therapy. In many, however, therapy must be continued for months to years. The erythematous component may be improved by therapy, but the telangiectasia persists.

Rhinophyma sometimes develops in patients with rosacea. As the name suggests, this disease involves hyperplasia of the sebaceous glands, connective tissue, and vascular bed of the nose. The hyperplasia can be striking, resulting in a bulbous nose. The nose of W. C. Fields was a prototype, but, contrary to popular belief, rosacea is not a sign of excessive alcohol intake. Ocular complications occur in some patients with rosacea. Eye findings range from blepharitis to conjunctivitis and even keratitis. The latter can be severe and has been known to result in visual impairment. Oral doxycycline is helpful for the ocular complications.

Pathogenesis

The pathogenetic mechanisms in this disease are not well understood. For the vascular component, investigators have suggested that sun exposure damages the collagen support of the vascular network, thereby resulting in vasodilatation. Other aggravating factors that have been incriminated, but not well proved, include the ingestion of foods that cause vasodilatation (e.g., hot liquids, alcohol, and spicy foods) and psychologic stress. Immune mechanisms have also been implicated, with immunoglobulin deposition occurring at the dermal–epidermal interface. The pathogenetic significance of this finding remains unclear. The cause of the pustular component is not known, although the pathogenesis may be similar to that of acne vulgaris. Clearly, genetics play a role as a family history for rosacea is often positive in a patient with rosacea.

UNCOMMON CAUSES OF PUSTULES

DEEP FUNGAL INFECTION – COCCIDIOIDOMYCOSIS

Coccidioidomycosis is a rare deep fungal infection presenting with skin manifestations. It is caused by the dimorphic fungus, *Coccidioides immitis*. Most cases result from inhalation of spores with subsequent dissemination to skin and other organs. Immunocompromised patients, especially HIV-infected individuals, are at highest risk. Clinical features of most deep fungal infections, including blastomycosis, are initial formation of pustules, plaques, and nodules evolving into verrucous plaques (**Fig. 12.28**). Biopsy and tissue culture confirm the diagnosis.

DERMATOPHYTE (KERION)

Dermatophytes can infect hair follicles and may result in pustules (**Fig. 12.29**). This condition sometimes is

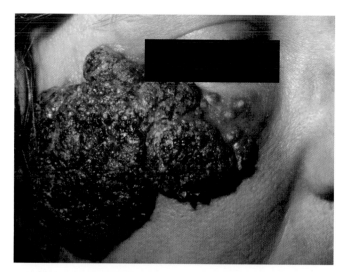

FIGURE 12.28 **Coccidioidomycosis** – large verrucous plaque with pustules.

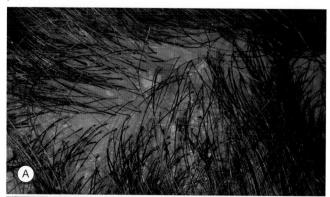

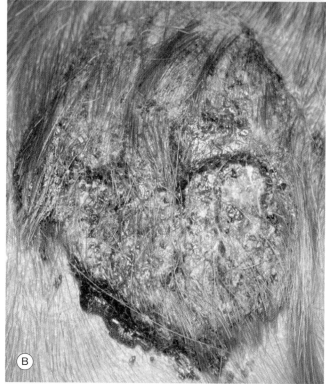

FIGURE 12.29 **Dermatophyte. A.** Pustules infecting hair follicle (culture necessary for diagnosis). **B.** Kerion – boggy plaque representing severe immunologic reaction to dermatophyte infecting hair follicles.

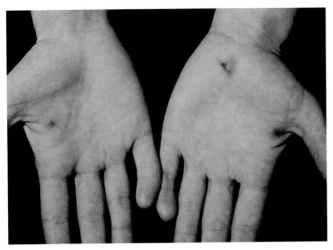

FIGURE 12.30 Gonococcemia – few hemorrhagic pustules in characteristic acral distribution.

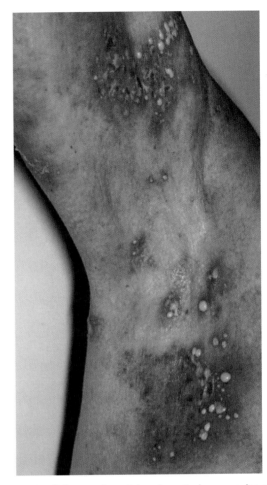

FIGURE 12.31 Subcorneal pustular dermatosis – annular plaques studded with pustules in axilla; flexural location is characteristic.

confused with bacterial folliculitis. A *kerion* is a dermatophytic infection, frequently of the scalp, that appears as an indurated, boggy, inflammatory plaque studded with pustules. Kerions are frequently confused with bacterial pyodermas. The most common organism causing a kerion is *Trichophyton rubrum*. Systemic antifungal therapy is necessary.

GONOCOCCEMIA

Gonococcemia (gonococcal arthritis-dermatitis syndrome) represents a systemic infection characterized by fever, arthralgia, tenosynovitis, septic arthritis, and hemorrhagic (or purpuric) pustules. The hemorrhagic pustules appear in an acral distribution and are few in number (**Fig. 12.30**). The disease results from dissemination of gonococci from an infected mucosal site. Diagnosis is confirmed by bacterial culture of the affected mucosal site. Treatment is with intravenous or intramuscular antibiotics, most commonly ceftriaxone.

Pustules in bacterial sepsis are purpuric.

SUBCORNEAL PUSTULAR DERMATOSIS

Sterile pustules are the hallmark of subcorneal pustular dermatosis. The disease is characterized by annular or expanding, polycyclic collections of pustules on a red base (**Fig. 12.31**). Flexural accentuation is common. The disease has a waxing and waning course. Monoclonal gammopathies have been reported with this condition. Skin biopsy confirms clinical suspicion of the disease. Dapsone is the treatment of choice.

13 White Spots

Chapter Contents

Key Points

1. Examine for partial versus complete pigment loss and presence or absence of scale
2. A Wood's light examination accentuates white spots, especially in fair-skinned individuals
3. Vitiligo is a common cause of depigmentation

ABSTRACT

White spots in the skin result from decreased melanin pigmentation. This can be caused by a reduction in the number of melanocytes or a decrease in their melanin production. Inflammatory events are frequently responsible, even though the inflammation may not be clinically appreciated. **Table 13.1** lists the four most common causes of white spots as well as one uncommon cause. Determination of the degree (partial versus complete) of pigment loss and identification of the presence or absence of scale are helpful distinguishing clinical features.

White spots should be examined for:
1. Partial versus complete pigment loss
2. Presence or absence of scale

The degree of pigment loss can be assessed roughly with a Wood's light examination, which helps to accentuate pigment contrast. In a darkened room with a Wood's light, lesions that are completely depigmented appear almost chalk white. This finding is characteristic in vitiligo. The Wood's light examination is also helpful in identifying white spots in lightly pigmented individuals; in patients with extremely fair complexions, white spots may not be evident under bright illumination (**Fig. 13.1**).

White spots are seen more easily by Wood's light examination.

The admonition, 'If it scales, scrape it!' also pertains to white spots. The two common hypopigmentary conditions that scale (i.e., tinea versicolor and pityriasis alba) can be distinguished with a potassium hydroxide (KOH) preparation.

PITYRIASIS ALBA

Key Points

1. Characterized by hypopigmented, white patches
2. More commonly seen in darkly pigmented children
3. Probably a low-grade 'eczematous' reaction

Definition

Pityriasis alba is an idiopathic hypopigmentary condition that appears clinically as white (alba) patches surmounted by fine, 'bran-like' (*pityron*, Greek for bran) scales (**Fig. 13.2**).

Incidence

The disease is extremely common but usually not sufficiently disturbing for most patients to seek medical attention. It affects mainly children between the ages of 3 and 16 years and is most common (or most noticeable) in dark-skinned individuals. Individuals with atopic dermatitis have a predilection for pityriasis alba.

TABLE 13.1 White spots

	Frequency (%)[a]	Etiology	Physical Examination			Differential Diagnosis	Laboratory Test
			Degree of Pigment Loss[b]	Presence of Scale	Distribution		
Pityriasis alba	0.4	Unknown	Partial	+	Face, upper arms	Tinea versicolor	–
Post-inflammatory hypopigmentation		Nonspecific sequelae of skin inflammation	Partial	–	Anywhere (sites of prior inflammation)	Vitiligo	–
Tinea versicolor	1.4	Fungus	Partial	+	Trunk	Vitiligo	KOH preparation
Vitiligo	0.6	Unknown	Complete	–	Anywhere		–
Tuberous sclerosis	Rare	Genetic	Partial	–	Trunk	Vitiligo	CNS imaging

[a]Percentage of new dermatology patients with this diagnosis seen in the Hershey Medical Center Dermatology Clinic, Hershey, PA.
[b]As assessed by Wood's light examination.
KOH, potassium hydroxide; CNS, central nervous system.

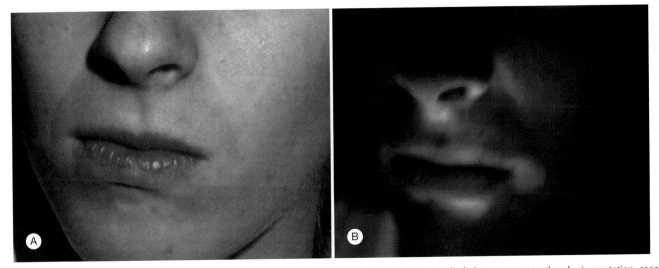

FIGURE 13.1 **A.** Periorificial vitiligo is difficult to appreciate in fair-skinned individuals. **B.** Wood's light accentuates the depigmentation seen in vitiligo.

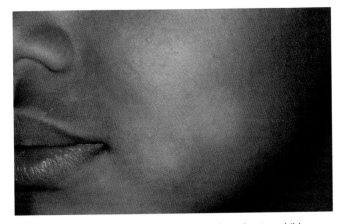

FIGURE 13.2 **Pityriasis alba** – hypopigmented patches in a child.

Pityriasis alba is most commonly recognized in darkly pigmented children.

History

Pityriasis alba is usually asymptomatic, although an occasional patient may complain of mild itching. Patients or parents are most concerned about the appearance of the lesions.

Physical Examination

The early lesion is a mildly erythematous, slightly scaling patch with an indistinct margin. Most often, only the subsequent lesion is seen – a 1–4 cm white patch with a

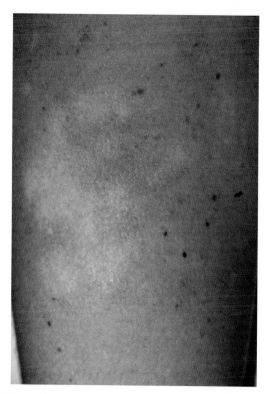

FIGURE 13.3 **Pityriasis alba** – hypopigmented patches on upper arms in an adult.

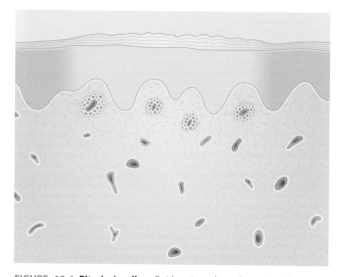

FIGURE 13.4 **Pityriasis alba.** Epidermis – hyperkeratosis; decreased pigmentation. Dermis – mild inflammation around superficial blood vessels.

fine, powdery scale. In children, the face is the most common area of involvement and may have one to several lesions. Pityriasis alba can occur in other locations. In young women, the most common area is the upper arms (**Fig. 13.3**). Rarely, widespread involvement occurs.

Differential Diagnosis

The disease is most often misdiagnosed as *tinea versicolor*. In temperate climates, adults with tinea versicolor seldom

have facial involvement, but in children (in whom the disease is much less common) the face is affected in approximately one-third of cases. Accordingly, a KOH preparation should be performed on all scaling white spots to rule out tinea versicolor. The white spots in *vitiligo* are distinguished by sharp demarcation, complete depigmentation, and lack of scale.

Laboratory and Biopsy

No specific laboratory test is available to establish the diagnosis. The KOH preparation is negative. The histologic picture is nonspecific, showing slight hyperkeratosis, decreased pigmentation in the basal cell layer, and a mild inflammatory reaction in the upper dermis (Fig. 13.4).

Therapy

Treatment is not often necessary as spontaneous resolution occurs. Emollients can be used for the dry scaling, and 1% hydrocortisone cream is used for the inflammatory reaction. For more severe disease, a trial of triamcinolone 0.1% cream twice daily for several weeks may be beneficial for involvement on the trunk.

Therapy for Pityriasis Alba

Initial
- Emollients (e.g., Eucerin cream)
- 1% Hydrocortisone cream daily

Alternative
- Triamcinolone 0.1% twice daily (avoid application to face)

Course and Complications

The patient must understand that repigmentation will be slow. In most patients, the disease resolves spontaneously, but this takes months and, sometimes, years. For affected children, the disease rarely persists into adulthood. The disorder has no complications.

Pathogenesis

The origin of this common disorder is unknown. Most investigators believe that the decreased pigment is a post-inflammatory phenomenon and that the initial event is a low-grade eczematous reaction. It may be a manifestation of inflammation related to decreased barrier protection from dry skin. The fact that the condition is commonly seen in children with atopic dermatitis lends credence to this dry skin association.

Pityriasis alba may be a low-grade eczema.

POST-INFLAMMATORY HYPOPIGMENTATION

Key Points

1. Inflammation suppresses or destroys melanocytes
2. Characterized by white macules without scale
3. Repigmentation takes months to years

Definition

Post-inflammatory hypopigmentation is the result of melanocyte destruction or suppressed melanin production secondary to inflammation of the skin (**Fig. 13.5**). It appears as a hypopigmented macule. The inflammation may be due to physical trauma, a chemical agent, or a primary skin disease.

Causes of post-inflammatory hypopigmentation:
1. Physical trauma
2. Chemicals
3. Skin diseases

Incidence

Inflammation-induced white spots are common incidental findings. Occasionally, they are the patient's primary complaint.

History

The inflammatory event responsible for the white spots is almost always remembered by the patient. Physical agents that often induce white spots include X-irradiation and frostbite. Industrial exposure to chemicals such as phenolic and sulfhydryl compounds can also produce hypopigmentation. Some inflammatory skin diseases can leave residual hypopigmentation. Common examples are discoid lupus erythematosus, eczematous dermatitis (particularly atopic dermatitis and seborrheic dermatitis in a darker-skinned individual), and psoriasis (**Fig. 13.6**). Uncommon causes are cutaneous sarcoidosis and mycosis fungoides, a form of cutaneous T-cell lymphoma.

Physical Examination

White macules, with or without scale, conform to areas of prior inflammation.

Differential Diagnosis

Post-inflammatory hypopigmentation may be confused with *vitiligo*, particularly when hypopigmentation is profound. However, the pigment loss is rarely complete, as it is in vitiligo. Moreover, in vitiligo, the depigmentation is only rarely preceded by recognizable inflammation.

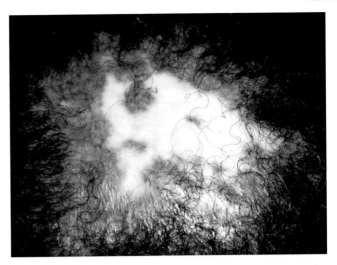

FIGURE 13.5 **Post-inflammatory hypopigmentation** – white macules on scalp secondary to 'burned out' discoid lupus erythematosus.

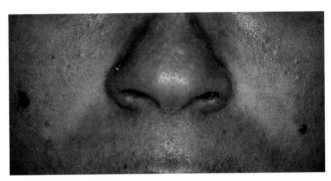

FIGURE 13.6 **Post-inflammatory hypopigmentation** – subtle white patches secondary to seborrheic dermatitis, more commonly seen in darker-skinned individuals. Note characteristic nasolabial involvement.

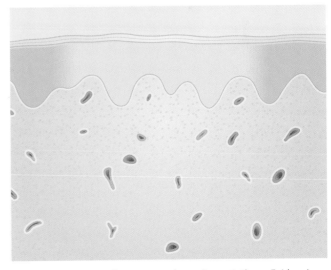

FIGURE 13.7 **Post-inflammatory hypopigmentation.** Epidermis – hypopigmented. Dermis – may show some residual inflammation.

Laboratory and Biopsy

No specific laboratory test is available. The biopsy is not specific, showing decreased pigmentation in the epidermis and occasional mild residual inflammation in the dermis (**Fig. 13.7**).

Therapy

Treatment is not usually required. No effective agent for repigmenting skin is available. Cosmetically troublesome areas can be disguised with an opaque cosmetic such as Covermark. To avoid future hypopigmentation, patients are advised to avoid contact with any responsible physical or chemical agents and to treat inflammatory skin disease promptly.

Therapy:
● None
● Cosmetic covering

Course and Complications

Usually, pigmentation returns gradually. Patients need to understand that this process takes months, and sometimes longer (**Fig. 13.8**). However, if the damage has been severe, the hypopigmentation may be permanent.

Repigmentation, if it occurs, takes months and, sometimes, years.

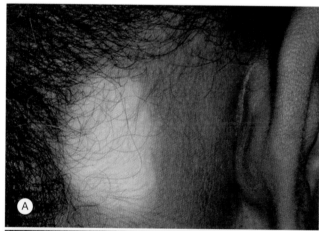
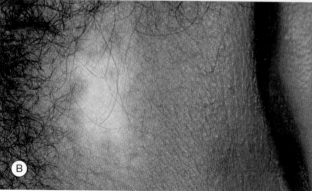

FIGURE 13.8 **A.** Post-inflammatory hypopigmentation secondary to the chemical squaric acid used to treat alopecia areata. **B.** Post-inflammatory hypopigmentation improving after 8 months of observation.

TINEA VERSICOLOR

Key Points

1. Common superficial fungal infection caused by *Malassezia* organisms
2. KOH preparation of subtle scale confirms the diagnosis
3. Appears on neck, trunk, and upper arms

Definition

Tinea versicolor is a superficial fungal infection of the stratum corneum that results in altered pigment in the epidermis. Clinically, the lesions appear as finely scaling patches, which, as the name versicolor implies, can be pink, tan, or white (**Figs 13.9, 13.10**). Of these, white is the most common.

Lesions in tinea versicolor can be of varying colors, the most common being white.

Incidence

Tinea versicolor is a common disease, affecting nearly 1% of the general population. In the authors' clinic, 1.4% of new patients are seen for tinea versicolor. The incidence is higher in tropical climates. Any age group may be affected, but the disease is most common in young adults. Immunosuppression, including that from systemic corticosteroids (either endogenous or exogenous), can be predisposing factors, but most patients are healthy.

History

Tinea versicolor is occasionally associated with mild pruritus, but more often it is asymptomatic. Most patients

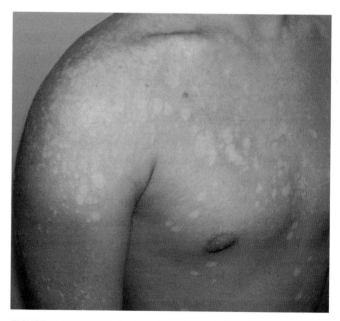

FIGURE 13.9 **Tinea versicolor** – hypopigmented patches.

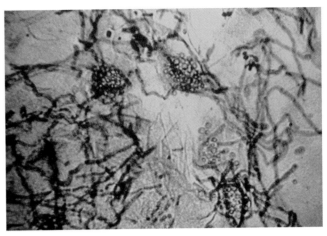

FIGURE 13.12 **KOH preparation** of tinea versicolor-diagnostic 'spaghetti (short hyphae) and meatballs (spores).'

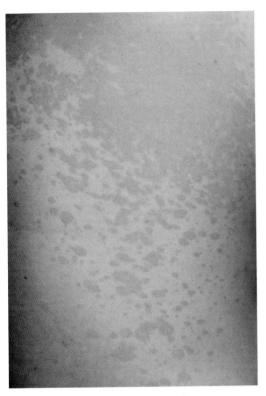

FIGURE 13.10 **Tinea versicolor** – pink-tan patches.

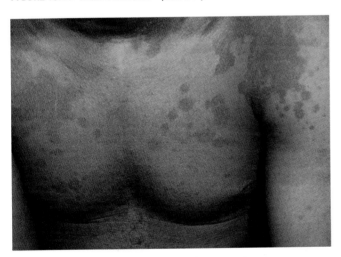

FIGURE 13.11 **Tinea versicolor** – darker brown patches.

seek medical attention because of its cosmetic appearance. Because the affected areas do not tan, the patient often first becomes aware of the condition after sun exposure. The surrounding normal skin tans, providing a contrast to the 'white spots.' During the winter months and in persons with darker complexions, the lesions appear more deeply pigmented than the normal skin (Fig. 13.11).

Physical Examination

The usual lesion is a round, hypopigmented, slightly scaling patch. It often starts as multiple small follicular macules, which subsequently become confluent. The scale usually is subtle and sometimes is appreciated only with gentle scraping of the skin, which reveals a fine,

crumbly scale. If a Wood's light examination is performed, the lesions will appear hypopigmented but not chalk white. With Wood's light examination, sometimes the scale fluoresces pale yellow or orange, but this finding is not universal and should not be relied on for diagnosis.

> In tinea versicolor, the scaling may be subtle.

The usual distribution for tinea versicolor is the neck, trunk, and upper arms, that is, the distribution of a short-sleeved turtleneck sweater. Distal extremity and facial involvement is uncommon, except in tropical climates.

Differential Diagnosis

In adults, the white spots of tinea versicolor are most often misdiagnosed as *vitiligo*. Tinea versicolor appearing as pink or tan scaling patches on the chest may be misdiagnosed as *seborrheic dermatitis*.

Laboratory Examination

The organism cannot be grown on routine fungal culture; therefore, the diagnosis rests with the KOH examination. Examination of the scale with a KOH preparation reveals short hyphae, which are often mixed with spores, giving an appearance of 'spaghetti (chopped-up spaghetti) and meatballs' or 'hot dogs and baked beans' (**Fig. 13.12**). Biopsy, seldom performed, shows abundant fungal organisms in a hyperkeratotic stratum corneum (**Fig. 13.13**).

Therapy

Topical selenium sulfide, zinc pyrithione (e.g., Head & Shoulders) shampoo, and ketoconazole (Nizoral) shampoo are commonly used. These agents are effective, easy to apply to a widespread area, and relatively inexpensive. The topical imidazole antifungal creams are effective against the organism, but this approach is expensive when the eruption is widespread – which it often is. Terbinafine (Lamisil) spray is also effective but expensive.

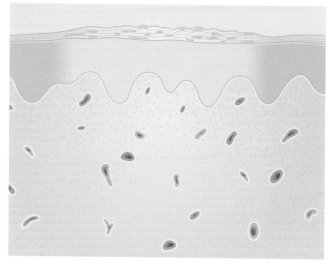

FIGURE 13.13 **Tinea versicolor.** Epidermis – slight hyperkeratosis; hyphae and spores, decreased pigmentation. Dermis – normal.

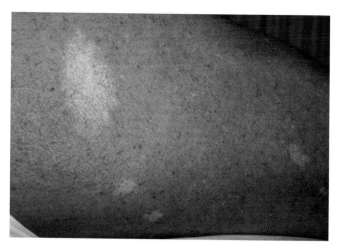

FIGURE 13.14 **Tuberous sclerosis** – white 'ash leaf' macule.

Oral fluconazole (Diflucan) is the simplest and most effective therapy. In most adult patients, the fungus is eradicated with a single 200-mg dose, which may be repeated in 2 weeks. Efficacy is enhanced if the patient works up a sweat 2 h after ingesting the fluconazole, thereby delivering the drug, which is concentrated in sweat, to the stratum corneum. For patients with recurrent disease, this regimen can be repeated every 3 months for 1 year.

Therapy for Tinea Versicolor

Initial

- Lather Selsun, Head & Shoulders, or Nizoral shampoo in a 'turtleneck sweater' distribution, preferably with a 'mesh puff'
- Rinse after 10 min
- Repeat this 3 days in a row, then 4 weeks in a row, then monthly to prevent recurrence
- Apply over-the-counter Lotrimin cream daily if just a couple of spots.

Alternative

- Fluconazole (Diflucan) one 200-mg tablet repeated again in 2 weeks
- Ketoconazole one 400-mg tablet repeated again in 2 weeks

Course and complications

The fungus is killed rapidly with therapy, but it takes months for the pigmentation to return to its normal color. It is important to explain this so that the patient will not view the treatment as a failure. After topical therapy, the recurrence rate is more than 50%, but this rate can be reduced to less than 15% with a monthly retreatment program using any of recommended treatment shampoos.

After the initial therapy, it takes months for the white spots to regain pigment.

Pathogenesis

Tinea versicolor is caused by infection with the fungus *Malassezia* species (*globosa*, *sympodialis*, and *furfur*). This organism is frequently present in its yeast form as a colonizer of normal skin. In tinea versicolor, the spores proliferate in the outer layers of the stratum corneum, often beginning in the areas of follicular openings. When the spore forms are transformed to hyphae, infection occurs as the hyphal structures invade more deeply into the stratum corneum, but they do not penetrate the viable epidermis. They cause thickening and disruption of the stratum corneum, expressed clinically as the fine scale. Fungal enzymes act on surface lipids and produce dicarboxylic acids that diffuse into the epidermis. These acids inhibit tyrosinase, the enzyme in melanocytes that is responsible for melanin production.

Not all patients exposed to this ubiquitous organism develop infection. In fact, conjugal cases are uncommon. Some individuals may be more susceptible by virtue of a genetic predisposition, the nature of which is not known.

TUBEROUS SCLEROSIS

Definition

Tuberous sclerosis is a rare, autosomal dominantly inherited, neurocutaneous disorder with several skin manifestations, including white macules, caused by mutations in one of two genes, hamartin (tsc1) and tuberin (tsc2). (Fig. 13.14). The classic triad of this disease consists of seizures, mental retardation, and adenoma sebaceum. *Adenoma sebaceum* is a misnamed disorder consisting of angiofibromas that begin in childhood and appear clinically as red papules on the face (**Fig. 13.15**).

White spots also often occur in this disease and are important diagnostically because they are usually present at birth. They appear as hypopigmented macules, ranging in size from 1 to 3 cm. They are often shaped like a 'thumbprint' or an 'ash leaf' – oval at one end and pointed at the other. They are most often found on the trunk and less often on the face and extremities. Patients may have as few as three or as many as 100 lesions. The spots are most easily seen with Wood's light examination; sometimes, particularly in infants with extremely fair

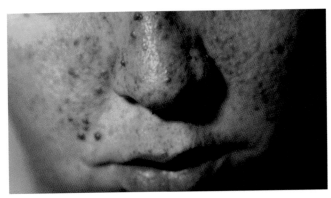

FIGURE 13.15 **Tuberous sclerosis** – adenoma sebaceum (angiofibromas) of the face.

skin, this is the only method of detection. Therefore, all infants with a seizure disorder should be screened for white spots with a Wood's light examination. Tuberous sclerosis is strongly suspected if more than three white spots are detected.

> The skin of all infants with seizures should be examined for white spots by Wood's light examination.

The nervous system is often affected. Calcification of intracranial nodules ('tubers') is common and can be detected early in patients and in apparently unaffected carriers with computed tomography or magnetic resonance imaging. Central nervous system involvement is the most debilitating. Mental retardation may be severe, and seizure disorders may be severe and difficult to control. Brain tumors occur in some patients. More than 10% of affected individuals die from internal organ involvement, including brain tumors, renal cysts and tumors, heart rhabdomyomas, and lung lymphangiomas. More mildly affected patients have slow progression of their disease over years.

VITILIGO

Key Points

1. Wood's light accentuates completely depigmented macules without scale
2. Commonly seen in periorificial and dorsal hands, elbows, and knees
3. Vitiligo is a common cause of depigmentation

Definition

Vitiligo is an acquired condition in which functional melanocytes disappear from affected skin. The cause is unknown. Lesions clinically appear as totally white, non-scaling, sharply demarcated macules (**Fig. 13.16**).

Incidence

The reported incidence of vitiligo varies with the population studied. Higher incidence rates in dark-skinned individuals may reflect the observation that vitiligo is more

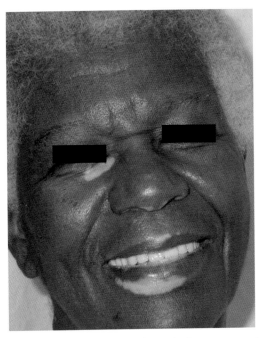

FIGURE 13.16 **Vitiligo** – depigmented macules in common periorificial distribution.

noticeable in more darkly pigmented skin. In the USA, vitiligo is estimated to occur in almost 1% of the general population. Vitiligo represents the presenting complaint in 0.6% of the authors' new patients. The disease can begin at any age, but the peak incidence is in the 10–30-year age group.

History

Vitiligo is usually asymptomatic. It begins as one or more small spots that gradually enlarge. The affected areas sunburn easily. Most patients seek medical help because of cosmetic disfigurement.

Physical Examination

The primary lesion is a white macule that is usually totally depigmented. This feature can be appreciated best by Wood's light examination, which accentuates the pigment contrast and also may make evident previously undetected areas in lightly pigmented skin. The skin otherwise is normal; specifically, no scale is present. Macules of vitiligo are round or oval. They may become confluent as they enlarge, resulting in a large macule that has an irregular border but remains sharply demarcated from the surrounding normal skin.

> In vitiligo, depigmentation is complete; this is best seen by Wood's light examination.

Vitiligo can affect any area of the skin and mucous membranes, but the most common areas are the extensor bony surfaces (backs of the hands, elbows, and knees) and the periorificial areas (around the mouth, eyes, rectum, and genitalia) (**Fig. 13.17**). Involvement of hairy areas often results in depigmentation of the hair (**Fig. 13.18**).

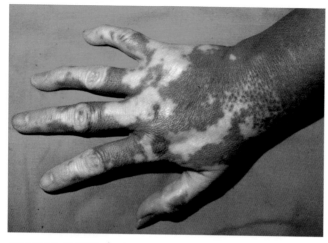

FIGURE 13.17 **Vitiligo** – depigmented macules in acral distribution are difficult to treat.

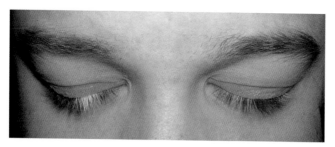

FIGURE 13.18 **Vitiligo** – hair turns white with follicular involvement.

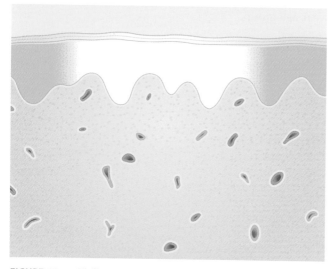

FIGURE 13.19 **Vitiligo.** Epidermis – complete absence of pigment and melanocytes. Dermis – normal.

Differential Diagnosis

Vitiligo is more often overdiagnosed than underdiagnosed. Any of the conditions listed in **Table 13.1** may be misdiagnosed as vitiligo. Less often, vitiligo is misdiagnosed as one of these conditions. However, vitiligo is the only one of the common white spot diseases that results in total depigmentation. In addition, it can be differentiated clinically from *tinea versicolor* and *pityriasis alba* by the absence of scale.

Laboratory and Biopsy

The laboratory is not helpful for diagnosing vitiligo. Serum thyroid tests and a complete blood count with differential may be ordered to screen for occasionally associated thyroid disease and rarely associated pernicious anemia and Addison's disease. Biopsy is not usually necessary. If performed, it will show an absence of melanocytes, sometimes with accompanying inflammation (**Fig. 13.19**). The presence or absence of melanocytes may be difficult to appreciate with routine hematoxylin and eosin staining. Special stains and techniques are required for definitive identification.

Therapy

There is no cure for vitiligo. Emotional support is a top priority. The goal of therapy is to deal with the cosmetic disfigurement caused by the disease. Therapy for repigmentation is prolonged, and the results are often suboptimal. For limited disease, topical high-potency steroids (e.g., clobetasol [Temovate]) have been successful in some patients. To avoid skin atrophy, the authors like to use the treatment in intervals (e.g., alternating twice daily for 1 week and then 1 week off). Topical macrolides (e.g., Protopic or Elidel) are gaining popularity for use in facial vitiligo. These agents do not cause skin atrophy. Facial and truncal vitiligo responds more favorably to medical therapy than vitiligo located on the extremities. For extensive involvement, the administration of ultraviolet (UV) light is recommended. The current treatment of choice is narrow-band UVB for adults and children over 6 years of age. The excimer laser, which emits light at 308 nm (close to narrow-band UVB wavelength), is a new form of phototherapy and has the advantage of delivering laser light to affected skin only. Long-term effects are unknown. Another phototherapy, which is more difficult for the patient, is the administration of a psoralen medication (trimethylpsoralen or 8 methoxypsoralen) followed by exposure to long-wave ultraviolet A light (PUVA). The psoralens can be administered topically or systemically (more frequently the latter), especially for widespread disease. Some 100 or more treatments are often required to achieve the end result, which in some patients is complete repigmentation; in others only partial pigmentation occurs, and in the remainder treatment fails.

Initial therapy: narrow-band UVB or topical steroids.

Surgical therapies have also been employed occasionally. Normally pigmented skin is harvested (by suction blisters or punch biopsies) and transplanted into vitiliginous areas. Experimental transplantation of cultured melanocytes has also been reported.

An alternative is to cover the lesions with a cosmetic that is blended to match the color of the patient's normal skin. The products most frequently used for this are Covermark and Dermablend.

Cosmetic covering agents may be helpful.

In selected patients with extensive disease, the best cosmetic result may be obtained by depigmenting the remaining normal skin. Topical application of 20% monobenzyl ether of hydroquinone (Benoquin) is used for this, but the patient must be aware that the resulting depigmentation is irreversible.

Therapy for Vitiligo

Initial
- Emotional support and covering cosmetics:
  - Covermark
  - Dermablend
- Topical steroids:
  - Clobetasol cream twice daily alternating one week on/off
- Narrow-band UVB
- Topical macrolides:
  - Protopic twice daily for 3 months

Alternative
- PUVA, topical or systemic
- Surgical: Epidermal grafting or autologous minigrafting

Course and Complications

The course of vitiligo is unpredictable. In most patients, it is chronic and often slowly progressive. Occasionally, it involves the total body surface, resulting in complete depigmentation. Spontaneous repigmentation occurs in a minority of patients but usually is incomplete. Repigmentation begins around the hair follicles, so it appears as freckles that become confluent as they enlarge.

Associated systemic disorders occur in some patients with vitiligo. Thyroid abnormalities, including Graves' disease and thyroiditis, are the most common, with a frequency ranging from 1% to 30%, depending on the series. Addison's disease, pernicious anemia, and alopecia areata are other 'autoimmune' disorders uncommonly found in association with vitiligo. Recent experiments indicate polymorphisms located in NALP1, which is involved in the regulation of innate immune responses, play a role in these other disease susceptibilities in a subset of patients with vitiligo.

Many patients with vitiligo, particularly deeply pigmented patients, suffer social stigmatization. In some cultures, vitiligo has been confused with the white spots of leprosy and has resulted in social ostracism.

Pathogenesis

Melanocytes are absent in vitiligo. The mechanism for their disappearance is not known. Three proposed theories, not necessarily mutually exclusive, are highlighted:

Proposed pathologic mechanisms:
1. Autoimmune
2. Neural
3. Self-destruction

1. *Autoimmune*. Investigators have proposed that melanocytes are destroyed by an immune mechanism. Antibodies against melanocyte antigens have been detected in patients with vitiligo. These may be the primary cause of the disease, or they may occur secondary to an initial injury to the melanocytes that results in the production of antigens with subsequent antibody formation. Cellular immune mechanisms have also been implicated in melanocyte destruction.
2. *Neural*. This theory proposes that a neurochemical mediator is responsible for the destruction of the melanocytes. Some animal models have clear-cut neural control mechanisms for pigment formation.
3. *Self-destruction*. The intermediate compounds in melanin synthesis are cytotoxic when present in sufficient concentrations. The self-destruction theory holds that, in vitiligo, these compounds accumulate in melanocytes and eventually destroy them.

UNCOMMON CAUSES OF WHITE SPOTS

HYPOPIGMENTED MYCOSIS FUNGOIDES

Mycosis fungoides is the most common type of cutaneous T-cell lymphoma. Patients often present with

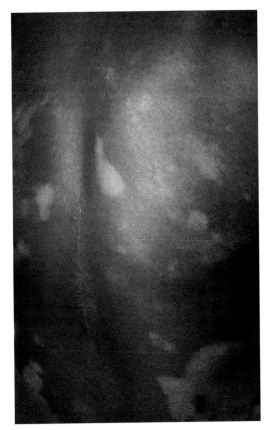

FIGURE 13.20 Hypopigmented mycosis fungoides – hypopigmented patches located on trunk.

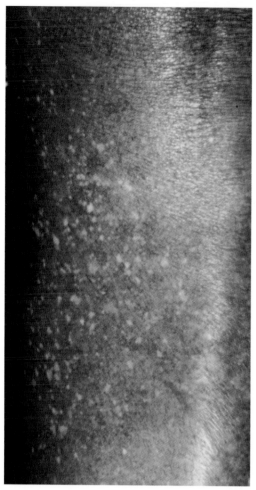

FIGURE 13.21 **Idiopathic guttate hypomelanosis** – 'confetti-like' white macules on anterior shin.

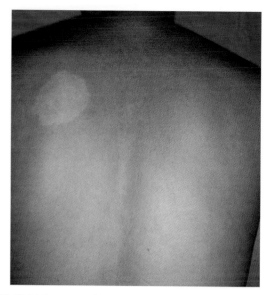

FIGURE 13.22 **Leprosy** – hypopigmented patch. *(Courtesy of Shyam B. Verma, MBBS, DVD, Baroda, India.)*

IDIOPATHIC GUTTATE HYPOMELANOSIS

Although this is a relatively common condition, it is under-recognized by physicians. Women are affected more commonly than men. The lesions appear as well demarcated, small macules, like 'sprinkled confetti' (**Fig. 13.21**). They appear most commonly on the shins, but may also be found on the forearms. There is no effective treatment.

LEPROSY

Leprosy is endemic in south-eastern USA and Hawaii. It is caused by the acid-fast organism *Mycobacterium leprae*. The diagnosis is frequently delayed by 1 year in the USA. Often the earliest sign is a solitary hypopigmented macule (**Fig. 13.22**). The earliest sensory change is loss of feeling to light touch and cold in the hands and feet. Nerve involvement is a disease hallmark. A biopsy with special stains (Fite stain) for the organism confirms the diagnosis.

patches that have been diagnosed as 'nonspecific eczema.' Although the patches of mycosis fungoides are characteristically erythematous with fine scale, they can appear as hypopigmented patches. The skin lesions have a predilection for the buttocks and trunk (**Fig. 13.20**), and can evolve into plaques or tumors. If a dermatitis fails to respond to topical steroids, especially when located on the trunk, a skin biopsy should be performed to confirm the suspicion of mycosis fungoides.

Generalized Erythema 14

Chapter Contents

- Drug Eruptions
- Viral Exanthems
- Uncommon Causes of Generalized Erythema
  - Systemic Lupus Erythematosus
  - Toxic Erythema
- Other Uncommon Causes – Generalized Erythema
  - Erythroderma
  - Sézary Syndrome

Key Points

1. Drug reactions and viral exanthems are the most common causes of a generalized erythema
2. Rule out infection first in a patient with generalized erythema
3. Correct diagnosis requires complete history, physical exam with attention to sites of skin involvement, skin biopsy consideration, and appropriate laboratory work-up

ABSTRACT

The rashes discussed in this chapter are composed of erythematous macules and papules that are widespread and sometimes confluent. Various terms have been used to describe this type of eruption, including maculopapular, exanthematous, and morbilliform (measles-like). In order to correctly diagnose generalized erythema, one must focus primarily on a complete history and physical, with special attention to sites of skin involvement. Skin biopsies tend to show nonspecific findings and fail to distinguish the causes of generalized erythema, except in the cases of systemic lupus erythematosus and Sézary syndrome. The majority of causes of generalized erythematous eruptions are listed in **Table 14.1** in the order of relative frequency.

DRUG ERUPTIONS

Key Points

1. Appear suddenly and with symmetry
2. Antibiotics, especially penicillins and sulfonamides, are common culprits
3. Discontinuation of offending drugs leads to quick resolution

Definition

The expression: 'For any rash, think drug!' reflects the finding that drug eruptions can appear similar to many inflammatory skin diseases. Think drug reaction for any symmetric rash of sudden onset. The two most common eruptions for drug reactions are hives (discussed in Ch. 16) and morbilliform rashes. Of these two, morbilliform rashes are more common. A morbilliform drug rash appears as a generalized eruption of erythematous macules and papules, often confluent in large areas (**Fig. 14.1**).

Incidence

Only 0.6% of the authors' new outpatients are seen for a drug eruption. The frequency, however, is much higher among hospitalized patients, most of whom are elderly and who receive an average of nine drugs. Drug rashes head the list for our hospital consultations and account for 7% of all dermatology consultations. It is estimated that 7% of inpatients experience an adverse drug reaction and that 2.3% of inpatients have skin reactions related to medications. Common offenders are:

- Antibiotics:
  - β-Lactam antibiotics-penicillins, cephalosporins
  - Sulfonamides-trimethoprim-sulfamethoxazole (be aware of cross-reactivity with sulfonamide derivatives, especially in the following drug classes: diuretics, hypoglycemic, and anti-inflammatories)
- Diuretics:
  - Furosemide (contains a sulfonamide)
  - Hydrochlorothiazide (contains a sulfonamide)
- Nonsteroidal anti-inflammatory drugs (NSAIDs)

TABLE 14.1 Generalized erythema

	Frequency[a]	Etiology	History	Physical Examination	Differential Diagnosis	Laboratory Test
Drug eruption	0.6[b]	Drug	Recent new drug Pruritus Usually no fever	Rash bright red and confluent	Exfoliative erythroderma (chronic)	–
Viral exanthem	0.2	Rubeola Rubella Enteroviruses, etc.	Associated 'viral' symptoms	Erythema mild to moderate Mucous membranes occasionally involved	Drug reaction	Acute and convalescent viral titers
'Toxic' erythema	<0.1	Group A streptococci S. aureus Unknown	Patient feels extremely ill ('toxic') No pruritus	Rash accentuated in flexural folds and often feels like sandpaper Mucous membranes often involved	Drug reaction	Bacterial cultures
Systemic lupus erythematosus (SLE)	<0.1	Autoimmune	Other symptoms of SLE	'Butterfly' distribution on face Sun-exposed areas favored Rarely total body	Drug reaction	Antinuclear antibody Anti-DNA antibodies Complete blood count Urinalysis

[a]Percentage of new dermatology patients with this diagnosis seen in the Hershey Medical Center Dermatology Clinic, Hershey, PA.
[b]Frequency in outpatients. For an inpatient, a drug eruption is the most common dermatologic problem acquired in hospital.

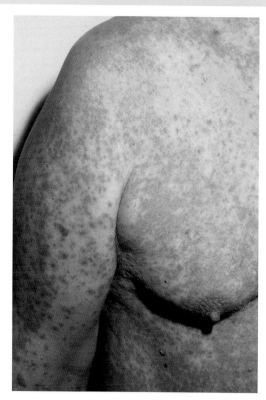

FIGURE 14.1 Drug eruption – bright red macules and papules confluent in large areas.

Approximately 2% of all medical inpatients experience drug-induced skin reactions.

History

The onset of a drug-induced morbilliform eruption is usually not immediate but rather begins within several days of the initiation of the drug. Onset is sometimes delayed for as long as 1 week, but seldom longer. Because no laboratory tests are available by which to identify the responsible drug, reliance is placed on the history. For patients receiving multiple drugs, this presents a problem. In selecting a single drug from a list of many, the two variables to be considered are: the temporal relationship between the initiation of the drug and the onset of the rash; and the likelihood that a given drug is likely to cause a drug eruption. In selecting a putative drug, it is helpful to construct a graph that depicts the patient's drug history (**Fig. 14.2**). In the example in **Figure 14.2**, drugs 'a', 'b', and 'c' are unlikely to be implicated because the patient had been receiving these agents for months. Drug 'd' was stopped 4 days before the rash began, thus making it a less likely cause. Drug 'g' was started 6 h *after* the rash appeared, and drug 'h' was started the following day. Drugs 'e' and 'f' were started 2 days before the rash and therefore have the best temporal relationship. Drug 'e' is a cephalosporin, a well known cause of rash, and drug 'f' is codeine, a rare cause of morbilliform eruptions. Therefore, drug 'e' is the probable cause and is the first to be discontinued. Remember to include over-the-counter medications such as vitamins in your exposure list as well as PRN medications for inpatients, such as furosemide which contains a sulfonamide, a common cause of inpatient drug reactions.

Suspect drugs that are:
1. New (started within 1 week of the rash)
2. Frequent offenders

In patients with drug rashes, itching is usually present but is not helpful as a diagnostic marker. Fever is rarely found.

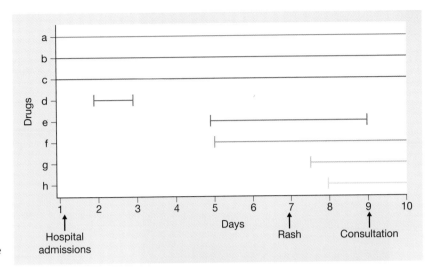

FIGURE 14.2 **Graphic depiction** of drug history (see text for discussion of drugs 'a–h').

TABLE 14.2 Other patterns of drug reactions

Type of Reaction	Drugs
Acneiform	Lithium
Pustules	β-Lactam antibiotics
Erythroderma	Allopurinol
Erythema multiforme, Stevens–Johnson syndrome, toxic epidermolysis necrosis	Anticonvulsants, allopurinol, NSAIDs, sulfonamides
Vasculitis	NSAIDs
Psoriasiform dermatitis	Interferon and granulocyte colony-stimulating factor (G-CSF), tumor necrosis factor inhibitors
Angioedema	ACE Inhibitors

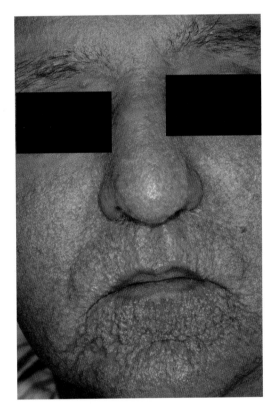

FIGURE 14.3 **Pustular drug eruption** – note symmetric distribution of minute pustules.

Physical Examination

The eruption is generalized and composed of brightly erythematous macules and papules that tend to be confluent in large areas. Characteristically, the erythema is intense or 'drug red'. Drug rashes usually start proximally and proceed distally, with the legs being the last to be involved as well as the last to clear. See **Table 14.2** for typical medications associated with other drug reaction patterns that are important to recognize clinically (**Fig. 14.3**).

Drug rashes are usually:
1. Bright red
2. Confluent in large areas

Differential Diagnosis

The differential diagnosis includes viral exanthem, toxic erythema, and chronic exfoliative erythroderma.

Differential diagnosis for acute morbilliform eruptions:
1. Drug
2. Viral
3. 'Toxic'

A *viral exanthem* and a drug eruption can be indistinguishable clinically. Often, a drug eruption is much more erythematous, more confluent, and more *pruritic*. The presence of viral signs and symptoms favors a diagnosis of a viral exanthem.

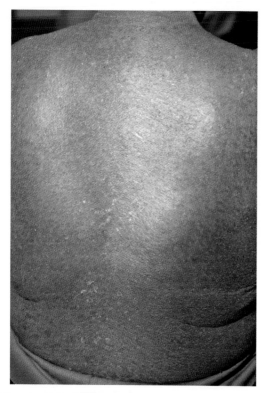

FIGURE 14.4 Exfoliative erythroderma.

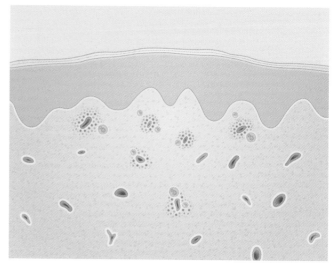

FIGURE 14.5 Epidermis – normal. Dermis – superficial and deep perivascular inflammatory cell infiltrate that includes eosinophils.

Toxic erythemas include scarlet fever, staphylococcal scarlatiniform eruptions, and Kawasaki syndrome (mucocutaneous lymph node syndrome). Features that help to distinguish these rashes from drug eruptions include a sandpaper-like texture of the 'toxic' rash, mucous membrane involvement (scarlet fever and Kawasaki syndrome), the presence of fever, and a focus of infection or the presence of lymphadenopathy.

When a generalized erythema becomes chronic, it is called an *exfoliative* erythroderma – exfoliative because of the prominent desquamation (**Fig. 14.4**). Long-term administration of an offending drug is one cause. The other three causes are generalization of a benign dermatosis (most often, psoriasis or atopic dermatitis), malignancy (most often, the Sézary variant of cutaneous T-cell lymphoma; see Ch. 9), and an idiopathic disorder.

Laboratory and Biopsy

No laboratory tests can enable the diagnosis of a drug eruption or the incrimination of a specific drug. Peripheral blood eosinophilia is sometimes present and may heighten the suspicion of a drug reaction. Skin biopsy is most often performed in patients with chronic exfoliative erythrodermas. A drug eruption shows a superficial and deep perivascular inflammatory cell infiltrate (**Fig. 14.5**). The presence of eosinophils in the infiltrate is an important clue suggesting a drug-related cause. Skin tests for penicillin may be useful for the diagnosis of immediate hypersensitivity reactions (hives and anaphylaxis) but not for morbilliform eruptions.

Therapy

When the offending drug is identified, it should be discontinued. If the patient is taking multiple drugs and it is not possible to be certain of the offending drug, the number of administered drugs should be reduced to an absolute minimum, and any remaining possible offenders should be changed to alternative agents when possible.

Therapy otherwise is symptomatic, with antihistamines (e.g., hydroxyzine 10–25 mg four times daily) most often used for the pruritus. Moisturizing lotions are helpful during the late desquamative phase of the reaction. Topical steroids are of little value. Systemic steroids are rarely required but are helpful for the patient experiencing intense pruritus.

Therapy for Drug Eruptions

Initial
- Discontinuance of the offending drug
- Antihistamines:
  - Hydroxyzine (Atarax) 10–25 mg q.i.d.
  - Diphenhydramine (Benadryl) 25–50 mg q.i.d.
- Moisturizers:
  - Eucerin cream b.i.d.

Alternative
- Systemic steroids: Prednisone 1 mg/kg then taper dose over 7–10 days

---

Course and Complications

Drug eruptions clear slowly with *time* after discontinuation of the responsible agent. The time required for total clearing is usually 1–2 weeks. For several days after the offending drug has been stopped, the eruption may actually worsen.

> Drug eruptions take 1–2 weeks to clear.

Complications are uncommon and primarily cutaneous. When large areas of skin are inflamed, increased body heat and water loss occur. In a patient already seriously ill, this could be a problem, but for most patients it is not.

One main risk of continuing an offending agent in the presence of a drug eruption involves progressive worsening of the rash, possibly eventuating in toxic epidermal necrolysis, which is characterized by the loss of large sheets of epidermis. Fortunately, this complication rarely occurs. In fact, sometimes a drug eruption clears despite continued treatment with the offending agent, although this approach is not desirable if an alternative drug is available. If the responsible drug has been identified, the patient should be advised to avoid the drug in the future, and the medical record should be clearly labeled.

> Potential consequences of continuing the offending drug – worsening rash.

Pathogenesis

Although specific immunologic and non-immunologic mechanisms have been documented for some types of drug-induced cutaneous reaction (e.g., hives and vasculitis), the mechanism for the morbilliform eruption remains unclear. Increasing experimental evidence points to a major role for cellular immune (type IV) processes. The clinical course with delayed onset and prolonged duration of the rash also favors this mechanism.

VIRAL EXANTHEMS

> ### Key Points
>
> 1. Caused by hematogenous dissemination of virus to skin
> 2. Preceded by prodrome of fever and constitutional symptoms
> 3. Treatment is symptomatic

Definition

Viral exanthems are caused by hematogenous dissemination of virus to the skin, in which a vascular response is elicited (**Fig. 14.6**). The clinical appearance of a virus-induced generalized erythema is not specific for a given virus; other signs and symptoms, however, may indicate a particular etiologic agent. The viruses that are most often associated with exanthems are rubeola (measles), rubella (German measles), herpesvirus type 6 (roseola), parvovirus B19 (erythema infectiosum), and the enteroviruses (ECHO and coxsackievirus).

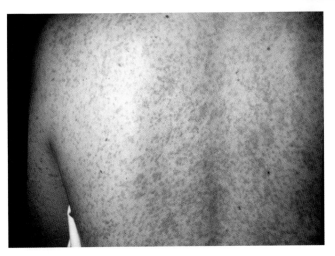

FIGURE 14.6 Viral exanthema – symmetric red macules and papules.

> Major viruses producing exanthems:
> 1. Measles (rubeola)
> 2. German measles (rubella)
> 3. Herpesvirus type 6 (roseola)
> 4. Parvovirus B19 (erythema infectiosum)
> 5. Enteroviruses (ECHO and coxsackievirus)

Incidence

Exanthem-producing viral infections rank high among the classic 'common childhood diseases'. Widespread immunization for rubella and rubeola has significantly reduced the incidence of these diseases. Most cases of measles in the USA are importation associated.

Viral exanthems occur in adults, but much less often than in children. In children aged less than 2 years, roseola is the most common viral exanthem. Erythema infectiosum ('fifth' disease) occurs in young school-aged children, often in epidemics. Enteroviral infections are most common in the summer and fall.

History

Most viral exanthems are preceded by a prodrome of fever and constitutional symptoms. In *measles*, the prodrome is characterized by the three Cs: cough, coryza, and conjunctivitis. A history of previous exposure to infected individuals may be elicited. Incubation times vary from days to weeks, depending on the virus. *Mononucleosis* alone is associated with rash only about 3% of the time, but with the administration of ampicillin the frequency of rash approaches 100%.

> In patients with infectious mononucleosis, ampicillin increases the likelihood of rash from 3% to nearly 100%.

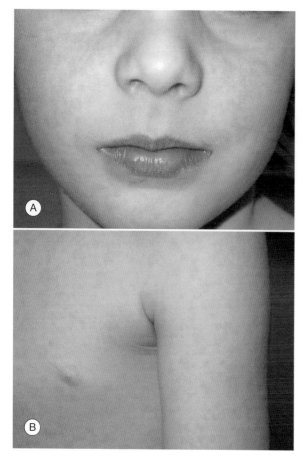

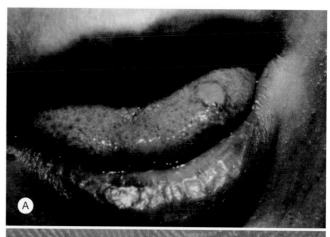

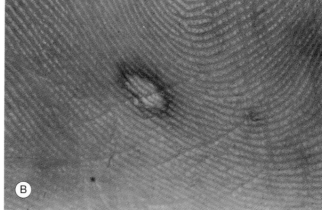

FIGURE 14.7 Erythema infectiosum. A. Characteristic 'slapped' cheeks. **B.** Reticulated (net-like) erythema on upper arm.

FIGURE 14.8 Hand-foot-mouth disease. A. Erosion with fibrinous base on tongue. **B.** Pustule with peripheral erythema oriented along skin lines on palm.

Physical Examination

The generalized eruption is composed of erythematous macules and papules. In *measles* and German measles, the rash typically begins on the head (characteristically behind the ears in measles) and proceeds to involve the trunk and extremities. In measles, individual lesions tend to become confluent on the face and trunk but remain discrete on the extremities. The macules and papules in *rubella* are discrete, even on the trunk and have a cephalo-caudad spread of exanthema, like measles. In *roseola* (exanthem subitum), rose-red macules and papules develop primarily on the trunk and proximal extremities. *Erythema infectiosum* characteristically begins with red cheeks that have a 'slapped' appearance followed by a reticulated (net-like) erythema on the trunk and proximal extremities (**Fig. 14.7**). The rashes associated with *enterovirus infections* are most often rubella-like, but occasionally purpuric. Vesicular eruptions also occur with some types of enterovirus infections, e.g., hand, foot, and mouth disease from coxsackievirus A-16 infection (**Fig. 14.8**).

Mucous membranes are sometimes involved. In rubella, red spots occur on the soft palate. In measles, Koplik's spots are characteristic and often precede the rash. *Koplik's spots* are found on the buccal mucosa and appear as tiny gray-white papules on an erythematous base. In roseola, erythematous macules develop on the soft palate 48 h before the exanthem.

Fever is almost always present. In patients with roseola caused by human herpesvirus type 6, the fever characteristically subsides abruptly just before the rash appears. The rash lasts 24–48 h and appears as discrete rose-red macules or maculopapules, similar to rubella and rubeola. (**Fig. 14.9**) In rubella, the most strikingly enlarged lymph nodes are found in the head and neck; in measles, lymphadenopathy is often generalized. Aseptic meningitis occasionally occurs in enterovirus infections.

> In roseola, fever subsides just before the rash appears.

Differential Diagnosis

Drug rashes are usually pruritic and are redder and more confluent than viral exanthems. *Toxic erythemas* favor flexural folds, may feel like sandpaper, and often have more extensive mucous membrane involvement. The rash in *Rocky Mountain spotted fever* begins as erythematous macules and papules but typically starts distally (hands and feet) and becomes *purpuric* as it progresses (see Ch. 17).

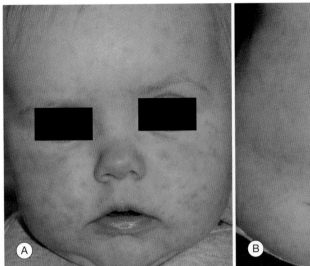
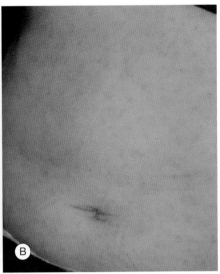

FIGURE 14.9 Roseola. A. Discrete rose red macules and papules on face. **B.** Discrete rose red macules and papules on trunk in same infant.

Laboratory and Biopsy

Routine laboratory tests are of no help. Usually, no tests are ordered; however, serologic tests can confirm the diagnosis by detecting a rise in antibody titer in convalescent compared with acute serum samples. Viral cultures are available but are not often obtained.

Skin biopsy is not indicated; histologic examination usually shows a nonspecific lymphocytic perivascular infiltrate. In measles, the infection also involves the epidermal cells, resulting in intranuclear inclusions, multinucleated giant cells, and individual cell necrosis.

Therapy

Treatment of acute disease is symptomatic. Rubeola and rubella can be prevented through vaccination with live attenuated virus.

Therapy for Viral Exanthems

Initial
- Antipyretics and analgesics: acetaminophen or ibuprofen
- Hydration
- Vaccine

Course and Complications

Spontaneous, complete resolution usually occurs over several days to a week. Systemic complications are uncommon. Encephalitis is the most serious, occurring in patients with measles at a rate of approximately 1 in 1000; it results in death in 10–20% of affected patients. The rate is much higher in some developing countries, where encephalitis remains a leading cause of death in children. Worldwide, measles continues to cause about 1 million deaths per year among children less than 5 years of age.

Encephalitis is the most serious complication of measles.

Rubella and erythema infectiosum are frequently complicated by arthritis in adults. Infection with parvovirus B19 has also been associated with acute aplastic crises in patients with a history of prior chronic hemolytic anemia, such as sickle cell disease. The most important complication of rubella is the *congenital rubella syndrome*, which occurs in babies born of mothers who were infected during the first trimester of pregnancy. With rubella vaccination in widespread use, this condition is rare. Herpesvirus type 6 is a major precipitant of febrile seizures in infants.

Pathogenesis

In all the viral exanthems, the virus gains entry through the upper respiratory (e.g., rubella and rubeola) or gastrointestinal (enteroviruses) route, incubates 'silently' for a period of days to weeks, and then enters a viremic phase that causes the febrile prodrome and results in dissemination of virus to other tissues, including the skin.

UNCOMMON CAUSES OF GENERALIZED ERYTHEMA

SYSTEMIC LUPUS ERYTHEMATOSUS

Key Points

1. An 'autoimmune' disorder
2. Malar rash is characteristic
3. Screen for systemic involvement
4. Stress sun protection

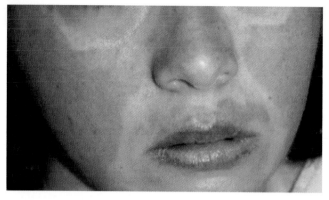

FIGURE 14.10 Systemic lupus erythematosus – 'butterfly' rash characterized by erythema with or without telangiectasia.

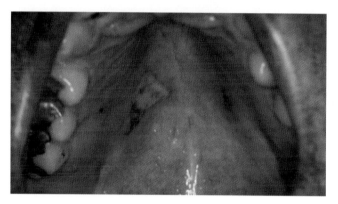

FIGURE 14.11 Systemic lupus erythematosus – erosion on hard palate.

Definition

Systemic lupus erythematosus (SLE) is an 'autoimmune' disorder in which virtually any kind of skin lesion can occur, including macules, papules, plaques, bullae, purpura, subcutaneous nodules, and ulcers (**Fig. 14.10**). The face is frequently involved. Discoid lupus erythematosus and subacute cutaneous lupus erythematosus are scaling disorders, discussed in Chapter 9. For generalized erythematous eruptions, SLE should be considered a possible (although uncommon) cause, particularly when other signs and symptoms of the disease are present.

Incidence

In the USA, the number of women with SLE outnumber men with the condition, by approximately 6 : 1. African-American women have a 2.5–6-fold higher risk of developing SLE compared with Caucasian women. Women of childbearing age are most commonly affected.

History

With active SLE, fatigue, fever, arthralgia, and weight change are the most common constitutional symptoms. Mucocutaneous symptoms of SLE include nasal and oral ulcerations, photosensitivity, alopecia, and Raynaud's phenomenon (**Fig. 14.11**). Arthritis is common. Serositis (with pleuritis or pericarditis) and neurologic manifestations (e.g., headache and seizures) also occur.

Because SLE can be drug induced, a careful drug history is important. The drugs most often implicated are procainamide, hydralazine, quinidine, and isoniazid. Drug induced lupus tends to occur in patients over 50 years old, has a male to female ratio of 1 : 1, and symptoms resolve after drug discontinuation.

Physical Examination

The erythematous rash of lupus often has a violaceous hue. It is frequently accentuated in sun-exposed areas, but in some patients, is generalized. The malar area of the face is a common location, where it produces the 'butterfly rash'. The malar rash in lupus tends to spare the nasolabial folds and is frequently accompanied by telangiectasia.

Differential Diagnosis

The diagnosis of SLE is established by a combination of historic, physical, and laboratory findings. The American Rheumatism Association criteria for lupus are listed below. In this listing, the definitions of the disorders are as follows: persistent heavy proteinuria or cellular casts for renal; seizures or psychosis for neurologic; hemolytic anemia, leukopenia, lymphopenia, or thrombocytopenia for hematologic; and positive lupus anticoagulant, anti-double-stranded DNA antibody, anti-Smith (Sm) antibody, or anti-cardiolipin antibody (false-positive serologic test for syphilis) for immunologic. Patients with four or more of the criteria are diagnosed as having SLE.

American Rheumatism Association criteria for SLE[a]:
1. Malar rash
2. Discoid rash
3. Photosensitivity
4. Oral ulcers
5. Arthritis
6. Serositis
7. Renal disorder
8. Neurologic disorder
9. Hematologic disorder
10. Immunologic disorder
11. Antinuclear antibody

[a]SLE is diagnosed if four or more are present.

Other *collagen vascular diseases* may be considered in the differential diagnosis, and sometimes an overlap occurs among several of these disorders; mixed connective tissue disease is an example. In *dermatomyositis*, the characteristic skin findings are violaceous ('heliotrope') edema of the eyelids (**Fig. 14.12**), flat-topped papules over the knuckles (Gottron's papules) (**Fig. 14.13**), and reticulated patches of pigment, erythema, and telangiectasia (poikiloderma). Periungual erythema with telangiectasia is virtually diagnostic of a collagen vascular disease, most often dermatomyositis (**Fig. 14.14**). *Scleroderma* is less likely to be confused with SLE, but Raynaud's phenomenon, although less common in SLE, occurs in both conditions, and some patients have features that overlap the two diseases.

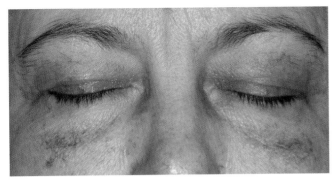

FIGURE 14.12 Dermatomyositis – violaceous ('heliotrope') macules of eyelids.

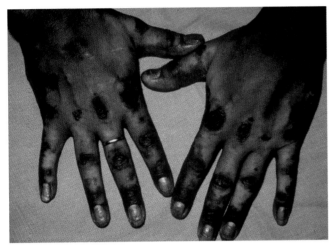

FIGURE 14.13 Dermatomyositis – Gottron's papules; hyperpigmented papules over the knuckles.

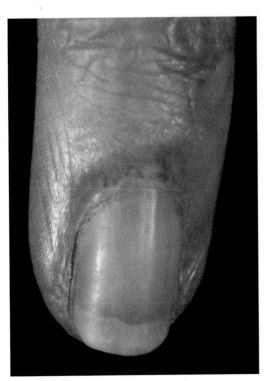

FIGURE 14.14 Periungual telangiectasia in a patient with dermatomyositis.

In patients with *photosensitivity*, causes other than lupus should be considered. The major causes are drugs, porphyria, and polymorphous light eruption (see Ch. 23).

The most common cause of a butterfly rash is not SLE but rather *seborrheic dermatitis*. Seborrheic dermatitis usually can be distinguished by the presence of the fine, yellowish scale, involvement of the nasolabial folds, and coexistence of a similar scaling rash on the scalp, behind the ears, on the eyebrows, and, often, in the presternal area. Also, rosacea is commonly mistaken for lupus. Like lupus, rosacea flares with sun exposure. The presence of papules and pustules on convex surfaces of the face and the lack of systemic symptoms in rosacea distinguish it from lupus.

Laboratory and Biopsy

The screening tests for SLE are complete blood count, platelet count, urinalysis, and antinuclear antibody (ANA) test. If the ANA test is positive, an anti-DNA antibody test is ordered because it is more specific for SLE. Antibodies to the Sm antigen are also highly specific for SLE but are found less frequently than are the antibodies to double-stranded DNA (dsDNA). Serum complement is often depressed in patients with active SLE. Antibodies to DNA histones are positive in patients with drug-induced lupus.

SLE initial screen:
1. Complete blood count with platelet count
2. Urinalysis
3. Antinuclear antibody test

Confirmatory autoantibody tests for lupus:
1. Double-stranded DNA
2. Smith

Skin biopsy findings in lupus include vacuolar degeneration of the basal cell layer with a perivascular and periappendageal lymphocytic infiltrate. With immunofluorescence staining, immunoglobulin and complement depositions are found at the dermal-epidermal junction (lupus band test), not only in involved skin but often also in clinically uninvolved skin in patients with SLE (**Fig. 14.15**). The lupus band test is also positive in involved skin but is negative in clinically uninvolved skin in patients with purely cutaneous lupus. Although still used occasionally, the lupus band test has now been largely replaced by serologic testing (ANA, anti-DNA, anti-Sm).

Therapy

Cutaneous involvement can be treated with moderate- to high-potency topical steroids or topical macrolides (tacrolimus) and sunscreens that filter out both short- and long-wave ultraviolet light (e.g., sunscreens that contain zinc oxide or titanium dioxide). An antimalarial such as hydroxychloroquine (Plaquenil) at a dosage of 200 mg

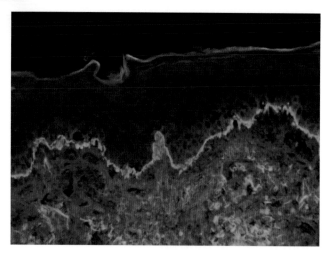

FIGURE 14.15 Systemic lupus erythematosus – lupus band test; immunoglobulin G deposition at the dermal-epidermal junction. *(Reprinted from Helm KF, Marks JG Jr. 1998. Atlas of Differential Dermatology, 1st edn, p. 36. Copyright 1998, with permission of Elsevier.)*

daily or twice daily is used for more severe cutaneous disease that is unresponsive to topical therapy. Antimalarials are also helpful for fatigue and arthritis. In patients with systemic disease including renal involvement, systemic steroids and other immunosuppressants are used.

Therapy for Cutaneous Lupus

Initial
- Sunscreens and protective clothing
- Topical steroids:
  - Triamcinolone cream 0.1% (medium)
  - Fluocinonide cream 0.05% (strong)
- Topical macrolides:
  - Tacrolimus
  - Pimecrolimus
- Antimalarials (for more severe disease):
  - Hydroxychloroquine 200 mg b.i.d.

Alternative
- Immunosuppressants:
  - Mycophenolate mofetil
  - Azathioprine
  - Methotrexate
- Systemic steroids

Course and Complications

In patients with SLE, the 5-year survival rate is now greater than 90%, and more than 80% of patients survive at least 10 years. Patients with nephritis have a worse prognosis than those without the complication. Men do worse than women. Patients less than 16 years of age who have no renal involvement have an excellent prognosis. In one large series, the most common causes of death were renal disease and sepsis, often secondary to iatrogenic immunosuppression.

Pathogenesis

The pathogenesis of the skin lesions in lupus is discussed in Chapter 9. Patients with subacute cutaneous lupus erythematosus often have extensive skin disease but limited systemic involvement. These patients are frequently ANA negative but have circulating antibodies to cytoplasmic antigens, designated Ro (Sjögren's syndrome A) and La (Sjögren's syndrome B) antigens. In SLE, autoantibodies are formed to nuclear antigens (ANA and anti-DNA). Autoantibodies are involved in the formation of immune complexes, followed by complement activation, and this process contributes to the inflammatory response in many tissues, including skin and kidney. The degree of complement consumption is reflected by the finding of diminished serum levels of complement in patients with active disease.

In lupus, the autoantibodies are produced by B cells, which appear to be stimulated by activated T cells (higher ratio of CD4+ to CD8+ T cells) that have escaped from the normal mechanisms of tolerance to self-antigens.

Genetic factors play a role in many patients with lupus. Familial lupus is well documented. Concordant disease is approximately 30% in monozygotic twins compared with 5% in dizygotic twins.

Environmental factors also have been implicated in lupus. For example, SLE is rare in Black Africans. Sunlight is definitely involved.

TOXIC ERYTHEMA

Key Points

1. Infection is usually the cause
2. Flexural accentuation of exanthem is often present
3. Treat underlying infection

Definition

Toxic erythema is a cutaneous response to a circulating toxin. In scarlet fever, erythrogenic toxin is elaborated by group A streptococci (*Streptococcus pyogenes*), usually infecting the pharynx. In staphylococcal scarlatiniform eruption, staphylococcal scalded skin syndrome (SSSS), and toxic shock syndrome, the responsible toxins are elaborated by a focus of *Staphylococcus aureus* infection or colonization. Cases of toxic shock-like syndrome have also been reported in association with severe infections with group A streptococci. In mucocutaneous lymph node syndrome (**Fig. 14.16**), a toxin is presumed but has not been identified. For all toxic erythemas, the skin becomes generally red, often feels like sandpaper, and undergoes post-inflammatory desquamation. Mucous membrane involvement is also common.

Toxic erythemas:
1. Scarlet fever
2. Staphylococcal scalded skin syndrome

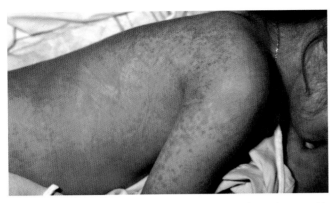

FIGURE 14.16 **Kawasaki syndrome** – generalized erythema with sandpaper texture.

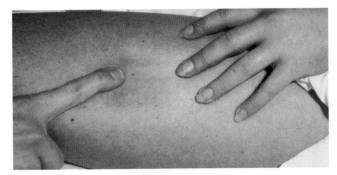

FIGURE 14.17 **Toxic shock syndrome** – generalized erythema that blanches.

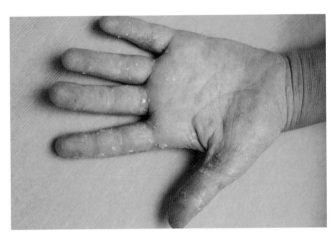

FIGURE 14.18 **Kawasaki syndrome** – desquamation follows erythema and edema of the hands, a typical finding.

3. Toxic shock syndrome
4. Kawasaki syndrome

Incidence

Toxic erythemas are still uncommon, although they have been increasing in frequency in recent years. Children are affected most often, except for toxic shock syndrome, which usually occurs in adults. After the advent of antibiotics, scarlet fever became a less common and generally less serious disease, although this trend has been reversing in recent years. Neonates are at highest risk for SSSS because of decreased toxin clearance by kidneys and lack of antibody to the toxin.

> Except for toxic shock syndrome, toxic erythemas occur most often in children.

History

Fever is common to all toxic erythemas. Patients with scarlet fever have a history of a sore throat preceding the rash by 1–2 days. In SSSS, patients may have a history of a local staphylococcal infection causing conjunctivitis, cutaneous abscess, or external otitis. Patients with toxic shock syndrome and mucocutaneous lymph node syndrome look and feel the most seriously ill. Staphylococcal toxic shock syndrome was first described in menstruating women who used occlusive tampons that allowed staphylococcal organisms to proliferate in the occluded vaginal tract. This disorder is now more frequently found in postoperative patients. The focus of infection for staphylococcal toxic shock syndrome is usually the skin, most commonly an area of painful cellulitis on an extremity. The onset of toxic shock syndrome is abrupt. As the name suggests, hypotension is common, as are vomiting, diarrhea, severe myalgia, and encephalopathy with mental confusion. Patients with Kawasaki syndrome frequently experience abdominal pain, diarrhea, arthralgia, and other systemic symptoms.

Physical Examination

Toxic erythemas are characterized by a generalized, usually brightly erythematous eruption that frequently feels sandpapery and is accentuated in flexural folds (**Fig. 14.17**). Post-inflammatory desquamation, particularly of the hands and feet, is common but not pathognomonic (**Fig. 14.18**).

> Toxic erythemas are usually:
> 1. Sandpapery
> 2. Accentuated in flexural folds
> 3. Followed by desquamation

Mucous membrane involvement is usually striking, occurring in all toxic eruptions except SSSS. Patients with scarlet fever have acute streptococcal pharyngitis and a 'strawberry tongue', which starts with a white exudate studded with prominent red papillae ('white strawberry'). After several days, the tongue becomes 'beefy red' ('red strawberry'). In toxic shock syndrome, mucous membrane hyperemia frequently affects the conjunctivae, oral pharynx, or vagina. In Kawasaki syndrome, patients usually have marked erythema of the lips ('cherry-red' lips), tongue ('strawberry' tongue), and conjunctivae. In this disease, asymmetric lymphadenopathy occurs in approximately 75% of patients – hence the name mucocutaneous lymph node syndrome.

> Mucous membrane involvement accompanies all toxic erythemas except staphylococcal scalded skin syndrome.

TABLE 14.3 Diagnostic criteria for toxic shock syndrome and Kawasaki syndrome

Toxic Shock Syndrome	Kawasaki Syndrome
Fever of 38.9°C or higher	Fever for 5 days or more
Scarlatiniform rash	Red palms and soles with edema, then desquamation
Desquamation of skin 1–2 weeks after onset	Exanthem on trunk
Hypotension	Conjunctivitis
Clinical or laboratory abnormalities of at least three organ systems	Mucosal erythema (lips, tongue, or pharynx)
Absence of other causes of the illness	Cervical lymphadenopathy
(All six are required for diagnosis)	(Fever plus four of the remaining five criteria are required for diagnosis)

Differential Diagnosis

The differential diagnosis includes *drug eruption, viral exanthem,* and *toxic epidermal necrolysis.* Toxic epidermal necrolysis is a severe, generalized form of erythema multiforme (see Ch. 16) characterized by intense erythema and extensive blistering that occurs in sheets. Skin biopsy in this disease shows the blister to be subepidermal, rather than intraepidermal. In SSSS, the skin split is intraepidermal, specifically in the granular layer.

Group A streptococci are recovered from the pharynx in patients with scarlet fever. Absence of mucous membrane involvement suggests staphylococcal scarlatiniform or scalded skin eruption. Multisystem involvement including hypotension in a menstruating female patient strongly suggests toxic shock syndrome. Striking mucous membrane involvement and lymphadenopathy in a child who appears seriously ill are features of Kawasaki syndrome. The diagnostic criteria for toxic shock syndrome and Kawasaki syndrome are listed in **Table 14.3**.

Laboratory and Biopsy

Bacterial cultures from potential foci of infection are mandatory. In suspected cases of scarlet fever, a throat culture should be taken. Less often, streptococcal impetigo serves as the focus of infection. For staphylococcal toxic erythemas, a focus of bacterial colonization or infection should be sought and cultured. In women with suspected toxic shock syndrome, vaginal cultures should be obtained. In seriously ill patients, blood cultures should also be drawn because some patients with staphylococcal toxic shock syndrome are septic. The focus of infection in patients with streptococcal toxic shock syndrome most often is a severe, necrotizing cellulitis, which should be cultured. These patients often also have positive blood cultures. Laboratory evaluation of other organ systems is appropriate in toxic shock syndrome and Kawasaki

disease. These include tests of hematopoietic, hepatic, cardiac, and renal functions. In toxic shock syndrome, thrombocytopenia occurs early; in Kawasaki disease, thrombocytosis occurs late.

Cultures should be obtained from potential bacterial reservoirs:
1. Throat
2. Skin
3. Vagina
4. Blood

The biopsy is nonspecific in toxic erythemas, except in SSSS, in which an intraepidermal separation is found.

Therapy

Initial management of toxic erythemas often require inpatient hospitalization, except for scarlet fever, in order to provide intensive supportive care. Streptococcal disease is usually treated with penicillin, although penicillin-resistant strains of streptococci are beginning to be reported. Staphylococcal infections are treated with penicillinase-resistant antibiotics such as oral dicloxacillin or intravenous nafcillin. Intravenous γ-globulin and aspirin are used to treat Kawasaki syndrome.

Initial treatment:
1. Hospitalization for supportive and ancillary care
2. Antibiotics for infections
3. Aspirin and γ-globulin for Kawasaki syndrome

Course and Complications

Scarlet fever follows a relatively benign course, with complete recovery usually within 5–10 days. Penicillin has dramatically altered the course of scarlet fever in both duration and severity. Complications are uncommon with scarlet fever, although post-streptococcal glomerulonephritis may occur. Death has occurred in patients with toxic shock syndrome as a result of severe hypotension, sepsis, or multisystem organ failure. The death rate for streptococcal toxic shock syndrome is higher than that for staphylococcal toxic shock syndrome (70% versus 30%, respectively).

Fever is most prolonged in Kawasaki syndrome, usually lasting for more than 5 days. Death can result from Kawasaki syndrome, usually the result of coronary artery aneurysm and thrombosis, which is striking given the young age of these patients. Cardiology consultation and follow-up are critical. This complication occurs in up to 20% of patients and can be delayed by 1 year or more after the acute episode. It can often be prevented with the acute-phase therapy mentioned above.

For all of these disorders, post-inflammatory desquamation usually occurs in 1–2 weeks. It is most striking on the hands and feet, where stratum corneum often sheds in large sheets.

Pathogenesis

The toxins involved in toxic erythemas act as 'superantigens' that directly activate T cells, thus causing the release of massive amounts of cytokines, especially tumor necrosis factor-α, interleukin 1, and interleukin 6. These cytokines are thought to be responsible for the clinical manifestations. An erythrogenic toxin is produced by a lysogenic bacteriophage found in most strains of group A β-hemolytic streptococci. Although repeated streptococcal infections may occur, scarlet fever usually does not recur because of specific antitoxin antibodies that are formed from the first episode.

SSSS is caused by a toxin produced by phage group II *S. aureus*. This toxin binds to and disrupts the desmosomal protein, desmoglein 1, which is heavily concentrated in the granular layer of the epidermis. This is why skin biopsy in SSSS shows separation in the granular layer of the epidermis. In toxic shock syndrome, several staphylococcal toxins have been isolated, although the one most often implicated is an exoprotein designated toxic shock syndrome toxin 1. Other toxins (e.g., *Streptococcus pyogenes* exotoxin), as well as the host responses to the toxins, probably also play a role in the pathogenesis of toxic shock syndrome.

OTHER UNCOMMON CAUSES – GENERALIZED ERYTHEMA

ERYTHRODERMA

Erythroderma is a generalized, inflammatory skin condition involving more than 90% of the skin surface area (**Fig. 14.19**). Erythema is remarkable and when significant scaling is present, the term exfoliative erythroderma is often used. The causes of erythroderma fall into four broad categories: (1) Primary skin disease (e.g. psoriasis, atopic dermatitis); (2) Medication reactions; (3) Reaction to underlying malignancy; and (4) Idiopathic. Work-up of an erythrodermic patient requires a complete history and physical, with special attention to age-related malignancy screens, and appropriate laboratory and imaging evaluation. Skin biopsies rarely help distinguish the multiple causes of erythroderma. Unfortunately, a large proportion of cases of erythroderma are of unknown trigger, labeled idiopathic, and require periodic evaluation to search for underlying causes.

SÉZARY SYNDROME

Sézary syndrome is a specific cause of erythroderma, being labeled as a malignancy (cutaneous T-cell lymphoma) and a primary skin disease (**Fig. 14.20**). It is

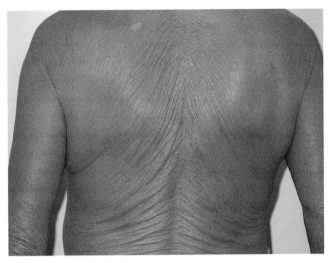

FIGURE 14.19 Erythroderma – generalized erythema that despite intensive work-up remained idiopathic in nature.

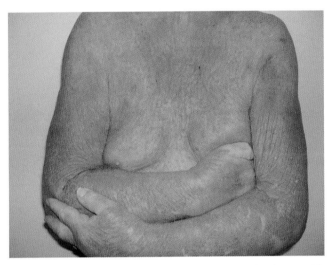

FIGURE 14.20 Sézary syndrome – exfoliative erythroderma with palpable lymphadenopathy.

characterized by erythroderma, generalized lymphadenopathy, and circulating malignant T cells, called Sézary cells, in the blood. Immunophenotypic analysis reveals CD4:CD8 ratio that exceeds 10 : 1 because the malignant T cells that expand are CD4 positive. Skin and lymph node biopsy shows the malignant T cells infiltrating the epidermis and lymph node, respectively. Sézary syndrome has a high mortality rate, with the majority of patients dying from infection secondary to immunosuppression.

15 Localized Erythema

Key Points

1. Dermal inflammation often presents as localized erythema
2. Localized erythema is most commonly due to infection (e.g., cellulitis or abscess) or inflammation (e.g., erythema nodosum)

ABSTRACT

In the disorders described in this chapter, the erythema is confined to discrete lesions and is localized to a small area of the body surface. Characteristically the epidermis is spared, but the dermal inflammation may extend into the subcutaneous fat. The three most common examples of localized erythema are: *cellulitis*, an indurated plaque; *abscess* and *furuncle*, each of which is a fluctuant mass; and *erythema nodosum*, a nodule (**Table 15.1**).

ABSCESS AND FURUNCLE

Key Points

1. *Staphylococcus aureus* is a common pathogen
2. Recurrent furunculosis often associated with nasal colonization of *S. aureus*
3. Check bacterial culture and sensitivity for methicillin-resistant *S. aureus*

Definition

Abscesses and furuncles (boils) are pus-filled nodules in the dermis. *S. aureus* is the usual pathogen, but Gram-negative organisms and anaerobic bacteria may also be causes. Abscesses often arise from traumatic inoculation of bacteria into the skin, whereas furuncles arise from infected hair follicles. The clinical lesion is a red, tender, fluctuant nodule (**Fig. 15.1**).

> *Staphylococcus aureus* is the usual pathogen.

Incidence

In one survey, cutaneous abscesses accounted for 2% of all patient visits to the emergency department of a large city hospital. Patients with recurrent furuncles are seen more often by a dermatologist.

History

Patients with abscesses may give a history of preceding trauma, including surgery. Some patients with furuncles give a history of recurrent lesions. Immunodeficiency, intravenous drug abuse, and perhaps diabetes mellitus predispose some patients to bacterial infections, but most patients with a furuncle or an abscess have no underlying medical disease.

Physical Examination

Furuncles and abscesses often begin as hard, tender, red nodules that become more fluctuant and more painful with time. Abscesses tend to be larger and deeper than furuncles. Regional lymph nodes are sometimes enlarged, but fever is rarely present.

Differential Diagnosis

Abscesses and furuncles are rarely confused with other entities. Acne and hidradenitis suppurativa can cause pus-filled nodules and cysts. In both conditions, the distribution of the lesions usually provides the diagnostic clue. In *cystic acne*, multiple lesions are distributed on the face and upper trunk, and other acne lesions (e.g., comedones, papules, pustules) are usually present. In *hidradenitis suppurativa*, draining nodules are present in

TABLE 15.1 Localized erythema

	Frequency (%)[a]	Etiology	History	Physical Examination	Differential Diagnosis	Laboratory Test
Abscess and furuncle	0.4	*S. aureus* (usually)	–	Red, tender, fluctuant mass	Cystic acne Hidradenitis suppurativa	Culture
Cellulitis	0.1	Group A streptococci (usually)	Fever	Red, warm, indurated, tender area of skin	Contact dermatitis Superficial thrombophlebitis Erythema infectiosum	Culture: 1. Skin aspirate 2. Blood
Erythema nodosum	0.3	Hypersensitivity reaction	Search for associated conditions, including drug history	Red, tender, deep nodules, usually on lower legs	Thrombophlebitis Subcutaneous fat necrosis	Chest radiography Throat culture Antistreptolysin-O titers PPD skin test ± skin biopsy

[a]Percentage of new dermatology outpatients with this diagnosis seen in the Hershey Medical Center Dermatology Clinic, Hershey, PA. PPD, purified protein derivative.

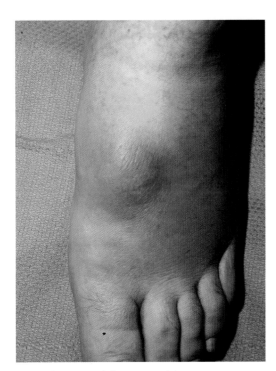

FIGURE 15.1 **Abscess** – red, fluctuant nodule.

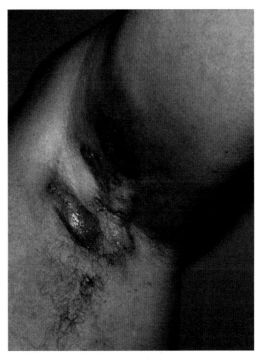

FIGURE 15.2 **Hidradenitis suppurativa** – recurrent, draining nodules and scarring in axilla.

the axillary, inguinal, and perineal areas. These nodules are often accompanied by open comedones and scars (**Fig. 15.2**).

The most commonly mistaken diagnosis for an abscess is a ruptured *epidermal inclusion cyst*. The intense inflammatory reaction to keratin, usually contained by the cyst lining, creates a fluctuant nodule, most commonly located on the back. Lack of fever and prior history of a cyst are distinguishing factors. Incision and drainage is the primary treatment (**Fig. 15.3**).

Laboratory and Biopsy

The diagnosis is usually made clinically and confirmed by routine culture of the purulent material that has been

obtained from incision and drainage. Methicillin-resistant *S. aureus* (MRSA) is an emerging pathogen in hospitals and communities, and needs to be checked by requesting a culture and sensitivity. In immunocompromised patients, anaerobic cultures may be desired. Blood cultures are rarely positive and are not indicated unless the patient has signs of sepsis.

Biopsy is rarely indicated. If biopsy is performed, a large, dense collection of neutrophils will be found in necrotic dermis (**Fig. 15.4**).

Therapy

The principal therapy consists of incision and drainage. In a study of 135 patients, this approach resulted in

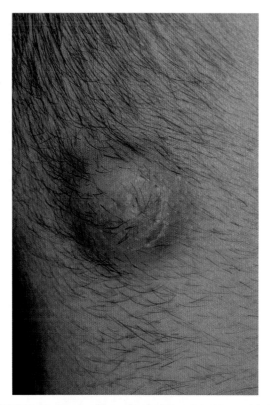

FIGURE 15.3 Ruptured epidermal inclusion cyst. Incision and drainage provide immediate relief.

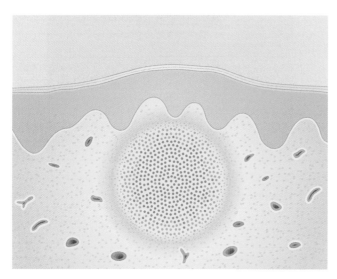

FIGURE 15.4 Abscess. Epidermis – normal. Dermis – dense aggregate of acute inflammatory cells replacing necrotic dermis.

complete healing in all patients, including those who did not receive systemic antibiotics. Systemic antibiotics, however, may result in involution of early lesions, may prevent progression of nodular lesions to fluctuant ones, and may decrease contagiousness. Because *S. aureus* is the organism usually responsible, the antibiotic of choice is cephalexin (Keflex) or dicloxacillin, in doses of 250–500 mg four times daily for 1 week. Choice of antibiotic is also based on the culture and sensitivity of the organism, especially with the emergence of MRSA. If the clinical response is poor, a change in antibiotic therapy can be considered. For this, culture results are helpful.

Therapy for Abscesses

Initial
- Incision and drainage
- Antibiotics:
  - Beta-lactamase-resistant penicillin (e.g., dicloxacillin 250 mg q.i.d.)
  - First-generation cephalosporin (e.g., cephalexin 250 mg q.i.d.)

Alternative – for MRSA Most Commonly
- Antibiotics:
  - Trimethoprim-sulfamethoxazole
  - Doxycycline
  - Parenteral antibiotics

Course and Complications

Untreated lesions often rupture and drain spontaneously. After surgical or spontaneous drainage, healing usually occurs. Large lesions may leave scars.

In patients with recurrent furunculosis, an underlying predisposing systemic defect may be considered but usually is not found. Many such patients, however, harbor *S. aureus* in sequestered mucocutaneous sites, the most common of which is the nose. A total of 1.5% of US residents are carriers for MRSA, harboring the bacteria in the anterior nares. In such patients, the regular use of antiseptic agents may decrease bacterial colonization and thereby prevent furuncles from recurring. The authors recommend a total body scrub every other day with an antiseptic cleansing agent such as chlorhexidine and twice-daily nasal application of an antibiotic ointment such as mupirocin.

Patients with recurrent furuncles are often staphylococcal carriers.

Pathogenesis

For abscesses and furuncles, the bacteria usually gain entry to the dermis by an external route. For abscesses, this may be a traumatic inoculation such as a puncture wound, laceration, or surgical incision.

For furuncles, the bacteria enter by a hair follicle, in which they form deep folliculitis and extend into the surrounding dermis. In both instances, the presence of a large number of bacteria in the dermis elicits a vigorous inflammatory response and eventuates in a massive collection of inflammatory cells, primarily neutrophils.

CELLULITIS

Key Points

1. Frequently caused by *Staphylococcus aureus* and group A streptococci
2. Fever is often present
3. Resolves with antibiotics

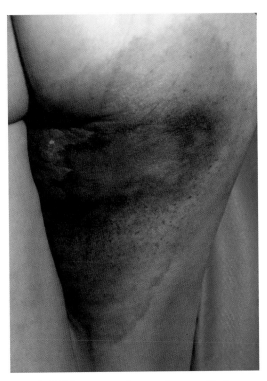

FIGURE 15.5 **Cellulitis** – note erythema, edema, and bulla.

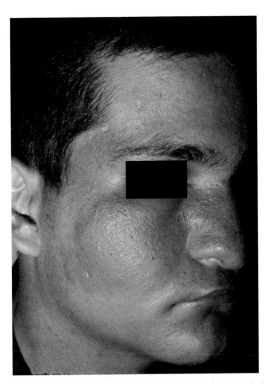

FIGURE 15.6 **Erysipelas** – sharply demarcated, edematous, red plaque.

Definition

Cellulitis is a deep infection of the skin resulting in a localized area of erythema (**Fig. 15.5**). Group A streptococci (*Streptococcus pyogenes*) and *Staphylococcus aureus* are the organisms most often responsible. MRSA is becoming a prevalent pathogen. Before the introduction of the *Haemophilus influenzae* vaccine, facial cellulitis in extremely young children was frequently caused by this bacterium. Streptococcal infection is now the most common cause, even in this age group. Rarely, other aerobic and anaerobic bacteria, as well as deep fungi such as *Cryptococcus neoformans*, cause cellulitis, particularly in patients who are immunosuppressed. In immunocompetent hosts, bacteria gain entry into the skin by a break in the skin's barrier while in immunosuppressed hosts bacteria or other organisms seed the skin from the blood.

> Cellulitis is most frequently caused by infection with group A streptococci and *Staphylococcus aureus*.

Erysipelas is sometimes considered separately from cellulitis, but the distinction between the two entities may be a matter of semantics. The border of the involved area is more sharply demarcated in classic erysipelas than in cellulitis, and the surface looks more like an orange peel (**Fig. 15.6**). However, both disorders are caused by bacteria, most often group A streptococci; for diagnostic and therapeutic purposes, they can be considered the same.

Incidence

Patients with this acute febrile disease are seen most often by their primary physician or an emergency physician. Only 0.1% of the present authors' new patients are seen for cellulitis.

History

Patients usually feel ill and febrile. The fever may precede the physical appearance of the skin involvement. A history of trauma or a preceding infected skin lesion is sometimes elicited. Saphenous venectomy for coronary bypass surgery can predispose patients to recurrent cellulitis of the legs. Buccal cellulitis in children often accompanies otitis media, and symptoms of an ear infection may be present.

> Fever is almost always present.

Physical Examination

The involved skin shows all four cardinal signs of inflammation: redness (rubor), warmth (calor), swelling (tumor), and tenderness and pain (dolor). The epidermis usually is unaltered, although, rarely, blisters are present. The erythema in *H. influenzae* facial cellulitis is characteristically violaceous. Perianal fissures in children predisposed to perianal are cellulitis caused by group A streptococci (**Fig. 15.7**).

> The skin shows all four signs of inflammation:
> 1. Rubor
> 2. Calor
> 3. Tumor
> 4. Dolor

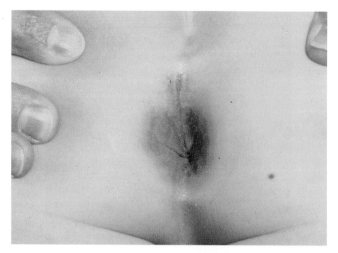

FIGURE 15.7 Perianal streptococcal infection in a child – well demarcated erythema with fissures.

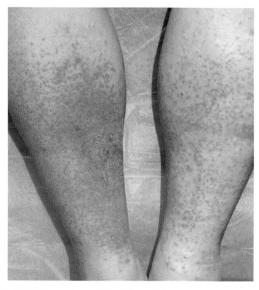

FIGURE 15.8 Stasis dermatitis. Bilateral lower leg involvement with significant epidermal change.

In adults, cellulitis most often affects the lower legs, especially when lymphatic obstruction is present. In these patients, fissures between the toes owing to tinea pedis often serve as the initial portal of entry of bacteria.

Differential Diagnosis

Contact dermatitis, when severe, can mimic the erythema and swelling of cellulitis, but important distinguishing characteristics of contact dermatitis are the more marked epidermal involvement with vesicles, the symptom of itch rather than of tenderness, and the absence of fever.

Stasis dermatitis is often confused with cellulitis. Distinguishing features include chronicity, bilateral involvement, epidermal involvement with crust and scale, and absence of fever (**Fig. 15.8**).

Superficial thrombophlebitis of the lower legs can cause redness and tenderness, and is sometimes difficult to distinguish from cellulitis. Fever is not present in

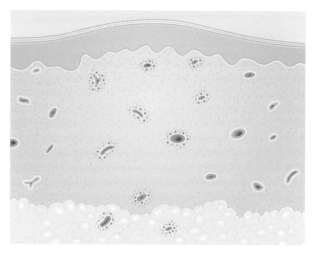

FIGURE 15.9 Cellulitis. Epidermis – normal. Dermis – inflammation diffusely through the dermis, extending into the subcutaneous fat.

superficial thrombophlebitis, however, and the involved vein often can be palpated as a hard cord.

Facial cellulitis in children can be confused with the 'slapped cheek' appearance seen in *erythema infectiosum*. In erythema infectiosum, however, the erythema is bilateral and usually non-tender, and the patient's condition does not appear toxic.

Laboratory and Biopsy

Skin and blood cultures may be obtained, but the responsible bacterial pathogen is not always recovered. A skin culture may be taken from the leading edge of the lesion by injecting and then aspirating 0.5 mL non-bacteriostatic saline. The aspirate is Gram-stained and cultured. Unfortunately, the highest reported yield from this procedure is only 50%, and in most series is much less than this. Culture of a skin biopsy increases the yield, but not to 100%.

Skin cultures are often negative.

A skin biopsy is usually not needed in ambulatory, immunocompetent patients. However, a biopsy is often done to identify a responsible organism in an immunocompromised patient whose cellulitis has not responded to antibiotic therapy. If a biopsy is performed, the examiner will see an inflammatory infiltrate composed primarily of neutrophils throughout the dermis, occasionally extending into the subcutaneous fat. Edema and dilatation of lymphatics and small blood vessels are also present (**Fig. 15.9**). Special stains for bacteria may be positive. Fungal stains to search for cryptococcal organisms also should be done, particularly on tissue from immunocompromised patients.

Complete blood count reveals leukocytosis in immunocompetent patients.

Therapy

Systemic antibiotics are the mainstay of therapy. It is important to identify the organism and then tailor the antibiotic therapy. In most cases of cellulitis in immuno-competent hosts, empiric antibiotics are started along with warm wet compresses, bed rest, and close outpatient follow-up. Cephalexin (Keflex) or dicloxacillin, in doses of 500 mg four times daily, is prescribed for a 10-day course. Remember to account for MRSA if the patient is not responding to the antibiotics. Patients who are more seriously ill, particularly those with facial cellulitis, should be hospitalized and administered parenteral anti-biotics, such as 2 g nafcillin intravenously every 4 h. In immunocompromised patients, coverage may be needed for Gram-negative bacteria or fungal organisms. In young children with facial cellulitis, antibiotic therapy must include coverage for *H. influenzae*, with amoxicillin com-bined with trimethoprim-sulfamethoxazole (Bactrim) or amoxicillin-clavulanate (Augmentin) combined with a third-generation cephalosporin such as ceftriaxone.

Therapy for Cellulitis

Initial
- Oral antibiotics
  - Cephalexin 500 mg q.i.d.
  - Dicloxacillin 500 mg q.i.d.
  - Doxycycline 100 mg b.i.d. or trimethoprim-sulfamethoxazole for MRSA

Alternative
- Intravenous antibiotics (if severe)
  - Nafcillin 2.0 g every 4 h
  - Or appropriate antimicrobial agent in an immunocompromised host

Course and Complications

With antibiotic therapy, the fever usually resolves within 24 h. If it persists beyond 48 h, a change in antimicrobial therapy should be considered, optimally guided by the initial culture results. The skin inflammation resolves more slowly than the fever, sometimes taking 1 or 2 weeks to subside completely. For most patients, complete recovery can be expected.

Cutaneous inflammation is slow to subside.

Mortality is rare but can occur in neglected cases or in cases due to a virulent organism, such as *Pseudomonas aeruginosa*. Illnesses such as congestive heart failure, renal insufficiency, and morbid obesity predispose to more serious complications. Facial cellulitis caused by *H. influenzae* is often accompanied by otitis media and less often by meningitis. Osteomyelitis due to cellulitis is a rare sequela.

Cellulitis once was a serious and sometimes life-threatening disease, but the use of antibiotics has reduced the mortality rate to near zero in immunocompetent hosts. In immunosuppressed patients, cellulitis from usual as well as unusual pathogens still may be a serious, sometimes life-threatening, infection (**Fig. 15.10**).

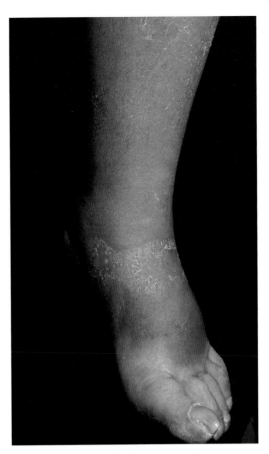

FIGURE 15.10 Cryptococcal cellulitis in setting of immunosuppression patient. Organism discovered by biopsy after patient failed to respond to standard antibiotics.

Pathogenesis

In cellulitis, the bacteria may enter the dermis by an external or a hematogenous route. In immunocompetent hosts, the source is usually external. In immunosup-pressed hosts, the source is usually internal. Tissue edema predisposes to bacterial proliferation. Proteolytic enzymes elaborated by bacteria such as group A streptococci con-tribute to the spread of inflammation. Host defense mechanisms involve cellular infiltrates and elaboration of cytokines, which rapidly kill the bacteria and thereby contribute to the inflammation. Damage to local lym-phatics during an acute episode can result in residual lymphedema and may predispose the patient to recurrent episodes.

ERYTHEMA NODOSUM

Key Points

1. Inflammatory reaction in subcutaneous fat
2. Tender nodules on lower legs
3. Treat underlying disease

Definition

Erythema nodosum is an inflammatory reaction in the subcutaneous fat that, in most cases, represents a

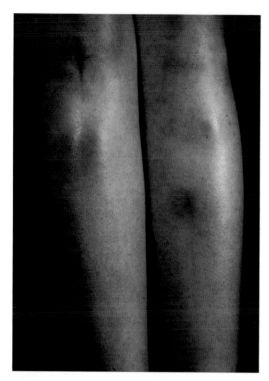

FIGURE 15.11 **Erythema nodosum** – multiple, deep, tender nodules.

Causes:
1. Post-streptococcal infection
2. Sarcoidosis
3. Deep fungal infection: coccidioidomycosis, histoplasmosis
4. Tuberculosis
5. Inflammatory bowel disease
6. *Yersinia* enterocolitis
7. Pregnancy
8. Drugs
9. Idiopathic

Physical Examination

Lesions of erythema nodosum appear as erythematous, well localized, extremely tender, deep nodules that are 1–5 cm in diameter and have indistinct borders. As lesions evolve, they become yellowish-purple and look like bruises. Multiple lesions are usually present, with the typical location being the pretibial areas. Much less often, lesions occur on the thighs and arms. Ulceration rarely occurs.

Typical nodules are:
1. On lower legs
2. Tender
3. Deep

Differential Diagnosis

The diagnosis is usually evident, clinically. Lesions of erythema nodosum may appear as *traumatic bruises*, but the history should discriminate between the two. *Superficial thrombophlebitis* also produces tender lesions on the lower legs, but these lesions are usually more linear and not multiple. *Subcutaneous fat necrosis* is a rare condition that produces tender nodules on the lower legs and occurs in the setting of pancreatitis or pancreatic carcinoma. Patients with this disorder usually have raised serum amylase and lipase levels, and a diagnostic skin biopsy.

Laboratory and Biopsy

Laboratory testing takes into consideration the possible causes, and a few simple tests can screen for most of these conditions. Appropriate tests include a throat culture, antistreptolysin-O titer, tuberculosis skin test, and chest radiography. The chest radiograph is used to screen for both pulmonary infection and sarcoidosis. In patients with bowel symptoms, further gastrointestinal tract evaluation should be pursued.

Laboratory tests:
1. Throat culture
2. Antistreptolysin-O titer
3. Chest radiography
4. Tuberculosis skin test

hypersensitivity response to a remote focus of infection or inflammation. Clinically, erythema nodosum appears as deep, tender, red nodules that are usually located on the lower legs (**Fig. 15.11**).

Incidence

Erythema nodosum is an uncommon disorder, representing 0.3% of the authors' new dermatology patients. It occurs most often in young adults, with females outnumbering males by a ratio of 3:1.

History

The history is guided by consideration of the etiologic possibilities. In erythema nodosum precipitated by streptococcal infection, the nodules occur within 3 weeks of pharyngitis. Fever and lower respiratory symptoms may be elicited from patients with pulmonary infections caused by deep fungi or tuberculosis. A history of abdominal pain and diarrhea suggests an inflammatory bowel disorder. Ulcerative colitis is the most common inflammatory bowel disease associated with erythema nodosum. Regional enteritis and *Yersinia* enterocolitis are encountered less frequently. Inquiry should be made regarding pregnancy. A complete drug history should be elicited, although, with the exception of birth control pills, drugs are uncommon causes. Most cases are of unknown cause and labeled 'idiopathic.'

Pain and tenderness are usually associated with the skin nodules. Fever and arthralgias may also be present regardless of the cause. Joint symptoms most often affect the ankles and sometimes the knees and may precede the rash.

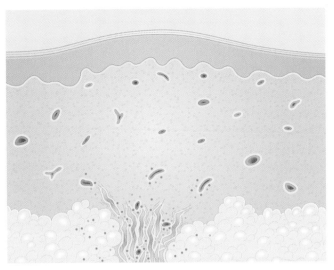

FIGURE 15.12 **Erythema nodosum.** Epidermis – normal. Dermis – inflammation in the lower dermis and in widened septa in the subcutaneous fat.

A skin biopsy is usually not required. If biopsy is performed, the changes will be found primarily in the subcutaneous fat, where vascular and perivascular inflammation is present in the fibrous septa separating the fat lobules. The septa become widened by edema and, subsequently, by fibrosis (**Fig. 15.12**). Acutely, the inflammation shows numerous neutrophils and also involves the lower dermis. Hemorrhage may be present. In older lesions, a granulomatous infiltrate may be found.

Therapy

Therapy is aimed at the underlying disease, if one is identified. Symptomatic therapy may be achieved with aspirin or other non-steroidal anti-inflammatory drugs (NSAIDs) (e.g., 25 mg indomethacin three times daily). Bed rest is also helpful. In patients with extensive involvement and marked discomfort, a short course of systemic steroids (e.g., prednisone, starting with 40 mg daily and tapered over 2–3 weeks) often provides dramatic relief, provided the cause is not infectious. Some patients with chronic idiopathic erythema nodosum have been treated successfully with oral saturated solution of potassium iodide. The mechanisms of action for these drugs are not known. Support stockings may be helpful in patients with chronic or recurrent disease.

Therapy for Erythema Nodosum

Initial
- Identification of the precipitating disease, if any
- Bed rest or support stockings
- Non-steroidal anti-inflammatory drugs:
  - Indomethacin – 25 mg t.i.d.

Alternative
- Prednisone (if severe)
- Immunosuppressants if recurrent (mycophenolate mofetil or cyclosporine)
- Potassium iodide

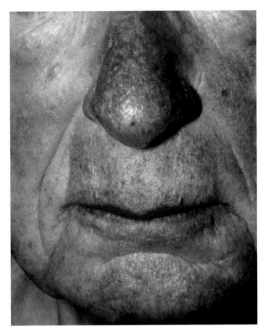

FIGURE 15.13 **Carcinoid** – persistent erythema and flushing of face in a patient with liver metastases.

Course and Complications

The course is usually self-limiting, typically lasting 3–6 weeks. Erythema nodosum associated with inflammatory bowel disease may parallel the course of the underlying disorder, relapsing with the bowel disease. Erythema nodosum in most other settings does not often recur.

Cutaneous complications are infrequent and inconsequential. Although ulceration does not occur, slightly depressed scars may result.

Pathogenesis

Evidence suggests that erythema nodosum is mediated by immune complexes. Deposition of immunoglobulins and complement has been demonstrated in the blood vessels in early lesions of erythema nodosum. In addition, many patients have circulating immune complexes, presumably related to the underlying disorder. The usual localization of the disease to the skin of the lower legs may be related to hemodynamic factors. The relatively sluggish circulation in the dependent lower extremities predisposes patients to the deposition of immune complexes in those blood vessels.

UNCOMMON CAUSES OF LOCALIZED ERYTHEMA

CARCINOID SYNDROME

Carcinoid syndrome is associated with cutaneous flushing and erythema, commonly located on the face (**Fig. 15.13**). This clinical feature becomes apparent only after hepatic metastases have occurred or when the primary tumor is in the lung (the venous drainage bypasses the liver). The diagnosis is established by high levels of 5-hydroxyindoleacetic acid (5-HIAA) in the urine.

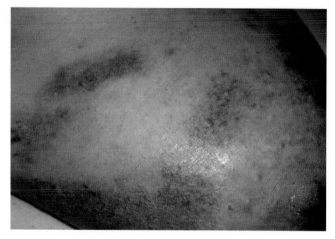

FIGURE 15.14 **Carcinoma erysipeloids** – initially treated as cellulitis, biopsy of these red, slightly purpuric, patches confirmed the diagnosis.

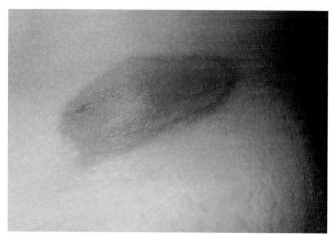

FIGURE 15.15 **Fixed drug eruption** – well demarcated red plaque that recurred after each exposure to trimethoprim-sulfamethoxazole.

Treatment involves resection of the primary tumor or liver metastases, or chemotherapy.

CARCINOMA ERYSIPELOIDS

Cutaneous metastases can resemble erysipelas and cellulitis. Tumor cells infiltrate the superficial lymphatics and cause the appearance of a warm, red patch or plaque (**Fig. 15.14**). This occurs most commonly on the anterior chest wall in association with breast carcinoma. Patients fail to respond to antibiotics for a presumptive infection. Biopsy confirms the diagnosis.

FIXED DRUG ERUPTION

Fixed drug eruptions appear as sharply demarcated red plaques (**Fig. 15.15**) that later take on a dusky hue. With first exposure to the drug, the lesion appears in 1–2 weeks. Upon subsequent re-exposures, the lesion appears within 24 h at exactly the same location. The lesions can affect any part of the body but are most common on the distal extremities, face, lips, and genitalia. Biopsy confirms the diagnosis. The most common offenders are NSAIDs, sulfonamides, tetracyclines, and carbamazepine.

Specialized Erythema 16

Chapter Contents

- Erythema Migrans
- Erythema Multiforme
- Urticaria (Hives)
- Uncommon Causes of Specialized Erythema
  - Erythema Ab Igne
  - Erythema Annulare Centrifugum
  - Erythema Gyratum Repens

Key Points

1. The distinctive morphology of the specialized erythemas is key to the diagnosis (e.g., erythema multiforme)
2. Specialized erythemas represent a reactive pattern to an underlying cause (e.g., erythema multiforme caused by herpes simplex infection)

ABSTRACT

Urticaria and erythema multiforme are characterized by lesions that are so distinctive that they are assigned special names. In urticaria, the lesion is a *hive* (or wheal), which is defined, in Chapter 3, as a papule or plaque of dermal edema, often with central pallor and an irregular, erythematous border. The *target lesion*, when present, is diagnostic of erythema multiforme and is characterized by three concentric zones of color. The third disease described in this chapter is erythema migrans, an expanding annular erythematous skin lesion found in Lyme disease. Additional features of these disorders are outlined in **Table 16.1** and in the discussion that follows.

ERYTHEMA MIGRANS

Key Points

1. Hallmark sign of Lyme disease, the most common tick-borne disease in the USA
2. Caused by *Borrelia burgdorferi*, which is transmitted by a tick, *Ixodes* spp.
3. Treatment with antibiotics avoids late complications, notably arthritis

Definition

Erythema migrans represents the skin lesion associated with Lyme disease, a tick-borne illness caused by the spirochete *Borrelia burgdorferi*. Erythema migrans begins as a small, erythematous macule or papule that expands slowly over days to weeks. It must achieve a diameter of at least 5 cm to qualify as erythema migrans (**Fig. 16.1**). Erythema migrans occurs in 60–80% of patients with Lyme disease. The late manifestations include involvement of the musculoskeletal, nervous, or cardiovascular system.

> The size criterion for erythema migrans is a diameter of 5 cm.

> Erythema migrans occurs in 60–80% of patients with Lyme disease.

Incidence

Lyme disease was first described in 1977, when it was diagnosed in a cluster of children living near Lyme, Connecticut, who were initially thought to have juvenile rheumatoid arthritis. Since then, the numbers of reported cases and their geographic distribution have increased steadily. Although still found most often in north-eastern USA, cases have been reported from nearly every state in the country. Lyme disease is the most frequently reported arthropod-borne disease in the USA. Most cases occur between May and September.

> Lyme disease is the most frequent arthropod-borne disease in the USA.

History

Erythema migrans begins 3–30 days after a tick bite (**Fig. 16.2**). Because the tick is so small, many patients do not recall having received a bite. Most patients, however, do have a history of recent exposure to potential tick habitats such as woodlands or grassy areas. Many patients with erythema migrans have accompanying systemic symptoms such as fever, myalgia, arthralgia, headache, malaise, or fatigue. The skin lesion itself is usually asymptomatic but is noted by the patient to expand slowly over time.

TABLE 16.1 Specialized erythema

	Frequency (%)[a]	Etiology	History	Physical Examination	Differential Diagnosis	Laboratory Test
Erythema migrans	<0.1	Tick-borne spirochete (*B. burgdorferi*)	Constitutional symptoms accompany rash Prior tick bite	One or more *expanding* red, annular macules at least 5 cm in diameter	Cellulitis Tinea corporis Granuloma annulare Fixed drug reaction Other insect bite reaction	Serology Skin biopsy
Erythema multiforme	0.3	Drugs Infection Idiopathic	Constitutional prodrome Prior herpes simplex infection	Erythematous plaques Bullae Target lesions Mucous membrane involvement	Viral exanthem Scalded skin syndrome Pemphigus Pemphigoid	May be indicated: Chest radiography Skin biopsy
Urticaria	2	Ingestants Drugs Foods Infection Physical agents ?Emotions Idiopathic	Lesions last less than 24 h	Wheals Generalized distribution	Erythema multiforme Juvenile rheumatoid arthritis Erythema marginatum	–

[a]Percentage of new dermatology patients with this diagnosis seen in the Hershey Medical Center Dermatology Clinic, Hershey, PA.

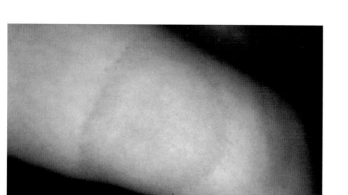

FIGURE 16.1 Erythema migrans – expanding red patch with central clearing.

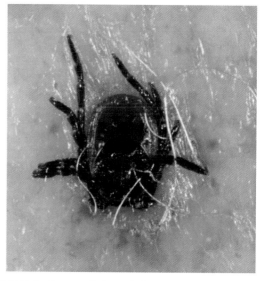

FIGURE 16.2 *Ixodes scapularis* – tick that transmits Lyme disease.

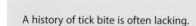

A history of tick bite is often lacking.

Physical Findings

The erythema migrans lesion is located at a body site favored by a feeding tick, such as the waistband and intertriginous areas, as well as the extremities (**Fig. 16.3**). The diameter of the lesion must be at least 5 cm to qualify as erythema migrans. From reported cases, the average diameter has been found to be 15 cm, but a diameter of 68 cm has been reported.

A central punctum from the tick bite may be evident but often is not. Typical erythema migrans has a macular border and a clearing center, but less classic features are common and include a papular border, alternating rings of erythema and clearing, and a center that is intensely erythematous, vesicular, purpuric, necrotic, or even ulcerated. However, all erythema migrans lesions have in common an expanding border. Multiple skin lesions occur in 15% of patients.

Erythema migrans lesions expand slowly over days to weeks.

Differential Diagnosis

The differential diagnosis includes cellulitis, tinea corporis, granuloma annulare, fixed drug reaction, and other

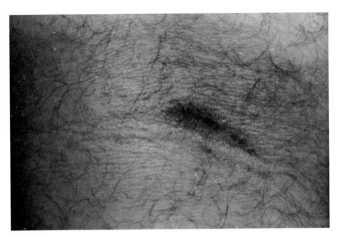

FIGURE 16.3 Lyme disease – tick bite occurred in popliteal fossa resulting in central purpura and red patch >5 cm. Patient developed stage 2 Lyme disease.

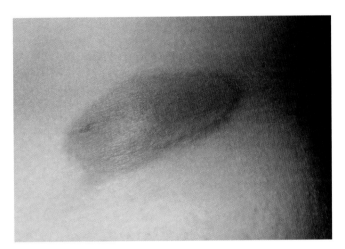

FIGURE 16.4 Fixed drug eruption.

insect bite reactions. Except for cellulitis, these conditions are not accompanied by systemic symptoms. In addition, compared with erythema migrans, the cellulitis is more tender and usually more acute, warmer, and redder; *tinea corporis* has a scaling border that is potassium hydroxide-positive for fungal elements and is more chronic; granuloma annulare, an idiopathic dermal granulomatous process, has a firm, elevated border and persists for months to years; *fixed drug eruption* has no central clearing, is violaceous, and characteristically recurs in the same spot within hours of ingestion of the offending agent (**Fig. 16.4**); other insect bite reactions often have more prominent central puncta, are smaller, and usually more transient than erythema migrans.

Laboratory and Biopsy

Lyme disease is diagnosed clinically, especially in endemic areas. Serologic tests (e.g., enzyme-linked immunosorbent assay; ELISA) for IgM and IgG anti-*B. burgdorferi* antibodies are commonly used, but this test is neither sensitive (antibodies do not appear until after the first 2–4 weeks of illness) nor specific (false-negative results in infected individuals and false-positive results in

persons with other diseases including systemic lupus erythematosus and rheumatoid arthritis). Positive or equivocal tests should be followed up with a standardized western blot. An unequivocal diagnosis is established by culturing *Borrelia*. This is a low-yield procedure. Polymerase chain reaction (PCR) testing for *Borrelia* DNA is best done on cerebrospinal or synovial fluid, but is expensive and not widely available.

Serologic tests have limited usefulness.

Therapy

The ideal treatment is prevention, including tick avoidance, protective clothing, DEET (*N,N*-diethyl-m-toluamide) repellent, and prompt removal of ticks within 24 h. All patients with erythema migrans are defined as having Lyme disease and thus require antibiotic therapy. The preferred agent is doxycycline, 100 mg twice daily for 10–21 days. Alternatively, amoxicillin 500 mg three times daily for 10–21 days can be used. Erythromycin 250 mg four times daily for 10–21 days is a third but less preferable alternative. Manifestations and therapy of early disseminated infection and late persistent infection are discussed below.

Therapy for Erythema Migrans (Early Localized Lyme)

Initial
- Antibiotics for 10–21 days:
  - Doxycycline 100 mg b.i.d.; or
  - Amoxicillin 500 mg t.i.d.
- For children aged <12 years:
  - Amoxicillin 50 mg/kg daily divided t.i.d.

Course and Complications

The course and manifestations of Lyme disease share many similarities with syphilis. In Lyme disease, even without therapy, the erythema migrans lesion usually resolves spontaneously within a month. However, without treatment of early localized infection (stage 1), the disease may progress to stage 2 or 3.

Stages:
1. Localized
2. Early disseminated
3. Late persistent

In stage 2 (early disseminated infection), the *B. burgdorferi* spirochete is spread hematogenously to distant sites. The skin is affected in approximately 50% of patients with annular lesions, which usually are smaller than the primary one. Patients are systemically ill with fever, chills, headache, arthralgia, and fatigue. Infection of other organ systems can result in a variety of symptoms, including arthritis, meningitis, cranial neuritis

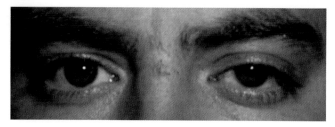

FIGURE 16.5 Lyme disease – stage 2 Bell's palsy. Note that patient cannot lift left upper eyelid.

(particularly Bell's palsy) (**Fig. 16.5**), lymphadenopathy, carditis, and atrioventricular conduction defects. After inoculation, neurologic involvement occurs weeks to months later and affects approximately 15–20% of patients; cardiac involvement occurs within weeks and affects 4–8%. Arthritis is the most common manifestation and occurs at a mean of 6 months, with a range of 2 weeks to 2 years. It affects 60% of patients with intermittent asymmetric arthritis that affects primarily large joints, especially the knee.

> Arthritis is the most common manifestation of disseminated disease.

Without treatment, the disease may enter stage 3, with late persistent infection. The major manifestation of this stage is *continual* arthritis, lasting for more than 1 year. Chronic central nervous system involvement also may occur with manifestations that include ataxia and mental disorder.

Treatment of cardiac and neurologic manifestations requires parenteral therapy with 2 g ceftriaxone intravenously daily for 14–21 days. Lyme arthritis can be treated orally with 100 mg doxycycline twice daily for 30 days, or amoxicillin 500 mg orally four times daily for 30 days.

> Cardiac and neurologic manifestations require parenteral antibiotic therapy.

Pathogenesis

The disease is caused by *B. burgdorferi*, a spirochete carried by *Ixodes* ticks. In the north-eastern and mid-western USA, the tick species is *I. dammini* (deer tick). In the western USA, the species is *I. pacificus*, and in Europe, it is *I. ricinus*. These ticks have a 2-year life cycle, and their preferred host in North America is the white-footed mouse, which asymptomatically carries the *Borrelia* infection and transmits it to a feeding larval tick. The white-tailed deer is the preferred host for the infected adult tick, hence the name deer tick. Deer, however, are not involved in the life cycle of the spirochete. The *Borrelia* infection is transmitted to humans when an infected tick feeds, thereby injecting the spirochete from its salivary glands into the skin. Once injected, the spirochete produces a local infection with an inflammatory reaction that produces a visible skin lesion – erythema migrans.

Untreated, the infection often disseminates, spreading hematogenously to internal organs.

ERYTHEMA MULTIFORME

> ### Key Points
>
> 1. Target lesions have concentric rings that are diagnostic
> 2. Recurrent disease is most often precipitated by herpes simplex virus infection
> 3. Involvement of two or more mucosal surfaces signifies a poorer prognosis (Stevens–Johnson syndrome)

Definition

Erythema multiforme is an immunologic reaction in the skin possibly triggered by circulating immune complexes. As its name suggests, the eruption is characterized clinically by a variety of lesions, including erythematous plaques, blisters, and 'target' lesions (**Fig. 16.6**). Recurrent disease is caused most often by herpes simplex infection and termed erythema multiforme minor. Mucous membrane involvement also occurs in the severe form of the disease – *erythema multiforme major* or *Stevens–Johnson syndrome* – and is usually caused by drugs or infection.

> The most common causes of erythema multiforme:
> 1. Drugs
> 2. Infection

Incidence

Erythema multiforme, although not rare, is uncommon. Fewer than 1% of the authors' new dermatology patients are seen for this condition. The disorder most often affects older children and young adults.

History

The lesions usually appear abruptly within a 24-h period. Some 50% of patients give a history of coincident herpes infection. The lesions are pruritic and may have a burning sensation.

Recurrent herpes simplex infection is the precipitating event in the majority of patients with *recurrent* erythema multiforme (**Fig. 16.7**). The herpetic lesion usually precedes the erythema multiforme by a few days to 1 week or more. For the most extended intervals, the herpetic lesions may have healed by the time the patient presents for treatment, so the history is important.

> Recurrent herpes simplex is the most common cause of recurrent disease.

Mycoplasma pneumoniae infection is the precipitating event in some patients; a history of fever and cough is usually found. *Mycoplasma*-related and drug-induced

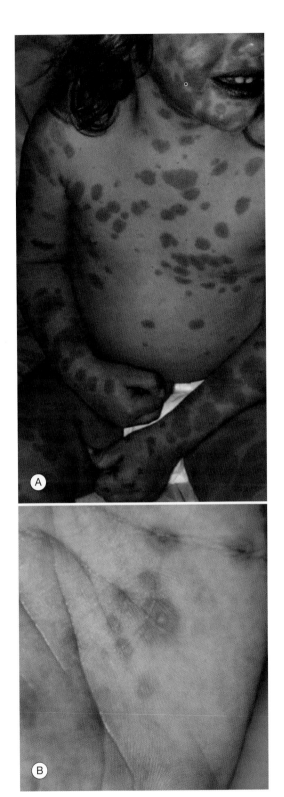

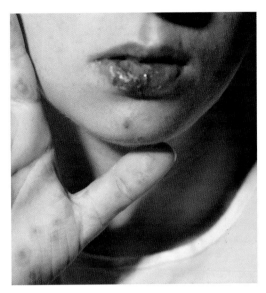

FIGURE 16.7 **Recurrent erythema multiforme** secondary to herpes simplex virus.

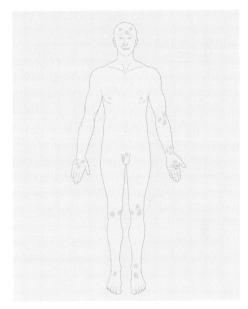

FIGURE 16.8 **Distribution of erythema multiforme** is symmetric and favors the extremities.

FIGURE 16.6 **Erythema multiforme. A.** Generalized, circular plaques with dusky centers secondary to upper respiratory infection. **B.** Classic target lesions with *three zones* of color.

erythema multiforme reactions are often severe (Stevens–Johnson syndrome), but they do not usually recur.

A cause is not always identifiable, particularly in patients with a single episode of erythema multiforme. In some patients, a febrile prodrome with upper respiratory symptoms precedes the cutaneous eruption by 1–14 days. Treatment of the prodrome with antibiotics probably led in the past to a falsely high rate of incrimination of these drugs as etiologic agents.

Physical Findings

The disorder ranges in severity from mild to severe. In the mild form of the disease (*erythema multiforme minor*), erythematous papules and plaques predominate. Characteristically, the distribution of the lesions favors the extremities and is strikingly symmetric (**Fig. 16.8**). Target lesions are often present and are diagnostic. To meet the criteria for a target lesion, *three* zones of color must be present: (1) a central dark area or a blister surrounded by (2) a pale edematous zone surrounded by (3) a

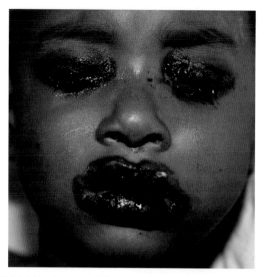

FIGURE 16.9 Erythema multiforme major (Stevens–Johnson syndrome) secondary to *Mycoplasma*. Distribution of erythema multiforme is symmetric and favors the extremities.

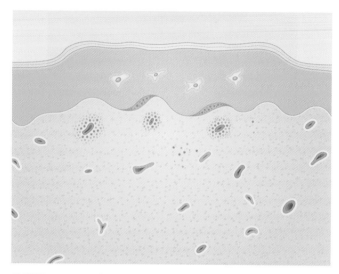

FIGURE 16.10 Erythema multiforme. Epidermis – normal or may have individual cell necrosis or exocytosis of mononuclear cells. Dermis – subepidermal separation (center of target lesion); inflammation in the papillary dermis.

peripheral rim of erythema. Target lesions are seen most often on the palms and soles but may occur anywhere. Patients with erythema multiforme minor are not usually systemically ill. In the severe form of erythema multiforme (*erythema multiforme major* or *Stevens–Johnson syndrome*), the skin disease is more widespread, blisters develop frequently, and mucous membrane involvement is characteristic. The oral mucosa, lips, and conjunctivae are usually the most severely affected (**Fig. 16.9**). Blisters inside the mouth cause painful erosions that make eating difficult or even impossible when involvement is extensive. Purulent conjunctivitis may become so severe that the eyes swell shut. Patients with Stevens–Johnson syndrome look and feel systemically ill, with fever and prostration.

> Target lesions have three zones of color and are diagnostic for erythema multiforme.

Differential Diagnosis

For the minor form of erythema multiforme, the usual differential diagnosis includes urticaria and viral exanthems. *Hives* may be confused with target lesions, but hives have only two zones of color (a central pale area surrounded by erythema), and individual lesions last for <24 h. *Viral exanthems* are usually monomorphous, less red, more confluent, and more centrally distributed than erythema multiforme. Conditions to be considered in the differential diagnosis of the major form of erythema multiforme are the other blistering disorders, including the *staphylococcal scalded skin syndrome*, in which the skin is diffusely red and the superficial epidermis strips off easily; pemphigus, in which histological examination shows an intraepidermal blister; and *pemphigoid*, in which blisters often arise on clinically uninflamed skin and mucous membrane involvement is uncommon. As in erythema multiforme, the blister in bullous pemphigoid is subepidermal, but immunofluorescent studies of a skin

biopsy specimen enable distinction between the two. IgG is present at the dermal-epidermal interface in pemphigoid but not in erythema multiforme.

Laboratory and Biopsy

For herpes simplex-precipitated disease, if the responsible vesicular lesion is still present, a Tzanck preparation or viral culture can be obtained. Chest radiography is appropriate to screen for pulmonary infection. *Mycoplasma* infection can be further confirmed with acute and convalescent cold agglutinin titers. For drug-induced cases, the laboratory is not helpful.

The disease is so clinically distinctive, particularly when target lesions are present, that a skin biopsy is usually not required for diagnosis. Biopsy of an erythematous plaque shows dermal changes with a lymphohistiocytic perivascular infiltrate and edema in the papillary dermis. Histologically, the epidermis may also be involved, with changes ranging from spongiosis and individual cell necrosis to full-thickness epidermal necrosis. Subepidermal separation is found in blisters and in the center of target lesions (**Fig. 16.10**).

Therapy

No convincing evidence indicates that medical therapy favorably alters the course of this disease once the disease is established. Treatment of a precipitating infection is appropriate: erythromycin, azithromycin, or clarithromycin is recommended for *M. pneumoniae*, and a 5-day course of oral valacyclovir (Valtrex) 500 mg twice daily or famciclovir (Famvir) 125 mg twice daily for herpes simplex infection. Recurrent herpes-associated erythema multiforme can be prevented with maintenance antiviral therapy. This is expensive and is reserved for patients with frequently recurring disease.

> Initial therapy: treat infection, if present.

For Stevens–Johnson syndrome, systemic steroids often have been used, but their value remains controversial; one retrospective study found that steroid treatment of children with Stevens–Johnson syndrome resulted in longer hospitalization and more frequent complications than no treatment. Nevertheless, systemic prednisone in doses ranging from 40 to 80 mg/m^2 is still used frequently in patients with severe erythema multiforme. A prospective study is needed to evaluate the wisdom of this approach more thoroughly. For patients with Stevens–Johnson syndrome, supportive measures are also important. These are directed toward restoring and maintaining hydration, preventing secondary infection, and providing pain relief. Intravenous fluids are required in patients with severe oral involvement. Local therapy with antiseptics and dressings may help to prevent secondary infections, and systemic analgesics are used for pain. The intraoral use of topical anesthetics helps to provide temporary relief for patients with painful mouth lesions; viscous lidocaine or dyclonine liquid can be used.

Systemic steroids are controversial but used frequently.

Therapy for Erythema Multiforme

Initial

- Treat infection, if present
  - For *Mycoplasma pneumoniae*: erythromycin, azithromycin, or clarithromycin
  - For recurrent herpes simplex: valacyclovir 500 mg b.i.d., or famciclovir 125 mg b.i.d.
- Discontinue responsible drug, if any

For Stevens–Johnson Syndrome:

- Supportive care
- Systemic steroids

Course and Complications

The mild form of erythema multiforme usually resolves spontaneously within 2–3 weeks. The time course is longer in patients with more severe involvement, lasting up to 6 weeks.

Spontaneous resolution occurs in 2–6 weeks.

Death occurs occasionally in patients with Stevens–Johnson syndrome; reported mortality rates range from 0% to 15%. Pneumonia and renal involvement can complicate the cutaneous picture but are uncommon. The major complications result from infection and fluid loss. The entire skin surface can become involved, resulting in a clinical presentation that resembles an extensive burn; this process is called *toxic epidermal necrolysis*. Dehydration results from both decreased oral intake and increased transcutaneous fluid loss. Conjunctivitis can be complicated by secondary bacterial infection and may result in corneal scarring.

Pathogenesis

Circulating immune complexes have been found in patients with erythema multiforme. The antigen is presumed to be derived from the implicated drug or infectious agent. Evidence supporting a pathogenic role for immune complexes includes the localization of IgM deposits around dermal blood vessels in affected skin and the finding of immune complexes containing herpes antigen in the serum in patients with herpes-associated recurrent erythema multiforme but not in patients with recurrent herpes simplex alone or in those with drug-induced erythema multiforme.

Some investigators favor a cellular immune mechanism. The predominance of mononuclear cells and the absence of leukocytoclastic vasculitis in the skin biopsy favor this mechanism.

URTICARIA (HIVES)

Key Points

1. Characterized by evanescent, edematous papules and plaques
2. Acute urticaria is often caused by upper respiratory infection
3. A cause is rarely found in chronic urticaria (>6 weeks)
4. Treat with antihistamines

Definition

Urticaria is a condition characterized by pruritic, transient wheals in the skin resulting from acute dermal edema (**Fig. 16.11**). Acute urticaria is often caused by upper respiratory infections and drugs. For chronic (lasting more than 6 weeks) urticaria, a cause is usually not found.

Incidence

Urticaria is common, with the highest incidence in young adults. Some 20% of the general population will have hives at some point. Two percent of the authors' new clinic patients were seen for this condition. Patients with acute urticaria often present to the emergency department.

History

Acute urticaria presents with new onset of pruritus and urticaria. In addition to pruritus and urticaria, patients with chronic urticaria are distressed owing to the longevity of signs and symptoms. Itching is nearly always present. Diagnosis is based mainly on history. For example, in acute urticaria the most common cause is upper respiratory infection, so associated symptoms such as cough and fever may be present. The drug history is the most important, including over-the-counter medications, which the patients may perceive as being unimportant.

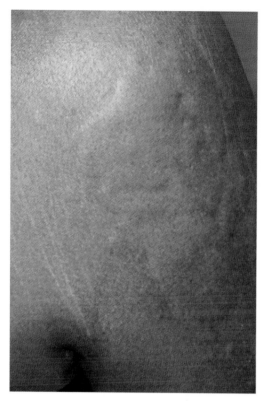

FIGURE 16.11 **Urticaria** (hives) – edematous plaques with scratch marks on the shoulder.

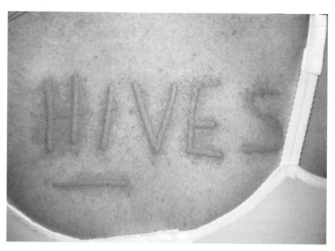

FIGURE 16.12 **Dermographism.**

Inquiry regarding specific medications (e.g., vitamins, analgesics, and laxatives) may help to jog the patient's memory. A history of aspirin and other non-steroidal anti-inflammatory drug (NSAID) ingestion, for example, is particularly important because salicylates cause hives in some patients and aggravate them in as many as one-third of all patients with urticaria, regardless of the cause.

> Itching is a prominent symptom.

> Ask about over-the-counter medications as well as prescription drugs.

For chronic urticaria, occult infections (e.g., dental and sinus) and physical modalities of urticaria (e.g., cold, pressure, sunlight, physical exercise, and heat and stress) should be evaluated. Foods are a rare cause of acute and chronic urticaria. A history of obstructive airway or other anaphylactic symptoms imparts greater seriousness to the problem. Urticaria accompanied by fever and arthralgia occurs in serum sickness reactions and in prodromal viral hepatitis.

Although allergy to an external allergen is most often manifest by contact dermatitis, in some patients contact of the skin to certain chemicals can cause an urticarial

response, such as contact urticaria. For example, the latex in rubber gloves and other rubber objects is a relatively common cause of contact urticaria in medical and dental personnel.

Physical Findings

Hives are skin lesions that are easily recognized. They appear as edematous plaques, often with pale centers and red borders. They frequently assume geographic shapes and are sometimes confluent. The lesions may be scattered but usually are generalized. By definition, an individual hive is transient, lasting less than 24 h, although new hives may develop continuously. Serum sickness reactions include lymphadenopathy, fever, and arthralgias.

> An individual hive lasts less than 24 h.

Dermographism can be elicited in many patients with urticaria, including patients who have no visible hives at the time. This 'writing with wheals' reaction represents a wheal and flare response to scratching the skin (**Fig. 16.12**). It indicates that the cutaneous mast cells are unstable and are easily provoked to release their histamine content. Many healthy patients develop erythema after stroking the skin, but wheal formation is limited mainly to patients with urticaria. In eliciting this reaction, one should realize that it takes several minutes for the wheal to develop after the skin has been scratched.

Differential Diagnosis

Lesions sometimes mistaken for urticaria include those seen in erythema multiforme, juvenile rheumatoid arthritis, erythema marginatum, and urticarial vasculitis. In *erythema multiforme*, erythematous plaques are often seen, but they last much longer than 24 h. The individual lesions in *juvenile rheumatoid arthritis* are transient, like hives, but they differ in size (only 2–3 mm), color

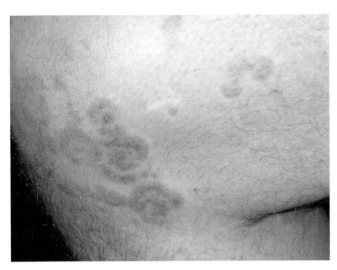

FIGURE 16.13 **Urticarial vasculitis** – annular urticarial plaques with residual purpura.

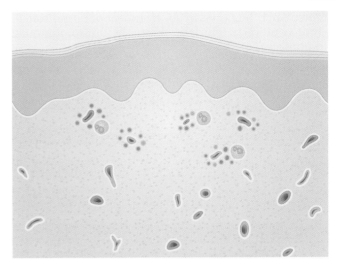

FIGURE 16.15 **Urticaria.** Epidermis – normal. Dermis – papillary dermal edema; sparse inflammatory cell infiltrate around dilated vessels; eosinophils sometimes present.

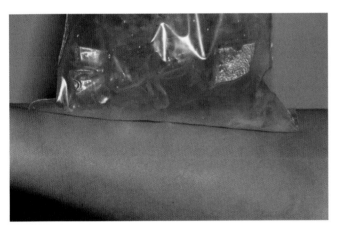

FIGURE 16.14 **Physical urticaria** – cold induced.

(typically salmon), and timing (usually appearing with fever spikes). *Erythema marginatum* is associated with acute rheumatic fever. The skin lesions are erythematous, annular, and either macular or papular. They are also often transient but rarely itch. *Urticarial* vasculitis is associated with hives that last longer than 24 h, typically have a burning sensation, and resolve with residual purpura (**Fig. 16.13**).

Biopsy shows evidence of vasculitis, and work-up for systemic involvement is important.

Laboratory and Biopsy

History confirms the diagnosis and is supported by appropriate investigations. In acute urticaria, 40% of cases are caused by upper respiratory infections, 9% by drugs, 1% by foods and 50% by unknown causes. In chronic urticaria, 60% are idiopathic (most of these cases are likely due to autoimmune factors), 35% are physical, and 5% are vasculitic. For chronic urticarias, it is important to always rule out physical causes of urticaria (e.g., cold, solar, cholinergic, heat and stress and pressure) (**Fig. 16.14**). Rarely chronic urticaria can be associated

with malignancy, so a complete history and physical examination are recommended. Liver function tests are appropriate in patients with urticaria and fever to rule out hepatitis. However, for most patients, the laboratory is rarely helpful in eliciting a cause. A biopsy is rarely required. If biopsy is performed, the pathologic findings are minimal, with vasodilation, dermal edema, and a sparse perivascular inflammatory infiltrate composed mainly of lymphocytes, sometimes admixed with eosinophils (**Fig. 16.15**).

Therapy

Any suspected medication, including aspirin, should be discontinued. Avoidance may be helpful for some of the physical urticarias, such as solar and cold urticaria. Symptomatic therapy is usually achieved with H1 antihistamines given on a regular, rather than an intermittent as-necessary, basis. Taking an antihistamine after the hives break out, as in the as-necessary schedule, is analogous to closing the barn door after the horses have escaped. Hydroxyzine (Atarax) is often used in doses of 10–25 mg four times daily for 1–2 weeks in acute urticaria. For chronic disease, long-term therapy (months to years) may be required, with frequent attempts to taper the dose. Patients who are bothered by sedation from hydroxyzine can be treated with the non-sedating (but more expensive) antihistamines: loratadine (Claritin) or cetirizine (Zyrtec) 10 mg daily, or fexofenadine (Allegra) 180 mg daily.

Initial therapy: antihistamines.

The tricyclic antidepressant doxepin (Sinequan), in a dose of 25 mg once or twice daily, is also effective and has been shown to have both H1 and H2 antihistamine activity. Prednisone is effective but not usually needed and is to be avoided in long-term therapy. Immunosuppressants, such as azathioprine or mycophenolate mofetil, may be necessary for treatment of uncontrolled, chronic urticaria which is driven by an autoimmune response.

Therapy for Urticaria

Initial
- Discontinue drugs suspected to be responsible
- Avoid aspirin and other non-steroidal anti-inflammatory drugs
- Antihistamines:
  - Hydroxyzine 10–25 mg q.i.d.
  - Loratadine 10 mg daily
  - Fexofenadine 180 mg q.d.

Alternative
- Tricyclic drugs:
  - Doxepin 25 mg b.i.d.
- Less frequently used agents:
  - Prednisone 0.5 mg/kg daily
  - Immunosuppressants

Course and Complications

Acute urticaria usually resolves within 2 weeks, whereas chronic urticaria can last several years. Drug-induced urticaria usually clears within several days of discontinuation of the responsible medication. Physical urticarias often have a prolonged course. Hives have no complications other than discomfort from intense itching. Hives, however, may precede or accompany a potentially life-threatening anaphylactic response in patients with a severe reaction.

Chronic urticaria may last for years.

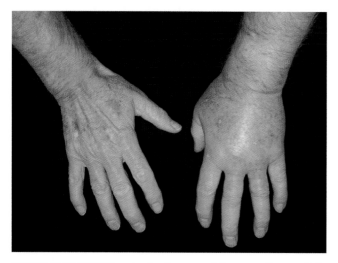

FIGURE 16.16 Hereditary angioedema – soft tissue swelling results in loss of vein markings of affected hand.

Pathogenesis

As summarized below, hives can be mediated immunologically or non-immunologically. Immunoglobulin E (IgE) mediation is the most common immunologic mechanism. In this pathway, a sensitized individual possesses IgE antibodies against a specific antigen, such as penicillin. These IgE antibodies are attached to the surface of mast cells and, when rechallenged, are bridged by the antigen. This results in a sequence of reactions leading ultimately to the release of numerous biologically active products from the mast cells, the most important of which appears to be histamine.

Mechanisms for the Production of Hives

- Immunologic
  - Immunoglobulin E mediated
  - Complement mediated
- Non-immunologic
  - Agents that directly cause mast cell degranulation (e.g., opiates and radiocontrast media)
  - Agents that cause alteration in arachidonic acid metabolism (e.g., aspirin and other non-steroidal anti-inflammatory agents)
- Idiopathic

Autoantibodies to the high-infinity IgE receptor or to IgE itself have been identified in some patients with chronic idiopathic urticaria. These autoantibodies possess histamine releasing activity, and this activity may play a role in this disorder.

Complement-mediated urticaria occurs in several settings, the most spectacular of which is the syndrome of hereditary or acquired *angioedema*, in which patients have a deficiency of the inhibitor of the activated first component of the complement system (C1 esterase). Trauma often precipitates attacks that result clinically in massive local swelling and, occasionally, fatal laryngeal edema (**Fig. 16.16**). The complement system also participates in the hives that occur in *serum sickness*. The postulated mechanism is deposition of immune complexes in blood vessel walls, with fixation of complement and ensuing inflammation. Several drugs can cause direct release of histamine from mast cells. The most commonly encountered are opiates and radiocontrast media.

The mechanism by which aspirin and other NSAIDs causes hives is thought to be their effect on arachidonic acid metabolism. By blocking the production of prostaglandins from arachidonic acid, the pathway is shifted to the production of other metabolites, including the leukotrienes, a family of compounds that includes the previously designated slow-reacting substance of anaphylaxis. As that name suggests, this chemical has the ability to induce urticarial reactions. All of these pathways ultimately result in the release of vasoactive substances (e.g., histamine) that alter vascular permeability and produce dermal edema, which appears clinically as a hive.

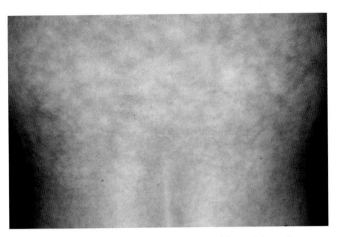

FIGURE 16.17 **Erythema ab igne** – reticulated brownish erythema on back secondary to heating pad.

UNCOMMON CAUSES OF SPECIALIZED ERYTHEMA

ERYTHEMA AB IGNE

Erythema ab igne (EAI) results from chronic exposure to a heating source, most commonly a space heater (affects lower anterior legs) and a heating pad (affects lower back). The pathophysiology is unknown. The skin lesions have a net-like (reticulated) erythema and hyperpigmentation (**Fig. 16.17**). There is a low risk of developing squamous cell carcinoma within the lesion. Treatment involves removal of the heating source.

ERYTHEMA ANNULARE CENTRIFUGUM

Erythema annulare centrifugum is characterized by annular red plaques that expand centrifugally (**Fig. 16.18**). There are two forms of the disease: (1) a superficial form with a trailing edge of white scale, and (2) a deep form with infiltrated borders and no scale. The most common locations for involvement are the axillae, hips, and thighs. The lesions can be episodic and last for months. The cause remains unknown and treatment is often unsatisfactory. Some investigators believe the condition to be a cutaneous response to a distant infection, most often tinea pedis.

ERYTHEMA GYRATUM REPENS

Erythema gyratum repens (EGR) most often represents a paraneoplastic figurate erythema. The most common underlying neoplasms are lung, breast, or esophagus. The rash can appear either before or after detection of the malignancy. The rash is striking, characterized by gyrate red plaques (**Fig. 16.19**) that can advance their edges by up to 1 cm per day. The skin lesions resolve when the malignancy is treated.

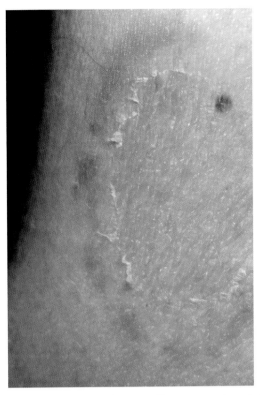

FIGURE 16.18 **Erythema annulare centrifugum** – annular red plaques with characteristic trailing edge of scale.

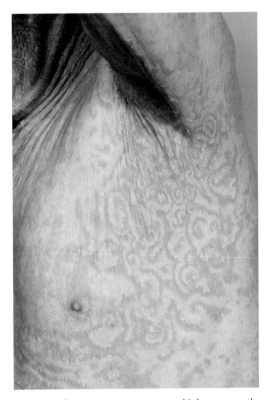

FIGURE 16.19 **Erythema gyratum repens** – multiple gyrate erythematous plaques (wood grain appearance).

17 Purpura

Key Points

1. Purpura (Latin purple) is extravasated blood outside blood vessels and therefore does not blanch
2. Distinguish palpable from non-palpable purpura
3. Palpable purpura represents vasculitis
4. Always rule out infection first in a patient with purpura

ABSTRACT

The word *purpura* is derived from the Latin word for 'purple,' a clinical characteristic that helps to differentiate the lesion from erythema, which is red. Blanchability is the clinical sign that best distinguishes the two. Purpura is non-blanchable because the blood is extravasated outside the vessel walls.

Purpura is purple and non-blanchable.

Purpura is divided into two major categories: non-palpable (macular) and palpable (papular). Non-palpable purpura results from bleeding into the skin without inflammation of the vessels and is due to either a bleeding disorder or blood vessel fragility. Non-palpable purpura is divided further according to the size of the lesion. Purpuric macules smaller than 3 mm are called petechiae; those larger than 3 mm are called ecchymoses. Thrombocytopenia is manifested by petechiae. Ecchymoses are due to blood vessel fragility. Necrotic ecchymoses are found in disseminated intravascular coagulation (DIC), in which thrombi in dermal vessels lead to infarction and hemorrhage.

Non-palpable purpura:
1. Petechiae are found in thrombocytopenia
2. Ecchymoses result from fragile blood vessels
3. Necrotic ecchymoses occur in DIC

Palpable purpura results from inflammatory damage of blood vessels (vasculitis). The inflammation accounts for the elevation of the lesions and allows leakage of blood through the vessel wall. Features of these disorders are outlined in **Table 17.1**. Infection needs to be ruled out in patients with purpura, especially in those with accompanying fever. Most causes of purpura, except for actinic purpura, are uncommon. Other uncommon causes of purpura are highlighted in the differential diagnosis sections.

Palpable purpura represents vasculitis in the skin.

ACTINIC PURPURA

Key Points

1. Incidental finding in the elderly
2. Appears as purpuric macules on forearms secondary to minor trauma
3. Caused by dermal atrophy from sun exposure and age
4. There is no specific treatment

Definition

Purpura resulting from blood vessel fragility appears clinically as ecchymoses, that is, purpuric macules of more than 3 mm in diameter (**Fig. 17.1**). Dermal tissue atrophy resulting from sun exposure and aging is the most common cause. Blood thinners such as low dose aspirin also lead to additive susceptibility.

Incidence

Actinic purpura is extremely common in elderly people, in whom it is usually noted only as an incidental finding.

TABLE 17.1 Purpura

	Frequency (%)[a]	Etiology	History	Physical Examination	Differential Diagnosis	Laboratory Test
Thrombocytopenic purpura	Uncommon	Drugs Malignancy 'Autoimmune'	Drugs Fever	Petechiae, often on legs Mucosal bleeding	Valsalva maneuver Schamberg's disease Hypergammaglobulinemic purpura Venous stasis	Complete blood count with platelet count
Actinic purpura	Uncommon	Blood vessel fragility from sun and aging	Sun exposure Steroid use	Ecchymoses confined to hands and arms	Steroid purpura Amyloidosis	Skin biopsy if amyloid is suspected
Disseminated intravascular coagulation (DIC)	Rare	Sepsis Malignancy Obstetric complications Idiopathic Warfarin	Fever (sepsis) Antecedent viral or streptococcal infection	Necrotic ecchymoses and/or: Petechiae Acral cyanosis Palpable purpura Mucosal bleeding Bleeding from venipuncture site	Vasculitis	Coagulation studies Protein C levels
Vasculitis	0.3[b]	Sepsis Collagen vascular disease Cryoglobulinemia Drugs Malignancy	–	Purpuric papules, nodules, or bullae Legs most commonly affected	DIC	Skin biopsy Screening tests for systemic involvement

[a]Percentage of new dermatology outpatients with this diagnosis seen in the Hershey Medical Center Dermatology Clinic, Hershey, PA.
[b]Of inpatient dermatology consultations, 2% are for vasculitis.

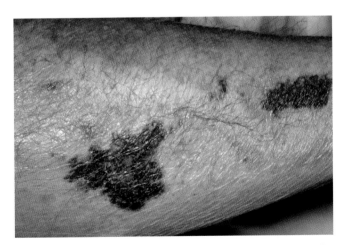

FIGURE 17.1 Actinic purpura – macular purpura with a regular border (ecchymosis).

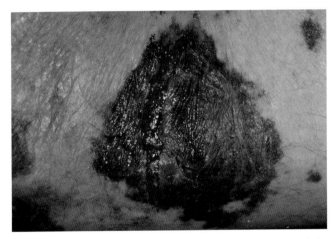

FIGURE 17.2 Actinic purpura with tear in skin secondary to slight trauma.

History

The trauma that induces the purpura is often so minor that it is not remembered by the patient. The patient has no symptoms, and health is unaffected.

Physical Findings

Ecchymoses are usually round or oval macules. In actinic purpura, they are characteristically confined to the dorsa of the hands and forearms. The skin itself in these areas may also be more fragile and may tear easily (**Fig. 17.2**).

Actinic purpura occurs only on the hands and forearms.

Another clinical finding is the development of stellate pseudoscars (**Fig. 17.3**). These thin line scars result from the healing of the skin tears.

Differential Diagnosis

Other causes of blood vessel fragility, in declining order of frequency, are corticosteroid use, amyloidosis, and

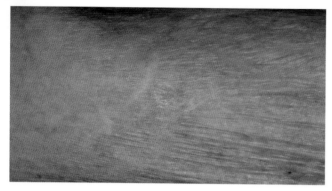

FIGURE 17.3 **Stellate pseudoscars on forearm** – thin white scars resulting from healing of skin tears, commonly seen with actinic purpura.

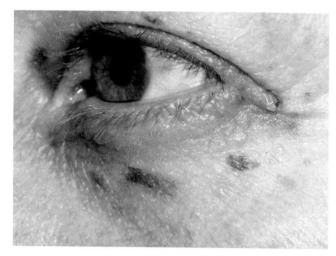

FIGURE 17.4 **Amyloidosis** – 'pinch' purpura.

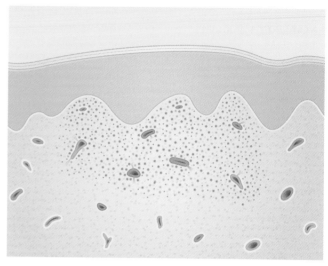

FIGURE 17.5 **Actinic purpura.** Epidermis – normal. Dermis – confluent hemorrhage in the superficial dermis; damaged collagen.

Ehlers–Danlos syndrome. Steroid purpura with skin atrophy can result from topically or systemically administered corticosteroids. Patients with excessive systemic steroids also have a moon facies, a 'buffalo hump' on the upper back, purple striae, and, in younger patients, steroid acne.

Causes of blood vessel fragility:
1. Actinic damage
2. Steroid use
3. Amyloidosis
4. Ehlers–Danlos syndrome

In patients with amyloidosis, the amyloid may infiltrate the skin and result in papules and nodules, which are most often present on the face, particularly the eyelids. These characteristically bleed easily. Purpura also occurs in the absence of papules and can be precipitated by minor trauma or the Valsalva maneuver, referred to as 'pinch' purpura (**Fig. 17.4**). The tongue may also be enlarged.

Ehlers–Danlos syndrome is the least common cause of blood vessel fragility. Several variants of this syndrome are known, in which joint hyperextensibility, skin hyperelasticity, increased fragility of the skin, and increased tendency to bruise occur in varying combinations. Ecchymoses resulting from blood vessel fragility are distinguished from vasculitis by being macular and from the ecchymoses in DIC by their usually smooth rather than ragged contour and by the absence of necrosis.

Ecchymoses resulting from fragile blood vessels have a smooth border and are not necrotic.

Laboratory and Biopsy

Because the diagnosis of actinic purpura is obvious clinically, a biopsy is not required. If a biopsy is done, hemorrhage without inflammation will be noted in the dermis, along with actinically damaged collagen, which appears disorganized, smudged, fragmented, and more basophilic than normal collagen on routine hematoxylin and eosin staining (**Fig. 17.5**).

Therapy

No therapy exists for actinic purpura. Protection against sun exposure with sunscreens is advisable to prevent further damage. Avoidance of prolonged topical steroid use is recommended.

Course and Complications

Ecchymoses slowly fade, leaving brown macules from residual hemosiderin. New ecchymoses, however, continue to develop. Scars frequently occur after tearing of the skin, and are referred to as stellate pseudoscars.

Pathogenesis

The diseases of blood vessel fragility have in common the problem of defective collagen, which weakens the vessels and makes them more susceptible to bleeding from minor trauma. In actinic purpura, blood vessel fragility results from both aging and the damaging effect of sunlight on connective tissue support to blood vessels in sun-exposed skin. Steroid purpura results from inhibition of collagen metabolism by high-dose corticosteroids. In amyloidosis, amyloid material infiltrates and weakens the vessel walls. In Ehlers–Danlos syndrome, fragility of blood vessels results from an intrinsic abnormality in collagen biosynthesis.

DISSEMINATED INTRAVASCULAR COAGULATION

Key Points

1. Life-threatening
2. Seen in bacterial sepsis (meningococcemia)
3. Stellate purpura with central necrosis is characteristic
4. Treat underlying condition

Definition

DIC is a condition in which uncontrolled clotting results in diffuse thrombus formation. The skin is frequently affected, with thrombosed vessels causing skin necrosis. Hemorrhage from these vessels appears as ecchymoses (**Fig. 17.6**). Petechiae also occur as a result of the thrombocytopenia from platelet consumption.

Incidence

DIC is an uncommon, life-threatening disease. It usually occurs in the setting of bacterial sepsis (particularly meningococcemia). DIC may also be associated with malignancy, particularly prostatic carcinoma and acute promyelocytic leukemia. It can also be precipitated by massive trauma. Occasionally, it may result from amniotic fluid embolism, or it may occur as an idiopathic or 'post-infection' phenomenon (purpura fulminans). Localized intravascular coagulation occurs in patients with protein C deficiency who are given warfarin (Coumadin necrosis).

Causes of DIC:
1. Bacterial sepsis
2. Malignancy
3. Amniotic fluid embolism
4. Trauma
5. Idiopathic (purpura fulminans)

History

Patients with DIC are usually systemically ill, often severely so. Fever and shock are frequently present. Symptoms of infection (e.g., headache and stiff neck with meningococcal meningitis) should be sought. A history of a malignancy may be important. Patients with purpura fulminans often have a prodrome of upper respiratory tract symptoms from viral or streptococcal infection. Patients with Coumadin necrosis are not affected systemically, but rather develop localized areas of skin hemorrhage and necrosis approximately 1 week after starting warfarin.

Physical Findings

Various hemorrhagic skin lesions may be present. The most distinctive is a purpuric, stellate ecchymosis, which often appears to be necrotic in the center. The stellate shape is characteristic of blood vessel thrombosis with infarction. Dark gray central areas indicate necrosis and impending slough. Most lesions are flat, but palpable purpura occurs in approximately 20% of patients as a result of edema associated with skin infarction. Petechiae are common, and hemorrhagic bullae, acral cyanosis, mucosal bleeding, dissecting hematomas, and prolonged bleeding from wound sites can also occur. Coumadin necrosis is usually limited to one or a few localized areas, but the skin involvement is severe and results in a full-thickness slough (**Fig. 17.7**) and is localized to fatty areas such as the breasts and thighs.

Stellate purpura with dark gray central areas indicates thrombosis and infarction.

Differential Diagnosis

Ecchymoses from fragile blood vessels are round or oval, have smooth borders, and are not necrotic; DIC-related ecchymoses are irregular (stellate) in outline and often become necrotic. In addition, patients with DIC are usually severely systemically ill. In contrast to vasculitic lesions, the purpura in DIC is usually flat but may occasionally be palpable. Elevated lesions in DIC can be distinguished from those of vasculitis by a skin biopsy. In bacterial sepsis, vasculitis and DIC can coexist.

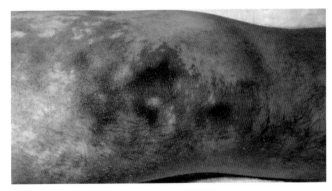

FIGURE 17.6 Disseminated intravascular coagulation – stellate purpura. Dark gray areas are necrotic and eventually slough; petechiae are also present.

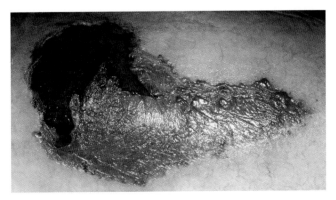

FIGURE 17.7 Warfarin (Coumadin) necrosis.

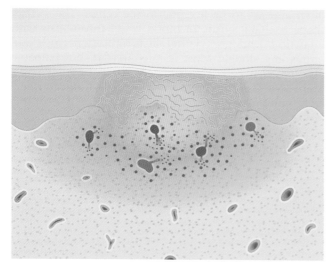

FIGURE 17.8 Disseminated intravascular coagulation. Epidermis – central necrosis. Dermis – fibrin thrombi in the capillaries in the middle to upper dermis; hemorrhage from necrotic vessels; no inflammation.

Laboratory and Biopsy

The laboratory findings characteristic for DIC are thrombocytopenia, prolonged prothrombin time, hypofibrinogenemia, and the presence of fibrin and fibrinogen degradation products. Of these tests, the platelet count and fibrinogen levels are the most useful for diagnosing and following patients with DIC.

Skin biopsy reveals the presence of intravascular thrombi, blood vessel necrosis, and extravasated red blood cells with little or no associated inflammation. Epidermal and dermal necrosis may result from infarction (**Fig. 17.8**).

Therapy

In DIC, the most important principle is to treat the underlying condition. Clotting factors should be repleted with infusions of platelets, cryoprecipitate (for fibrinogen and factor VIII), and fresh plasma (for factor V). Clinical thromboses, which occur particularly in patients with malignancy-associated DIC, are additionally treated with heparin to help control the clotting. Patients with Coumadin necrosis are also treated with heparin. Full-thickness skin necrosis may occur, particularly in Coumadin necrosis, and requires skin grafting for repair.

> **Therapy for Disseminated Intravascular Coagulation**
>
> **Initial**
> 1. Treatment of underlying condition
> 2. Repletion of clotting factors
> 3. Heparin (in select patients with intravascular thromboses)

Course and Complications

DIC is a serious disorder, with an overall mortality rate of about 50%. Early diagnosis and prompt therapy improve survival. Cutaneous complications result from infarction, causing necrosis of skin and the tips of digits.

Pathogenesis

The primary process appears to be widespread thrombus formation in which coagulation factors are consumed. Fibrinogen, the target protein, is acted on by thrombin and plasmin, and fibrin clots are formed. In DIC associated with Gram-negative bacterial sepsis, bacterial endotoxins are thought to induce this process. Cytokines such as tumor necrosis factor may also play a role. The clotting process also produces fibrinogen and fibrin degradation products that act as anticoagulants. These anticoagulants compound the bleeding diathesis produced by consumption of clotting factors.

Patients with inherited or acquired protein C deficiency are also susceptible to intravascular coagulation. Protein C is a vitamin K-dependent anticoagulant. Patients with congenital absence of protein C die early in life from purpura fulminans with internal thromboses. Patients who have inherited or acquired protein C deficiency are susceptible to recurrent venous thromboses and to skin necrosis if warfarin is administered. Warfarin causes necrosis in these patients by depleting their marginal reserves of protein C before depleting the vitamin K-dependent clotting factors. The resultant imbalance in the anticoagulation-to-coagulation ratio allows the formation of clots with subsequent skin necrosis.

THROMBOCYTOPENIC PURPURA

> **Key Points**
>
> 1. Petechiae are a major clinical finding
> 2. Drugs are a common cause
> 3. Check platelet count
> 4. Treatment depends on cause

Definition

Petechiae are purpuric macules <3 mm in diameter (**Fig. 17.9**). They are frequently caused by thrombocytopenia, which can result from drugs, preceding viral infection, acquired immune deficiency syndrome (AIDS), collagen vascular disease, hematologic malignancy, idiopathic (or immune) thrombocytopenic purpura (ITP), and thrombotic thrombocytopenic purpura (TTP).

> Causes of thrombocytopenic purpura:
> 1. Drugs
> 2. Viral infections
> 3. AIDS
> 4. Collagen vascular disease
> 5. Hematologic malignancy
> 6. ITP
> 7. TTP

Incidence

Of the causes listed, drugs most often cause thrombocytopenic purpura in adults. In children, acute

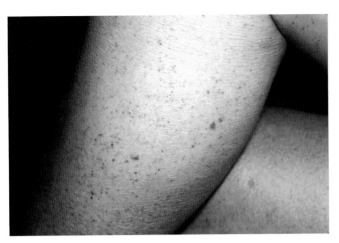

FIGURE 17.9 **Petechiae** – small (<3 mm) purpuric macules.

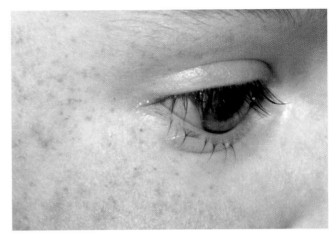

FIGURE 17.10 **Petechiae on the cheek** in a 2-year-old child after forceful retching.

thrombocytopenic purpura most often is precipitated by a viral infection and has an annual incidence of 4 per 100 000 children. About 15 000 new cases of ITP are diagnosed in the USA each year. TTP is uncommon.

History

In patients with petechiae, a drug history is important. Systemic symptoms should also be sought. For example, children with acute thrombocytopenic purpura usually have a history of a viral infection within the preceding 1–3 weeks. TTP is accompanied by fever, hemolytic anemia, and neurologic symptoms. Petechiae and purpura accompany TTP.

Physical Findings

Petechiae may be generalized but are usually most pronounced in areas of dependency. Easy bruising may be noted, and mucosal bleeding may also be present, so the conjunctivae and oral cavity should be examined carefully. Splenomegaly is frequent in patients with hematologic malignancies or chronic ITP.

Differential Diagnosis

Petechiae can also result from increased intravascular pressure with forceful retching or coughing (**Fig. 17.10**). This Valsalva maneuver results in petechiae on the face, neck, and upper trunk. Leakage of blood from capillaries also occurs in Schamberg's disease, an idiopathic capillaritis, in which inflammation (although not sufficient to cause elevation of the lesion) weakens the capillaries so they leak (**Fig. 17.11**). Schamberg's disease is one of the most commonly encountered petechial diseases in dermatology. This causes petechial lesions of the lower legs that have been likened in appearance to cayenne pepper. Petechiae in the lower extremities can also occur in the setting of venous stasis, particularly if the patient also has dermatitis.

Laboratory and Biopsy

In patients with petechiae, a complete blood cell count and platelet count should be ordered. Bleeding from thrombocytopenia usually does not occur unless the

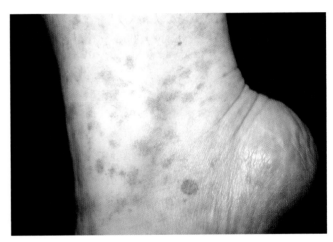

FIGURE 17.11 **Schamberg's disease** – patches of petechiae best seen under magnification on lower leg.

platelet count is <50 000/mm^3. A platelet count of <20 000/mm^3 results in bleeding from even minor trauma, and a count of <10 000/mm^3 predisposes the patient to internal bleeding.

Urinalysis and guaiac testing of the stool help to screen for bleeding from the urinary and gastrointestinal tracts. Skin biopsy enables non-inflammatory petechiae to be distinguished from vasculitis, although the clinical picture is usually so distinctive that a biopsy is not required (**Fig. 17.12**).

Screening tests:
1. Complete blood cell count
2. Platelet count
3. Urinalysis
4. Stool guaiac

Therapy

Therapy is aimed at the underlying disorder. If a drug is the cause, its discontinuation solves the problem, usually within several days. Therapy is not always needed in

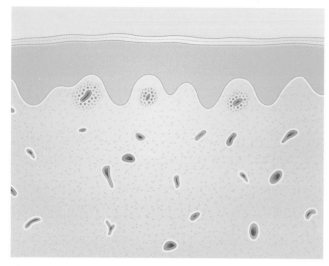

FIGURE 17.12 Petechiae. Epidermis – normal. Dermis – hemorrhage around superficial vessels.

children with acute thrombocytopenic purpura, although both prednisone and intravenous γ-globulin have been used with good effect. Adults with ITP are treated initially with prednisone to increase platelet production. Chronic ITP (defined by a platelet count of <100 000 cells/mm³ for more than 6 months) is often treated with splenectomy. Intravenous γ-globulin is often used to prepare patients for this surgery. Splenectomy prolongs platelet survival and results in sustained remission in 85% of patients with chronic ITP. Treatment failure may require immunosuppressant therapy. Plasmapheresis with plasma replacement is used, with good success, in the treatment of TTP.

Therapy for Thrombocytopenic Purpura

Initial
- Discontinue drug (if drug induced)
- Plasmapheresis (for TTP)
- Prednisone (for ITP)

Alternative
- Splenectomy (for TTP)
- Immunosuppressants (for TTP and ITP)
- IVIG (ITP)

Course and Complications

The course and complications depend on the nature of the underlying disease. Drug-induced thrombocytopenia can produce bleeding at other sites, particularly the gastrointestinal tract. Virus-induced acute thrombocytopenia resolves without therapy and without complications in 90% of children. ITP in adults may resolve spontaneously, but more often becomes chronic with a waxing and waning course that requires splenectomy in many patients. ITP is the presenting problem in some patients with underlying 'autoimmune' diseases such as systemic lupus erythematosus. TTP is the most severe disorder and was associated with a 75% mortality rate. With plasma exchange and infusion therapy, this rate has been reduced to 25%.

Pathogenesis

Platelets normally plug small defects in capillary walls and also help to initiate the clotting mechanism. Deficiency or dysfunction of platelets leads to 'leaky' vessels.

Drugs can cause both thrombocytopenia and platelet dysfunction. Drug-induced thrombocytopenia results from either a toxic or an antibody-mediated mechanism. Drugs causing immunologic platelet destruction include quinidine, quinine, sulfonamides, heparin, digitoxin, phenytoin (Dilantin), and methyldopa.

Drugs that can cause thrombocytopenia:
1. Quinidine
2. Quinine
3. Sulfonamides
4. Heparin
5. Digitoxin
6. Phenytoin
7. Methyldopa

Cancer chemotherapy causes thrombocytopenia through inhibition of marrow production. Aspirin causes platelet dysfunction through inhibition of thromboxane production. Decreased platelet production occurs in hematologic malignancies as a result of bone marrow replacement with malignant cells.

An autoimmune mechanism is operative in virus-induced acute childhood thrombocytopenia, AIDS-associated thrombocytopenia, and chronic ITP. In these disorders, immunoglobulin G (IgG) antiplatelet antibodies bind to specific platelet membrane glycoproteins. The immunoglobulin-coated platelets are then recognized and removed by the reticuloendothelial system, especially the spleen.

The cause of TTP remains unknown.

VASCULITIS

Key Points

1. Palpable purpura represents vasculitis
2. Rule out systemic involvement
3. Biopsy confirms the diagnosis
4. Treatment depends on the cause

Definition

Strictly speaking, any inflammation of blood vessels could be called 'vasculitis,' although the term is generally used to describe a necrotizing reaction in blood vessels. Numerous vasculitic disorders have been described, classified, and reclassified, and this has led to much confusion. When the skin is affected by vasculitis, the result is purpuric papules (palpable purpura) (**Fig. 17.13**). The

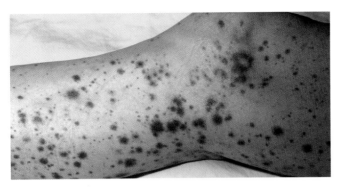

FIGURE 17.13 Vasculitis – purpuric papules.

lesions are elevated (palpable) because of inflammation and edema, and purpuric because of extravasation of blood from damaged blood vessels.

Palpable purpura indicates vasculitis.

Most often, cutaneous vasculitis affects only small vessels and results in purpuric papules. This process is mediated by neutrophils and is often termed leukocytoclastic vasculitis. Leukocytoclastic vasculitis can occur in a variety of settings, including sepsis, collagen vascular disease (particularly systemic lupus erythematosus and rheumatoid arthritis), cryoglobulinemia, drug reactions, and, occasionally, malignant lymphoma and myeloma. Henoch–Schönlein purpura is an idiopathic syndrome of cutaneous vasculitis associated with arthritis and abdominal pain, accompanied by gastrointestinal and renal vasculitis. Vasculitis confined to the skin in which an underlying cause cannot be found has been called allergic cutaneous vasculitis or hypersensitivity vasculitis. This is a common type of vasculitis, but a diagnosis of exclusion.

Causes of cutaneous vasculitis:
1. Infections
   - Bacterial
   - Rickettsial
   - Viral (hepatitis C virus)
2. Collagen vascular diseases
   - Systemic lupus erythematosus
   - Rheumatoid arthritis
3. Cryoglobulinemia
4. Drugs
5. Lymphoma and myeloma
6. Idiopathic
   - Henoch–Schönlein purpura
   - 'Hypersensitivity'

Incidence

Cutaneous vasculitis is uncommon. Of new patients seen in the authors' dermatology clinic, 0.3% had cutaneous vasculitis. It was more common in their hospital practice: 2% of the dermatology consultations were for vasculitis.

History

Systemic disease must be ruled out, and the history is the first step in doing so. In patients with a history of fever and cutaneous vasculitis, sepsis must be considered. Bacteria causing septic vasculitis include: *Neisseria meningitidis, Neisseria gonorrhoeae, Staphylococcus aureus, Streptococcus pneumoniae,* Viridans streptococci, and *Pseudomonas aeruginosa*. Fever may also occur in patients with viral infection, collagen vascular disease, and even drug reactions, but the first responsibility is to rule out sepsis. This includes rickettsial sepsis (Rocky Mountain spotted fever), in which the abrupt onset of fever is accompanied by headache and myalgia, and is followed several days later by an erythematous rash, which characteristically begins on the wrists and ankles and then involves the palms and soles as it becomes generalized and purpuric. The history and appearance of the rash permit an early clinical diagnosis of this disease, which is fatal if not treated promptly.

First, rule out sepsis as the cause of vasculitis.

The rash in Rocky Mountain spotted fever starts on the wrists and ankles.

Symptoms of multisystem involvement in vasculitis may include arthritis, hematuria, abdominal pain and melena, cough and hemoptysis, and neurologic involvement with headaches and peripheral neuropathy. Although drug-induced vasculitis is uncommon, drug history is important. The drugs most frequently implicated include aspirin, phenothiazines, penicillin, sulfonamides, and thiazides.

Physical Examination

The primary lesion in cutaneous vasculitis is a purpuric papule (palpable purpura). Necrosis sometimes follows; it is heralded by the appearance of a dark gray color in the center of a lesion, followed by slough. In the absence of necrosis, lesions evolve by flattening and fading. The flattening may occur surprisingly quickly, so a lesion that is palpable on the first day may be flat by the second. As lesions fade, hemosiderin remains, leaving the affected skin brown. In gonococcemia, lesions are distinctive in that they are pustular as well as purpuric, sparse, and distributed distally on the extremities (**Fig. 17.14**). Lesions of vasculitis are most often located on the lower extremities, but they may be generalized in patients with extensive disease.

Gonococcemia is characterized by purpuric pustules in acral distribution.

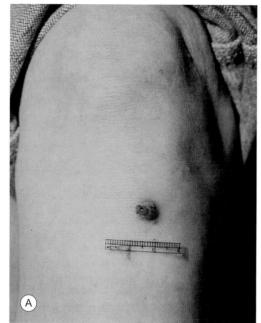

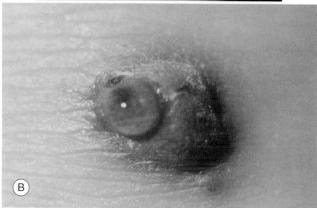

FIGURE 17.14 Gonococcemia. A. Hemorrhagic (purpuric) pustules sparsely distributed on distal extremities. **B.** Close-up of hemorrhagic pustule.

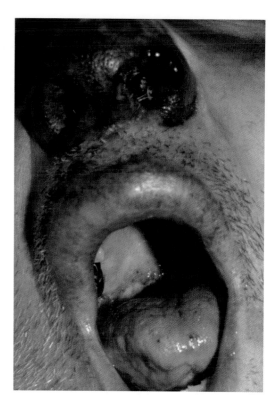

FIGURE 17.15 Wegener's granulomatosis – necrotic lesions of the nose and ulcerations in the mouth are due to vasculitis of larger vessels.

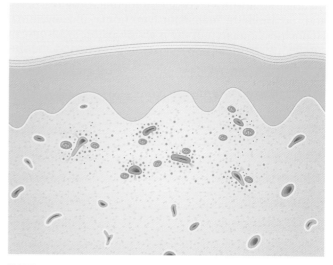

FIGURE 17.16 Vasculitis. Epidermis – normal. Dermis – neutrophils and nuclear debris in and around blood vessels; endothelial swelling and necrosis of blood vessel walls; hemorrhage.

Differential Diagnosis

For purpuric lesions, the first step is to determine whether they are palpable. The causes of non-palpable purpura were listed above. Lesions in DIC may be flat or elevated. Those that are elevated are so because of edema that acutely accompanies necrosis. Vasculitis may coexist with DIC in some patients who have bacterial sepsis (e.g., meningococcemia) – bacterial emboli cause the vasculitis, and endotoxin initiates the DIC. Candidal sepsis produces papular skin lesions that usually are erythematous but may also be purpuric when accompanied by thrombocytopenia. Patients with large vessel vasculitis (e.g., polyarteritis nodosa and Wegener's granulomatosis) frequently experience ulcerations of the skin as a manifestation of obliterative necrosis of vessels that are larger than those involved in the vasculitis lesions discussed above (**Fig. 17.15**).

Laboratory and Biopsy

The diagnosis of necrotizing vasculitis is confirmed by skin biopsy. The histologic features are: (1) the presence in and around the blood vessel walls of neutrophils with leukocytoclasis (i.e., destruction of neutrophils leaving nuclear debris); (2) hemorrhage; (3) endothelial cell swelling; and (4) fibrinoid necrosis of the vessel wall (**Fig. 17.16**). Immunofluorescent stains may show immunoglobulin deposition in the vessel walls in early lesions, but this is not diagnostically helpful, except in Henoch–Schönlein purpura, in which the immunoglobulin deposited is characteristically IgA rather than the IgG or IgM seen in all other types of vasculitis.

Laboratory tests are used to rule out systemic involvement or specific systemic diseases. Blood cultures should be obtained in all patients with vasculitis and fever. Acute and convalescent serologic titers confirm (posthumously, if treatment is not instituted early in the disease) a diagnosis of Rocky Mountain spotted fever. Other laboratory work includes a complete urinalysis, guaiac test of stool, complete blood count with differential and platelet count, sedimentation rate, serum creatinine, serum protein electrophoresis, cryoglobulins, antinuclear antibody test, rheumatoid factor, hepatitis-associated antigen, and chest radiography.

> Obtain blood cultures in patients with vasculitis and fever.

Therapy

Treatment is of the underlying disease, if one is found. In patients with suspected bacterial sepsis, treatment should be instituted immediately, not after culture results are returned. Meningococcemia is a dramatic example in which a treatment delay of a few hours can mean the difference between a favorable and a fatal outcome. The same is true for Rocky Mountain spotted fever, in which early treatment (with tetracycline) is life-saving and must be instituted on the basis of clinical suspicion.

If a drug reaction is suspected, the drug should be discontinued. Most other forms of vasculitis are treated with prednisone or immunosuppressant therapy. Patients with idiopathic vasculitis limited to the skin respond well to prednisone, but dapsone also frequently controls the process and is safer for long-term administration. Colchicine has also been used with success in some patients. One should not be overzealous in the treatment of cutaneous vasculitis because this condition is chronic and often does not affect the viscera.

Therapy for Vasculitis

Initial
- Treat infection if suspected
- Discontinue implicated drugs, if any
- For acute non-infectious vasculitis: prednisone

Alternative
- For chronic cutaneous vasculitis:
  - Dapsone
  - Colchicine
  - Immunosuppressants

Course and Complications

The course and complications depend on the underlying disease and extent of organ involvement by the vasculitis. Vasculitis associated with bacterial or rickettsial sepsis responds promptly to antibiotic therapy. If a drug is responsible, its withdrawal solves the problem. Purpuric lesions associated with viral diseases (e.g., enterovirus infections and atypical measles) resolve spontaneously. The skin disease in Henoch–Schönlein purpura is usually self-limiting, but renal impairment persists in nearly 30% of these patients. Rheumatoid vasculitis is usually associated with a high titer of rheumatoid factor; a reduction in rheumatoid factor is usually accompanied by improvement in the vasculitis. Idiopathic cutaneous vasculitis has a tendency to wax and wane, frequently over a period of years, and is not usually a harbinger of serious internal involvement.

Serious complications are related less to the skin than to internal organ involvement, with the kidney most often and usually most seriously affected.

> The kidney is the most frequently involved internal organ.

Pathogenesis

Vasculitis is thought to be an immune complex-mediated disease. The antigen in the immune complex may be exogenous (e.g., bacterial, drug) or endogenous (e.g., another antibody, as in rheumatoid factor; or nuclear antigens, as in lupus). These circulating immune complexes lodge in the walls of blood vessels; in the skin, small venules are most often involved. The propensity for involvement in the lower legs may relate to hydrostatic forces that predispose to sluggish blood flow and immune complex deposition. The complement cascade is then activated, producing chemotactic factors that attract polymorphonuclear leukocytes into the vessel wall. Lysosomes are released from the leukocytes and cause sufficient damage to the vessel wall to permit extravasation of red blood cells.

> Vasculitis is a type III immune complex reaction.

The antibodies in the immune complexes are usually of the IgG or IgM class, with the exception of Henoch–Schönlein purpura, in which they are characteristically IgA.

18 Dermal Induration

Key Points

1. Dermal induration presents with firm and thickened skin
2. Skin biopsy is often necessary for diagnosis
3. Diseases tend to run a natural course despite treatment intervention

ABSTRACT

Induration represents dermal thickening resulting in skin that feels thicker or firmer than normal. Scleroderma is the disease that best exemplifies this process. All of the diseases included in this chapter are uncommon conditions, except for granuloma annulare. Stasis dermatitis, a cause of dermal induration of the lower extremities, has a significant epidermal component and is discussed in Chapter 8. For all causes of dermal induration, skin biopsy is often necessary for confirmation of the diagnosis, where the degree of dermal inflammation varies depending on whether the biopsy is performed at an early or late ('burned out') stage of the disease process. Treatment options are limited and usually have minimal impact on the disease course.

GRANULOMA ANNULARE

Key Points

1. Self-limiting, asymptomatic condition with papules arranged in annular configuration
2. Commonly affects children and young adults
3. Occurs mostly on dorsal hands and feet

Definition

Granuloma annulare is an asymptomatic skin condition characterized by dermal papules (no overlying epidermal change), forming annular plaques and commonly arising on the dorsal hands and feet (**Fig. 18.1**). Although the center of the plaques becomes depressed, the leading edge of papules represents dermal induration. Granuloma annulare is most often localized but can be generalized.

Incidence

Granuloma annulare appears most commonly in children and young adults, and affects females more commonly than males.

History

The lesions are usually asymptomatic and come to the attention of the physician because of cosmetic concerns. Some patients mistakenly treat the condition for tinea corporis because of the annular configuration.

Physical Examination

The localized variant appears as shiny dermal papules and annular plaques that are centrally depressed. Granuloma annulare can be skin colored, violaceous, or erythematous. Generalized granuloma annulare can affect the entire body (**Fig. 18.2**). Other, less common, variants are subcutaneous (deep dermal solitary nodules) (**Fig. 18.3**) and perforating (papules with central umbilication that is crusted and ulcerated). Both the subcutaneous and perforating variant of granuloma annulare appear on the distal extremities.

Clinical variants of granuloma annulare:
1. Localized
2. Generalized
3. Subcutaneous
4. Perforating

Differential diagnosis

Granuloma annulare can be confused with other, often more serious, conditions. Papular granuloma annulare can appear similar to papular *sarcoidosis* (**Fig. 18.4**) and *lichen planus*. A skin biopsy easily distinguishes between these conditions. Necrobiosis lipoidica diabeticorum (NLD) can appear clinically and histologically similar to

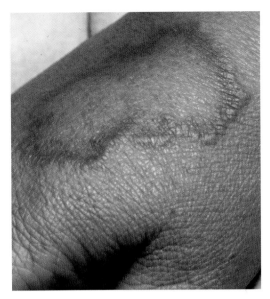

FIGURE 18.1 **Granuloma annulare** – annular dermal plaque.

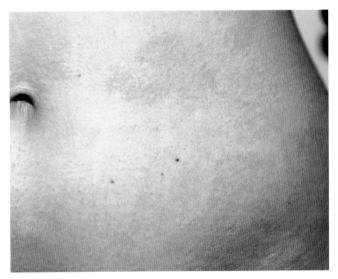

FIGURE 18.2 **Generalized granuloma annulare** – brownish plaques with serpiginous borders.

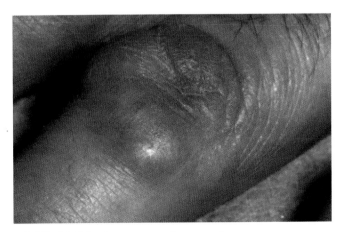

FIGURE 18.3 **Subcutaneous granuloma annulare.**

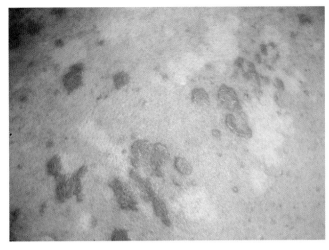

FIGURE 18.4 **Cutaneous sarcoidosis** – reddish brown, annular plaques.

granuloma annulare. NLD often has a yellowish hue, and telangiectasias present centrally within the depressed plaques on the lower legs. NLD has a stronger association with diabetes mellitus than does granuloma annulare. Subcutaneous granuloma annulare can appear similar to rheumatoid nodule, both clinically and histologically. Arthritis is not present with granuloma annulare. Annular granuloma annulare is most often confused with tinea corporis, but lack of scale in granuloma annulare should enable the clinician to distinguish between the two.

> Annular plaques of granuloma annulare have no scale; tinea corporis has scale.

Laboratory and Biopsy

Laboratory work-up with granuloma annulare is not usually necessary. Diabetes mellitus has been reported to be associated with generalized granuloma annulare. Skin biopsy shows necrobiosis (degenerative collagen) in the dermis with a predominantly histiocytic (i.e., macrophages) and multinucleated giant cell infiltrate on the periphery.

Therapy

Treatment of granuloma annulare is unsatisfactory. For young children, spontaneous resolution occurs. Therefore, no treatment is the best treatment (i.e., benign neglect). For cosmetically disfiguring lesions, treatment with potent topical corticosteroids, such as fluocinonide 0.05% cream, or intralesional triamcinolone 5–10 mg/mL may be effective. Skin atrophy is always a concern with prolonged topical or intralesional corticosteroid use. Psoralen plus ultraviolet A radiation (PUVA) and the antimalarial hydroxychloroquine (200 mg b.i.d.) are reserved for patients with generalized granuloma annulare. No well designed studies favor any systemic therapy.

> Localized granuloma annulare often resolves spontaneously.

Therapy for Granuloma Annulare

Initial
- Observation
- Topical steroids (fluocinonide 0.05% cream)
- Intralesional steroids (triamcinolone 5–10 mg/mL)

Alternative (for Generalized Variant)
- PUVA
- Antimalarial (hydroxychloroquine 200 mg b.i.d.)

Course and Complications

After 2 years, approximately 75% of granuloma annulare lesions will disappear. Recurrences are not uncommon. This is a self-limiting disease.

Pathogenesis

The cause remains unknown.

LICHEN SCLEROSUS ET ATROPHICUS

Key Points

1. Sclerotic white plaques
2. Often affects genital skin
3. Pruritic

Definition

Lichen sclerosus et atrophicus is a chronic inflammatory condition that results in sclerotic white plaques due to thickening of the superficial dermis with overlying, thinned, finely wrinkled epidermis (**Fig. 18.5**). Genital involvement of lichen sclerosus et atrophicus is more common than non-genital involvement and it can coexist with morphea, suggesting that the two diseases are related. Pruritus is often a major complaint.

Incidence

Lichen sclerosus et atrophicus is an uncommon disease. Females are reportedly more commonly affected, but this is unproven.

History

Lichen sclerosus et atrophicus involving non-genital skin is mostly asymptomatic, but can be dry and pruritic. The lesions can be cosmetically disfiguring. Involvement of the genitalia can result in intractable pruritus, leading to the development of dyspareunia in women and phimosis in men. In young females the initial appearance of lichen sclerosus et atrophicus can have a bruise-like quality (resembling traumatic hemorrhage) and lead to the misdiagnosis of child abuse.

Bruise-like quality of lichen sclerosus et atrophicus in young females can lead to misdiagnosis of child abuse.

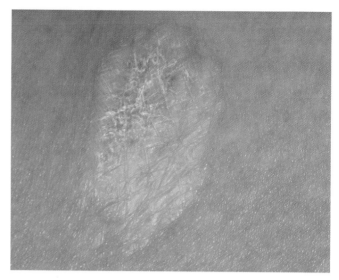

FIGURE 18.5 Lichen sclerosus et atrophicus – sclerotic white plaque with wrinkled, atrophic epidermis.

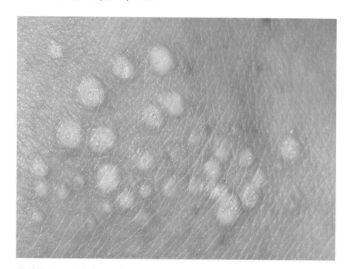

FIGURE 18.6 Lichen sclerosus et atrophicus – guttate papules.

Physical Examination

Non-genital disease occurs primarily on the trunk and extremities. The initial lesions appear as guttate (i.e., drop-like), white papules that can coalesce into larger plaques (**Fig. 18.6**). The sclerotic plaques are covered by a finely wrinkled (often referred to as cigarette paper- or parchment-like) epidermis. In women, the vulva and perianal area are often involved, resulting in a figure-of-eight configuration. The initial erythema evolves into a hypopigmented sclerotic plaque that may erode and scar, making sexual intercourse difficult (**Fig. 18.7**). The corollary in men is foreskin involvement leading to phimosis.

Guttate white papules are characteristic of early lichen sclerosus et atrophicus.

Differential Diagnosis

The two key differential diagnoses are morphea for non-genital lichen sclerosus et atrophicus and sexual abuse

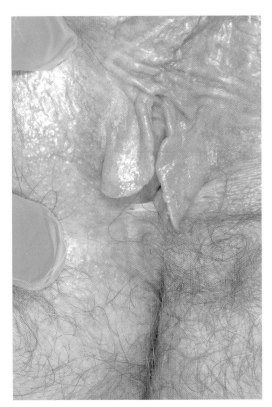

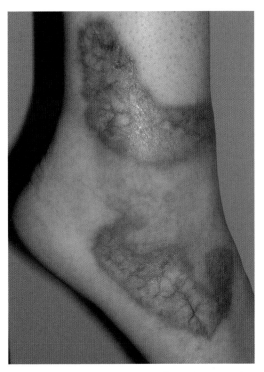

FIGURE 18.8 Necrobiosis lipoidica – yellow plaques with atrophic centers and prominent blood vessels.

FIGURE 18.7 Lichen sclerosus et atrophicus – Note adhesion developing at lower vaginal introitus and faint pinkness. Skin biopsy confirmed diagnosis.

with genital lichen sclerosus et atrophicus. Early squamous cell carcinoma (erythroplasia of Queyrat) can mimic erosive genital lichen sclerosus et atrophicus, and biopsy is mandatory.

> Biopsy erosive lichen sclerosus et atrophicus of the genitals to rule out squamous cell carcinoma.

Laboratory and Biopsy

Lichen sclerosus et atrophicus is not associated with any systemic disease. Biopsy shows a homogenized (smudgy collagen) superficial dermis with a flattened dermoepidermal junction.

Therapy

Emollients and ultra-potent steroids are the treatment of choice in genital lichen sclerosus et atrophicus for both children and adults. Clobetasol propionate 0.05% cream or foam needs to be applied for 12–24 weeks. Even with long-term use, no major side-effects, including atrophy, have been reported in these studies. The author recommends use on alternate days to avoid skin breakdown. Topical macrolides used twice daily for 3–6 months have been shown to be effective. For non-genital lichen sclerosus et atrophicus judicious use of ultra-potent topical corticosteroids is recommended. For severe, generalized disease, acitretin at a dose of 25–50 mg/day for 3–4 months has anecdotally been reported to be effective. Recurrence of disease with treatment discontinuation is always a concern.

Therapy for Lichen Sclerosus Et Atrophicus

Initial
- Emollients
- Topical ultra-potent steroids (clobetasol propionate 0.05% cream or foam)

Alternative
- Topical macrolides (tacrolimus or pimecrolimus b.i.d.)
- Acitretin 25–50 mg/day for generalized disease

NECROBIOSIS LIPOIDICA

Key Points

1. Plaques with reddish brown active border and yellowish depressed center with telangiectasias
2. Involves anterior shins
3. Two-thirds of patients have abnormal glucose tolerance

Definition

Necrobiosis lipoidica is characterized by distinctive, well circumscribed, yellowish plaques with a yellow center commonly affecting the anterior lower legs (**Fig. 18.8**). It is often associated with diabetes mellitus.

> Necrobiosis lipoidica is strongly associated with diabetes.

Incidence

Necrobiosis lipoidica occurs more commonly in females than in males, with a 3:1 ratio. Approximately 0.3% of diabetics suffer from necrobiosis lipoidica. Young adults are most commonly affected.

History

The plaques of necrobiosis lipoidica evolve slowly over a number of years and are often brought to the attention of the physician because of cosmetic disfigurement. Rarely, the condition ulcerates and becomes painful.

Physical Examination

Necrobiosis lipoidica is a brownish-red (early) papule that evolves into a plaque. With time, the center of the plaque becomes atrophic, takes on a yellowish hue, and develops prominent telangiectasias. An elevated and sharply defined border is present. The lesion is firm to touch. Uncommonly ulcers and erosions develop within the plaques, often following trauma. Necrobiosis lipoidica is commonly distributed symmetrically on the anterior shins. Rarely, it appears in a generalized distribution.

> Rarely, ulceration develops within necrobiosis lipoidica following trauma.

Differential Diagnosis

Usually the clinical appearance is sufficient to make the diagnosis. Skin biopsy is sometimes needed to distinguish from granuloma annulare and sarcoidosis.

Laboratory and Biopsy

Abnormal glucose tolerance is detected in two-thirds of patients with necrobiosis lipoidica, hence the historic name of necrobiosis lipoidica diabeticorum. A general rule of thumb to follow for patients with necrobiosis lipoidica is: one-third have diabetes, one-third have abnormal glucose tolerance, and one-third have normal glucose tolerance. Skin biopsy confirms the diagnosis by showing layered granulomatous inflammation in the dermis that is parallel to the epidermis, areas of connective tissue degeneration, and destruction of blood vessels.

> Two-thirds of patients with necrobiosis lipoidica have abnormal glucose tolerance.

Therapy

There is no known effective treatment for necrobiosis lipoidica. Smoking cessation as well as optimizing diabetic control may halt disease progression and decrease the likelihood of ulceration. Potent topical steroids, such as fluocinonide 0.05% cream, can be applied to the active borders. Alternatively, intralesional triamcinolone 10 mg/mL can be injected into the active borders to help halt disease expansion. Limited success has been reported with pentoxifylline (Trental; 400 mg b.i.d.) and a host of other agents.

Therapy for Necrobiosis Lipoidica

Initial
- Optimize diabetic control
- Topical steroid: fluocinonide 0.05% cream b.i.d.

Alternative
- Intralesional steroids: triamcinolone 10 mg/mL
- Pentoxifylline 400 mg b.i.d.

SCLERODERMA/MORPHEA

Key Points

1. Morphea is localized scleroderma confined to skin
2. Systemic scleroderma involves skin and internal organs, especially the esophagus
3. Raynaud's phenomenon is often present in systemic scleroderma
4. Treatment for systemic scleroderma is supportive, not curative

Definition

In scleroderma, an increase in the number and activity of fibroblasts produces excessive collagen, which results in thickening of the dermis (**Fig. 18.9**). Localized scleroderma is confined to the skin and is called *morphea*. It is distinct from systemic scleroderma, which is also called *progressive systemic sclerosus* (PSS). In PSS, fibrosis affects the skin more diffusely, and also affects some internal organs. Scleroderma is classified as an 'autoimmune' collagen vascular disease.

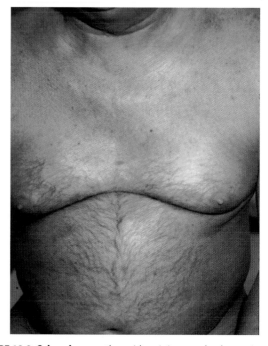

FIGURE 18.9 Scleroderma – the epidermis is normal or hyperpigmented and the dermis is thickened and feels indurated.

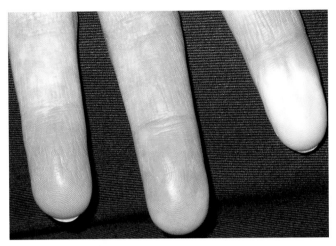

FIGURE 18.10 **Raynaud's phenomenon in a patient with CREST syndrome.** Note characteristic red, white, and blue color changes that occurred with exposure to low temperature.

> Morphea is localized scleroderma, confined to the skin; systemic scleroderma affects skin and viscera.

Incidence

Both forms of scleroderma are uncommon. The annual incidence of PSS has been estimated at fewer than three new patients per 1 million population. About 20% of cases occur in children and teenagers. A linear variant of morphea affects children. Otherwise, morphea and PSS are diseases of adults, with women affected three times more often than men.

History

Morphea is usually asymptomatic; patients present for treatment because of concern over the appearance of the lesions.

Patients with PSS frequently have symptoms. Early in the disease, the most common symptom is Raynaud's phenomenon, which is characterized by pain and color change of the digits on exposure to cold (**Fig. 18.10**). The classic color changes are, in sequence, white, purple, and red, but the most important is white, which is caused by cold-induced vasoconstriction. Patients with more advanced disease also notice tightening of the skin, manifested by an inability to open the mouth widely (their dentist may comment on this) and contractures of fingers causing decreased manual dexterity. Ulcerations of the fingertips also occur frequently. Systemic symptoms include difficulty in swallowing, joint pain, and shortness of breath.

> White is the most diagnostic color in Raynaud's phenomenon.

Physical Examination

Morphea appears as a sclerotic, asymmetrically distributed, sharply demarcated plaque, which may be flat, slightly elevated, or slightly depressed. Most importantly, it *feels* indurated. Early lesions have a lilac border, indicating inflammatory activity, and a whitish center.

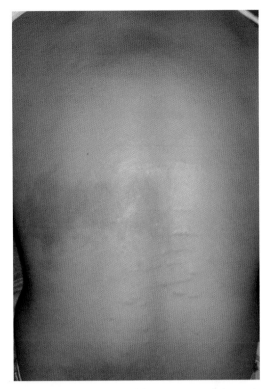

FIGURE 18.11 **Morphea** – indurated, hyperpigmented plaques in mature lesions.

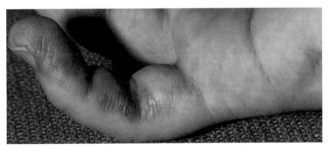

FIGURE 18.12 **Linear morphea** – more common in children.

Mature lesions are hyperpigmented (**Fig. 18.11**). Lesions of morphea most often affect the trunk, except for the linear variant, which usually involves the head or an extremity (**Fig. 18.12**).

The thickened skin in PSS is not sharply separated from normal skin, although some areas, such as the hands and face (acrosclerosus), may be more thickened than others. Thickened facial skin appears unusually smooth, except around the mouth, where it is furrowed and has a purse-string appearance. Involvement of the digits produces thickened, sausage-shaped digits (sclerodactyly; **Fig. 18.13**). Ulcerations followed by pitted scars occur on the fingertips. In generalized involvement, the skin is often hyperpigmented and may have areas that are speckled light and dark ('salt and pepper'). Patients with marked generalized thickening of the skin (see **Fig. 18.9**) appear to have the worst prognosis.

Telangiectasia is prominent in some patients with scleroderma. It appears as multiple, small, punctate macules that are particularly prominent on the face and hands (**Fig. 18.14**). Cutaneous calcinosis and impaired

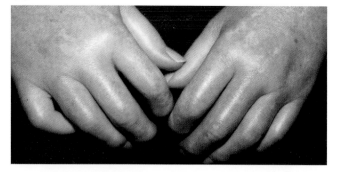

FIGURE 18.13 **Sclerodactyly** in a patient with systemic scleroderma.

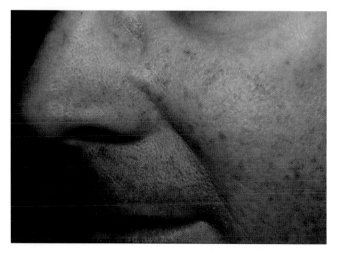

FIGURE 18.14 **Telangiectasias** in a patient with scleroderma.

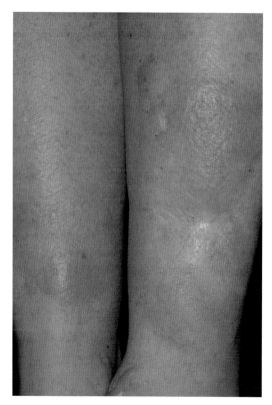

FIGURE 18.15 **Myxedema** – indurated red plaques on shins.

esophageal motility also occur in patients with the CREST syndrome (*c*alcinosis, *R*aynaud's phenomenon, *e*sophageal dysfunction, *s*clerodactyly, and *t*elangiectasia).

Differential Diagnosis

The differential diagnosis of morphea includes two uncommon disorders. *Lichen sclerosus et atrophicus* is an idiopathic disorder that appears as a porcelain-white, dermal, indurated plaque with an atrophic, slightly wrinkled epidermis. It most often affects the vulvar area but sometimes occurs in scattered patches on the trunk. Occasionally, lichen sclerosus et atrophicus and morphea coexist. *Necrobiosis lipoidica diabeticorum* most often (but not always) occurs on the lower legs in diabetic patients as an orange-red, indurated plaque with an atrophic epidermis through which large telangiectatic blood vessels are seen.

The generalized thickened skin in PSS may be confused with several uncommon disorders. In *myxedema* from hypothyroidism, the skin may be markedly thickened, but it feels more doughy than hard (**Fig. 18.15**). *Scleromyxedema* is a rare disease characterized by mucin deposition in the skin. It can mimic scleroderma clinically, but the biopsy is diagnostic, and the skin involvement is accompanied by a serum monoclonal immunoglobulin G (IgG) protein. *Mixed connective tissue disease* is an 'overlap' syndrome with features of several collagen vascular diseases: scleroderma, dermatomyositis, and lupus erythematosus. This syndrome is characterized serologically by high levels of antibodies against ribonuclear

protein in extractable nuclear antigen. In chronic *graft-versus-host disease*, skin manifestations are prominent and may be strikingly similar to those of generalized scleroderma. *Porphyria cutanea tarda* occasionally is accompanied by diffusely thickened, hyperpigmented, 'sclerodermoid' skin. The more usual manifestations, however, are blisters and fragility of the skin on the dorsa of the hands, and hyperpigmentation and hypertrichosis of the upper lateral cheeks. The anticancer drug *bleomycin* can cause sclerodermatous skin changes that are indistinguishable from those of systemic sclerosus. *Nephrogenic fibrosing dermopathy* is a newly described entity seen in patients with renal insufficiency, including those on dialysis, and presents with indurated skin, most commonly affecting the extremities.

Laboratory and Biopsy

Laboratory tests are not needed in patients with morphea, except for a skin biopsy if the diagnosis is in question. Patients with generalized scleroderma require laboratory and radiographic evaluation for systemic involvement that includes a complete blood count, urinalysis, renal function tests, chest radiography, pulmonary function testing, and barium swallow. An antinuclear antibody test is positive in 95% of patients with systemic scleroderma. Human epithelial (HEp-2) cells are used as the substrate for the antinuclear antibody test. The pattern of positive staining on these cells correlates with the type of systemic scleroderma as follows: nucleolar staining is associated with mixed connective tissue disease; anticentromere staining is associated with CREST syndrome; and a pattern of diffuse fine speckles is associated with a positive Scl-70 antibody found in diffuse scleroderma.

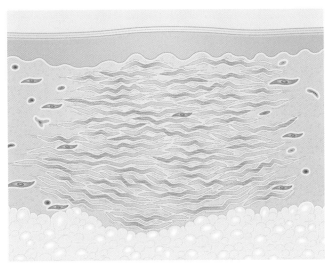

FIGURE 18.16 Scleroderma. Epidermis – normal. Dermis – thickened; fibroblasts are increased in number; collagen bundles are increased in thickness and number.

Laboratory and radiologic tests for systemic scleroderma:
1. Complete blood count
2. Urinalysis
3. Renal function tests
4. Chest radiography
5. Antinuclear antibody test
6. Pulmonary function tests
7. Barium swallow

Morphea and PSS show the same histologic changes in the skin (**Fig. 18.16**) Collagen bundles are increased in number and thickness, and appear more eosinophilic on hematoxylin and eosin staining. These changes are most marked in the lower two-thirds of the dermis and extend into the subcutaneous fat. Inflammation is present in the early stages, when the diagnosis is easily missed histologically because the collagen changes may not be appreciated. In later stages, the sclerotic process entraps, and finally obliterates, the dermal appendages, with an end result that may resemble a scar. In addition, in the late stages blood vessels appear thickened, hyalinized, and decreased in number.

Therapy

Treatment of scleroderma is frustrating. Topical, intralesional, and even systemic steroids have been used for morphea, usually with disappointing results. Topical macrolides and calcipotriene have also been used with limited success. For severe cases, especially cosmetically and physically debilitating linear variants, methotrexate is often used. Long lists of drugs have been used in PSS, most with little or no proven effect. D-penicillamine, which prevents cross-linking of collagen fibers, and immunosuppressive agents such as prednisone and azathioprine or methotrexate, are other systemic therapies. D-penicillamine is the agent of first choice for systemic

scleroderma, but monitoring (e.g., monthly complete blood counts and urinalyses) must be done because of potential resulting toxicity. For patients with sclerodactyly and linear variants of morphea, physical therapy should not be overlooked. Daily range-of-motion exercises are important to help limit the flexion contractures that often develop over time.

Therapy for Scleroderma

Morphea
Initial
- Topical and intralesional steroids (clobetasol 0.05% b.i.d.)
- Topical macrolide (tacrolimus 0.1% b.i.d.)
- Topical calcipotriene with or without steroids

Alternative (for Widespread Disease)
- Systemic steroids
- Methotrexate
- Physical therapy for linear variants

Systemic Sclerosus
Initial
- Penicillamine
- Prednisone

Alternative
- Immunosuppressants
- Physical therapy (for contractures)

Course and complications

Morphea is usually limited to a few plaques, although it may be more widespread. Linear morphea in children may be accompanied by involvement of underlying muscle and even bone, with resulting atrophy of these tissues. Morphea often 'burns out' over time (usually years), with subsequent softening of the affected skin. Residual hypopigmentation or hyperpigmentation is common. Although rare cases of progression to systemic scleroderma have been reported, in most patients morphea is a benign disease.

Systemic scleroderma is frequently progressive, and death from systemic involvement is not uncommon. Reported 5-year survival rates range from 50% to 90%, depending on the type and extent of visceral involvement. Renal failure, often accompanied by severe hypertension, is a frequent cause of death. Cardiac complications include conduction defects, pericarditis, and heart failure. Pulmonary fibrosis is another serious complication. Involvement of the smooth muscle of the lower part of the esophagus produces impaired esophageal motility with reflux, causing strictures. Weight loss and malnutrition can result.

The skin thickening often begins with an early, edematous phase followed by hardening and increasing thickening. Cutaneous complications include ulcerations of fingertips, sometimes complicated by infection with osteomyelitis. Flexion contractures of the hands and fingers can result from sclerosus.

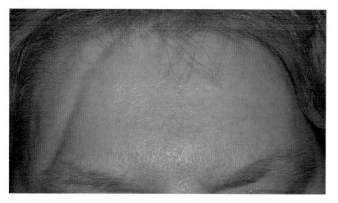

FIGURE 18.17 **En coup de sabre** – indurated linear depression commonly affecting forehead.

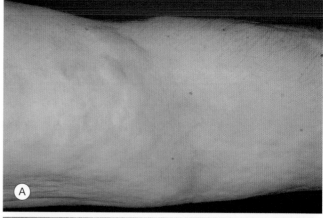

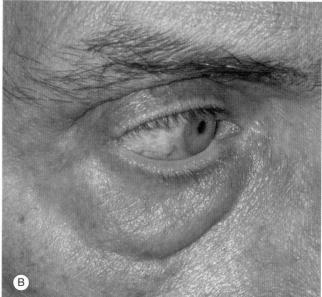

FIGURE 18.18 **Nephrogenic systemic fibrosis. A.** Indurated plaques. **B.** Yellow sclera.

Pathogenesis

Patients with scleroderma have increased numbers of fibroblasts and an increased rate of collagen biosynthesis in the skin. Although the primary causes are unknown, increasing evidence suggests that the process is immunologically mediated. Several European studies have implicated the spirochete *Borrelia burgdorferi* in the pathogenesis of morphea, and have reported success with penicillin treatment in some patients. These results have not been duplicated in the USA. The role, if any, of antinuclear antibodies in the pathogenesis of scleroderma is unknown. They may be a result, rather than a cause, of the disease.

UNCOMMON CAUSES OF DERMAL INDURATION

EN COUP DE SABRE

Paramedian sclerotic depressions of the forehead represent a linear variant of morphea (**Fig. 18.17**) Similar to morphea, purplish borders signal disease activity. It can extend to the eyebrows, nose, or cheek. A severe variant can lead to hemifacial atrophy and is called Parry–Romberg syndrome. High titers of antinuclear antibody are frequently present. Treatment is challenging and methotrexate is often used when cosmetic disfigurement is a concern.

NEPHROGENIC SYSTEMIC FIBROSIS

Nephrogenic systemic fibrosis affects persons with renal impairment who are exposed to magnetic resonance imaging contrast containing gadolinium. Indurated plaques can develop on the trunk and extremities. Diffuse skin thickening and tightening can develop and lead to joint contractures. Yellowing of the sclera is another clinical clue (**Fig. 18.18**). Treatment remains a challenge.

Ulcers 19

Key Points

1. Ulcers have many causes
2. Good wound care promotes healing
3. Cure requires resolution of the underlying etiology

History:
1. Onset
2. Symptoms
3. Neoplasm
4. Family history
5. Social history
6. Travel
7. Medications

ABSTRACT

Ulcers have multiple causes, including vascular diseases, neoplasms, hematologic disorders, drug-induced, connective tissue diseases, neurologic disorders, infections, physical etiologies, and idiopathic. The history and physical may point to the cause. However, laboratory testing is frequently necessary to confirm the diagnosis. Treatment is focused on removing the underlying cause of the ulcer along with good wound care that promotes healing.

Definition

An ulcer is an open sore that results from loss of the epidermis and part or all of the dermis (**Fig. 19.1**). Ulcers have numerous causes (**Table 19.1**). A detailed history and physical examination are often sufficient to establish a diagnosis; however, laboratory tests may be necessary to confirm the initial clinical impression.

Incidence

An ulcer is the chief complaint in 0.5% of the authors' new patients. The frequency of different types of ulcer depends in part on the circumstances of the patient population. For example, decubitus ulcers are a common problem in bedridden patients, whereas leprosy might be considered in a patient from a tropical environment.

History

The history begins with the mode of onset. Is the ulcer acute or chronic? The sudden appearance of severe pain in an extremity suggests *arterial occlusion* due to an embolus or thrombus. The gradual onset of pain with exertion relieved by rest is characteristic of intermittent claudication due to *arteriosclerosis*. A history of lower leg heaviness, aching, and swelling, particularly after periods of inactive standing or sitting, is typical of *venous stasis*.

Patients with *neoplastic* ulcers often have a history of a growth that preceded the ulceration. A family history is important in the diagnosis of ulcers caused by *hemoglobinopathies* such as thalassemia and sickle cell anemia.

Factitial ulcers are suspected in patients with a history of emotional disorders and overly dramatic and reactive behavior or indifference. If an ulcer is painless, a *neurotrophic* ulcer should be suspected.

Various *infectious agents* cause ulceration. Acute onset after wildlife exposure in a patient with fever, chills, and malaise suggests a diagnosis of tularemia, plague, or anthrax. Travel history is particularly important in considering tropical diseases such as amebiasis or leishmaniasis. Sexual history is important if a venereal cause is suspected.

The *drug* history should not be overlooked. Medications alone, however, are a rare cause of ulcer. More often, ulcers are secondary to drug-induced epidermal necrolysis or vasculitis. Allopurinol, barbiturates, anticonvulsants, and antibiotics may cause these eruptions. The cause of a *physical* ulcer usually is not a diagnostic problem because it is readily apparent to the patient.

Physical Examination

The physical examination should include characteristics of the ulcer (e.g., size, shape, color), its location (e.g., leg, genitals, buttock), and associated physical findings (e.g., surrounding skin, pulses, neurologic findings). Changes in skin color, skin temperature, and pulse pattern suggest *arteriosclerotic* peripheral vascular disease. The skin is purplish red with dependency, but changes to pallor when the extremity is elevated. In chronic severe ischemia, the skin and muscles become atrophic in association with hair loss and brittle, opaque nails. The skin is cool, and **235**

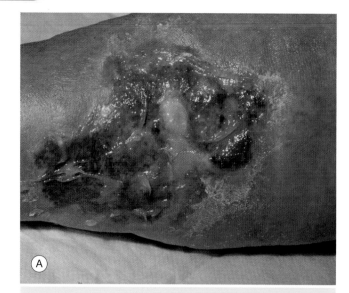

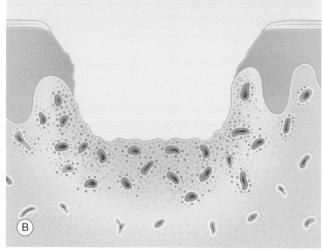

FIGURE 19.1 **Stasis ulcer. A.** Irregularly shaped ulcer surrounded by an erythematous, sclerotic plaque. **B.** Epidermis – absent. Dermis – chronic inflammation, dilated capillaries.

TABLE 19.1 Etiology of ulcers

Vascular	Neurologic
Venous stasis Arteriosclerosis Thromboangiitis obliterans Vasculitis Embolic – tumor, infections (SBE) Hypertension Calciphylaxis	Neuropathic – diabetes, syringomyelia, tabes dorsalis, leprosy, trigeminal trophic syndrome Factitial
Neoplastic	**Infectious**
Carcinoma – cutaneous or metastatic Lymphoma – mycosis fungoides Sarcoma – Kaposi's sarcoma	Bacteria – atypical mycobacteria, tuberculosis, diphtheria, anthrax, tularemia, chancroid, granuloma inguinale, syphilis Fungi – blastomycosis, histoplasmosis, chromomycosis, sporotrichosis, cryptococcosis, coccidioidomycosis, aspergillosis Protozoa – leishmaniasis, amebiasis Virus – herpes
Hematologic	
Hemoglobinopathy – sickle cell anemia, spherocytosis, thalassemia Dysglobulinemia – cryoglobulinemia, macroglobulinemia	
Drug-related	**Physical**
Methotrexate Bleomycin Ergot Coumarin Heparin Iodine Bromine	Chrome Coral Beryllium Radiation Trauma Cold Heat Pressure (decubitus) Bites (brown recluse spider)
Connective tissue disease	**Unknown**
Rheumatoid arthritis Lupus erythematosus Scleroderma Dermatomyositis	Pyoderma gangrenosum Necrobiosis lipoidica

SBE, subacute bacterial endocarditis.

peripheral pulses are lost. Patients with ischemic leg or ankle ulcers may also have ulceration of the toes.

Physical examination:
1. Size, shape, and color of ulcer
2. Location
3. Associated physical findings

Lower leg edema, brawny induration, brownish discoloration, petechiae, and dermatitis are typical of *venous insufficiency*. Stasis ulcers (**Fig. 19.1**) rarely occur below the level of the malleolus. Varicose veins may or may not be prominent.

Multiple small ulcers (0.5–2 cm) occurring predominantly on the lower legs suggest *vasculitis* (**Fig. 19.2**). The ulcer borders are usually purpuric, hemorrhagic, and necrotic. Crusted purpuric papules and nodules also occur.

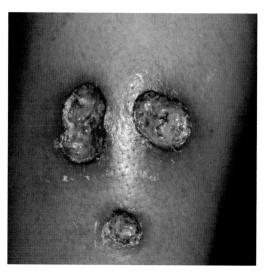

FIGURE 19.2 **Vasculitis** – multiple, punched out ulcers on the leg of a patient with rheumatoid arthritis.

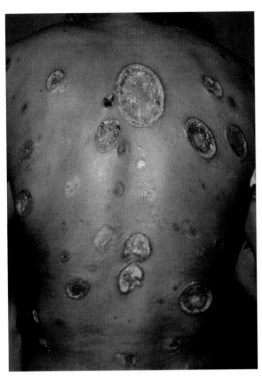

FIGURE 19.3 **Mycosis fungoides** – ulcerated plaques and tumors on the back.

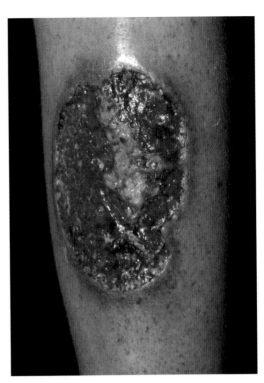

FIGURE 19.5 **Pyoderma gangrenosum** – leg ulcer in a patient with inflammatory bowel disease.

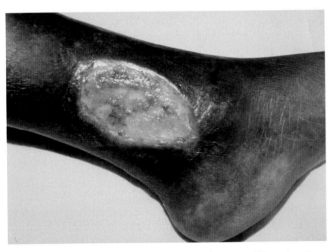

FIGURE 19.4 **Sickle cell anemia** – lower leg ulcer in an African-American patient.

The development of individual or multiple cutaneous nodules that become ulcerated is characteristic of an underlying *neoplasm* (**Fig. 19.3**). However, a preceding nodule is not always present in a malignant ulcer. Ulceration of the lower third of the leg above the ankle in an African-American adult patient is a major manifestation of homozygous *sickle cell disease* (**Fig. 19.4**).

Areas of pressure and trauma, particularly on an insensate foot, are susceptible to the development of a *neuropathic ulcer* (mal perforans), which occurs mainly in patients with diabetes or leprosy. The ulcer frequently has significant softened, macerated callus.

Geometric, bizarrely shaped, angular ulcers are characteristic of a self-inflicted *factitial* cause. Genital ulceration is highly suggestive of a venereal cause, which may be *herpes simplex*, *syphilis*, *chancroid*, or *granuloma inguinale*.

The most common physical ulcer (3% of hospitalized patients) is the *pressure sore* or *decubitus ulcer*. Shearing forces, friction, moisture, and pressure contribute to the development of these ulcers. Bedridden or wheelchair-bound patients unable to ambulate are most at risk. These patients are usually elderly and frequently incontinent. The most common sites are the sacral and coccygeal areas, ischial tuberosities, and greater trochanter. These ulcers begin as irregular, ill-defined, reddish, indurated areas that resemble abrasions. A full-thickness skin defect develops with extension into the subcutaneous tissue and ultimate penetration into the deep fascia and muscle.

A rapidly developing, painful ulcer with an undermined edge and gangrenous border is characteristic of *pyoderma gangrenosum* (**Fig. 19.5**). These ulcers usually occur on the lower legs. Pyoderma gangrenosum is frequently associated with ulcerative and granulomatous colitis, rheumatoid arthritis, and myeloproliferative diseases.

Laboratory and Biopsy

Laboratory tests are necessary to confirm the origin of some ulcers after the history and physical examination. Several *vascular studies* can be used to assess for peripheral vascular disease. Indirect and direct non-invasive testing is used initially to determine arterial competence. The ankle:brachial index is the best screening test to rule out peripheral arterial disease. When limb salvage is indicated, selective arteriography and/or arterial duplex ultrasonography can locate and define the extent of arterial obstruction. Photoplethysmography is performed in patients to delineate venous and arterial pathologic and physiologic abnormalities. In addition, photoplethysmography can be used to determine cutaneous blood perfusion at ulcer margins and thus help to predict the potential for healing. Venous duplex scanning is used to rule out venous insufficiency, deep vein thrombosis, and superficial thrombophlebitis.

Laboratory tests:
1. Vascular studies
2. Blood tests
3. Cultures
4. Biopsy

Several *blood tests* can be helpful in the workup of ulcers. Connective tissue diseases are diagnosed clinically with supportive serologic tests, including tests for antinuclear antibody, rheumatoid factor, anti-DNA antibody, antiphospholipid antibodies, and lupus anticoagulant. Patients with suspected hematologic disorders can be diagnosed with the appropriate tests for sickle cell anemia, spherocytosis, thalassemia, and dysglobulinemias.

Cultures are necessary for diagnosing tropical or unusual infections. Routine cultures of chronic ulcers generally grow out of a mixture of organisms. However, antibiotic therapy for secondarily infected ulcers without treatment of the underlying cause does not result in healing. Diagnostic radiography is indicated when underlying osteomyelitis is a potential complication.

A *biopsy* is indicated for all chronic ulcers of unknown origin, and is particularly helpful in ruling out neoplasms. Vascular causes of ulcers, including venous stasis and vasculitis, have characteristic histologic changes. Infectious ulcers are diagnosed by skin biopsy, with special stains used to demonstrate the causative organism. In addition, a portion of the biopsy specimen is sent to the microbiology laboratory for culture (**Fig. 19.6**).

Biopsy chronic ulcers of unknown origin, to rule out cancer.

Therapy

Appropriate treatment depends on correctly identifying and removing the cause. Venous or arterial insufficiency is the most common cause of ulceration in the ambulatory patient, and correcting the underlying vascular abnormality, if possible, is paramount. For example, *stasis ulcers* are unlikely to heal in a patient with persistent edema caused by incompetent veins. External compression of venous diseased legs is the most effective therapy. Initially, stasis ulcers and edema are treated with a compressive boot that is changed weekly. After healing, knee-high, medium-pressure elastic compression stockings are used to prevent recurrent stasis ulcers.

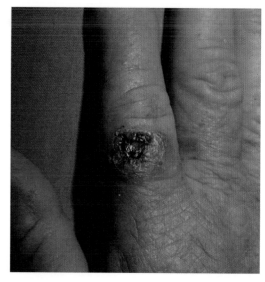

FIGURE 19.6 Sporotrichosis – finger ulcer developed after traumatic injury while gardening.

Surgery, chemotherapy, and radiotherapy are used to treat *neoplastic ulcers*. The most important treatment of *neuropathic* ulcers and *pressure sores* is prevention of pressure, friction, and trauma. Pressure is relieved with mechanical devices, such as orthotic shoes for a diabetic patient with a foot ulcer. *Infection* requires appropriate antibiotic therapy. Removal of the offending *drug* is the obvious remedy for ulcers caused by drugs.

The general management of ulcers includes measures that promote wound healing, such as medical or surgical debridement, occlusive dressings, treatment of infection, and good nutrition. Numerous agents are used to remove devitalized and purulent tissue from wounds, including moist to dry dressings with normal saline.

Occlusive dressings made from various polymers (e.g., polyethylene, polyurethane) have made a significant contribution to ulcer therapy. These dressings keep the ulcer moist, a feature that promotes epidermal repair through migration of epithelial cells over the ulcer. Initially, large amounts of exudate form under the occlusive dressing, which remove crust and necrotic debris through a process of autolytic digestion. The dressing must be changed every 2–3 days because of exudate build-up, but with healing the dressing may be changed less frequently (i.e., every 5–7 days). Another characteristic of occlusive dressings is significant pain relief.

The use of oral and topical antibiotics is often ineffective because of the development of resistant bacteria. Antibiotics should be reserved for ulcers that are complicated by cellulitis, lymphangitis, or septicemia.

Surgical intervention (bypass graft or thromboendarterectomy) is required in patients with peripheral vascular disease. In venous ulcers that have failed to respond to more conservative therapy, skin grafting is often necessary.

Complications such as cellulitis, lymphangitis, septicemia, and osteomyelitis may complicate healing and prolong the duration of the ulcer.

Complications:
1. Cellulitis
2. Lymphangitis
3. Septicemia
4. Osteomyelitis

Pathogenesis

Infectious agents, toxic chemicals, physical injury, and loss of nutrition from interruption of the cutaneous vasculature cause cell death, tissue loss, and ulceration. As long as cell death continues, the ulcer will persist.

Ulcer healing is a complex biologic process that requires an intact vascular supply, inflammation, and proliferation of fibroblasts, endothelial cells, and keratinocytes. Dermal integrity depends on the synthesis of collagen, elastin, and proteoglycans (ground substance) by fibroblasts. Epidermal repair requires the proliferation and migration of keratinocytes over a fibrin-fibronectin support matrix. Inflammation always accompanies the wound healing process, in which the macrophage is the essential and most important cell. Various growth factors (e.g., epidermal, platelet-derived, fibroblast, and transforming growth factor-β) appear to have a role in wound healing by enhancing re-epithelialization and granulation tissue.

Therapy for Ulcers

Initial

Correct or Treat the Underlying Cause
- Venous insufficiency – compression boot or stocking
- Arterial insufficiency – surgery
- Neoplasm – surgery, chemotherapy, radiotherapy
- Infection – antibiotics
- Neuropathic or decubitus ulcer – remove pressure
- Vasculitis or pyoderma gangrenosum – prednisone, dapsone, immunosuppressants, biologics, treatment of associated disease

Promote Wound Healing
- Cleanse and/or debridement – surgical, enzymes
- Dressings – non-adherent, occlusive, or moist to dry

Alternative
- Secondary infection control – antibiotics
- Skin grafting

Course and Complications

The healing rate of ulcers is related directly to successful treatment of the cause and aggravating factors, as well as prevention of complications. For example, a venous stasis ulcer may persist for years if it is treated inadequately. Removal of aggravating factors such as secondary infection and necrotic debris promotes ulcer healing.

Hair Disorders **20**

Key Points

1. Diagnosis requires a detailed history
2. Diagnose pattern as patchy or diffuse
3. Determine whether hair loss is scarring or non-scarring

ABSTRACT

The evaluation of a patient with hair loss requires a detailed history, physical examination, and, in some cases, laboratory tests and biopsy (**Table 20.1**). Important elements of the history include the time of onset, medications taken, recent emotional or physical stress, diet, grooming techniques, and family history of baldness or hair disorders.

The physical examination is helpful in making an accurate diagnosis by observing the pattern (patchy or diffuse) of hair loss and whether scarring is present as evidenced by loss of follicular openings. Patchy hair loss is readily apparent. However, diffuse hair loss may not be noticeable until the patient has more than 50% hair loss. The presence or absence of scarring is important diagnostically and prognostically. In non-scarring alopecia, the diagnosis is usually made without biopsy. In scarring alopecia, a biopsy is useful in establishing a prognosis and diagnosis and should be performed. Non-scarring alopecia may be a temporary phenomenon, whereas scarring indicates permanent hair loss. Except for discoid lupus, the main disorders discussed in this chapter are non-scarring.

> Observe the pattern of hair loss and whether scarring is present.

ALOPECIA AREATA

Key Points

1. Autoimmune disorder
2. Acute onset of well circumscribed, oval patches of non-scarring alopecia
3. No cure

Definition

Alopecia areata is an idiopathic disorder characterized by well circumscribed, round or oval patches of non-scarring hair loss (**Fig. 20.1**).

Incidence

Alopecia areata affects both sexes equally, with onset occurring most often in early adulthood. Almost 1% of the authors' new patients had this diagnosis. The incidence in Olmsted County, Minnesota was 20.2 per 100 000 person-years. Alopecia areata occurs in 1.7% of Americans by the age of 50 years.

History

Alopecia areata has an acute onset. It is sometimes associated with emotional stress, but in most patients the emotional stress seems to be caused by the hair loss. Approximately 25% of patients have other autoimmune disorders, such as type I diabetes mellitus, thyroid disease, and vitiligo. Atopic dermatitis is especially common in alopecia areata. Patients are generally healthy otherwise. Some 20–25% of patients have a family history of alopecia areata.

241

TABLE 20.1 Alopecia

	Incidence (%)[a]	History	Physical Examination	Scarring	Pattern	Differential Diagnosis	Laboratory Test (Biopsy)
Alopecia areata	0.9	Acute onset	Exclamation point hairs	Absent	Circular patches	Trichotillomania Secondary syphilis Fungal infection	None
Discoid lupus erythematosus	<0.1	Photosensitivity Other symptoms of lupus	Erythema Follicular plugs	Present	Patchy	Fungal infection Lichen planus Neoplasm	Biopsy
Androgenetic	0.6	Family history of baldness	Normal scalp	Absent	Male pattern	Androgen excess in women	None
Telogen effluvium	1.0	Physical or emotional stress 2–3 months previously	Positive hair pull >25% telogen hair	Absent	Diffuse	Diffuse Thyroid dysfunction Drug induced Nutritional deficiency	None
Trichotillomania	0.1	Emotional problems	Broken hair	Absent	Patchy	Alopecia areata Fungal infection	None
Fungal	0.1	Schoolmates with hair loss	Scaling, erythema, pustules	Absent	Patchy	Seborrheic dermatitis Alopecia areata Bacterial infection Trichotillomania	KOH preparation, culture

[a]Percentage of new dermatology patients with this diagnosis seen at the Hershey Medical Center Dermatology Clinic, Hershey, PA.
KOH, potassium hydroxide.

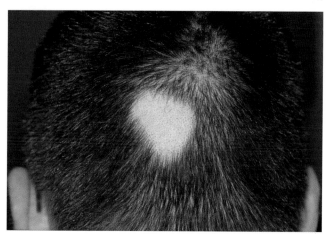

FIGURE 20.1 **Alopecia areata** – characteristic round patch of non-scarring alopecia.

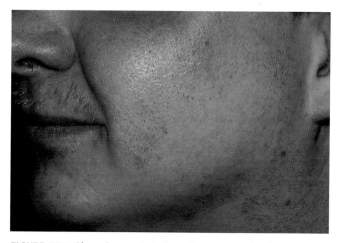

FIGURE 20.2 **Alopecia areata in beard area** – patch of non-scarring alopecia extending from chin to cheek.

Physical Examination

The disorder is characterized by well circumscribed, round or oval patches of hair loss, leaving a smooth, normal-appearing scalp. Erythema and slight tenderness may be present early in the course. Subsequently, the scalp may become slightly depressed. Characteristically, the periphery of the patches of hair loss is studded with *exclamation point hairs*, which are so named because of their resemblance to a punctuation mark. These fractured hairs are 2–3 mm long and tapered at the base.

Alopecia areata is characterized by non-scarring circular patches of alopecia with exclamation point hairs.

Alopecia areata most often affects the scalp, frequently with several 2–3-cm patches of hair loss. The eyebrows, eyelashes, and beard may also be affected, as may hair elsewhere on the body (**Fig. 20.2**). Approximately 1–2% of patients develop loss of all scalp hair (*alopecia totalis*) or loss of all body hair (*alopecia universalis*) (**Fig. 20.3**). Fine stippling and pitting of the nails are infrequent associated findings.

Differential Diagnosis

Other non-scarring forms of alopecia need to be considered in the differential diagnosis. *Secondary syphilis* can be ruled out by appropriate serologic examination. *Trichotillomania* and *fungal infection* should also be considered. Ill-marginated, irregular patches of alopecia containing

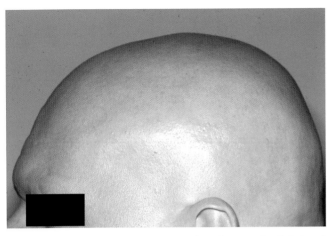

FIGURE 20.3 Alopecia universalis – complete absence of scalp hair and eyebrows and eyelashes.

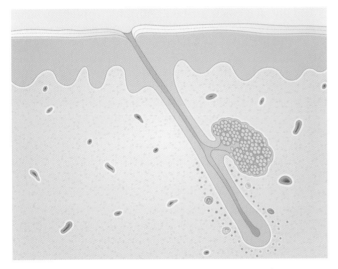

FIGURE 20.4 Dystrophic follicle without a hair shaft. Dermis – lymphocytes surrounding the hair bulb.

the stubble of broken hairs are typical of trichotillomania. If doubt exists, a biopsy helps to differentiate trichotillomania from alopecia areata. A potassium hydroxide (KOH) preparation and culture, and clinical evidence of redness and scale, enable the diagnosis of a fungal infection.

Laboratory and Biopsy

Histopathologic examination of alopecia areata reveals the presence of small, dystrophic hair structures. A lymphocytic infiltrate surrounds the early anagen hair bulbs like a 'swarm of bees' (**Fig. 20.4**).

Therapy

The treatment of alopecia areata depends on the extent of involvement and the patient's emotional need for regrowth of hair. There is no cure for alopecia areata. In localized disease, topical potent steroids such as clobetasol (Temovate) gel or intralesional injections of triamcinolone (Kenalog-10) are sometimes effective. In widespread disease, systemic steroids are sometimes used, but their hazards must be considered before starting treatment. Prompt hair loss after discontinuation of

oral steroids is discouraging. Other modes of therapy include immunotherapy by induction of allergic contact dermatitis (aka contact sensitization), phototherapy, topical minoxidil, and oral cyclosporine. Patients with alopecia areata need psychologic support, and all patients should visit the National Alopecia Areata Foundation's website (http://www.naaf.org) or Children's Alopecia Project (www.childrensalopeciaproject.org). A wig is recommended when the hair loss is extensive.

Therapy for Alopecia Areata

Initial
- Steroids
  - Topical – clobetasol b.i.d.
  - Intralesional – triamcinolone 5 mg/mL every 4–6 weeks
- Topical minoxidil

Alternative
- Contact sensitization
- Systemic – prednisone (short course only)

Course and Complications

Alopecia areata has a variable, unpredictable course. Most patients with localized disease have spontaneous recovery. However, relapses are not uncommon. Duration of more than 1 year and extensive hair loss are poor prognostic signs. Spontaneous regrowth of hair in alopecia totalis (scalp) and alopecia universalis (total body) may occur but is uncommon; fewer than 5% of patients show any tendency toward hair regrowth.

Poor prognosis:
1. Long duration
2. Large areas of alopecia

Pathogenesis

The pathogenesis of alopecia areata remains poorly understood, although an immunologic process is favored. Recent research shows the common initiation of the autoimmune response in alopecia areata, celiac disease, rheumatoid arthritis, and diabetes. A lymphocytic inflammatory infiltrate surrounds the affected bulbs and presumably has a role in the disease. In response to this autoimmune process, the hair matrices become arrested, but retain the capacity for normal hair regrowth after months or years.

LUPUS ERYTHEMATOSUS

Key Points

1. Alopecia can be scarring or non-scarring
2. Biopsy confirms diagnosis
3. Treat aggressively to prevent permanent hair loss

Definition

Lupus erythematosus is an autoimmune disorder that often affects the scalp and causes alopecia. The loss of hair may be diffuse and non-scarring (systemic lupus erythematosus, SLE) or patchy and scarring (discoid lupus erythematosus, DLE). A general discussion of lupus erythematosus is found in Chapters 9 and 14.

Physical Examination

Diffuse non-scarring alopecia of the scalp in the form of a telogen effluvium accompanies the acute phases of SLE in more than 20% of patients. In addition, short, broken hairs ('lupus hair') may be present, particularly in the frontal margin.

- SLE – non-scarring
- DLE – scarring

DLE is characterized by oval, scarring areas of alopecia. A typical plaque has an active erythematous margin and a white, atrophic, inactive center (**Fig. 20.5**). Within the plaques, telangiectasia and dilated keratin-filled follicles are present. Similar discoid lesions may be found on the ears, face, trunk, and extremities.

Differential Diagnosis

For the non-scarring alopecia caused by SLE, other causes of telogen effluvium, such as hypothyroidism, may be considered. However, in most patients with SLE, other manifestations of the disease are almost always evident.

Scarring alopecia caused by DLE must be differentiated from alopecia caused by *lichen planopilaris*, a form of lichen planus, *fungal infection*, or *neoplasm*. A biopsy helps to differentiate DLE from lichen planus and neoplasm. A KOH preparation and culture enable the diagnosis of a fungal infection.

Laboratory and Biopsy

A biopsy of the scalp for routine histologic examination is usually diagnostic of DLE. Atrophic epidermis, keratotic plugging of the follicles, hydropic degeneration of the basal cells, and patchy perivascular and perifollicular lymphocytic infiltrate are characteristic (**Fig. 20.6**). The lupus band test (direct immunofluorescence) is positive, but is usually not necessary to make the diagnosis. Appropriate laboratory tests, starting with a complete blood count, platelet count, antinuclear antibody test, renal profile, and urinalysis, should be ordered to rule out SLE.

Therapy

The goal of treatment in DLE is to prevent the follicular destruction that results in permanent alopecia. In many cases, the process can be arrested by the use of a potent topical (clobetasol, Temovate gel) or intralesional corticosteroids (triamcinolone, Kenalog-10). Topical macrolides can also be tried. When this therapy fails, the addition of an antimalarial agent (hydroxychloroquine, Plaquenil) or immunosuppressant (e.g. mycophenolate mofetil) is indicated.

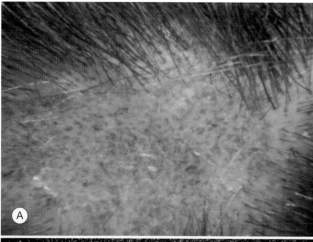
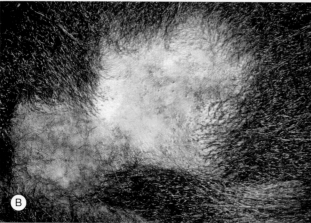

FIGURE 20.5 **Discoid lupus erythematosus. A.** Early lesion showing erythema and scarring. **B.** Late lesion showing hyperpigmentation and hypopigmentation within scarring alopecia in dark skin.

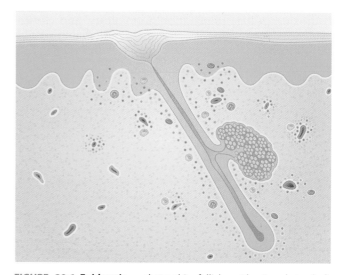

FIGURE 20.6 **Epidermis** – dystrophic follicle without a hair shaft; hyperkeratosis. Dermis – lymphocytic infiltrate at the dermal–epidermal junction and around hair follicles and blood vessels.

Course and Complications

Chronic scarring DLE causes permanent alopecia, whereas the diffuse alopecia associated with SLE is temporary and improves when the condition improves.

Pathogenesis

The pathogenesis of lupus erythematosus is discussed in Chapters 9 and 14.

MALE AND FEMALE PATTERN HAIR LOSS (ANDROGENETIC ALOPECIA)

Key Points

1. Non-scarring hair loss occurs in a patterned distribution
2. Occurs most often in genetically predisposed men and women
3. In males, dihydrotestosterone causes hair miniaturization

Definition

Male and female pattern hair loss (MPHL and FPHL, respectively) represents post-pubertal replacement of terminal hairs by miniaturized hairs and eventually completely atrophic follicles (**Fig. 20.7**). It occurs in individuals, both male and female, who are genetically predisposed. Clinically, the disorder is non-scarring and involves the vertex and frontotemporal regions of the scalp.

Incidence

The prevalence of common baldness varies with the population studied. Among male Caucasians, it approximates 100%, but age at onset is highly variable. In Native American, Japanese, and Chinese populations, baldness is less common. Patterned hair thinning occurs in approximately 50% of women aged over 40 years.

History

The process begins at any age after puberty, but temporal recession is often noticed between the ages of 20 and 30 years. The onset and progression are gradual. Women often report see-through hair where scalp skin is noticed. The patient usually has a family history of baldness.

Physical Examination

In areas of baldness, the coarse, dark terminal hairs are replaced by finer, miniaturized (e.g., vellus-like) hairs, which then become atrophic, leaving a smooth, shiny scalp with barely visible follicular orifices (**Fig. 20.8**). The number of hair follicles remains unchanged. Baldness characteristically occurs in a distinctive pattern that spares the posterior and lateral margins of the scalp. In men, the process begins with bitemporal recession, followed by balding of the vertex. In women, FPHL most often is manifest by diffuse thinning over the top of the scalp

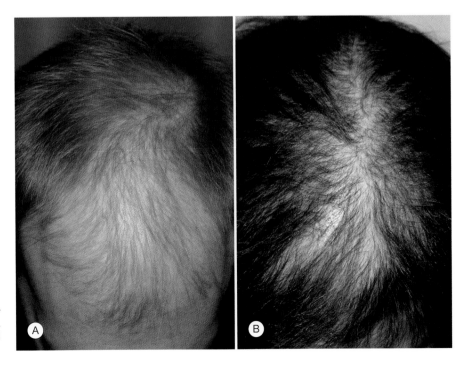

FIGURE 20.7 **Male and female pattern hair loss. A.** Frontal and vertex alopecia in a male. **B.** Diffuse thinning on crown with intact frontal hairline in a woman.

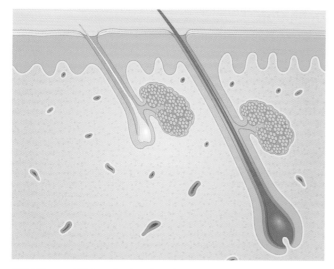

FIGURE 20.8 **Miniaturized** (vellus-like) hair (left) is found in areas of baldness. **Terminal** hair (right) is shown for comparison.

(e.g., the crown) and by an intact frontal hairline. The earliest sign in women is a gradual widening of the part width on the crown of the scalp when compared with the back of the scalp. Women experience thinning of hair, not baldness. In areas of baldness, the scalp appears completely normal, with no evidence of scarring or inflammation.

> Miniaturized hairs replace thicker terminal hairs in androgenetic alopecia.

Differential Diagnosis

In men, the diagnosis is usually straightforward. In women, the diagnosis of FPHL may be more difficult. In most women, it is simply an inherited trait. *Hormonal abnormality* should be considered in women with baldness, particularly when accompanied by acne or hirsutism. They should be asked about menstrual irregularities and infertility. In some women, hypothyroidism may also be present.

Laboratory and Biopsy

Ordinarily, no laboratory examination or biopsy is done. Biopsy would show increased numbers of miniaturized hairs. Androgen excess in women can be screened for with measurements of serum-free and total testosterone and dehydroepiandrosterone sulfate.

Therapy

Minoxidil, 2% solution (Rogaine) and 5% solution/foam (Rogaine Extra Strength for Men) applied twice daily, is a moderately effective treatment for men and women with androgenetic alopecia. It stops or reduces the rate of hair loss and reverses the process of hair miniaturization by prolonging anagen or growth phase of hair follicles. After 1 year of treatment, 20–40% of men achieve moderate to dense regrowth of terminal hairs with the 2% solution and some increased effectiveness with the 5% solution. Up to 60% of women experience hair regrowth with the 2% solution after 8 months of treatment. This new hair growth is not permanent. Cessation of treatment results in loss of hair within a few months. Even with continued therapy, hair regrowth plateaus after 1 year and slowly declines over subsequent years. Despite Food and Drug Administration approval for treating vertex thinning, minoxidil solution also works on the frontal scalp in both men and women, but not on bitemporal recession seen in men. For women, off-label treatment includes treatment with 5% topical minoxidil foam once nightly.

Finasteride, 1 mg (Propecia), a type II 5a-reductase inhibitor, is given once daily. Five-year data show that 90% of men maintain their present hair and two-thirds of men experience some degree of hair regrowth. Finasteride is contraindicated in women of child-bearing potential because of its teratogenic effects on male offspring.

Extensive areas of baldness can be covered with a hair-piece or wig. For selected patients, surgical treatment with hair transplantation is successful.

> **Therapy for Male and Female Pattern Hair Loss**
>
> **Initial**
> - Minoxidil 2% or 5% solution/foam b.i.d.
> - Finasteride 1 mg daily (males only)
>
> **Alternative**
> - Surgery – hair transplant
> - Wig

Course and Complications

The balding process is usually gradual and most evident between the ages of 30 and 50 years. Thereafter, it is much slower, although hair thinning continues into later life.

Pathogenesis

The development of common baldness is genetically predetermined and androgen dependent. Castration of males before puberty prevents the development of baldness. However, when testosterone is administered, a predisposed eunuch becomes bald. It seems contradictory that androgens cause scalp baldness but stimulate hair growth on the chest, face, and genital regions. This phenomenon may be explained by regional differences in androgen metabolism. Hair follicles in bald areas of the scalp have increased levels and activity of 5a-reductase, which causes increased levels of dihydrotestosterone that shortens the hair cycle and miniaturizes scalp follicles.

> Common baldness is androgen-dependent in males.

TELOGEN EFFLUVIUM (STRESS-INDUCED ALOPECIA)

Key Points

1. Identify trigger for increased shedding of telogen hairs
2. Triggering event occurs 3–6 months before onset of hair shedding
3. Gentle hair pull is positive for telogen hairs

Definition

Marked emotionally or physiologically stressful events may result in an alteration of the normal hair cycle and diffuse hair loss. The scalp is made up of a mosaic of anagen (growing) and telogen (resting) hairs. Telogen effluvium is characterized by excessive and early entry of hairs into the telogen phase. Causes of telogen effluvium include high fever, childbirth, chronic illness, major surgery, anemia, severe emotional disorders, crash diets, hypothyroidism, and drugs, such as birth control pills (starting, stopping, or changing).

> Telogen effluvium occurs most often postpartum.

Incidence

The incidence of telogen effluvium is probably greater than that seen by the dermatologist because most episodes are transient and minor.

History

Hair loss occurs 2–4 months after the physical or mental stress. Most patients are women who have diffuse hair thinning postpartum. They are concerned about going bald and characterize their hair loss as coming out by 'handfuls' after combing and shampooing. If the patient has not recently given birth, a history of other physical or emotional stress, dietary habits, and medications should be sought.

Physical Examination

The patient has diffuse thinning of the hair that at first is not readily apparent to the examiner (**Fig. 20.9**). The scalp is normal, with no scarring or erythema. The part width on the crown is equal in coverage compared to the back of the scalp. The remainder of the skin examination, including hair elsewhere on the body, nails, and teeth, is normal. Gentle pulling of the hair (hair-pull test) verifies excessive hair shedding. The hair pull is done by grasping a small lock of hair and applying gentle traction from the base to tip of the lock of hair. Normally, fewer than three hairs are pulled out with this maneuver. Pulling out more than three hairs consistently from different scalp areas confirms that excessive shedding is present (**Fig. 20.10**).

> The excessive loss of telogen hairs is characteristic and manifest by a positive hair-pull test.

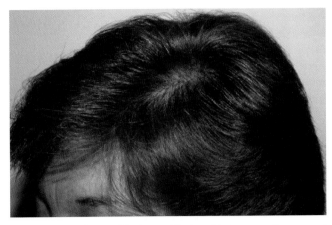

FIGURE 20.9 Telogen effluvium – thinning of hair not readily apparent to a casual observer.

In stress-induced alopecia, the number of telogen hairs is increased from a normal percentage of 10–20% to more than 25%. This results in as many as 400–500 lost hairs daily. Normally, fewer than 100 hairs are lost daily.

Differential Diagnosis

The challenge is to search for a cause of the telogen effluvium. *Abnormal thyroid function*, particularly hypothyroidism, produces hair that is dry and sparse diffusely, often with loss of the lateral third of each eyebrow. *Nutritional deficiencies* (e.g., lack of an essential fatty acid, biotin, or zinc), rarely seen in practice, also cause a telogen effluvium. *Toxic drugs*, particularly alkylating agents, cause loss of hair in the anagen phase and this is called an anagen effluvium.

Laboratory and Biopsy

The history and clinical examination are usually diagnostic. Minimum laboratory tests include complete blood count, thyroid stimulating hormone, and iron studies, including ferritin to assess for total body iron storage. Biopsy is rarely performed but would show an increased percentage (>25%) of telogen hairs in a 4-mm punch biopsy submitted for horizontal sectioning.

Therapy

In most patients, the stressful event has passed, and reassurance that the patient will not go bald is all that is required.

Therapy for Telogen Effluvium

Initial
- Reassurance

Course and Complications

This condition is usually a self-limiting, reversible problem that resolves within 2–6 months. It may be prolonged for years if the underlying stress continues.

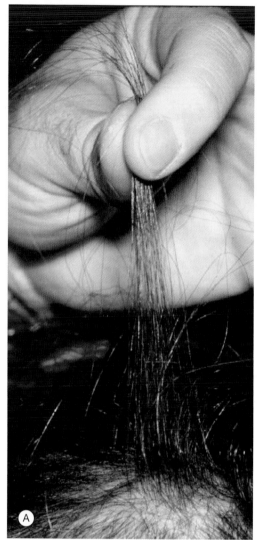

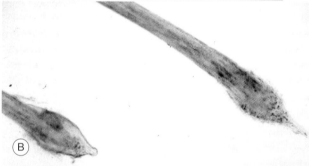

FIGURE 20.10 A. Demonstration of gentle hair-pull test. **B.** Microscopic examination shows telogen or club hairs.

A chronic telogen effluvium lasting for up to 5 years has been described to occur, particularly in middle-aged women, without a recognizable initiating factor.

Pathogenesis

The normal hair cycle is disturbed in telogen effluvium. Growing anagen hairs are prematurely converted to resting telogen hairs, which are subsequently shed. The mechanism for this alteration of the normal hair cycle is unknown.

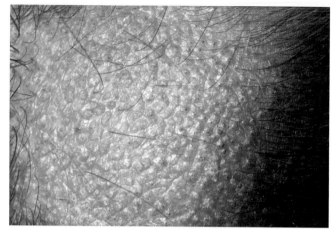

FIGURE 20.11 Tinea capitis – non-scarring patch of alopecia with black dots (broken hairs), erythema, and scale.

TINEA CAPITIS

Key Points

1. Superficial fungal infection (*Trichophyton tonsurans*) of scalp, most common in children
2. Diagnosis confirmed by KOH and fungal culture
3. Treat with systemic antifungals

Definition

Tinea capitis is a superficial fungal infection of the scalp (**Fig. 20.11**). The three most common dermatophytes that cause tinea capitis are *Trichophyton tonsurans*, *Microsporum canis*, and *M. audouinii*. The disease varies from non-inflamed scaling patches to inflamed, pustule-studded plaques (kerion) that may leave scars.

Incidence

Epidemic tinea capitis occurs worldwide, mostly in school-aged children. Males and females are equally affected. *T. tonsurans* is the predominant cause of tinea capitis in Blacks and Whites. *M. canis*, typically transmitted by a pet, is seen less frequently.

History

Often, the patient has a history of a family member, friend, or pet with hair loss.

Physical Examination

Tinea capitis can appear as seborrheic-like dermatitis with minimal inflammation, patchy alopecia with broken hair shafts leaving residual black stumps ('black dot' ringworm). Occipital lymph nodes are often present (**Fig. 20.12**). A more severe infection with indurated, boggy plaques (kerion) covered with pustules and crusting, accompanied by lymphadenopathy, can result in scarring.

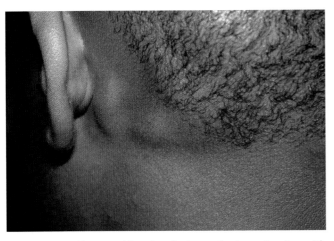

FIGURE 20.12 **Tinea capitis** – lymphadenopathy in conjunction with patches of alopecia is a typical sign.

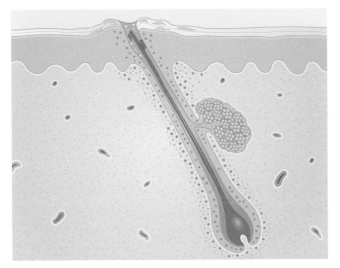

FIGURE 20.13 **Tinea capitis.** Epidermis – hyperkeratosis, broken hair; spores and hyphae in stratum corneum and hair shaft. Dermis – perifollicular inflammation.

Tinea capitis causes:
1. Seborrheic-like dermatitis
2. 'Black dot' ringworm
3. Kerion

Differential Diagnosis

Alopecia areata, seborrheic dermatitis, bacterial scalp infection, and *trichotillomania* should be considered in the differential diagnosis of tinea capitis. A KOH preparation or fungal culture confirms the diagnosis of tinea capitis.

Laboratory and Biopsy

Until recently, the Wood's lamp examination was a simple method of screening for tinea capitis. Hairs infected with *M. audouinii* and *M. canis* fluoresce bright green with this long-wave ultraviolet light. The Wood's lamp, however, has become much less useful because most cases of tinea capitis are now caused by non-fluorescing *T. tonsurans*.

The diagnosis is made by KOH microscopic examination and culture of broken hairs. The KOH preparation reveals spores surrounding the hair shaft (ectothrix), characteristic of *Microsporum* spp., or within the shaft (endothrix), characteristic of *T. tonsurans*. Although biopsy is not usually performed, histopathologic sections that are stained with periodic acid–Schiff or silver reveal spores and hyphae in the stratum corneum and hair shaft (**Fig. 20.13**).

Therapy

Topical agents are ineffective in treating tinea capitis. For children, microsize griseofulvin (Grifulvin V tablets or suspension), 20 mg/kg daily for 6–8 weeks, is the treatment of choice. In addition, shampooing with 2.5% selenium sulfide (Selsun) twice a week helps to reduce viable fungal spores and probably should be used by asymptomatic family members to reduce the carrier state. Oral terbinafine (Lamisil) or itraconazole (Sporanox) are alternative drugs if treatment with griseofulvin fails.

Therapy for Tinea Capitis

Initial
- Griseofulvin – 20–25 mg/kg daily
- Terbinafine
  - <20 kg: 62.5 mg daily
  - 20–40 kg: 125 mg daily
  - >40 kg: 250 mg daily

Alternative
- Itraconazole
  - <20 kg: 5 mg/kg daily
  - 20–40 kg: 100 mg daily
  - >40 kg: 200 mg daily

Course and Complications

With treatment, tinea capitis is cured in 1–3 months in most cases. Without treatment, the course is variable. In some children, particularly those with inflammatory tinea capitis, the course is self-limiting, with resolution within a few months. In others, the disease lasts for years, with resolution at puberty. Scarring and permanent hair loss may be the sequelae of a kerion, but often the permanent damage is surprisingly little, given the intense inflammation.

Pathogenesis

Epidemic tinea capitis is transmitted by human-to-human spread of the dermatophytes *M. audouinii* and *T. tonsurans*. Fungi have been cultured from fallen hairs, scales, and shared combs, hats, and brushes. *M. canis* is spread from animals (cats and dogs) to humans.

After an incubation period of several days, the fungal hyphae grow into the hair shaft and follicle. This growth causes broken hair, scaling, and a host inflammatory

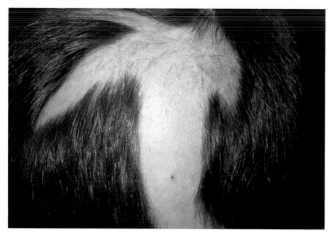

FIGURE 20.14 **Trichotillomania** – bizarre patch of broken hairs.

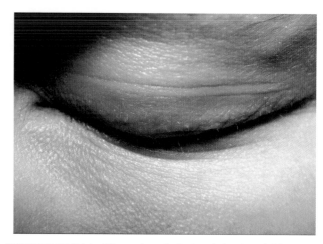

FIGURE 20.15 **Trichotillomania** – plucked eyelashes in a child.

response. The infection spreads centrifugally for 8–10 weeks, involving an area of scalp up to 7 cm in diameter. Spontaneous cure ensues, or a host–parasite equilibrium is maintained that results in a smoldering infection.

TRICHOTILLOMANIA

Key Points

1. Self-induced alopecia from compulsive hair pulling
2. Bizarre patterns of non-scarring alopecia
3. Poor prognosis in adults, better prognosis in children

Definition

Trichotillomania is a traumatic, self-induced alopecia. It results from compulsive plucking, twisting, and rubbing, which cause broken or epilated hair shafts (**Fig. 20.14**).

Incidence

Trichotillomania occurs in both children and adults. In children, it affects both sexes equally, and patients usually have no significant underlying emotional problem. In adults, it occurs predominantly among women and is often a sign of a personality disorder.

History

A history of emotional problems may be elicited, often with difficulty.

Physical Examination

The scalp is affected most often; much less often, the eyebrows and eyelashes are plucked (**Fig. 20.15**). Ill marginated, irregular, patchy areas of alopecia characterize trichotillomania. The scalp is normal, without inflammation or scarring. The patient has numerous twisted and broken hairs, which have a characteristic feel of coarse stubble.

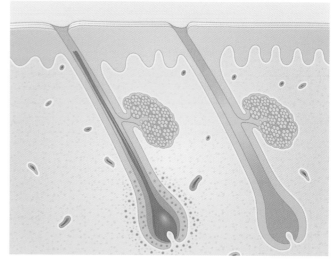

FIGURE 20.16 **Trichotillomania** – broken hair; empty follicle. Dermis – perifollicular hemorrhage.

Coarse-feeling, broken hairs are characteristic of trichotillomania.

Differential Diagnosis

Alopecia areata and *tinea capitis* should be considered in the differential diagnosis of trichotillomania. Exclamation point hairs, if present, are diagnostic of alopecia areata. Biopsy findings are also discriminating. KOH examination and fungal culture enable the diagnosis of fungal infection.

Laboratory and Biopsy

The biopsy (usually not required) reveals increased numbers of catagen (e.g., regressing) follicles, empty hair follicles in a non-inflammatory dermis, and traumatized follicles that have broken hair matrixes and perifollicular hemorrhage (**Fig. 20.16**).

Therapy

Treatment is based on the degree of underlying emotional disturbance. In children, the condition is usually self-limiting and is best termed 'trichotill,' because the habit of hair pulling is often not associated with psychiatric illness. When insight and reassurance are given to the child and parents, the process often resolves. In adults, the habit may be much more difficult to stop. Gentle probing into the stresses and anxieties that have led to the hair pulling can be explored. Referral for psychiatric evaluation should be considered in severely disturbed patients. Clomipramine (Anafranil), a tricyclic antidepressant with antiobsessional effects, appears to be an effective short-term treatment. Selective serotonin-reuptake inhibitors are also commonly used as adjunctive therapy, based on the rationale that trichotillomania is similar to obsessive compulsive disorder.

Therapy for Trichotillomania

Initial
- Emotional support
- Behavioral counseling

Alternative
- Referral to psychiatry:
  - Clomipramine 25–250 mg daily
- Selective serotonin-reuptake inhibitors (e.g., fluoxetine)

Course and complications

Trichotillomania is generally chronic and may be resistant to treatment, especially in adults, in whom it can be a serious problem. Symptoms may be severe enough to interfere with daily life; a patient's appearance may be sufficiently embarrassing to result in social isolation. In most children, hair pulling is a 'phase,' which improves and clears with time. Follow-up is required to establish rapport and to determine whether trichotillomania is a symptom of a serious underlying psychiatric disorder.

Pathogenesis

The obsessive urge to pull out one's own hair has been attributed to various psychodynamic conflicts. In children, problems at home or at school, sibling rivalry, mental retardation, and hospitalization can be psychosocial triggers for trichotillomania.

UNCOMMON HAIR DISORDERS

ACNE KELOIDALIS NUCHAE

This often pruritic condition occurs on the nape of the neck, most commonly in men who have darkly pigmented skin. Early lesions appear as dome-shaped papules with a central hair. Later, the papules may coalesce into large hypertrophic scars (**Fig. 20.17**). Multiple hairs entrapped by scar tissue can be seen exiting a single follicular opening (tufting). Despite common belief,

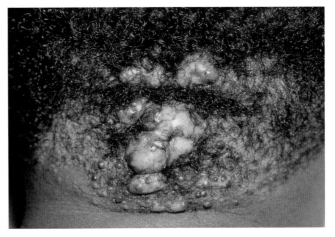

FIGURE 20.17 Acne keloidalis nuchae. Note dome-shaped papules on periphery and larger hypertrophic scars centrally.

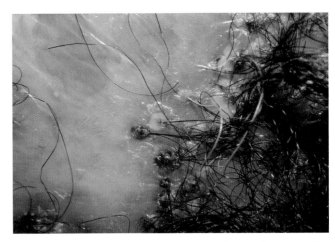

FIGURE 20.18 Folliculitis decalvans – scarring alopecia characterized by loss of follicular openings (slick surface) expanding centrifugally on the crown of the scalp. Note pustules at periphery.

acne keloidalis nuchae is not caused by ingrown hairs and most likely represents an abnormal inflammatory reaction to hairs. Anti-inflammatory treatments include intralesional and topical corticosteroids, and topical and oral antibiotics.

FOLLICULITIS DECALVANS

Folliculitis decalvans is characterized by an expanding patch of scarring alopecia with pustules at the periphery (**Fig. 20.18**). It occurs predominantly on the crown of the scalp. *Staphylococcus aureus* is often cultured from the pustules and may play a pathogenic role. Treatment is difficult, and includes appropriate systemic antibiotics.

LICHEN PLANOPILARIS

This scarring alopecia occurs more commonly in women than in men. Physical examination shows permanent loss of follicular openings and perifollicular erythema and scale (**Fig. 20.19**). The condition can be localized or widespread. Changes of lichen planus can be seen on

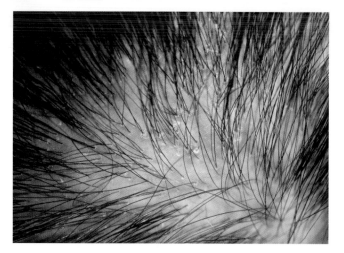

FIGURE 20.19 **Lichen planopilaris** – localized patch of scarring alopecia. Note widened spaces between follicles, and perifollicular erythema and scale.

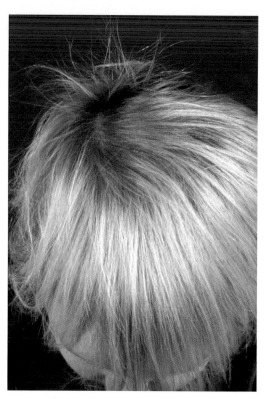

FIGURE 20.20 **Loose anagen syndrome** – a 2-year-old girl with classic phenotype of short blond hair that will not grow; in this case, hair thinning was diffuse.

glabrous skin and mucous membranes 50% of the time. A biopsy confirms the diagnosis. Lichen planopilaris is relatively resistant to treatment (e.g., antimalarial medications, oral and topical corticosteroids). Spontaneous resolution occurs on average in 18 months.

LOOSE ANAGEN SYNDROME

Loose anagen syndrome typically presents in a young girl with short blond hair (**Fig. 20.20**). The child seldom needs a haircut because the 'hair will not grow.' The hair thinning may be diffuse or patchy. Diagnosis is confirmed by the painless extraction of microscopically confirmed anagen hairs through gentle hair pulling. The cause remains unknown. Improvement occurs with age. The differential diagnosis includes telogen effluvium and trichotillomania.

Nail Disorders 21

Key Points

1. Appearance alone is usually not enough to make the diagnosis
2. Therapy is often difficult or unsuccessful

ABSTRACT

The nail is a specialized keratinized appendage found on the dorsum of each finger and toe. It protects the distal phalanx against trauma, is used for fine grasping and scratching, and has esthetic value. The diagnosis of nail diseases can be difficult because a single disease can cause widely varying changes of the nail and, conversely, because a given nail malformation can be the expression of a variety of diseases. Numerous disorders may affect the nail, including cutaneous and systemic diseases, tumors, infections, hereditary disorders, physical factors, and drugs. In this chapter, the four most common causes of nail disease are discussed: fungal infection, psoriasis, paronychia (**Table 21.1**), and ingrown toenail.

> The physical appearance of the nail cannot be used reliably to make a diagnosis.

FUNGAL INFECTION

Key Points

1. Confirm the diagnosis with culture or KOH preparation
2. Cure requires oral therapy

Definition

Onychomycosis and *tinea unguium* are synonyms for infection of the nail with dermatophytic fungi. The most common etiologic dermatophytes are *Trichophyton rubrum* and *T. mentagrophytes*.

Incidence

The prevalence of onychomycosis is 22 per 1000 population. Some 20% of persons in the USA between 40 and 60 years of age have onychomycosis. The most common sites of infection are the toenails, especially in the elderly.

History

The onset of onychomycosis is slow and insidious. The condition is often asymptomatic, but it can also cause pain in the affected toe, nail-trimming problems, discomfort when wearing shoes, and embarrassment because of the nail's distorted appearance.

Physical Examination

Infection of toenails is more frequent than infection of fingernails, and it is uncommon for all 10 nails to be involved. Dermatophytes most often infect the distal nail bed and undersurface of the distal nail, with resulting discoloration (white, yellow, or brown) of the nail plate and accumulation of subungual debris with separation of the plate from the nail bed (**Fig. 21.1A**). Less often, dermatophytes infect the top surface of the nail plate and cause a white, crumbly surface (superficial white onychomycosis) to develop. Neither type of infection produces much inflammatory reaction. Proximal white subungual onychomycosis, infection of the proximal nail plate, is a marker of human immunodeficiency virus (HIV) infection.

> Onychomycosis is associated with tinea pedis and tinea manuum.

Differential Diagnosis

Often, the nail changes of onychomycosis cannot be distinguished clinically from those of nail dystrophy caused by *psoriasis* (see **Fig. 21.4**), *eczema of the digits*, *trauma*, and *aging*. Associated skin findings and fungal studies differentiate these entities.

TABLE 21.1 Nail disorders

		Physical Examination			Laboratory Test	
	Frequency (%)[a]	Pits	Brown Stains	Differential Diagnosis	KOH	Culture
Fungal infection	0.4	Absent	Present	Psoriasis Trauma Aging Secondary to eczema	Positive	Positive
Psoriasis	<0.1	Present	Present	Fungus Trauma Aging Secondary to eczema Alopecia areata	Negative	Negative
Paronychia	0.3	Absent	Absent	Herpes simplex	Negative Positive	Bacterial *Candida albicans*

[a]Percentage of new dermatology patients with this diagnosis seen at the Hershey Medical Center Dermatology Clinic, Hershey, PA.
KOH, potassium hydroxide.

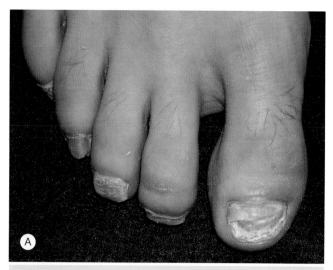

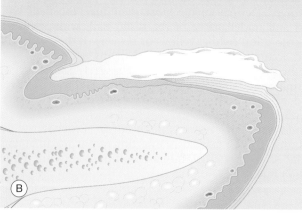

FIGURE 21.1 **Onychomycosis. A.** White, thick, and crumbly nail plate. **B.** Nail plate – irregular, thick, and containing fungal hyphae.

Laboratory and Biopsy

Documentation of nail fungal infection with a potassium hydroxide (KOH) preparation or fungal culture should be done because therapy is expensive and may have unwanted side-effects. Compared with skin scrapings, more time must be allowed for the KOH to dissolve thin nail specimens before microscopic examination. If the infection is in the nail bed or the deeper portion of the nail plate, scrapings should be obtained from as far back under the nail as possible. Occasionally, a nail biopsy is needed to obtain a positive result (**Fig. 21.1B**).

Therapy

Topical antifungal agents are ineffective in treating onychomycosis because of their poor penetration of the nail plate. Oral therapy with terbinafine (Lamisil) or itraconazole (Sporanox) should be given. Studies suggest that terbinafine is the most effective agent. The nail will not look completely normal at the end of treatment. Because terbinafine and itraconazole remain in the nail for months after therapy, retreatment should not be considered for approximately 6 months for fingernails and 12 months for toenails. In many individuals with asymptomatic onychomycosis of the toenails, systemic therapy is neither requested nor suggested. The risks and cost may outweigh any possible benefit.

> Asymptomatic onychomycosis of toenails needs no treatment.

Therapy for Onychomycosis

Initial
- Terbinafine: 6 weeks for fingernails, 12 weeks for toenails
  - <20 kg: 62.5 mg daily
  - 20–40 kg: 125 mg daily
  - >40 kg: 250 mg daily

Alternative
- Itraconazole: 2 pulses for fingernails, 3 pulses for toenails
  - <20 kg: 5 mg/kg daily for 1 week/month
  - 20–40 kg: 100 mg daily for 1 week/month
  - >40–50 kg: 200 mg daily for 1 week/month
  - >50 kg: 200 mg twice daily for 1 week/month

Course and Complications

Onychomycosis is a chronic infection that is difficult to eradicate permanently. Even with oral therapy, failure rates for treating toenail infections are 20–30%. Residual fungal spores present in the patient's shoes and environment are probably responsible for recurrence of the infection. For this reason, a topical antifungal (e.g., tolnaftate, Tinactin; miconazole, Micatin; or terbinafine, Lamisil) applied to the feet every week may be helpful for long-term prophylaxis.

Pathogenesis

Superficial fungal infection of the nail is probably a direct extension of involvement of the surrounding digital skin. Invasion and deformity of the nail are facilitated by fungal keratinases, which disrupt the keratin structure of the plate.

INGROWN TOENAIL

Key Points

1. Ingrown toenail causes a foreign body reaction
2. Nail avulsion and matrix destruction are curative

Definition

Ingrown toenail occurs when the lateral portion of the nail plate grows into the lateral nail fold, resulting in an inflammatory response.

Incidence

Ingrown toenail is a fairly common occurrence, with the great toenails most commonly affected.

History

Pain and swelling are the symptoms that cause patients to seek medical attention. Usually, the problem has been present for weeks or months with an acute flare, which may signal a secondary infection.

Physical Examination

The lateral nail fold is red, swollen, and usually has weeping granulation tissue (**Fig. 21.2**). The nail plate is penetrating into the lateral nail fold.

Differential Diagnosis

The diagnosis of ingrown toenail seldom causes difficulty because of its typical presentation.

Laboratory and Biopsy

Because the diagnosis is straightforward, no laboratory testing or biopsy is necessary

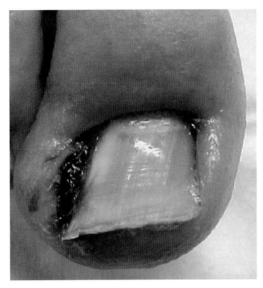

FIGURE 21.2 **Ingrown toenail** – red, swollen, lateral nail fold with granulation tissue.

Therapy

For mild to moderate ingrown toenail, wearing sufficiently wide shoes, trimming the nail plate straight across, antiseptic application, and inserting a cotton pledget under the nail edge may be successful. Operative intervention is necessary when conservative treatment fails or for severely ingrown toenails. Partial or total nail plate avulsion followed by surgical or chemical (85% aqueous phenol) nail matrix destruction is usually curative. Granulation tissue can be excised or cauterized.

Therapy for Ingrown Toenail

Initial
- Well-fitting shoes
- Trim nail plate straight across
- Topical antiseptics
- Cotton pledget insertion

Alternative
- Nail avulsion with matrix destruction

Course and Complications

Ingrown toenail is a chronic process, which causes pain and swelling that interfere with ambulation. Occasionally, cellulitis of the toe can be a complication.

Pathogenesis

The ingrown nail plate acts as a foreign body, causing an inflammatory reaction in the lateral nail fold.

PARONYCHIA

> ## Key Points
>
> 1. Acute paronychia is a primary bacterial infection
> 2. Chronic paronychia is a secondary candidal infection

Definition

Paronychia is an inflammatory process of the nail fold (**Fig. 21.3A**). Acute paronychia is most often the result of bacterial infection, commonly from *Staphylococcus aureus*. Chronic paronychia is usually caused by *Candida albicans*. The predisposing factor in the production of chronic paronychia is trauma or maceration producing a break in the seal (cuticle) between the nail fold and the nail plate. This break produces a pocket that holds moisture and promotes the growth of microorganisms.

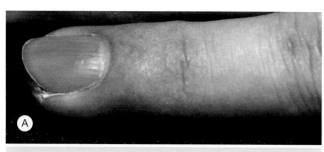

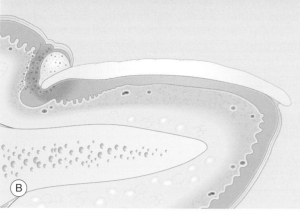

FIGURE 21.3 **A.** Acute paronychia – erythematous, swollen nail fold. **B.** Chronic paronychia – edema and inflammation, deformed cuticle with pocket with pus and candidal hyphae.

> Acute paronychia is usually caused by *Staphylococcus aureus*; chronic paronychia is caused by *Candida albicans*.

Incidence

Chronic paronychia occurs in children who habitually suck their thumbs and in adults who do 'wet' work.

Particularly vulnerable are adults (non-diabetic, 3.4%; diabetic, 9.6%) who are exposed to a wet environment while they perform the chores of childrearing and house-work. Bartenders, janitors, and other workers in wet occupations are also at risk.

History

Acute paronychia develops rapidly, leading to marked tenderness of the nail fold. Chronic paronychia develops insidiously and initially often goes unnoticed by the patient. A history of manicuring or wet work in adults or of finger sucking in children is common.

Physical Examination

Although any finger may be involved with paronychia, the second and third digits are the most commonly affected. Acute paronychia is painful, red, and swollen, and may be accompanied by an abscess or cellulitis.

Chronic paronychia is characterized by loss of the cuticle, slight tenderness, swelling, erythema, and, sometimes, separation of the nail fold from the plate. A purulent or 'cheesy' discharge and deformity of the nail plate are frequently seen.

Differential Diagnosis

Acute bacterial paronychia can be confused with *herpetic whitlow*. Tzanck preparation and cultures help to distinguish the two. Chronic paronychia is a distinctive clinical entity and should not be confused with other inflammatory processes.

Laboratory and Biopsy

Acute paronychia that does not respond to appropriate antibiotic therapy should be cultured and possibly radiographed, to rule out osteomyelitis. For chronic paronychia, a candidal origin can be confirmed with a KOH examination of debris taken from under the cuticle (**Fig. 21.3B**). Culture, if taken, often reveals mixed flora, including bacteria and *Candida* species.

Therapy

Acute paronychia should be incised and drained when it is fluctuant. Appropriate antibiotic therapy for the causative agent should be instituted. In most cases, this therapy consists of cephalexin (Keflex), erythromycin (Ilosone), or dicloxacillin (Dynapen).

Chronic paronychia requires the avoidance of prolonged exposure to wetness. Wearing gloves is mandatory, preferably cotton under rubber or vinyl gloves. Frequent washings and manicuring should be avoided. Broad-spectrum topical preparations, such as Lotrisone (clotrimazole and betamethasone dipropionate) applied twice daily, are helpful.

> Trauma and exposure to water must be stopped to cure chronic paronychia.

Course and Complications

Acute paronychia is usually not a precursor of chronic paronychia. It resolves after appropriate antibiotic therapy and, if needed, incision and drainage.

By definition, chronic paronychia continues for a long time because repeated mechanical trauma and exposure to water predispose to the chronic infectious and inflammatory process.

Pathogenesis

Chronic paronychia is caused by microorganisms that produce swelling and inflammation of the nail fold. Interruption of the cuticle and wetness create an environment that fosters the growth of yeast and bacteria. These microorganisms also cause inflammation of the nail matrix, resulting in abnormal nail formation and subsequent nail dystrophy.

PSORIASIS

Key Points

1. Psoriatic nails can mimic onychomycosis
2. Treatment is unsatisfactory

Definition

Nail dystrophy caused by psoriasis is the result of abnormal keratinization of the nail matrix and bed secondary to involvement of these structures with psoriasis.

Incidence

Nail involvement in patients with psoriasis is common. Reported incidences range from 10% to 50%.

History

Psoriasis of the nail is usually asymptomatic. However, involvement of the fingernails may be a significant cosmetic liability, and deformity of the toenails may cause pain secondary to pressure from shoes.

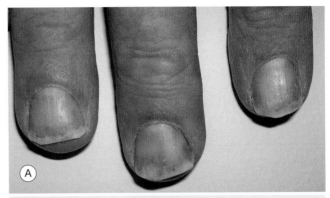

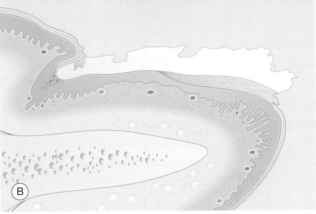

FIGURE 21.4 Psoriasis. A. Brown, discolored nail with distal separation. **B.** Nail plate – thick and pitted. Epidermis – thick, hyperkeratosis.

Physical Examination

In psoriasis, fingernails are affected more often than toenails. All, or a few, nails may be involved. It is unusual for psoriasis to involve only the nails; fewer than 5% of patients have involvement of the nails alone without cutaneous disease. The examiner should look elsewhere to confirm the diagnosis, especially other areas frequently affected by psoriasis: the scalp, elbows, knees, and intergluteal fold. In the nails, the most characteristic lesions are small, multiple pits produced by punctate psoriatic lesions in the nail matrix. Involvement of the nail bed produces brownish discoloration (oil stain), thickening of the nail plate, separation of the nail plate from the nail bed (onycholysis), distal crumbling, and splinter hemorrhages (**Fig. 21.4A**).

Psoriatic nails have:
1. Pits
2. Oil stain
3. Onycholysis
4. Thickening

Differential Diagnosis

The differential diagnosis of psoriasis of the nails includes *onychomycosis, trauma, aging,* and *dystrophy secondary to eczema,* or some other inflammatory process in the nail fold area. Fungal infections of the nail can be ruled out by a KOH preparation and culture. Otherwise, psoriatic nails can be diagnosed with confidence only when other typical lesions of psoriasis are found elsewhere. Although nail pitting is the finding most characteristic for psoriasis, it is also occasionally associated with *alopecia areata*.

Laboratory and Biopsy

Nails are rarely examined by biopsy to confirm the diagnosis of psoriasis (**Fig. 21.4B**).

Therapy

Treatment of psoriasis of the nails is difficult and usually unsatisfactory. Consequently, therapy is often not recommended. Injection of steroids into the proximal nail fold is painful, and the results are often disappointing. Topical preparations are ineffective.

Systemic medications used for psoriasis often help the nail involvement, but nail disease alone does not justify the use of these potent therapies. Trimming and paring of deformed nails reduce discomfort caused by pressure. Fingernails may be cosmetically improved by the use of sculptured plastic nails and the application of fingernail polish.

Therapy for Nail Psoriasis

- Trimming
- Cosmetics

Course and Complications

Psoriasis of the nail is a chronic condition and has a waxing and waning course. Frequently, distal interphalangeal joint arthritis is associated with nail involvement. The nail is sometimes secondarily infected with *Candida albicans* or *Pseudomonas aeruginosa*. *Pseudomonas* infection is easily recognized by green discoloration and is treated with 2% thymol in alcohol, one or two drops three times daily.

Pathogenesis

Psoriasis is characterized by a marked acceleration of the rate of epidermal cell replication, resulting in proliferation of keratinocytes. When this occurs in the nail bed, excess keratin is trapped under the nail plate, and onycholysis results. The 'oil stain' appearance is produced by keratinous debris and inflammation in the nail bed. The nail pits result from involvement of the nail matrix, in which the psoriasis presumably produces small defective foci in the nail plate. As the nail plate advances, these defective portions fall out, leaving behind the characteristic pits.

UNCOMMON NAIL DISORDERS

ALLERGIC CONTACT DERMATITIS TO SCULPTURED NAILS

The artificial sculptured nails are made by mixing a liquid monomer with a powder polymer and then molding this acrylate compound onto the natural nail. Polymerization of these acrylate plastics can be initiated by ultraviolet light which is frequently used in the nail saloon. The acrylate monomer is the sensitizer causing red, pruritic and painful paronychial inflammation a day or two after application. The resulting nail bed inflammation causes nail dystrophy as well as removal of the sculpted nail (**Fig. 21.5**).

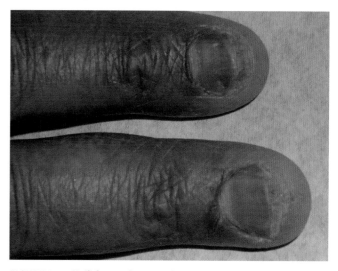

FIGURE 21.5 Nail dystrophy secondary to allergic contact dermatitis to sculptured nails.

Mucous Membrane Disorders **22**

Key Points

1. Often present as white lesions or ulcers/erosions
2. Biopsy white lesions and non-healing ulcers/erosions to rule out malignancy

Mucous membrane disorders:
1. Erosions and ulcerations
2. White lesions

White spots are hyperkeratotic lesions of the oral mucosa. Thickened stratum corneum of mucous membranes appears white because of maceration from continuous wetness. Malignancy must be ruled out as a cause.

White lesions represent hyperkeratosis.

APHTHOUS STOMATITIS

Key Points

1. Most common cause of recurrent oral ulcers
2. Ulcers have a yellow base and peripheral erythema
3. Multiple therapies indicate lack of effective treatment

ABSTRACT

Examination of the oral cavity can provide important diagnostic information for dermatologic diagnosis and therefore should be included in every skin examination. A variety of skin disorders can be accompanied by mucous membrane involvement. For example, erythema multiforme and systemic lupus erythematosus can cause erosions in the mouth, nose, or eyes. However, this chapter focuses on disorders either exclusively or predominantly confined to mucous membranes, usually of the oral cavity.

Mucous membrane disorders are divided into two broad categories: (1) erosions and ulcerations and (2) white lesions (**Table 22.1**). Erosions are lesions in which the mucosal epithelium is partly denuded. Ulcerations extend through the epidermis into the underlying tissue, which in mucous membranes is called lamina propria rather than dermis. Erosive and ulcerative diseases range in frequency from common (aphthous stomatitis) to rare (pemphigus), and their causes are idiopathic, immunologic, infectious, and malignant.

Definition

Aphthous stomatitis is a common, recurrent, idiopathic disorder of the mouth most often manifest by multiple small, 'punched-out' ulcers (**Fig. 22.1**).

Incidence

Recurrent aphthous stomatitis is a common disease, occurring in 20–60% of the general population. It is most common in young adults; the 60% prevalence was found in a survey of students attending professional schools.

History

A history of previous episodes is invariable. Recurrences are sometimes precipitated by trauma from biting or misguided toothbrushes. Some patients correlate outbreaks with emotional stress. Lesions are usually preceded by a 1-day prodrome of discomfort in the area of involvement. The ulcers are painful and sometimes interfere with eating.

TABLE 22.1 Mucous membrane disorders

	Etiology	History	Physical Examination	Differential Diagnosis	Laboratory Test
Ulcers					
Aphthous stomatitis (common cause)	Unknown	Recurrent disease	Sharply demarcated, round, yellowish erosions surrounded by erythema	Herpes simplex Behçet's syndrome Inflammatory bowel disease Erythema multiforme	–
Pemphigus and pemphigoid (uncommon causes)	Autoimmune	May have associated skin lesions	Ragged erosions and ulcerations; intact blisters rarely present	Aphthous stomatitis Erythema multiforme	Biopsy with immunofluorescence
Viral infections	Primary herpes simplex Coxsackie	Fever, malaise	Gingivitis; blisters also on lips	Aphthous stomatitis Erythema multiforme	Tzanck smear or culture
		Fever	Vesicles in *posterior* oral cavity	Aphthous stomatitis	–
Syphilis	*Treponema pallidum*	Sexual contact	*Indurated*, painless ulcer	Malignancy	Serologic test for syphilis
Deep fungal infection	Histoplasmosis	Immunosuppressed	Systemically ill; indurated ulcer	Malignancy	Biopsy with culture
Malignancy		Non-healing ulcer	Indurated ulcer	Major aphthous ulcer	Biopsy
White lesions					
Thrush	*Candida albicans*	Found in newborns and immunosuppressed patients	'Curd-like' papules, easily scraped off	Lichen planus	KOH preparation
Lichen planus	Unknown	Chronic disease; may have associated skin lesions	Reticulated white lines; sometimes erosions are present	Candidiasis Leukoplakia Secondary syphilis	Biopsy
Leukoplakia	Chronic irritation	Smoking Denture trauma	White patches and plaques	Lichen planus Secondary syphilis White sponge nevus Leukokeratosis	Biopsy
Squamous cell carcinoma		Smoking Alcohol Prior leukoplakia	*Indurated* or *ulcerated* plaque	Leukoplakia Major aphthous ulcer Erosive lichen planus Chancre Deep fungal infection	Biopsy

KOH, potassium hydroxide.

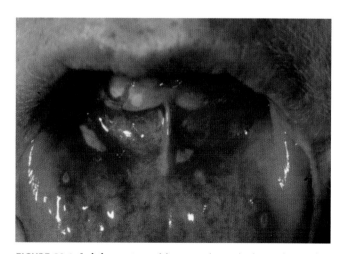

FIGURE 22.1 Aphthous stomatitis – round, punched-out ulcer with a white-yellow necrotic surface.

Physical Examination

Lesions in aphthous stomatitis appear as 2–5-mm, round, punched-out ulcers with a yellowish necrotic surface and surrounding erythema. Lesions may be single but more often are multiple. The buccal and labial mucosae are the most common locations.

Aphthous stomatitis is the most common cause of oral ulceration.

Differential Diagnosis

Recurrent aphthous stomatitis is most often confused with *herpes simplex infection*. Recurrent herpes simplex rarely occurs inside the mouth. When it does, it appears as grouped small vesicles or erosions on an erythematous base. A Tzanck preparation or culture proves the diagnosis of herpes infection.

> Herpes simplex rarely recurs inside the mouth.

The oral ulcerations in *Behçet's syndrome* are indistinguishable from those of aphthous stomatitis. However, Behçet's syndrome is distinguished by its extraoral manifestations. The classic triad consists of oral ulcerations, genital ulcerations, and ocular inflammation (iridocyclitis). Erythema nodosum, thrombophlebitis, arthritis, and neurologic and intestinal involvement may also occur. Patients with inflammatory bowel disease, particularly *ulcerative colitis*, occasionally have oral ulcerations that resemble aphthous stomatitis.

> Oral ulcerations in Behçet's syndrome look like aphthous stomatitis.

Laboratory and Biopsy

Usually, a biopsy is not required. If a biopsy is performed, the findings will not be diagnostic and will show only ulceration and nonspecific inflammation, composed primarily of lymphocytes. The only other laboratory test to consider is a complete blood count, to screen for the questionable association of iron or folate deficiency anemia in some patients with aphthous stomatitis.

Therapy

The variety of therapies that have been recommended for this disease indicates that a highly successful treatment is lacking. If an underlying iron or folate deficiency is detected, it should be corrected. The ulcerations are usually treated topically. Tetracycline suspension (250 mg/5 mL) 'swished and swallowed' four times daily helps in some patients. Patients in whom tetracycline therapy fails are treated with topical steroids in a gel (e.g., fluocinonide, Lidex gel) or a special adherent base (e.g., triamcinolone, Kenalog in Orabase) applied three times daily or with a spray preparation (e.g., beclomethasone, Vanceril) applied three to four times daily. Intralesional steroids (triamcinolone, Kenalog-10) are useful in patients with large aphthous ulcerations. Oral prednisone is effective in aphthous stomatitis but should be used for only a short course in patients with severe, incapacitating disease. Colchicine and pentoxifylline (Trental) have also been reported to be helpful in preventing recurrent disease, but the clinical trials were not controlled.

Pain relief can be obtained with topical anesthetics such as dyclonine hydrochloride (Dyclone liquid) or topical lidocaine (viscous Xylocaine) used 20 min before meals. These preparations numb the entire mouth, including the taste buds, for 1–2 h and allow for pain-free, albeit taste-free, dining.

Therapy for Aphthous Stomatitis

Initial
- Topical steroids
  - Fluocinonide gel 0.05%
  - Triamcinolone in Orabase
- Tetracycline 'swish and swallow'
- Dyclonine hydrochloride 1% solution
- Lidocaine jelly 2%

Alternative
- Intralesional triamcinolone
- Systemic treatment (colchicine/pentoxifylline)

Course and Complications

For minor aphthous stomatitis, spontaneous healing occurs within 4–14 days. Large aphthous ulcers (major aphthous ulcers) take as long as 6 weeks to heal. Individual ulcers lasting much longer than that should be examined by biopsy to rule out malignancy. Recurrences are common and range in frequency from occasional to almost continuous. In most patients, the disease eventually remits, but the time course is highly variable – from 5 to 15 years or longer.

Pathogenesis

Factors implicated in the pathogenesis include emotional and physical stress, hormones, infection, and autoimmunity. An immune mechanism is the most favored cause. Circulating T lymphocytes cytotoxic against oral mucosa have been identified and appear to play a role.

LEUKOPLAKIA

Key Points

1. White plaques can signify cancer
2. Indurated white plaques require biopsy
3. Smoking is most frequent cause

Definition

Leukoplakia literally means 'white plaque' (**Fig. 22.2**). Some clinicians simply use that as the definition of the disease, defining leukoplakia as 'a white patch or plaque that cannot be characterized clinically or pathologically as any other disease.' Others use the term *leukokeratosis* to describe a white patch that is histologically benign, and reserve the term *leukoplakia* for a white patch or plaque in which epithelial dysplasia is present pathologically. The authors prefer the second definition. Either way, the important point to remember is that, for white plaques on mucous membranes, a dysplastic change should be considered a possible cause.

The white color is due to macerated hyperkeratosis, which, in most cases, is caused by chronic irritation.

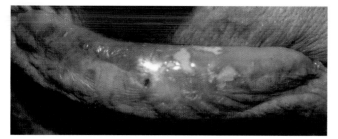

FIGURE 22.2 **Leukoplakia** – white patch or plaque that requires biopsy to rule out malignancy.

Smoking is the most frequent origin, but physical irritation from dentures or ragged teeth may also be causative.

> Smoking is a frequent cause.

Incidence

Leukoplakia is an uncommon disorder affecting primarily middle-aged and elderly adults. The incidence depends, of course, on the definition. The disease is about one-tenth as common when dysplastic histologic changes are required criteria.

History

The onset is gradual and usually asymptomatic. Accordingly, leukoplakia is sometimes an incidental finding during a routine physical examination. Some patients seek medical attention because of irritation, which may be the original cause of the problem. Many patients are smokers or have used smokeless tobacco.

Physical Findings

Leukoplakia appears as a white patch or plaque on the mucous membrane. The surface may be flat or verrucous, and the color varies from pure white to gray. It can be located anywhere in the mouth. The tongue is a common location, but leukoplakia can occur on the tonsils, pharynx, or larynx. Leukoplakia may also be found on genital mucosa.

All white lesions should be palpated for induration. Induration and ulceration are important physical findings that strongly suggest carcinoma (**Fig. 22.3**). Sometimes, only part of a white plaque is indurated, and this area should be examined by biopsy to rule out cancer.

> All white plaques should be palpated; indurated areas must be examined by biopsy to rule out cancer.

Differential Diagnosis

The differential diagnosis of white lesions in the mouth is given in **Table 22.1**. The reticulated form of oral *lichen planus* is usually clinically distinctive. Mucous patches in *secondary syphilis* are accompanied by other manifestations of that disease, including skin rash and constitutional symptoms. *White sponge nevus* is a hereditary

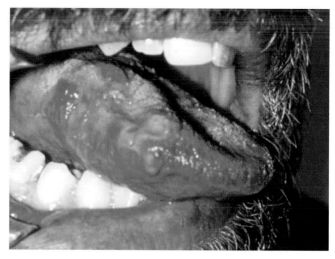

FIGURE 22.3 **Squamous cell carcinoma of the tongue** – the surface of this large nodule is white (hyperkeratotic) and ulcerated, and the base feels hard and indurated.

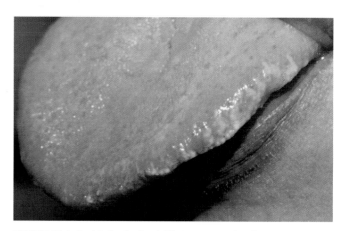

FIGURE 22.4 **Oral hairy leukoplakia** is associated with AIDS.

condition that begins in childhood and results in a white lesion that appears 'spongy.' *Leukokeratosis* is a diagnosis of exclusion that clinically does not fit another known entity and histopathologically shows no dysplastic changes. The diagnosis then often rests with the biopsy.

> Diagnosis depends on the biopsy.

Oral hairy leukoplakia affects the sides of the tongue with white papules and plaques that sometimes have a filiform ('hairy') surface (**Fig. 22.4**). This disorder occurs almost exclusively in patients with acquired immune deficiency syndrome (AIDS) and may be the first sign of human immunodeficiency virus (HIV) infection. Ultimately, as many as 30% of patients with AIDS are affected with oral hairy leukoplakia. It is asymptomatic, not premalignant, and is now known to be caused by infection with Epstein–Barr virus. Treatment with acyclovir and other antiviral agents can cause the condition to regress.

Laboratory and Biopsy

The histopathologic findings include hyperkeratosis, acanthosis, and underlying inflammation in the lamina propria composed of lymphocytes and plasma cells (plasma cells are common in inflammatory reactions of mucous membranes). In leukoplakia, the epithelial dysplastic changes are similar to those found in actinic keratosis and include cellular pleomorphism, increased numbers of mitotic figures, and derangement of the usual orderly architectural pattern of stratified epithelium. The dysplastic changes may be mild, moderate, or severe. When they are severe (carcinoma *in situ*), the entire thickness of epithelium is involved with marked dysplastic changes. Invasion of these cells into the underlying lamina propria signifies squamous cell carcinoma.

Therapy

The goals of therapy are to eliminate the cause and surgically remove persistent lesions. Smoking or the use of smokeless tobacco should be eliminated and sources of physical trauma corrected. Lesions may then resolve spontaneously, particularly when only mildly dysplastic. For lesions that are persistent or more severely dysplastic, active intervention is recommended. Superficial mucosal lesions can be removed with cryosurgery, carbon dioxide laser ablation, or shave excision. Medical therapies include topical bleomycin and systemic retinoids. Lesions suggestive of squamous cell carcinoma should be excised.

Therapy for Leukoplakia

Initial
- Biopsy
- Cessation of tobacco use
- Elimination of sources of physical trauma
- Excision (if cancer is suspected)

Alternative
- Ablation of superficial lesions
  - Cryosurgery
  - Carbon dioxide laser
  - Shave excision
- Topical bleomycin
- Systemic retinoids

Course and Complications

Spontaneous involution may occur, especially when the aggravating factors are withdrawn. Some lesions may become stationary, whereas others progress to squamous cell carcinoma.

The frequency of development of squamous cell carcinoma in lesions of leukoplakia depends in part on the definition. If dysplasia is among the diagnostic criteria, approximately 30% of leukoplakia lesions will progress to squamous cell carcinoma. If the broader definition (not requiring dysplasia) is used, invasive carcinoma will occur in only 3–6%.

> Squamous cell carcinoma develops in 30% of patients with 'dysplastic leukoplakia.'

Pathogenesis

Usually, leukoplakia appears to be induced by chronic, mild irritation from physical, chemical, or inflammatory processes. Smoking is the most frequent and important cause. Chemical agents in smoking include polycyclic hydrocarbons and phenolic oils. Heat may also contribute. Physical trauma from ill-fitting dentures, long-term use of toothpicks, and irritation from jagged teeth can also cause leukoplakia. Most recently, human papillomavirus infection has been implicated in the pathogenesis of some cases of leukoplakia.

LICHEN PLANUS

Key Points

1. Characteristic lace-like pattern on buccal mucosa
2. Diagnosis confirmed by biopsy
3. Resistant to treatment

Definition

Oral lesions in lichen planus occur alone or in association with skin lesions. The oral lesions are characterized by inflammation and hyperkeratosis, which appears clinically as white lesions, most commonly in the form of reticulated papules and lines that assume a lace-like pattern (**Fig. 22.5**). *Erosive lichen planus* is a less common variant. The origin of lichen planus is unknown.

Incidence

Lichen planus is probably the most common cause of white lesions in the mouth. It has been found in 0.5–1% of patients in dental clinics. The highest incidence occurs in adults aged 40–60 years.

> Lichen planus is the most common cause of white lesions in the mouth.

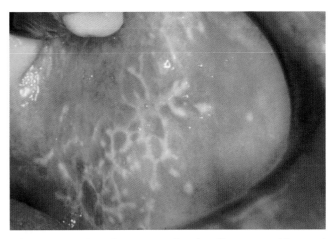

FIGURE 22.5 Lichen planus – reticulate, lace-like pattern of lines and papules on buccal mucosa.

History

Drugs can also cause a lichen planus type of eruption in the mouth. Most often implicated are quinidine, quinacrine, sulfonylureas, and tetracycline.

> Drugs can be causative.

Usually, no symptoms are associated with the hyperkeratotic type of oral lichen planus. Erosive lichen planus is painful and may make eating difficult. If the patient has accompanying skin lesions, they usually are pruritic.

Physical Examination

Patches of oral lichen planus usually appear as white lines and puncta in a reticulated (lace-like) pattern. Occasionally, these patches become confluent, producing a solid plaque. Blisters and erosions occur less often and are the result of an intense dermal inflammatory reaction occurring at the dermal–epidermal junction.

> The reticulated (lace-like) pattern is characteristic.

The most common site of involvement is the buccal mucosa, which is affected bilaterally in virtually 100% of patients. The tongue, gingiva, and lips may also be affected. Skin lesions (described in Ch. 11) accompany oral lichen planus in 10–40% of cases.

Differential Diagnosis

Candidiasis is distinguished from lichen planus by the ease with which white material can be scraped off and by finding hyphae on potassium hydroxide (KOH) examination. The two conditions can coexist, so a scraping is often worthwhile because the candidal component is easily treatable. *Leukoplakia* should be considered in patients with the plaque form of lichen planus – a biopsy enables distinction between the two. Mucous patches in *secondary syphilis* are usually accompanied by other manifestations of this disease (e.g., rash, fever, lymphadenopathy), and the disease is diagnosed with a serologic test for syphilis.

Laboratory and Biopsy

The diagnosis is generally made clinically for lesions in the usual reticulate pattern. If doubt exists or if the patient has plaques, blisters, or erosions, a biopsy is diagnostic. The histologic findings are similar to those in lichen planus in the skin. Even a thin keratinized layer represents *hyper*keratosis in areas that are not normally keratinized, such as the buccal mucosa. In addition, a dense, band-like, inflammatory infiltrate in the papillary dermis obscures the basement membrane zone and is accompanied by degenerative changes in the basal cell layer. If the reaction is intense, separation may occur at this area and may result in blisters and erosions.

> Biopsy is diagnostic.

Therapy

Oral lesions in lichen planus tend to be even more resistant to therapy than skin lesions. Asymptomatic involvement requires no therapy. In patients with symptoms (e.g., those with erosive disease), various agents have been tried with limited success. Some patients benefit from twice-daily applications of a potent (e.g., Lidex) topical steroid gel or ointment. Long-term use, however, predisposes to candidiasis and causes tissue atrophy. Intralesional triamcinolone (Kenalog) in a concentration of 5 mg/mL can be injected into local lesions, sometimes with long-lasting effect. Systemic corticosteroids are effective but should generally be avoided for this chronic disease. Topical tretinoin (Retin-A) gel 0.025%, applied twice daily, helps occasionally. A higher success rate is achieved with the orally administered retinoid, acitretin, in a dose of 25 mg daily. This drug is associated with many side-effects, so its use should be reserved for patients with severe, refractory disease. Such patients have also been successfully treated with oral cyclosporine. Improvement has also been reported with the use of a cyclosporine 'swish and spit' regimen in a dose of 5 mL (500 mg) three times daily. The extraordinary expense of this therapy can be reduced by applying smaller amounts of the medication directly to the lesions.

> **Therapy for Oral Lichen Planus**
>
> **Initial**
> - Topical therapy
>   - Steroids (e.g., fluocinonide gel 0.05%)
>
> **Alternative**
> - Topical
>   - Tretinoin gel 0.025%
>   - Cyclosporine solution
> - Intralesional steroids
> - Systemic therapy (reserved for extremely severe disease)
>   - Prednisone
>   - Acitretin
>   - Cyclosporine

Course and Complications

The course is measured in terms of months to decades. In patients with white lesions, approximately 50% experience remittance within 2 years, and of these, approximately 20% experience recurrence. The course is more prolonged in patients with blistering and erosive disease.

> The course is usually chronic.

Secondary candidal infection occurs in some patients with oral lichen planus. Cases of squamous cell carcinoma have been reported in association with oral lichen planus. Although this complication is uncommon, it appears to be more than coincidental. Therefore, patients with chronic erosive oral lichen planus should be followed; if an indurated lesion develops, a biopsy should be performed to rule out squamous cell carcinoma.

Patients with erosive oral lichen planus are at risk for squamous cell carcinoma.

Pathogenesis

The pathogenesis of lichen planus is discussed in Chapter 11.

THRUSH (ORAL CANDIDIASIS)

Key Points

1. Common in newborns and immunosuppressed adults
2. Appears as white patches that easily scrape off
3. Treat with topical or oral antifungals

Definition

Thrush is caused by infection of the oral epithelium with *Candida albicans*. The infected epithelium appears white and can be scraped off, leaving an inflamed base (**Fig. 22.6**).

Incidence

Thrush is most common in newborns, with one-third of neonates affected by the first week after birth. In adults, this disorder is uncommon and usually occurs in denture-wearing patients or in the setting of local or systemic immunosuppression. For example, oral candidiasis is frequent in patients with AIDS; in these patients, it may extend to involve the esophagus. Thrush also occurs in patients with chronic mucocutaneous candidiasis, a rare disorder in which chronic mucous membrane infection is accompanied by skin and nail involvement most likely secondary to a T-cell defect (**Fig. 22.7**).

Thrush is most common in newborns and immunosuppressed patients.

History

Mothers of infected newborns usually have a history of vaginal candidiasis during the latter part of their pregnancy. For older patients acquiring thrush, predisposing factors include the following: dentures; intraoral steroids, such as the aerosolized preparations used to treat asthma; broad-spectrum systemic antibiotics; and systemic immunosuppression from disease or drugs, including systemic corticosteroids.

Predisposing factors:
1. Dentures
2. Steroids
3. Antibiotics
4. Immunosuppression

Physical Examination

The lesions appear as white, curd-like papules and patches that sometimes resemble 'cottage cheese.' Much of this material can be scraped off, leaving an erythematous base. The tongue and buccal mucosa are affected most often. In denture-wearing patients, the mucosal surfaces under the dentures are involved, so the dentures must be removed for the mucosa to be evaluated. The angles of the mouth also may be involved (*angular cheilitis*), particularly when this area remains moist, such as in patients with ill-fitting dentures that cause excessive overlap of the upper lip (**Fig. 22.8**).

The curd-like material can be scraped off easily.

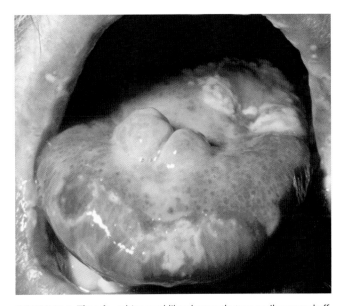

FIGURE 22.6 Thrush – white, curd-like plaques that are easily scraped off.

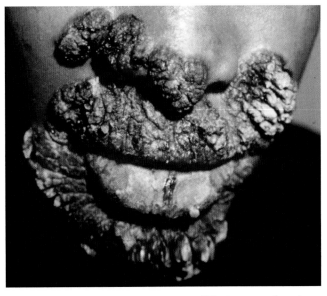

FIGURE 22.7 Chronic mucocutaneous candidiasis – warty, hyperkeratotic plaques; culture grew *Candida*.

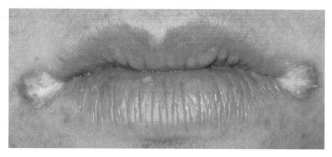

FIGURE 22.8 Angular cheilitis – moist white papules at corners of mouth; potassium hydroxide confirms clinical suspicion.

Differential Diagnosis

Lichen planus may be confused with thrush. However, thrush is differentiated from this and the other white lesion diseases in that the white material in thrush is scraped off easily.

Laboratory and Biopsy

The diagnostic test is a KOH examination of material from a scraping. With thrush, there is usually no difficulty in finding hyphae and pseudohyphae. These same elements would be found in the surface epithelium were a biopsy to be done, but because the KOH preparation is diagnostic, biopsy is not required. A culture is not helpful because *C. albicans* may be found in normal flora in the mouth. Candidiasis affecting adults who do not have predisposing factors, such as dentures or antibiotics or corticosteroid use, should prompt consideration of immunosuppressive conditions, such as AIDS.

> The KOH examination is diagnostic.

Therapy

Infants are treated with nystatin suspension by applying 1 mL (100 000 units) to each side of the mouth four times daily for 5–7 days. Adults can be treated with a 'swish and swallow' nystatin suspension in a dose of 5 mL (500 000 units) four times daily. An alternative topical therapy is clotrimazole (Mycelex) troches dissolved in the mouth five times daily for 1–2 weeks. Itraconazole (Sporanox) solution can also be used in a 'swish and swallow' regimen. Other systemic therapies include fluconazole (Diflucan) and ketoconazole (Nizoral) taken for 1–2 weeks.

In denture-wearing patients, candidal colonization of the dentures also must be treated. Acrylic dentures can be soaked overnight in a dilute (1 : 10) sodium hypochlorite (Clorox) solution, and a 0.12% chlorhexidine solution (Peridex) can be used for soaking metal plates.

Course and Complications

In newborns, thrush often clears spontaneously, but healing is hastened with therapy. In immunosuppressed patients, the disease can become recurrent and chronic. The most chronic infections are encountered in patients

---

Therapy for Thrush

Infants and Children
Initial
- None
- Nystatin suspension 2 mL (200 000 units) q.i.d.

Alternative
- Fluconazole oral suspension 2–3 mg/kg daily

Adults
Initial
- 'Swish and swallow'
  - Nystatin suspension 5 mL (500 000 µL) q.i.d.
  - Itraconazole solution 10 mL (100 mg) b.i.d.

Alternative
- Oral
  - Fluconazole 100 mg daily
  - Ketoconazole 200 mg daily

---

with the syndrome of chronic mucocutaneous candidiasis who are deficient in cellular immunity for *C. albicans*. Even in these patients, however, systemic therapy results in clearing, although recurrences usually follow cessation of therapy.

Complications are uncommon. In severely immunosuppressed patients, esophageal involvement can occur; rarely, the infection spreads systemically, causing disseminated candidiasis, which frequently is a fatal infection.

Pathogenesis

The pathogenesis of candidal infections is discussed in Chapter 12.

UNCOMMON CAUSES OF ORAL ULCERS

Numerous uncommon causes of oral ulcerations exist; several are listed in **Table 22.1**. Causes include autoimmunity, infection, and malignancy.

AUTOIMMUNE DISEASES

Pemphigus vulgaris and mucous membrane pemphigoid are autoimmune chronic blistering diseases with prominent or predominant mucosal involvement. Some 90% of patients with *pemphigus vulgaris* have oral involvement, and in 50%, the disease begins in the mouth (**Fig. 22.9**). Fragile blisters are easily broken, so erosions are the usual finding. The erosions are larger than those of aphthous stomatitis and are present continuously. Further details of this disease are discussed in Chapter 10. *Cicatricial pemphigoid* is a subepidermal blistering process confined to mucous membranes (**Fig. 22.10A**). Mucosae of the mouth, eyes, and conjunctivae are most frequently affected. Eye involvement may lead to scarring and blindness (**Fig. 22.10B**).

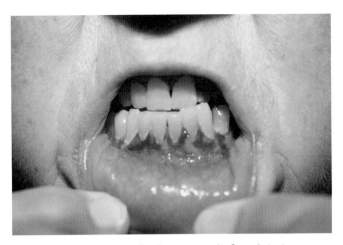

FIGURE 22.9 Pemphigus vulgaris. Erosive and inflamed gingiva present.

In both diseases, autoantibodies are directed against mucosal epithelia and are detected by direct immunofluorescence of biopsied mucosa (**Fig. 22.10C**). In pemphigus vulgaris, the antibodies are deposited between the cells in the epithelium; in mucous membrane pemphigoid, as in bullous pemphigoid, the deposition occurs in the basement membrane zone.

CANCER

Malignant tumors inside the mouth can erode and result in ulceration. Characteristically, these lesions are indurated. The most common cause is *squamous cell carcinoma*, but lymphomas and leukemias can also cause oral ulcers (**Fig. 22.11**). A biopsy is diagnostic. Intraoral squamous cell carcinoma is more likely to metastasize than cutaneous squamous cell carcinoma.

INFECTIONS

Infectious diseases causing oral ulcerations include, in decreasing order of frequency, viruses (herpesvirus and coxsackievirus), *Treponema* (syphilis), and systemic fungi (histoplasmosis). As already mentioned, herpes simplex rarely recurs inside the mouth, but the initial episode often involves the oral mucosa with *herpetic gingivostomatitis*. Erosive gingivitis is characteristic of primary oral herpetic infection and is usually accompanied by lesions on the lips and perioral skin (**Fig. 22.12**). It is accompanied by fever and regional lymphadenopathy and lasts for 2–3 weeks. Infection with coxsackievirus A-4 causes *herpangina*, which appears as a vesicular eruption in the posterior oral cavity lasting 7–10 days. Coxsackievirus A-16 causes *hand, foot, and mouth disease*, a distinctive disorder characterized by small vesicles in the posterior portion of the mouth and accompanied by similar lesions on the palms and soles (**Fig. 22.13**).

The lesion in primary *syphilis* is a *chancre*, which appears as a single, painless, punched-out ulcer and characteristically feels indurated. A darkfield examination of an oral chancre must be interpreted with caution because non-treponemal spirochetes normally colonize the mouth. If doubt exists, a serologic test for syphilis should

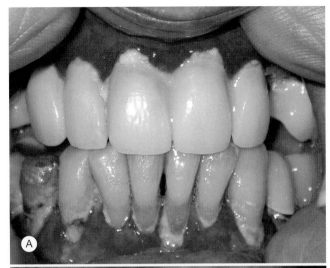
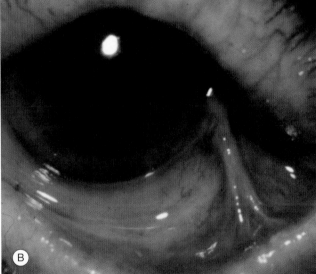
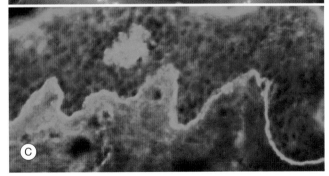

FIGURE 22.10 Cicatricial pemphigoid (mucous membrane pemphigoid). A. Shallow, inflamed ulcerations of gingiva. **B.** Eye involvement can lead to scarring and symblepharon formation. **C.** Immunoglobulin G deposition at the basement membrane zone.

be performed. If the result is negative, the test should be repeated in 1 month.

Indurated oral ulcerations occur rarely in patients with disseminated systemic fungal infections such as *histoplasmosis*. A biopsy with special stains and cultures confirms the diagnosis.

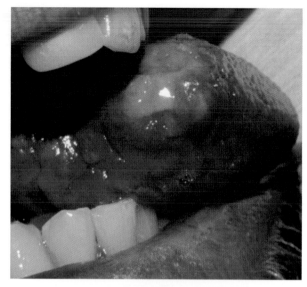

FIGURE 22.11 **Squamous cell carcinoma** – indurated nodule on the side of the tongue; biopsy is mandatory.

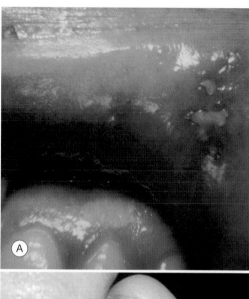

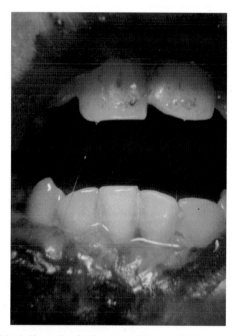

FIGURE 22.12 **Herpetic gingivostomatitis** – multiple painful erosions on labial mucosa and inflamed gingiva.

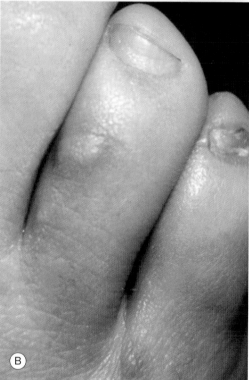

FIGURE 22.13 **Hand, foot, and mouth disease. A.** Erosions on upper labial mucosa. **B.** Pustule with red flare on toe.

Skin Signs of Systemic Disease **23**

Chapter Contents

- Fever and Rash
- Itching Patient
- Skin Signs of AIDS
- Skin Signs of Cancer
- Sun Sensitivity

ABSTRACT

The skin can be the window to systemic diseases. The presenting cutaneous symptoms and signs will lead the clinician to a more focused differential diagnosis and thus aid in the ordering of laboratory tests. In some cases, e.g., lymphoma, the skin biopsy is diagnostic.

FEVER AND RASH

Key Points

1. Characterize the rash to limit the differential diagnosis
2. Do laboratory tests based on the history and physical examination

A wide spectrum of diseases can present with fever and rash, including infections, drug reactions, collagen vascular diseases, and vasculitis. These causes are listed in **Table 23.1**, according to the primary cutaneous lesions: macules and papules, purpura, nodules and plaques, vesicles and bullae, and pustules. Some of these diseases (e.g., meningococcemia; **Fig. 23.1**) are life-threatening and require prompt diagnosis and treatment.

The methods used to diagnose the cause of fever and rash are similar to those used for fever of unknown origin. Clues are sought in the history and physical examination (**Fig. 23.2**). The type of eruption is particularly important, as noted in **Table 23.1**.

Diagnostic laboratory tests are directed by the history and physical examination. Simple procedures such as a potassium hydroxide preparation, a Gram-stain, and a Tzanck smear should not be overlooked. These 'bedside' tests can quickly establish an infectious cause. A skin biopsy with appropriate stains and cultures may be diagnostic. Further work-up is dictated by the clinical setting.

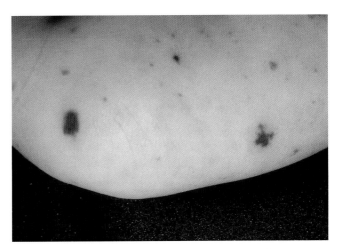

FIGURE 23.1 **Meningococcemia** – purpura in an acutely ill patient.

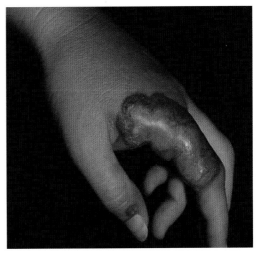

FIGURE 23.2 **Sweet syndrome** (acute febrile neutrophilic dermatosis) manifest by a bullous appearing hemorrhagic plaque. This patient had fever, neutrophilia, and acute myelogenous leukemia.

269

TABLE 23.1 Fever and Rash

Macules and papules (erythematous rashes)

Infections
  Viral
    Measles (rubella, rubeola)
    Adenovirus
    Echovirus
    Infectious mononucleosis
    Human immunodeficiency virus (HIV)
    West Nile
  Bacterial
    Staphylococcus – toxic shock syndrome
    Streptococcus – erysipelas, rheumatic and scarlet fever
    Typhoid fever
    Typhus – endemic
    Rat-bite fever
  Treponemal
    Erythema migrans (Lyme disease)
    Secondary syphilis
  Fungal
    Cryptococcosis
Drug reaction
Connective tissue disease
    Systemic lupus erythematosus
    Dermatomyositis
    Juvenile rheumatoid arthritis
Erythema multiforme
Kawasaki syndrome
Tumor necrosis factor receptor-associated periodic syndrome (TRAPS)
Familial Mediterranean fever
Hyperimmunoglobulinemia D syndrome (HIDS)

Purpura

Infections
  Viral
    Enterovirus
    Dengue
    Hepatitis
  Bacterial
    Gonococcemia
    Meningococcemia
    Pseudomonas septicemia
    Bacterial endocarditis
  Rickettsial
    Typhus – epidemic
    Rocky Mountain spotted fever
  Ehrlichiosis

  Fungal
    Candidal septicemia
Drug reaction
Vasculitis
Connective tissue disease
    Systemic lupus erythematosus
    Rheumatoid arthritis
Thrombotic thrombocytopenic purpura

Nodules and plaques

Infections
  Bacterial
    Tuberculosis
  Fungal
    Histoplasmosis
    Blastomycosis
    Coccidioidomycosis
Lymphoma
Erythema nodosum
Sweet syndrome

Vesicles and bullae

Infections
  Viral
    Herpes simplex (primary, disseminated)
    Herpes zoster (disseminated)
    Coxsackie (hand, foot, and mouth syndrome)
    Varicella
  Rickettsial
    Rickettsialpox
  Bacterial
    Staphylococcal scalded skin syndrome
Erythema multiforme

Pustules

Infections
  Viral
    Herpes simplex and zoster
    Varicella
  Treponemal
    Congenital syphilis
  Bacterial
    Gonococcemia
  Fungal
    Candidal septicemia
    Blastomycosis
Pustular psoriasis

ITCHING PATIENT

Key Points

1. Primary lesions suggest a dermatologic disorder
2. No primary lesions suggest a systemic cause

Because itching is a common symptom, it is often not diagnostically discriminatory. Chronic pruritus has a significant negative impact on quality of life similar to pain. **Table 23.2** lists two general categories in which itching is important: skin rashes in which itching is a *prominent* complaint, and systemic conditions causing generalized pruritus without primary skin lesions. For the itching patient, therefore, one must first decide whether the itching is caused by a skin disorder or a systemic disorder.

For skin disorders, primary lesions are present, and the type of primary lesion is used to identify the cause. Of the skin disorders listed, scabies (**Fig. 23.3**) is missed most often because of its nonspecific eczematous appearance and the difficulty of finding a mite. Dermatitis herpetiformis, a rare disorder, is also overlooked because the intensely pruritic vesicles are excoriated, leaving only nonspecific crusts. Xerotic (dry) skin is one of the most common causes of itching along with eczema and psoriasis.

TABLE 23.2 Pruritus

Primary Lesion (Skin Disease)	No Primary Lesion (Systemic Disease)
Macules	*Endocrine*
Urticaria pigmentosa (hives when stroked)	Hyperthyroidism
Erythroderma (Sézary syndrome)	Diabetes mellitus[a]
Drug eruptions	Hypothyroidism[a]
Papules and plaques	*Hepatic*
Scabies	Biliary obstruction
Lichen planus	*Renal*
Atopic dermatitis	Uremia
Psoriasis	*Hematologic*
Eczematous dermatitis	Lymphoma (especially Hodgkin's disease)
Insect bites	Polycythemia vera
Miliaria (heat rash)	Leukemia[a]
Drug eruption	Anemia[a]
Dry skin	*Carcinomas[a]*
Vesicles	Lung
Chickenpox	Gastrointestinal
Dermatitis herpetiformis	Breast
Urticaria	*Neuropsychogenic/ neuropathic*
	Delusions of parasitosis
	Neurodermatitis
	Infections
	Intestinal parasites

[a]Not well documented.

In pruritus resulting from systemic disease, primary skin lesions are absent (**Fig. 23.4**), although excoriations may be found. Patients with generalized pruritus require a medical history and physical examination. Screening tests include a complete blood count with differential, liver and renal function tests, thyroid profile, and chest radiography. Sometimes, however, a primary cutaneous or a systemic cause is not found.

SKIN SIGNS OF AIDS

Key Points

1. Chronic or unusual infection
2. Kaposi's sarcoma

Skin disorders are frequent in patients with acquired immune deficiency syndrome (AIDS). A generalized erythematous exanthem may accompany a febrile illness that occurs 3–6 weeks after the primary inoculation with human immunodeficiency virus (HIV). This symptomatic primary infection occurs in only approximately 10–20% of patients and is not diagnostic of early HIV infection. Skin signs are more frequent and more diagnostic later in the course of the disease. Immunosuppression predisposes to the infections, and probably also to some of the neoplastic manifestations. For example, infection with type 8 herpes simplex virus is strongly associated with Kaposi's sarcoma (**Fig. 23.5**), and human papillomavirus 16 has been implicated in oral squamous cell carcinoma. The cause of the miscellaneous disorders in patients with AIDS is unknown.

As noted in **Table 23.3**, some of the mucocutaneous findings are diagnostic for AIDS, as defined by the Centers for Disease Control and Prevention. HIV-infected individuals are diagnosed as having AIDS if they have any of the following mucocutaneous AIDS indicator conditions: Kaposi's sarcoma; herpes simplex ulcers lasting for more than 1 month; candidiasis of the esophagus

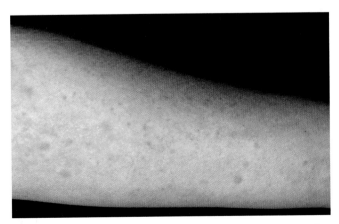

FIGURE 23.3 Scabies – markedly pruritic, nonspecific appearing papules.

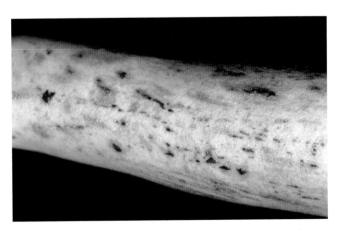

FIGURE 23.4 Hodgkin's disease – excoriations with no primary lesions in this patient with severe generalized pruritus.

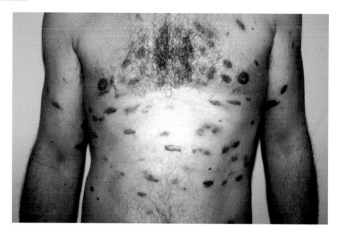

FIGURE 23.5 Kaposi's sarcoma – diffuse purple plaques in a patient with AIDS.

TABLE 23.3 Skin signs of AIDS

Skin Sign	Condition
Viral infection	Herpes simplex, chronic ulcerative[a]
	Herpes zoster, severe
	Oral hairy leukoplakia
	Genital warts
	Molluscum contagiosum, extensive
Fungal infection	Candidiasis (esophageal, tracheal, pulmonary)[a]
	Papules and nodules from systemic fungal infection[a]
	Seborrheic dermatitis (*Malassezia*), severe
Bacterial infection	Staphylococcal abscesses, recurrent and severe
	Papules, nodules, abscesses from mycobacterial infection[a]
	Bacillary angiomatosis
Neoplasm	Kaposi's sarcoma[a]
	Oral and rectal squamous cell carcinoma
	Lymphoma
Miscellaneous	Psoriasis, explosive and severe
	Acquired ichthyosis
	Pruritic papules/folliculitis

[a]AIDS-indicator conditions (see text).

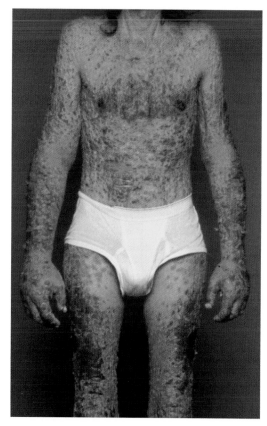

FIGURE 23.6 Psoriasis – severe and explosive onset in a patient with AIDS.

patient has more than one of them. For confirmation of HIV infection, blood testing is performed.

SKIN SIGNS OF CANCER

Key Points

1. Hard dermal nodules
2. Chronic chest 'cellulitis'

Numerous internal cancers have cutaneous manifestations that may be a clue to an underlying malignancy (**Table 23.4**). These lesions are produced by three mechanisms: infiltration of the skin with the cancer; changes in the skin produced by secretory products from the tumor; and unknown. The two most common infiltrative presentations of metastatic cancer are *hard* dermal nodules (**Fig. 23.7**) and chest 'cellulitis' from inflammatory breast carcinoma (**Fig. 23.8**). Examples of tumors with secretory products that cause skin changes include carcinoid tumors that produce vasoactive substances causing the classic flush, and tumors (most commonly small cell carcinomas of the lung) that produce polypeptides with melanocyte-stimulating activity. The necrolytic skin lesions that develop in patients with glucagon-secreting

or pulmonary tree; or extrapulmonary (e.g., skin) coccidioidomycosis, cryptococcosis, histoplasmosis, cytomegalovirus infection, or infection with a mycobacterial organism.

Of the disorders listed in **Table 23.3** that are not diagnostic for AIDS, oral hairy leukoplakia is the most suggestive because 83% of these patients develop AIDS within 3 years. For the other non-diagnostic disorders such as severe and explosive onset psoriasis (**Fig. 23.6**), the possibility of AIDS should be raised, especially if a

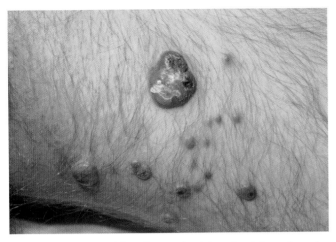

FIGURE 23.7 Metastatic lymphoma – hard dermal nodules and papules with some crusted.

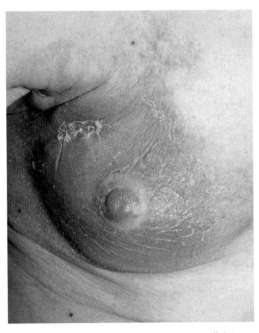

FIGURE 23.8 Inflammatory breast carcinoma – cellulitic appearing plaque.

SUN SENSITIVITY

Key Points

1. Sun-exposed distribution
2. The primary lesion helps to narrow the diagnosis

Table 23.5 outlines the small but important differential diagnosis for patients with photosensitivity. The eruption characteristically occurs on sun-exposed skin: the face, the 'V' of the neck, and the dorsal aspects of the arms and hands. A clear history of exacerbation by sunlight is present in all of these diseases except porphyria cutanea tarda.

TABLE 23.4 Skin signs of cancer

Skin Sign	Condition
Dermal nodules	Metastases – carcinoma, lymphoma, leukemia, myeloma
Erythema, macular, and generalized	Flushing – carcinoid
	Exfoliative erythroderma – cutaneous lymphoma
Erythema, localized plaques or nodules	'Cellulitis' – inflammatory breast carcinoma
	Subcutaneous fat necrosis – pancreatic carcinoma
Erythema with scaling patches	Erythema gyratum repens – carcinoma
	Neurolytic migratory erythema – glucagonoma
	Dermatomyositis – carcinoma
Pigmentation, macular and generalized	Addisonian pigmentation – ACTH/MSH-producing tumor
	Slate-gray pigmentation – melanoma
Pigmented patches and plaques	Acanthosis nigricans – carcinoma
	Eruptive seborrheic keratoses (Leser–Trélat) – carcinoma
Bullae/'juicy' plaques	Sweet syndrome – leukemia
	Paraneoplastic pemphigus – lymphoma, thymoma
Scaling (acquired ichthyosis)	Lymphoma (especially Hodgkin's disease)
	Excoriations (from generalized pruritus)
	Lymphoma (especially Hodgkin's disease)

ACTH, adrenocorticotropic hormone; MSH, melanocyte stimulating hormone.

TABLE 23.5 Sun sensitivity

Skin Sign	Condition
Macules, papules, plaques	Lupus erythematosus[a]
	Phototoxic – thiazide, quinidine, griseofulvin, doxycycline
	Photoallergic – sunscreens, fragrances
	Polymorphous light eruption – idiopathic[a]
Hives	Solar urticaria
Bullae	Porphyria cutanea tarda

[a]Most common causes.

pancreatic tumors may be due to the accompanying low levels of circulating amino acids that are normally needed for skin maintenance and repair. Acanthosis nigricans and acquired ichthyosis are examples of skin signs of cancer in which the pathogenesis is unknown.

Lupus erythematosus (**Fig. 23.9**), phototoxic drug eruption, and polymorphous light eruption are the most frequent causes of photosensitivity. Lupus erythematosus, whether cutaneous or systemic, has a diagnostic biopsy and patients with systemic lupus have positive serologic test results. The diagnosis of a phototoxic drug eruption is suggested by the history and confirmed by resolution of the eruption when the offending medication is discontinued. Polymorphous light eruption is a diagnosis of exclusion. It is an idiopathic disorder in which eczematous papules and plaques develop within 24 h after sun exposure and persist for a couple of days, despite sunlight avoidance. The skin biopsy has characteristic findings suggesting polymorphous light eruption. With repeated sunlight exposure, the eruption becomes less prominent, a phenomenon called 'hardening.'

Photoallergic contact dermatitis is an uncommon adverse effect of sunscreens. Photopatch testing can confirm this diagnosis. Solar urticaria is a rare idiopathic disorder that has a characteristic history of urticaria occurring within minutes of sun exposure and disappearing in approximately an hour with sunlight avoidance. Porphyria cutanea tarda typically presents as blisters and fragile skin affecting the dorsum of the hands (see Ch. 10).

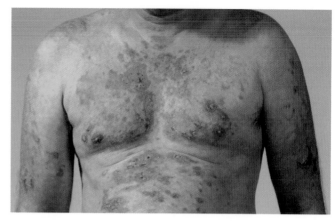

FIGURE 23.9 Subacute cutaneous lupus erythematosus – marked photosensitive eruption.

Self-Assessment 24

ABSTRACT

The following case studies are presented to reinforce what you have learned from reading *Principles of Dermatology*.

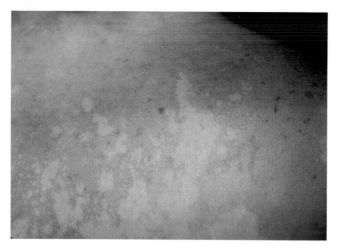

FIGURE 24.1 This 25-year-old woman was seen in the dermatology clinic in October, with a 4-month history of white spots on her upper trunk. With sun exposure over the summer, the spots had become more noticeable. They had not been red or symptomatic.

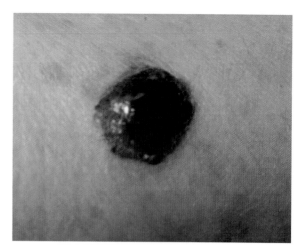

FIGURE 24.2 This 29-year-old Caucasian woman was seen in the dermatology clinic because of a bleeding growth. It had been present for 6 months and had grown rapidly. Her medical history was otherwise unremarkable.

CASE 1 – WHITE SPOTS (Fig. 24.1)

WHAT IS THE MOST LIKELY DIAGNOSIS?

This patient has a typical history for tinea versicolor. Scratching of the affected areas elicited a fine, crumbly scale, further heightening the suspicion of tinea versicolor.

WHAT TEST WOULD YOU DO?

The potassium hydroxide (KOH) preparation is diagnostic, revealing numerous short hyphae and spores.

HOW WOULD YOU TREAT THIS PATIENT?

Fluconazole was prescribed in a single 200 mg dose and repeated again in 2 weeks. The skin gradually repigmented over the following 3 months. Prevention of recurrence can be achieved with periodic washing of the affected areas with zinc pyrithione or selenium sulfide shampoo. Localized areas may be treated with Micatin cream.

> **Important Points**
>
> 1. If it scales, scrape it
> 2. It takes months for repigmentation to occur

CASE 2 – BLEEDING GROWTH (Fig. 24.2)

WHAT IS YOUR DIFFERENTIAL DIAGNOSIS OF THIS LESION?

This 6-mm nodule has the blue-black color and eroded surface typical of a nodular malignant melanoma. The differential diagnosis includes blue nevus, nodular pyogenic granuloma, and hemangioma.

WHAT WOULD YOU DO NOW?

An excisional biopsy revealed histopathologic changes typical of a nodular melanoma invading to a depth of 3.7 mm. The remainder of the skin examination and a general physical examination were normal. A sentinel lymph node biopsy was free of tumor. A 2.0-cm margin of normal skin was excised around the biopsy scar.

HOW WOULD YOU DETERMINE THE PROGNOSIS OF THIS PATIENT?

The prognosis of malignant melanoma is related to tumor thickness. Because this is a thick melanoma, the patient's prognosis is poor. Initial staging studies, including a complete blood count, liver function tests, and chest radiography, were negative.

> **Important Points**
>
> 1. All bleeding pigmented lesions should be examined by biopsy, not merely watched
> 2. Patients with thick melanomas have a poor prognosis
> 3. Most melanomas can be removed (and cured) when they are thin – if physicians and the public are alert to these diagnostic signs

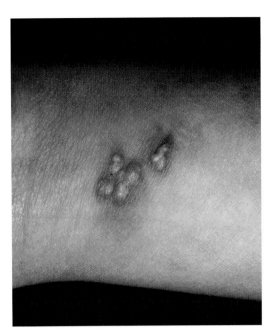

FIGURE 24.3 This 32-year-old woman had a history of a recurrent vesicular eruption. It started 5 years previously and recurs five or six times yearly. A tingling sensation precedes the onset of the rash.

CASE 3 – RECURRENT VESICLES
(Fig. 24.3)

WHAT IS YOUR DIAGNOSIS?

These grouped vesiculopustules on an erythematous base are typical of herpes simplex virus (HSV) infection. In addition, the history of a recurrent vesicular eruption in the same place is classic for this viral infection. No other diagnosis should be seriously considered.

WHAT LABORATORY TESTS WOULD YOU DO?

A Tzanck preparation is all that is necessary to confirm the clinical diagnosis. If still in doubt, a viral culture can be obtained.

WHAT ARE YOUR RECOMMENDATIONS TO THIS PATIENT?

Acyclovir, valacyclovir, or famciclovir may be used in patients with frequent recurrences. These medications reduce the duration of viral shedding and time to healing of lesions when administered early in the course of a recurrent episode.

Important Points

1. The Tzanck preparation is an easy laboratory test that confirms the diagnosis of HSV infection
2. Acyclovir, valacyclovir, and famciclovir are the current treatments of choice for HSV infection, but they are not curative

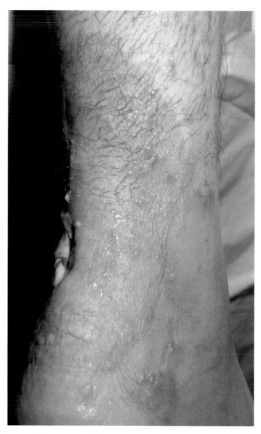

FIGURE 24.4 This 40-year-old man was using povidone-iodine ointment dressings on a non-healing wound. Two weeks after starting this therapy, he developed a markedly pruritic eruption under the dressing. The physical examination revealed a 3-cm necrotic ulcer with a surrounding erythematous, papulovesicular rash conforming to the rectangular area covered by the povidone-iodine dressing.

CASE 4 – PAPULOVESICULAR RASH
(Fig. 24.4)

WHAT IS YOUR DIFFERENTIAL DIAGNOSIS?

This acute eczematous eruption confined to the area beneath the dressing is typical of contact dermatitis. A less likely cause would be a fungal or bacterial infection since pustules are absent.

HOW WOULD YOU TREAT THIS PATIENT?

The dermatitis cleared when the povidone-iodine dressings were replaced with saline compresses and a topical steroid cream.

HOW WOULD YOU PROVE YOUR DIAGNOSIS?

The patient had no history of iodine sensitivity. However, he had been applying the povidone-iodine dressing for 2 weeks, which is sufficient time to develop sensitivity to this compound. A patch test to 10% povidone-iodine solution was positive, confirming the diagnosis of allergic contact dermatitis.

Important Points

1. Topical medicaments are an important cause of allergic contact dermatitis and should be suspected when an eczematous eruption occurs in areas that conform to application of the medication
2. Avoidance of the allergen is the treatment of choice. Topical steroids hasten resolution of allergic contact dermatitis
3. Patch testing confirms the diagnosis of allergic contact dermatitis

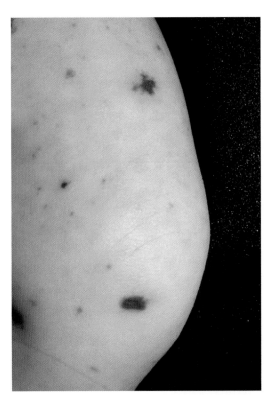

FIGURE 24.5 This 4-month-old infant was brought to the emergency room because of sudden onset of fever and irritability that progressed within hours to obtundation. On physical examination, hypotension, nuchal rigidity, and skin lesions were seen.

CASE 5 – FEVER AND PURPURA (Fig. 24.5)

WHAT DO YOU SEE?

The lesions (shown here on the thigh) are palpable and purpuric. Petechiae are also present.

WHAT IS THE MOST LIKELY DIAGNOSIS?

In a patient with fever and palpable purpura, sepsis is the first and most important diagnosis to consider. In an infant or young child, bacterial meningitis is the most likely diagnosis, particularly if the child has signs of meningeal irritation or altered consciousness.

HOW WOULD YOU PROVE IT?

Blood and cerebrospinal fluid (CSF) should be obtained immediately for bacterial cultures. In addition to culturing the CSF, a Gram-stain, cell count and differential, glucose, and protein should be performed.

HOW WOULD YOU TREAT IT?

This is a medical emergency and empiric antibiotic therapy must be administered promptly beginning with vancomycin plus cefotaxime or ceftriaxone.

Important Points

1. In a patient with fever and palpable purpura, sepsis must be considered first
2. If bacterial sepsis is *suspected*, antibiotic treatment should be initiated immediately

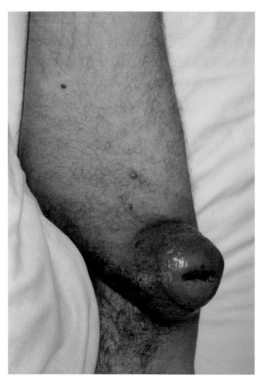

FIGURE 24.6 This 50-year-old man sought medical attention because of the large nodule on his right hip. Otherwise, he felt well. On examination, the nodule felt extremely firm. A healing excision from a recent biopsy was present.

CASE 6 – FIRM NODULE (Fig. 24.6)

WHAT IS THE MOST LIKELY DIAGNOSIS?

Malignancy must be suspected for all firm dermal nodules. A benign process would be particularly unlikely in this patient because of the size and firmness of the nodule.

WHAT SHOULD BE DONE NEXT?

All suspicious nodules must be examined by biopsy. Biopsy of this nodule was initially interpreted as undifferentiated metastatic malignancy, not further classifiable.

DO YOU SEE ANY OTHER SKIN LESIONS OF NOTE?

The patient was examined to search for the primary tumor. The physician noted on the patient's mid-thigh a small, darkly pigmented plaque with bluish color, irregular border, and white halo. Excision and histologic examination of this lesion revealed a primary malignant melanoma. Retrospective review of the original biopsy from the nodule showed it to be metastatic melanoma.

Important Points

1. For firm nodules in the skin, malignancy must be suspected, and biopsy must be performed
2. A complete skin examination is an important part of every physical examination. In this case, it revealed the source of the primary malignant disease

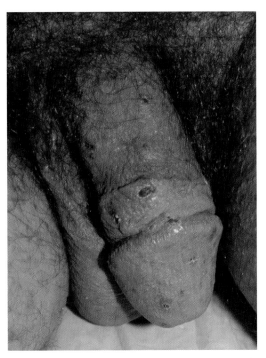

FIGURE 24.7 This 30-year-old man presented with a 2-month history of itching that had become progressively more severe. The itching spared the head but was otherwise generalized, including involvement of the genitalia.

CASE 7 – GENERALIZED ITCHING PAPULES (Fig. 24.7)

WHAT DO YOU SEE?

Physical examination revealed discrete papules, many of which were excoriated.

WHAT IS THE MOST LIKELY DIAGNOSIS?

The most likely diagnosis is scabies. Scabies should be suspected for any generalized pruritic process. For pruritic papules on the penis, the diagnosis is scabies until proved otherwise.

HOW WOULD YOU CONFIRM IT?

The diagnosis is secured if a mite can be found. For this, careful examination of the entire cutaneous surface should be carried out in the search for burrows. The patient's hands, particularly the finger webs, should be scrutinized. Even if a burrow is not found, scraping of several of the papules may reveal a mite or mite products. In this patient, scraping of the penile papules was positive.

Important Points

1. Suspect scabies for any generalized itching condition
2. The index of suspicion should be greatly heightened if pruritic papules are found on the penis
3. Although burrows are diagnostic and are the best place to scrape, the mite can also be recovered from scrapings of the papules

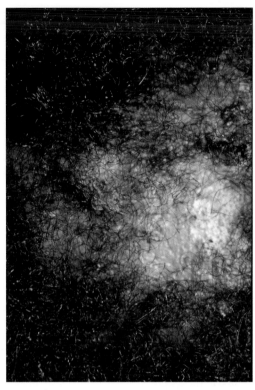

FIGURE 24.8 This 7-year-old girl developed itching of the scalp and progressive areas of hair loss 6 weeks before she was seen in the dermatology clinic. The use of an antiseborrheic shampoo, oral erythromycin, and a topical antifungal agent had not helped. The physical examination revealed circular areas of non-scarring alopecia. The scalp was erythematous, crusted, and scaling in the patches of hair loss.

CASE 8 – HAIR LOSS (Fig. 24.8)

WHAT IS YOUR DIFFERENTIAL DIAGNOSIS?

The differential diagnosis of non-scarring alopecia includes stress-induced alopecia, androgenic alopecia, trichotillomania, alopecia areata, lupus erythematosus, and fungal infection. The patchy nature of the hair loss ruled out stress-induced and androgenic alopecia and systemic lupus erythematosus. This was not discoid lupus erythematosus because the patient had no scarring or follicular plugging. Alopecia areata and trichotillomania do not scale. The inflammation and scaling of the scalp favored a fungal infection.

WHAT WOULD YOU DO NOW?

A KOH preparation of several plucked broken hairs was positive for spores and hyphae. If the KOH preparation had been negative or equivocal, a fungal culture would have been done. A biopsy with special stains also enables the diagnosis of a fungal infection, but usually is not needed.

HOW WOULD YOU TREAT THIS PATIENT?

The patient should be treated with oral griseofulvin or terbinafine for at least 4–6 weeks. Treatment is continued until the scalp appears normal, new hair regrowth appears, and the KOH preparation is negative.

Important Points

1. KOH preparations of tinea capitis require plucked hairs. The scale may be negative. When in doubt, do a fungal culture
2. Treatment of tinea capitis requires oral preparations; topical antifungals are ineffective

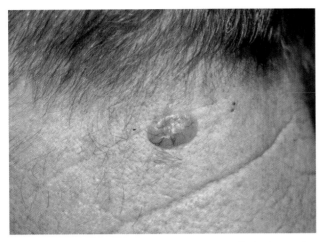

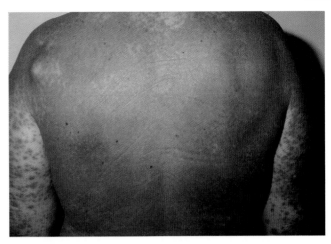

FIGURE 24.9 This 55-year-old Caucasian man was seen in the dermatology clinic because of a nodule on his neck. It had been present for the past year and was growing slowly. His occupation was farming. He had a history of tanning poorly and numerous sunburns. His past medical and dermatologic history was otherwise negative.

FIGURE 24.10 Two days after this patient's coronary artery bypass graft, he developed a pruritic, intensely erythematous eruption that began on his face and trunk, became confluent, and subsequently involved the extremities. He was afebrile and otherwise was recovering uneventfully from the surgical procedure.

CASE 9 – PEARLY NODULE (Fig. 24.9)

WHAT IS YOUR DIFFERENTIAL DIAGNOSIS?

This pearly nodule with telangiectasia and a central depression is characteristic of a nodular basal cell carcinoma. The surrounding skin is thickened and furrowed, and has a yellowish hue typical of sun damage. Also to be considered in the differential diagnosis is a squamous cell carcinoma. The relatively recent onset of the lesion rules out a flesh-colored nevus, and its size and color make sebaceous hyperplasia (yellow) unlikely.

HOW WOULD YOU TREAT IT?

Excisional surgery was chosen to remove this tumor. Histologic examination confirmed the clinical diagnosis of basal cell carcinoma and the margins of the excision were free of tumor.

WHAT PRECAUTIONS SHOULD THIS PATIENT TAKE IN THE FUTURE?

This patient should prevent further sun damage to the skin by wearing protective clothing, including a broad-brimmed hat and a long-sleeved shirt, when working outside. In addition, he should use a broad spectrum sunscreen with a sun protection factor (SPF) of ≥30. He should be seen again in the clinic for periodic examinations because his chances of developing skin cancer in the future are high: 30% in the next 5 years.

Important Points

1. The recent acquisition of a pearly nodule may indicate a skin cancer
2. Basal cell carcinoma is treatable and rarely metastasizes
3. Precautions should be started to prevent excessive ultraviolet radiation exposure, because this is the most common etiologic agent of basal cell carcinoma

CASE 10 – GENERALIZED ERYTHEMA (Fig. 24.10)

The patient had been taking furosemide and diazepam on a long-term basis. On the day of surgery, he was started on cefazolin, codeine, morphine, and flurazepam.

WHAT IS THE MOST LIKELY DIAGNOSIS?

A drug eruption is favored by virtue of the intensity of the erythema, the confluence of the rash, the presence of pruritus, and the absence of fever or other constitutional symptoms.

IF YOU SUSPECT A DRUG REACTION, WHAT IS THE MOST LIKELY DRUG?

The most likely drug is one that has been recently administered. From the list of this patient's recent drugs, cefazolin, a cephalosporin antibiotic, is statistically the most likely culprit.

HOW CAN YOU PROVE IT?

No confirmatory tests are available. The diagnosis is purely clinical. Only a rechallenge with the suspected drug (which is rarely done) could confirm your clinical suspicion.

Important Points

1. For any eruption, consider a drug etiology
2. In most cases, the history and physical suggest a drug eruption. There are no definitive diagnostic tests

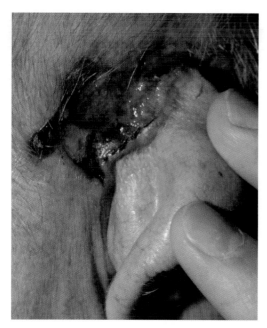

FIGURE 24.11 This 60-year-old man had a 1-year history of a non-healing ulcer. He had otherwise been in excellent health and had no previous history of ulcers. The general physical examination was normal. The skin examination revealed a fair-skinned Caucasian man with a 6-cm shallow ulcer behind his ear. The base of the ulcer was clean and the surrounding skin appeared normal. The patient had used a number of topical preparations and had been treated with systemic antibiotics without success.

CASE 11 – ULCER BEHIND THE EAR
(Fig. 24.11)

WHAT IS YOUR DIFFERENTIAL DIAGNOSIS OF THIS ULCER?

The differential diagnosis of an ulcer is extensive. Neither the history nor the physical examination gives us a clue to its origin. However, a negative medical history and normal general physical examination make a vascular, hematologic, neurologic, drug, connective tissue disease, or physical cause of this ulcer less likely. This leaves a neoplastic, infectious, or unknown origin.

WHAT WOULD YOU DO NOW?

The next step is a biopsy of the ulcer.

WHAT IS THE BEST TREATMENT?

The biopsy revealed a basal cell carcinoma. Treatment was excision of the tumor with the Mohs technique, which conserves as much normal skin as possible and ensures the greatest potential for cure.

Important Points

1. Ulcers of unknown origin must be examined by biopsy to rule out neoplasm
2. Appropriate therapy is dictated by correct identification of the cause

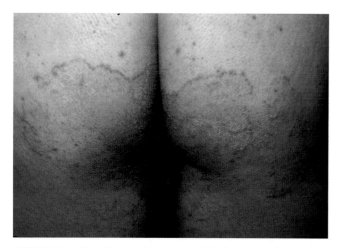

FIGURE 24.12 This 50-year-old man was initially seen in dermatology consultation for generalized dry, red, itchy skin of many years' duration. Three skin biopsies were performed and showed an inflammatory infiltrate with some atypical lymphocytes, but not in sufficient numbers to diagnose mycosis fungoides (Sézary syndrome). The patient was treated with a topical steroid cream applied to the entire skin surface. At follow-up 2 weeks later, much of the rash had improved, but a sharply demarcated, scaling eruption persisted on the buttocks and feet.

CASE 12 – SCALING RASH (Fig. 24.12)

WHAT IS YOUR DIFFERENTIAL DIAGNOSIS?

The differential diagnosis would include any of the papulosquamous disorders, although pityriasis rosea, secondary syphilis, and discoid lupus erythematosus are not likely. Mycosis fungoides must still be considered for these irregularly shaped, asymmetric plaques, especially in light of the patient's history. Partially treated psoriasis is also possible. For a scaling rash of uncertain origin (especially one in which the lesions have sharp, serpiginous borders), however, fungus infection is the first diagnosis to exclude.

WHAT TEST WOULD YOU DO NEXT?

A KOH preparation should be the first test. A positive result in this case is diagnostic for a superficial fungal infection.

Important Points

1. This case illustrates the general rule: if the diagnosis is uncertain and if the rash scales, scrape it
2. Because the eruption was widespread, a systemic antifungal agent was prescribed, and the rash cleared

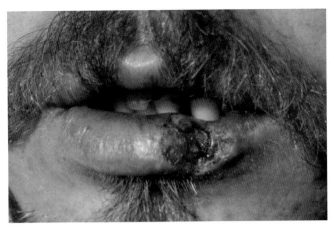

FIGURE 24.13 This 33-year-old man presented with a lesion on the lower lip that started with a 'cigarette burn' 1 year earlier. He remained a heavy smoker. On examination, you see a crusted and scaling ulcer.

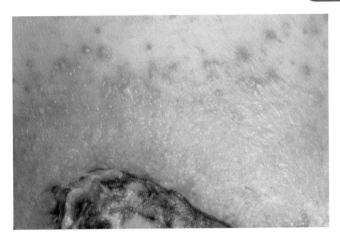

FIGURE 24.14 This 38-year-old woman was receiving wet dressings to her leg ulcer. After 1 week, a rash developed around the ulcer.

CASE 13 – LIP ULCER (Fig. 24.13)

HOW WOULD YOU COMPLETE THE PHYSICAL EXAMINATION?

Palpate the lesion and feel for local lymph nodes. This lesion felt firm and indurated. The patient's head and neck were examined for lymphadenopathy, but none was found.

WHAT IS YOUR MOST LIKELY DIAGNOSIS?

For a chronic mucous membrane ulcer, squamous cell carcinoma is the favored diagnosis. The suspicion is heightened by the finding of induration.

HOW WOULD YOU CONFIRM IT?

A biopsy is required. In this case, it confirmed the diagnosis of squamous cell carcinoma. The lesion was totally excised subsequently.

Important Points

1. Smoking is a risk factor for the development of mucous membrane squamous cell carcinoma
2. Biopsy is required for all chronic ulcers, especially when these lesions are indurated

CASE 14 – PUSTULES AND PAPULES SURROUNDING AN ULCER (Fig. 24.14)

DESCRIBE WHAT YOU SEE

Surrounding the ulcer is a pink, slightly scaling patch with satellite pustules and papules.

WHAT IS YOUR DIFFERENTIAL DIAGNOSIS?

The differential diagnosis includes contact dermatitis from the medications used in the dressings. However, with the satellite pustules and papules, candidiasis also needs to be considered.

WHAT IS THE FIRST DIAGNOSTIC TEST YOU WOULD DO?

The first diagnostic test should be a KOH examination of a scraping from the border of the lesion. In this patient's case, it was positive for hyphae. It is difficult to distinguish microscopically between candidal and dermatophytic hyphae, but the clinical picture favors candidiasis.

HOW WOULD YOU TREAT IT?

Local therapy with a topical imidazole cream, applied sparingly twice daily, and discontinuation of the wet dressings resulted in prompt clearing of the eruption.

Important Points

1. Do not forget a simple diagnostic test like a KOH
2. Azole antifungals such as miconazole treat both candida and dermatophytes. Nystatin only is effective against candida

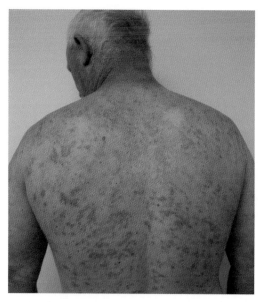

FIGURE 24.15 This 48-year-old man developed pruritic, pink, slightly scaling papules and plaques 3 years ago, on the head, neck, trunk, and arms. His review of systems and past medical history were unremarkable. It was uncertain whether the eruption was exacerbated by sunlight.

CASE 15 – SCALING RASH ON HEAD, TRUNK, AND ARMS (Fig. 24.15)

WHAT IS YOUR DIFFERENTIAL DIAGNOSIS?

A widespread scaling eruption suggests a differential diagnosis of psoriasis, tinea, pityriasis rosea, secondary syphilis, lupus, T-cell cutaneous lymphoma, and dermatitis. The chronic course eliminates pityriasis rosea and syphilis.

WHAT WOULD YOU DO NOW?

A KOH preparation was negative for fungal elements. A skin biopsy helped make the diagnosis and it revealed pathologic changes of lupus erythematosus. Further lab testing resulted in normal antinuclear antibody, double-stranded DNA, complete blood cell count with platelet count, urinalysis, and complete metabolic profile. Testing for SSA was positive and SSB was negative. All these tests confirm the diagnosis of cutaneous lupus erythematosus.

HOW WOULD YOU TREAT THIS PATIENT?

Sun protection is first and foremost, even with his questionable history of sun sensitivity. Topical steroids such as triamcinolone cream 0.1% in large volumes may suppress the lupus. The next step would be an antimalarial such as hydroxychloroquine 200 mg b.i.d. If these interventions fail, then systemic immunosuppressants are warranted.

Important Points

1. Scaling eruptions in a sun-exposed distribution suggest the possibility of lupus erythematosus
2. A skin biopsy is diagnostic of lupus
3. The medical history, general physical, and laboratory examination will separate cutaneous vs systemic involvement

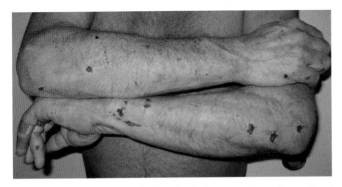

FIGURE 24.16 This 51-year-old man had a 10-year history of occasional blisters on his hands. In the past year, the blistering had become worse, with involvement of his arms, legs, and head. A trip to the beach flared the eruption.

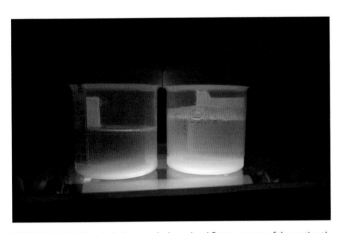

FIGURE 24.17 Wood's light revealed coral red fluorescence of the patient's urine (left) compared with the normal lime green urine (right).

CASE 16 – CRUSTED EROSIONS ON THE DORSUM OF THE HANDS AND FOREARMS (Figs 24.16, 24.17)

WHAT IS YOUR DIFFERENTIAL DIAGNOSIS?

Erosions suggest a blistering disease. The configuration, distribution, and history make an infectious cause such as herpes and impetigo unlikely. Acute contact dermatitis causes vesicles and bullae. However, there is no evidence of dermatitis surrounding the crusts. Uncommon blistering diseases such as pemphigus, bullous pemphigoid, epidermolysis bullosa, and porphyria should be considered. Hypertrichosis of his temples suggests the diagnosis of porphyria cutanea tarda.

WHAT WOULD YOU DO NOW?

A simple test is to fluoresce the patient's urine with a Wood's light (**Fig. 24.17**). This is a quick screen for detecting elevated urine uroporphyrins. His laboratory tests revealed elevated liver enzymes, iron levels, and urine uroporphyrins. He had negative tests for hepatitis C, hemochromatosis, and HIV. His diagnosis is porphyria cutanea tarda.

HOW WOULD YOU TREAT THIS PATIENT?

Treatment begins with preventing further liver and cutaneous damage by cessation of alcohol and precipitating medications, as well as starting sun protection. Phlebotomy is the first-line therapy. Low-dose antimalarials such as hydroxychloroquine can be used as an alternative treatment.

Important Points

1. When there is crusting, look for blisters
2. Consider a systemic disease in your differential diagnosis of skin symptoms

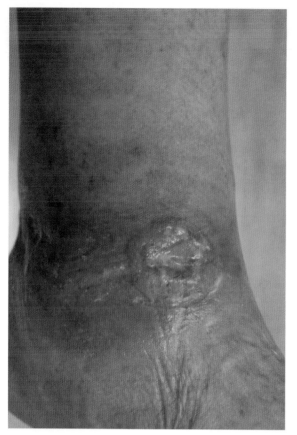

FIGURE 24.18 This 81-year-old man developed this painless, pink, ulcerated nodule on his lower leg a couple of months ago. He otherwise felt healthy and the general physical examination was normal.

CASE 17 – NODULE ON THE LOWER LEG (Fig. 24.18)

WHAT IS YOUR DIFFERENTIAL DIAGNOSIS?

The first concern is whether this nodule represents a malignancy. If the patient was immunosuppressed or had a history of trauma, then an infectious or physical etiology could be considered.

WHAT DIAGNOSTIC WORK-UP WOULD YOU DO NOW?

A skin biopsy is the next logical step. It revealed a dense dermal, hyperchromatic, lymphoid infiltrate of CD-20, BCL-2, and BCL-6-positive B cells. Further work-up revealed a normal complete blood count and metabolic profile. A positron emission tomography/computed tomography whole-body scan had enlarged lymph nodes in the neck.

WHAT IS YOUR DIAGNOSIS AND HOW WOULD YOU TREAT THIS?

The diagnosis is B-cell lymphoma, leg type. This lymphoma occurs in the elderly and has an overall 60% survival at 5 years. Treatment depends on the extent of the disease and can be local radiation, chemotherapy, and rituximab alone or in combination.

Important Points

1. Consider a malignant neoplasm as the cause of nodules, especially if they are firm, dermal, and eroded
2. A skin biopsy is an important diagnostic tool

Index

Page numbers followed by 'f' indicate figures, 't' indicate tables, and 'b' indicate boxes.

289

MEDIEVAL AMERICAN ART

Masterpieces of the New World before Columbus

BY

PÁL KELEMEN

Third Revised Edition

IN TWO VOLUMES

Volume Two

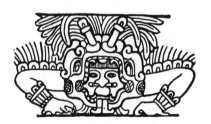

Dover Publications, Inc., New York

Published in Canada by General Publishing Company, Ltd.,
30 Lesmill Road, Don Mills, Toronto, Ontario.
Published in the United Kingdom by Constable and Company, Ltd.,
10 Orange Street, London WC 2.

This Dover edition, first published in 1969, is an unabridged
and revised republication of the second edition (Macmillan,
1956) of the work originally published by The Macmillan Company, New York, in 1943. The alterations made in the present edition are explained in detail in the author's new Preface to the
Dover Edition (see especially page xiii).

International Standard Book Number: 0-486-21994-1
Library of Congress Catalog Card Number: 68-28248

Manufactured in the United States of America

DOVER PUBLICATIONS, INC.
180 Varick Street
New York, N. Y. 10014

Contents

Illustrations in Volume Two

This compilation contains data, measurements, and various credits not included in the text or captions. Measurements denote height unless otherwise stated. When a museum or a collector owns the piece and has also furnished the photograph of it, the name is given only once. The following abbreviations have been used for names which occur most frequently.

AMNH. American Museum of Natural History, New York
BG. Brummer Gallery, Inc., New York
CIW. Carnegie Institution of Washington, Washington, D. C.
DO. Dumbarton Oaks Collection, Washington, D.C.
EZK. Elisabeth Zulauf Kelemen
FAM. Fogg Art Museum, Cambridge, Mass.
FM. Field Museum, Chicago, Ill.
INAH. Instituto Nacional de Antropología e Historia, Mexico, D.F.
JW. John Wise, Ltd., New York
LA. Laboratory of Anthropology, Santa Fé, N.M.
LAM. Los Angeles Museum of History, Science, and Art, Los Angeles, Calif.
M. Museum
MAG. Museo de Arqueología, Guatemala
MAI. Museum of the American Indian, Heye Foundation, New York
MAL. Museo Nacional de Arqueología, Lima, Peru
MARI. Middle American Research Institute, Tulane University, New Orleans, La.
MFA. Museum of Fine Arts, Boston, Mass.
MH. Musée de l'Homme, Paris, France
MN. Museo Nacional de Arqueología, Historia y Etnografia, Mexico, D.F.
MVBG. Museum für Völkerkunde, Berlin, Germany
MVBS. Museum für Völkerkunde, Basle, Switzerland
MVVA. Museum für Völkerkunde, Vienna, Austria
OSM. Ohio State Museum, Columbus, Ohio
Ph. Photograph
PM. Peabody Museum of Harvard University, Cambridge, Mass.
RC. Rossbach Collection, Chichicastenango, Guatemala
TM. Textile Museum of the District of Columbia, Washington, D.C.
UCAL. University of California Museum, Berkeley, Calif.
UMP. The University Museum, Philadelphia, Pa.
USNM. United States National Museum, Washington, D.C.

Weaving

Metal – Work

< x >

plaque representing a tower with four birds of prey. 6 in. TM. *c* and *d*) Quimbaya cast gold female idols, Antioquia. 6 and 9 in. respectively. PM and UMP.

219 Cast gold staff heads, Colombia. *a*) Quimbaya?, cast in several pieces. 5 in. MFA. *b*) Montería, Dept. of Bolívar, northwestern Colombia. About 8 in. long. MAI. *c*) Quimbaya? dog, about 2 in., and man blowing trumpet. Museo Preistorico ed Etnografico, Rome.

220 *a*) Quimbaya gold crown with soaring condor, Antioquia, Colombia. 6 in., including bird. UMP. *b*) Quimbaya gold helmet with human figure in repoussé. British M.

221 *a*) Gold helmet, Darién, Panama. 4¾ in., weight 11 oz. PM. *b*) Gold helmet, Sitio Conte, Coclé, Panama. Weight 7⅞ oz. PM.

222 *a*) Gold alligator or crocodile with human prey, Costa Rica. 4¼ in., weight 61½ grams. Museo Nacional, San José, Costa Rica. *b*) Gold shark pendant. Walters Art Gallery, Baltimore. *c*) Massive gold alligator carrying conventionalized object, Coclé, Panama. 7 in. long. TM. *d*) Twin alligators with conventionalized objects, Coclé, Panama. About 3½ in. PM.

223 Embossed gold plaques, Coclé, Panama. *a*) Diameter, 8 in. *b*) About 8½ in. UMP.

224 Masterpieces of the jeweler's art, Coclé, Panama. *a*) Insect of gold and quartz. 2 in. PM. *b*) Gold cuff with animals in repoussé. About 7 in. long. PM. *c*) Gold dogs or alligator cubs. About 2½ in. long. PM. *d*) Solid gold pendant with inset emerald, fashioned into a fantastic animal. 4¼ in. long. UMP.

225 Pendants with twin figures. *a*) *Tumbaga* (alloy of gold and copper), Coclé, Panama. About 3½ in. high and 5 wide. PM. *b*) Gold, Chiriquí?. About 4 in. wide. British M. *c*) Gold, Costa Rica. AMNH.

226 *a*) Gold bird pendant, Costa Rica. About 4 in. MFA. *b*) Gold bird pendant, Colombia. MAI. *c*) Gold figurine with pipe?, Panama. Peabody Museum of Yale

University. *d*) Gold rattle in human form, near volcano of Quarialba, Costa Rica. 3 in. MAI.

MAYA AND MEXICAN AREAS

227 *a*) Tarascan copper mask of Xipe-Totec. About 5½ in. MN. *b*) Copper bell in form of human face, Honduras. Over 3 in. MARI. *c*) Copper bell in form of turkey, Santa Barbara, British Honduras. About 3 in. PM.

228 Finger rings. *a*) Cast gold with descending eagle and pendant, Oaxaca, Mexico. About 2½ in. long. Oaxaca M. Ph: INAH. *b*) Copper with human head, Guatemala-Salvador border. About 1¼ in. Dr. E. O. Salazar Coll., San Salvador. *c*) Gold with feathered serpent, Oaxaca. About 1 in. MAI. *d*) Gold with glyphs, Oaxaca. Diameter, about ⅞ in. MN. *c*) Gold with feathered serpent, Oaxaca. About 1 in. UMP.

229 Gold articles of personal adornment, Oaxaca, Mexico. *a*) Labret, or lipplug, Ejutla. About 2½ in. long, including tongue. MAI. *b*) Gold diadem, diameter 6 in., and repoussé feather, about 13½ in., Monte Albán. Oaxaca M. Ph: INAH. *c*) Labret, Tlacolula. AMNH. *d*) Bracelet, Tomb 7, Monte Albán. Oaxaca M. Ph: Osuna.

230 Necklaces. *a*) Gold, Tomb 7, Monte Albán, Oaxaca, Mexico. About 2½ in. wide. Oaxaca M. Ph: INAH. *b*) Toltec silver and copper alloy, Texcoco, Mexico. FM. *c*) Gold, Tomb 7, Monte Albán. Oaxaca M. Ph: Osuna.

231 *a*) Mixtec cast gold pectoral of Jaguar Knight as God of Death, Tomb 7, Monte Albán, Oaxaca, Mexico. 4½ in., weight 3 oz. Oaxaca M. Ph: Osuna. *b*) Gold figure of the Aztec king, Tizoc, Texcoco, Mexico. 3½ in. MAI. *c*) Cast gold pectoral with fantastic animal, Costa Rica. AMNH.

232 *a*) Gold pendant made up of seven elements. 8½ in. long. *b*) Small gold mask of Xipe-Totec. 2¾ in. Both from Tomb 7, Monte Albán, Oaxaca, Mexico, and in Oaxaca M. Phs: Osuna.

< xi >

ILLUSTRATIONS IN VOLUME TWO

Jade and Other Semiprecious Stones

Murals and Manuscripts

Miscellaneous Applied Arts

perforated shell ornament, near Vera Cruz, Mexico. About 7 in. MARI.

282 *a*) Hohokam ring of glycimeris shell, Gila Valley, Ariz. Diameter, ¾ in. LAM. *b*) Xipe-Totec mask of reddish shell, Mexico. About 2½ in. BG. *c*) Mother-of-pearl pendant with seated Maya warrior, Tula, Hidalgo, Mexico. 3¾ in. FM.

283 Chimú shell mosaic-work. *a* and *c*) Earplugs. Diameter, about 2½ in. *b*) Cup with wooden base, Lambayeque, Peru. 9⅜ in. All MAI.

BONE-CARVING

284 *a* and *d*) Details of an incised peccary skull, showing two Maya priests and wild boars, Copán, Honduras. PM. *b* and *c*) Jaguar bone with glyphic carving, Tomb 7, Monte Albán, Oaxaca, Mexico. Between 6 and 8½ in. Oaxaca M. Ph: INAH.

285 *a*) Hohokam bone awl handle with mountain sheep surmounting rattlesnakes, Ariz. 1⁹⁄₁₀ in. LAM. *b* and *c*) Maya priest carved of jaguar bone, probably a staff head, provenience unknown. 2¾ in. MN.

FEATHER-WORK

286 *a*) Aztec feather headdress or cloak, gift of Mexico to Emperor Charles V. Greatest

height, over 4 ft. MVVA. *b*) Vignette from Sahagún's Codex (Florentino), showing craftsmen engaged in feather-work and merchant (top left) bringing in raw material. Ph: AMNH.

287 *a*) Aztec feather shield mounted on jaguar skin, Mexico. Diameter, about 2 ft. MN. *b*) Aztec ceremonial shield of feathers with gold outlining, showing the coyote Fire-god. *c*) Aztec feather standard with "fire-flower." Diameter, about 18 in. *b* and *c* were both gifts from Mexico to Charles V. MVVA.

288 Mitre and infula, Mexican feather-work, post-Columbian period. Pitti Gallery, Florence, Italy. Ph: Alinari.

289 *a*) Feather fan with woven framework, Central Coast? of Peru. About 10 in. MAI. *b*) Pair of Ica earplugs decorated with feather-work. Diameter, 2⅝ in. MAI. *c*) Chimú feather poncho, or shirt. AMNH.

290 *a*) Ica feather poncho with birds and feline figures. 33½ in. square. Ph: after Lehmann and Doering. *b*) Chimú feather poncho with geometric design. 51 x 42 in. Ph: after Schmidt.

< xix >

Facets of Daily Life

FACETS OF DAILY LIFE

Register of Museums and Collections

This list shows the location of most of the objects illustrated in this survey. In addition, there are twenty-five private collections represented which are not included here.

American Museum of Natural History, New York, N.Y.
28b, 33d, 62a, 69b, 89a, 97c, 98b, 101b, 104c, 114b, 115c, 115d, 117a, 118a, 118c, 119a, 134a, 140b, 142d, 150a, 156d, 158b, 162b, 164b, 164c, 165a, 166a, 166b, 167a, 169c, 171c, 172b, 176c, 183b, 185a, 190b, 191b, 191c, 191d, 192b, 196a, 204a, 204b, 207b, 213a, 225c, 229c, 231c, 243b, 245b, 276a, 276e, 289c, 293a, 294a, 294c, 294d, 294f, 296c, 298a, 299b.

British Museum, London, England
59a, 61a, 76b, 85b, 86a, 90, 111c, 117c, 126c, 131a, 144a, 153c, 174a, 174b, 203b, 205b, 206d, 209d, 210c, 211b, 214c, 217a, 220b, 225b, 238b, 242b, 246a, 255b, 275a, 278a, 278b, 278c, 279a, 292d, 299a.

Brooklyn Museum, Brooklyn, N.Y.
27b, 30b, 63b, 146a, 151h, 177a, 188a, 214a.

Brummer Gallery, New York, N.Y.
61b, 68c, 68d, 88c, 94a, 95b, 115a, 116c, 117e, 125a, 131d, 137a, 161a, 207a, 235b, 237c, 237d, 239f, 240b, 241g, 242d, 243c, 247b, 247c, 249b, 251d, 253a, 254b, 256a, 256d, 276c, 282b.

Buffalo Fine Arts Academy, Albright Art Gallery, Buffalo, N.Y.
135a.

Buffalo Museum of Science, Buffalo, N.Y.
106e.

Carnegie Institution of Washington, Washington, D.C.
262a, 263a.

City Art Museum, St. Louis, Mo.
132a.

Cleveland Museum of Art, Cleveland, Ohio
117b, 195c, 215a, 253d.

Copan Museum, Copan, Honduras
82a, 83b.

Cranbrook Academy of Art, Bloomfield, Mich.
66a, 156c, 199a, 202a.

Dartmouth College Museum, Hanover, N.H.
88b.

Denver Art Museum, Denver, Colo.
102b.

Dumbarton Oaks Collection, Washington, D.C.
66b, 206a, 206b, 206e, 241a, 250b, 250c, 252c, 252d.

Field Museum, Chicago, Ill.
108b, 109c, 111a, 111d, 111e, 112b, 114a, 114c, 125b, 126a, 133b, 149a, 156a, 156b, 161d, 162f, 184c, 191a, 193a, 193b, 200a, 204d, 230b, 243a, 244a, 258a, 272a, 276d, 277a, 282c, 296f.

Institute of Arts, Minneapolis, Minn.
64a.

Instituto Nacional de Antropología e Historia, Mexico, D.F.
264d.

Laboratory of Anthropology, Santa Fé, N.M.
101c, 102c, 103c, 105a, 105d.

Los Angeles Museum of History, Science, and Art, Los Angeles, Calif.
101e, 145c, 282a, 285a.

Metropolitan Museum of Art, New York, N.Y.
63b, 114b.

< xxiii >

Middle American Research Institute, Tulane University, New Orleans, La.
60b, 80d, 86d, 94b, 116d, 126b, 134d, 134e, 140a, 142e, 143a, 145b, 149c, 158c, 163a, 163b, 163c, 163d, 227b, 237a, 245h, 251f, 281b.

Montezuma Castle National Museum, Montezuma Castle, Ariz.
171a.

Musée de l'Homme, Paris, France
113c, 123b, 133a, 133c, 153d, 154c, 155a, 155d, 157b, 158d, 161b, 185b, 185c, 200b, 238a, 250a, 256b.

Museo Arqueológico, Guatemala, Guatemala
72a, 97a, 97b, 127a, 127b, 127c, 127d, 128a, 128b, 128c, 129a, 132b, 134b, 135c, 136a, 136c, 141a, 141d, 145d, 236b, 242c.

Museo Arqueológico Nacional, Madrid, Spain
81a, 214b.

Museo de la Universidad, Lima, Peru
99a.

Museo Nacional, San José, Costa Rica
97d, 148d, 222a, 294e.

Museo Nacional de Arqueología, Lima, Peru
99b, 198a, 198c, 199c, 201a, 202c, 258c.

Museo Nacional de Arqueología, Historia y Etnografia, Mexico, D.F.
58a, 58b, 65a, 65c, 67a, 67b, 67c, 69a, 75b, 78b, 82b, 82c, 84b, 93b, 110a, 110b, 110c, 111b, 111f, 112c, 113a, 115b, 119b, 121c, 122a, 122b, 124a, 124b, 227a, 228d, 233b, 234a, 237f, 241f, 246b, 248d, 249a, 249d, 254a, 257c, 257d, 260a, 260b, 261b, 269, 285b, 285c, 287a, 292a, 292b, 292e, 293c.

Museo Preistorico ed Etnografico, Rome, Italy
219c, 273a.

Museum für Völkerkunde, Basle, Switzerland
148b, 274.

Museum für Völkerkunde, Berlin, Germany
121a, 131b, 273c.

Museum für Völkerkunde, Vienna, Austria
59b, 65b, 68b, 189b, 239b, 240a, 249c, 251b, 286a, 287b, 287c.

Museum of Art, Providence, R.I.
201b.

Museum of Fine Arts, Boston, Mass.
192a, 202b, 216a, 219a, 226a.

Museum of New Mexico, Santa Fé, N.M.
4b, 170a.

Museum of the American Indian, Heye Foundation, New York, N.Y.
86c, 101a, 103f, 108c, 108d, 109b, 109d, 114d, 117d, 123a, 123c, 125c, 133d, 138a, 139d, 143c, 144c, 151e, 154a, 155b, 155c, 157c, 164a, 164d, 178a, 194a, 194b, 194c, 195b, 195d, 197a, 198b, 199b, 200c, 208a, 208b, 216b, 216c, 217b, 217c, 219b, 226b, 226d, 228c, 229a, 231b, 233a, 240c, 240d, 241b, 242a, 245e, 258b, 271a, 272b, 279b, 280a, 280b, 280c, 283a, 283b, 283c, 289a, 289b, 295a, 296e, 297b, 297c, 298b, 298c.

Oaxaca Museum, Oaxaca, Mexico
68a, 123d, 124c, 228a, 229b, 229d, 230a, 230c, 231a, 232a, 232b, 251e, 255a, 257a, 284b, 284c.

Ohio State Museum, Columbus, Ohio
194d, 295b, 295d, 296a, 296b, 296d.

Peabody Museum of Harvard University, Cambridge, Mass.
77a, 78a, 85a, 87, 88d, 89b, 102a, 106a, 106c, 106e, 107, 108a, 109a, 134c, 137b, 142c, 146b, 146c, 146d, 146e, 147a, 147b, 147c, 147d, 147e, 147f, 159a, 161c, 171b, 176b, 189c, 197b, 218c, 221a, 221b, 222d, 224a, 224b, 224c, 225a, 227c, 234b, 238c, 238d, 240e, 240f, 241d, 244b, 248a, 248b, 248c, 259a, 259b, 262b, 263c, 273b, 276f, 284a.

Peabody Museum of Yale University, New Haven, Conn.
148c, 148f, 149b, 205c, 226c, 295c.

Phillips Academy, Andover, Mass.
281a, 281c.

Pitti Gallery, Florence, Italy
288.

Puebla Museum, Puebla, Mexico
59c, 60c, 252a, 256c, 293b.

Rijksmuseum, Leyden, Holland
235a.

Rossbach Collection, Chichicastenango, Guatemala
96a, 136b, 141b, 141c, 208c, 208d, 237e, 241c, 241h.

Southwest Museum, Los Angeles, Calif.
170b.

Textile Museum of the District of Columbia, Washington, D.C.
165b, 175a, 175c, 178b, 178c, 179a, 180a, 182b, 183c, 187, 218b, 222c.

United States Department of the Interior, Park Service, Washington, D.C.
103e, 105b.

United States National Museum, Washington, D.C.
98c, 101d, 103a, 103b, 103d, 105c, 138b, 189a, 204c, 235d, 295e, 295f.

University of California, Berkeley, Calif.
162a, 162d, 162e, 167c, 167d, 175b, 179b, 181b, 183a, 184a.

University of Colorado, Boulder, Colo.
104b, 106b, 106d, 169b, 169d, 170d.

University of New Mexico, Albuquerque, N.M.
259c.

University of Pennsylvania, The University Museum, Philadelphia, Pa.
72b, 73a, 74a, 77b, 83a, 86b, 94d, 95a, 96b, 98a, 100a, 100b, 104a, 118b, 118d, 120, 121b, 129c, 130a, 130b, 130c, 130d, 139b, 149d, 150b, 150c, 150d, 152a, 152b, 154b, 158a, 160a, 167b, 168, 169a, 170c, 174c, 181a, 184b, 201c, 203a, 205a, 210a, 211a, 212, 213b, 215b, 218d, 220a, 223a, 223b, 224d, 228e, 239c, 244c, 245f, 251a, 271b, 272d, 272e, 297a.

Wadsworth Atheneum, Hartford, Conn.
253b.

Walters Art Gallery, Baltimore, Md.
60a, 62b, 222b.

Wise, John, Ltd., New York, N.Y.
176a, 177b, 179c, 180b, 180c, 182a, 182c, 186a, 186b, 190a, 196b, 239a, 241e, 245a, 245c, 275b.

Worcester Art Museum, Worcester, Mass.
157a.

SUPPLEMENT, 1968

The following items are now in the Cleveland Museum of Art: 61b*, 163a, 176a†, 179c†, 186a†, 186b†, 195a, 207a* (scraper and disk at right and necklace), 224c, 235b*, 237d*, 239f*, 240b*, 241g*, 247b*, 247d, 256d*. The items marked with an asterisk were acquired from the Brummer Gallery and should be considered as deleted from the Brummer listing; those marked with a dagger were acquired from John Wise, Ltd.; number 163a was formerly in the collection of the Middle American Research Institute; number 224c was formerly in the collection of the Peabody Museum at Harvard.

The following items are now in the Dumbarton Oaks Collection: 135b, 137a*, 207a* (scraper and disk at left), 213c, 237a, 237c*, 239a†, 243c*, 247c*, 254b*, 282b*. The asterisks and dagger have the same meaning as above; number 237a was formerly in the collection of the Middle American Research Institute. Numbers 241a, 250b, and 250c have been transferred from Dumbarton Oaks to private collections.

Numbers 242d and 253a of the Brummer Gallery listing are now in private collections.

< XXV >

VI

Weaving

IN THE 16th century three great civilizations of the Eastern Hemisphere simultaneously reached a high point in the textile art.[1] The silks of China were an item greatly prized in that commerce for which Columbus braved the unknown western sea. The rugs and fabrics of Persia, with metal threads frequently interwoven in their patterns, were goods eagerly sought in European trade. Europe saw the perfection of Venetian velvets and the rise of the great tapestry-weaving centers in the Low Countries and France.

Upon recognizing the skill of the native American weavers, the Spaniards made haste to employ it for their own ends, introducing new raw materials, looms of different construction, and patterns to imitate the fabrics popular in the market of their day. Thus, the textiles of medieval America were neglected and nothing was done toward their preservation at the time of the Conquest. What we know today of pre-Columbian weaving is gained largely from excavated material.

In many cases the soil has been unwilling to give back what was interred in it. A few beautiful fragments have been unearthed in the Southwest, preserved by the dry climate, but in the Mexican and Maya areas nearly nothing remains. The famous cities of these regions lay either in the subtropical belt, where there is heavy rainfall for many months each year, or in moist tropical lowlands. In either case the delicate fabrics generally disintegrated. Some bits of material were brought up in the diving activities at the Sacred Well at Chichén Itzá, but our clearest idea of the mature textile art in these areas is derived from the elaborate costume details faithfully recorded on stelae, stone and stucco reliefs, and vase paintings. In the Andean Area, however, where both an arid climate and peculiar burial customs—to be described later—were particularly favorable for the preservation of textiles, we find our greatest field for study.

The beginning of the art of weaving in general cannot be traced, for by the time recording had progressed far enough to picture details of the crafts, textiles were well advanced. In the Eastern Hemisphere it is possible to observe the development of various techniques to a certain extent. Babylon and Egypt produced a smooth plain cloth or linen weave, which was frequently decorated with embroidery. The early Greeks made a sort of bobbin weave, enlivening the web with a spatter of flowers of a different color. About the same time, tapestry in varicolored designs appeared in Egypt.[1]

In pre-Columbian America, however, where research in the higher cultures does not carry back more than two thousand years, this is not the case. Basketry was the forerunner of textile weaving in certain parts of the Southwest and will be discussed as such under *Pls. 169* and *170,* where examples of it are shown. Elsewhere there is no evidence of the beginnings, as the earliest pieces of woven fabric known, discovered in the Andean Area and coinciding in date with the beginning of the Christian era, show the same perfection and variety of techniques as the later ones; the only development that can be traced is in style and pattern preferences.[105] This is all the more remarkable because all the techniques known to the rest of the world plus several peculiar to the Peruvian weavers were employed in this region.

As was pointed out, the regions that used the true loom coincide in general with our five areas. This implement was the hand loom, one end of which—usually a half-polished stick—was hooked to a tree, fixed between two poles, or adjusted on a wall. The other end, with a belt attached, was placed around the waist of the weaver so that a movement of the body would slacken or tighten the warp. The width of the woven stuff could not be much broader than the convenient reach of the weaver, that is, about 30 inches. Such hand looms, called "girdle-back looms," can be seen in use today, especially in the more remote parts of Middle and South America (see *Pl. 173, fig. a*). It would appear that the women did a great part of the weaving, just as they made much of the pottery, another primarily "domestic" art.

Recently more intensive investigation into the techniques of pre-Columbian weaving has brought forward the opinion that these looms were not the only type in existence. Peruvian weavers sometimes produced a cloth over 5 feet wide, which must either have been set up on a larger loom or so arranged as to allow several persons to weave simultaneously on the same warp.[104]

The raw material for these textiles was primarily cotton, but human and animal hair and the feathers of birds were also woven into the fabric. In some regions the fiber of the maguey plant was utilized. The Andean Area was particu-

larly fortunate in having the wool of several members of the camel family, peculiar to the Andes—the llama, guanaco, alpaca, and vicuña. The finest in quality
is that of the vicuña, which in suppleness and sheen bears a resemblance to silk.[133]
This animal was protected by royal edict and only those of royal blood could use
its fleece.[139]

The numerous spindle whorls of clay, stone, and other materials found indicate that the thread was spun everywhere by the same general method: the strand
was twisted by hand and kept even by the revolving weight at the end of the
thread. Two- to seven-ply yarns have been found, far surpassing in fineness
those that a modern machine produces with the same materials. While Gobe-
lins seldom contain more than twenty warps to an inch, one Peruvian tapestry is
said to have had forty-two.[7]

The dyes used have been analyzed by modern research methods and found to
be of mineral, vegetable, and animal origin, depending on the shade desired and
the locality. They are always color fast. A rich carmine was obtained from the
cochineal, an insect which feeds upon a cactus common in Mexico and Peru.
Vast quantities of them had to be collected because of their minute size. Their
dried and pulverized bodies were highly valued as trade goods and provided one
of the most brilliant hues on the shining palette of medieval America.

Most of the textiles were probably used for apparel, but belts and carrying
straps were needed, as well as bags of various sizes and durability. In addition,
provision was made in the buildings for curtains and awnings, which may have
consisted of straw matting or strips of fabric. Doubtless the same taste and skill
that characterize their other applied arts were lavished upon their fiber ham-
mocks, an ingenious invention of pre-Columbian America. While most civilizations used from early times a sort of bedstead that rested on the ground, the Indian of many regions slung his sleeping outfit between two uprights of his hut.
Even today in tropical and subtropical districts there is great variety to be found
in this survival from medieval times.

Besides varied patterns and brilliant colors, embroidery and the addition of
fringe, tassels, and medallions embellished the textiles. Feathers were often incorporated into the stuff of shirts and mantles. Metal spangles, little bells, and
bits of colored stone, as well as mother-of-pearl and other shell where available,
were applied as trimming.

The costume of the pre-Columbian peoples appears not to have been tailored.
Rectangular pieces were woven to fit the individual requirement and the patterns
adapted to each. Besides the breechcloth, a man wore a loose tunic to cover the

upper part of the body. Sometimes it had no sleeves, but more often short ones made of simple rectangles were sewed to the sides at the shoulder and stitched together beneath the arm. The women wore a long tunic and mantle.

In the designs, both geometric and stylized nature motifs are used. The puma, fish, birds, and anthropomorphic figures occur the most frequently in the Andean Area, often in such strongly conventionalized forms that they are scarcely recognizable. Flower and plant motifs are exceptional.

Our European ancestors learned during the centuries of contact to enjoy the textiles of the Chinese and Persian civilizations, although these carried nothing of the Greek beauty ideal in their make-up. The mythical significance of their strange-looking human and animal forms or abstract patterns was disregarded, and the bit of silk, the rug, or embroidery prized for its exotic charm.

As yet, we have not had time enough to become so familiar with the figures in pre-Columbian textiles, and their stiffness still adds to our confusion in appraising them. Probably most of the patterns had religious and tribal significance that was traditional. Of all the arts, however, weaving tends to the most rapid conventionalization of pattern, and without a doubt designs were frequently chosen for their eye appeal without regard to any inner meaning.

As several erudite works specializing in the subject of medieval American textiles have been published here and abroad in the last decades, neither the presentation nor discussion of all the known techniques is undertaken here. A glossary, however, is included for convenient reference, defining the terms met with in this chapter.[168]

GLOSSARY

Bobbin, or *weft-pattern, weave* employs wefts of various colors upon the concealed warp, the pattern being carried only by the wefts. It may be single- or double-faced.

Brocade. A single-faced fabric in which the design is built up by alternating a pick of basic weft with a pick of decorative yarn, the greater diameter and softer twist of which allow the weft to be beaten up and buried under it. The decorative element appears in a raised pattern.

Crêpe. A fabric of crinkled texture, produced by using threads of exceedingly tight twist, often combined with other threads of reversed hard twist.

Damask weave has certain wefts floated upon the face of the fabric, their smooth unbroken surfaces forming a pattern against the background of the picked warps.

Double cloth. A fabric woven on two sets of warps of contrasting colors, usually natural light and dark wool or cotton, each with its own weft of self-color. In the process of weaving, pairs of wefts alternate to form the design so that it appears on both faces but in reverse coloring, the finished webs being separate except at the edges of the design.

Gauze. A lacelike web, not necessarily sheer, in which pairs of warp threads are twisted together and the crosses made permanent by the insertion of a pick of weft.

Loom, or *warp-pattern, weave.* The counterpart of bobbin, or weft-pattern, weave. It employs the more numerous warp threads to conceal the wefts and carry the design.

Meshed netting is fashioned without a loom, since one end must be free to make the knots and turns through the loops. There are many types.

Pile-knot fabric, or *simile velours,* was formed by enmeshing bunches of fiber or wool in a loosely knitted web. The knots, caught in the loops of the single thread as the fabric grows, are usually of different color to create a design, giving the effect of velvet or plush. *Pile-knot cord* was made by binding doubled tufts of wool of various colors mixed with hair to a core of three-ply cotton yarn twisted together.

Plain weave. A fabric made by picking warps singly with a single weft. Variations are achieved by the passing of a single weft under and over pairs of warps, or of two wefts under and over single warps. When two weft threads are interlaced with two warps, it is known as *basket weave.*

Rep. A corded fabric produced by wefts of smaller diameter beaten up upon less numerous rigid warps. Similar to unpatterned tapestry weave. A *warp rep* was made in Peru by employing a greater number of warps which, in close weave, concealed the wefts. This was sometimes striped or patterned, making a kind of false tapestry.

Tapestry. A close woven fabric, in which the wefts, always of lesser diameter and softer twist than the warps, are inserted slackly under and over equal units of the warp and are beaten up so as to cover them completely, each color going only so far as the design requires.

Kelim tapestry is distinguished by vertical slits where two colors meet and the component wefts turn back upon their respective warps.

Interlocking tapestry uses a manipulation of the wefts to avoid slits, either by looping the weft of one color into that of another or by slanting the design to engage successively the same warps by wefts of adjacent colors.

Limning, called also *eccentric weft,* is effected by leaving a bare warp between adjacent colors and introducing a weft, usually black, which wraps it
and, following the design, loops into both colored wefts.

Eccentric weave results from a manipulation of the wefts so that they cross
the hidden warps at various angles to produce curved designs.

Figure-8 stitch results from the passing of the yarn under and over the same
two warps or groups of warps.

Three-dimensional, or *needle, knitting.* A type of embroidery used for covering
seams, finishing edges, and creating three-dimensional figures that are built
up on a self-foundation by a chainlike adaptation of buttonhole stitch.

Tie-and-dye. A form of resist dye, in which parts of the cloth, usually a loosely
woven voile or crêpe, are bound round with a cord, which is waxed or otherwise treated to resist the penetration of dye. The cloth is then dipped. When
unwrapped, the parts which had been covered appear as rings, squares, or
stripes in natural color on a colored ground. Successive tying and dyeing in
different colors produces a multicolored patterned cloth.

Twill. A weave in which wefts are carried over one and under two or more
warp threads, producing a diagonal ribbed effect. The direction of the shift
may be reversed to form chevrons, diamonds, etc., in the cloth, either self-
colored or patterned.

Twined technique. A system of looping fibers in basketry.

Voile. A loosely woven cloth of hard-twisted threads in plain weave with either
or both elements paired.

Weft-loop, or *looped, weave* is a plain cloth of which one pick is inserted very
loosely at a given interval and the slack pulled out in loops after every ninth
warp or so.

Besides three-dimensional knitting and pile-knot cord, already described, the
following weaves are believed to be peculiar to ancient Peru: *discontinuous,* or
interlocking, weft weave, a method probably taken over from tapestry, in which
the weft is turned back on its own warp and looped into a weft of another color;
discontinuous, or *interlocking, warp weave,* in which the warps do not extend the
length of the fabric but are looped into those of another color; *warp-weft technique,* which contrived to fill an open space with warp and weft composed of the
same thread, and *skeleton weft technique,* a related weave, called by Lila O'Neale
"multicolored patchwork" and believed to have been built on a temporary scaf-
folding of wefts, later withdrawn.[105]

‹ 218 ›

THE SOUTHWEST

While weaving in the Andean Area appears before us already perfected, in the Southwest, an area known to have developed considerably later, we find interesting stages of the craft. The Basket Maker, the first figure to emerge from the archaic mists of this region, produced no textiles but was extraordinarily dexterous in fashioning baskets. That a satisfactory life can be made without either pottery or loom weaving is demonstrated by certain tribes living today in British Columbia.[103] Conceivably both pottery and weaving might branch from the skill of basketry, the former craft utilizing the shapes, the latter, the methods. Even after these other techniques were in practice, the Pueblo peoples, who followed the Basket Makers, retained a certain skill in basket-work.

There is a definite relationship between basketry and textile weaving. Before man raised the materials himself, reeds, vines, twigs, cane, rushes, leaves, and fiber offered themselves to be made into baskets, mats, and covers. Pre-Columbian baskets were usually made in one of two ways. Most were coiled; the second technique involved the intertwining of material about a set of radiating ribs. The twilled weave also occurs, but apparently not until the establishment of the Pueblo culture.[73]

The carrying or burden basket (*Pl. 169, fig. b*), 15 inches high and 32 in diameter, comes from Canyon del Muerto, Arizona, and is classified as Basket Maker III, or about A.D. 500 to 700. Fashioned with a remarkably even, beady surface, it carries both horizontal and vertical designs, each differing from the other. The colors used are red and black, making a sharp contrast with the ground.

The two Basket Maker sandals below it (*fig. d*), 9 inches long, are from northeastern Arizona and were woven some thirteen hundred years ago of fine cord made of yucca fiber. Each bears a complex pattern in red and black, fundamentally alike but differentiated in color and minor details. The Basket Makers seem to have made two types of sandals—one finely twined of cords, another fashioned of whole or partly shredded yucca leaves. They were perishable articles of clothing, yet much artistic finesse and maturity are manifest in these specimens, not only in the design but in the twined technique.

The three shallow baskets (*fig. c*), also from Canyon del Muerto, are all woven alike but have different decorative patterns. The two larger are Basket Maker III. The smallest, from Pueblo I Period, 800 to 950, is particularly gay with its several colors. Here the same ingenuity for working out a design is apparent that so skillfully adapted a geometric pattern to the rounded surface of pottery.

The "cradle" (*fig. a*) is a product of the Cliff-dweller people of Moki Canyon, Utah (Pueblo III, 1050 to 1300). It is 22½ inches high. The shape is highly complicated, but even so the two broad bands with their interlocking zigzag pattern are executed with absolute clarity. The fashioning of the legs shows extraordinary command of the technique. On the steep tricky paths among the canyons, this method of transporting and protecting young children must have been truly efficient.

The steady advance toward true textile technique is evident in *Pl. 170, fig. c,* a fragment of a burden strap woven of yucca cord, probably Basket Maker. It is 15 inches long and comes from Navaho Canyon in southwestern Colorado. The elaboration given to an article of such lowly purpose speaks well for the artistic feeling of these people. The bias zigzag is very effective on the narrow band.

The twined woven fabric of Basket Maker III (*fig. d*) shows still further advance, although it probably antedates the use of the true loom.[73] Stripes of various widths and patterns run across the unicolored material with no two of them alike. A similar fragment, now in the Southwest Museum in Los Angeles, is woven of the hair of buffalo and Rocky Mountain goat.

It was a general practice in the Southwest to apply strips of rabbit skin or feathers strung on a cord to a structural base such as that seen in *fig. b*. This foundation, made of yucca fiber, was for a small rabbit-skin blanket (Basket Maker or Early Pueblo), and traces of the strips of fur are still clinging to it. The solid workmanship in the piece is noteworthy.

In a much better state of preservation are the two feather blankets in *fig. a,* made in the same manner. They were found as shown, wrapped about the desiccated body of a child in Jemez Cave, New Mexico. The larger of the two, 34 inches long, inclosed the whole bundle, while the other covered the naked body of the child. Between were two deerskin robes, one heavier than the other. The three ears of corn were for the journey to the after-world. Both blankets show clearly the minute work involved in their manufacture. Infinite patience and a knowledge of all potentialities in the raw material were necessary to produce these articles, which after more than seven hundred years have still survived in good condition.[2]

About the 8th century cotton appears in the Southwest.[31] The introduction of this material furnished the early Pueblo peoples with a more workable fiber, and they made full use of it. It was undoubtedly raised in the locality where it was woven. The pieces illustrated on *Pl. 171* were probably made on the true loom.[38]

Our first cotton textile (*fig. a*) is a bag, 12½ inches long, found in a ruin near Montezuma Castle, Arizona. It is woven in damask technique with a white warp and black weft, the design produced by floating the warp thread. Here we meet again the interlocking motif that was seen in the pottery of this area. The date of the piece is approximately 14th century.

The larger lacelike fragment in *fig. b* is done in warp-weft openwork technique. It is 8 inches long, probably Pueblo III, and comes from Grant County, New Mexico. It shows a varied pattern composition in which oblique series of frets alternate with grille work. The narrow band above it is true lace.

The fragment in *fig. c,* dated in the 14th century, is unique, perhaps the finest extant piece of textile work from the medieval Southwest. It was about 48 inches by 30 originally and was a small robe or kilt found wrapped around a body in Grand Gulch, Utah. The piece is made in diagonal weave, producing a raised pattern in variations of frets, further accentuated by the use of yellow, black, and red.[38] Even in its fragmentary state, one can see how tightly the complicated pattern is knit into a single decorative scheme.

It seems appropriate to follow up these meager remnants with illustrations that show how persistently the talent of these peoples has continued. Although they now use different materials and new methods, it is safe to say that ancient traditions, even to some extent patterns, still survive.

A scene in Canyon de Chelly, Arizona (*Pl. 172, fig. a*), shows a group of Navaho women engaged in the manufacture of a blanket. The story goes that Antonio de Espejo, a Mexican merchant, obtained in 1581 four thousand cotton blankets in the Moqui (Hopi) towns.[36] The picture here is highly characteristic of the Southwest a few years ago. Unfortunately factory products have made a devastating inroad on the art during the last decades.

The sheep and goats in the background are Spanish introductions, but the standing loom, adopted from the Pueblos, and the other essentials are little changed. One woman is busy spinning, the girl beside her is carding, and the old woman with her back to us displays a finished blanket. The weaver is seated before the loom. She works without a sketch, carrying in her head the design, which, according to tradition, must be freshly inspired with each new web, for to repeat a successful pattern slavishly is to invite the gods to destroy one's inventive genius. The motifs generally have been handed down through generations, but they are strung together in an original pattern—as much a means of self-expression as words are to us.

An embroidered shirt from Acoma, New Mexico, dating from mid-19th century, is pictured in *fig. b.* This village, situated on a high table-land almost inaccessible, was one of the last strongholds of the Pueblo Indians, and here pre-Columbian patterns were preserved long after the Conquest. On the fine linen-like material of this shirt, motifs are worked which might have been copied from prehistoric baskets and pottery. The plain fabric with its colorful needlework is a mature expression of the textile art. Women's apparel from this same time shows a black base, with embroidery in red, blue, and green.

MEXICAN AND MAYA AREAS

The small fragments of textiles from the Mexican and Maya areas that have come to light in excavations are much too damaged to be representative of an art that must have been as highly advanced here as in other regions. There can be no doubt that these areas also had their beautifully woven and gorgeously colored vestments. Representations on stone and pottery should suffice as evidence, but we have additional proof, if needed, in letters, reports, and diaries of the *conquistadores,* which in many cases describe the attire of the dignitaries and chiefs in glowing terms. Lists also have been found of woven materials exported to Spain immediately after the Conquest. The cotton cloth of the Maya was so fine that it was at first mistaken for silk.[169]

The Tribute Roll of Montezuma pictures various types of blankets paid to him as taxes by certain districts of the country (*Pl. 173, fig. b*). From the sketches on this document, there would seem to have been stock patterns. Some carried involved all-over designs, others a central medallion on a solid color, while still others are spotted in imitation of a jaguar skin. Apparently the various types were differentiated with great care, a selective tendency that probably extended to the weaving of all articles of their clothing.

Although we have almost no pre-Columbian textile remnants from these regions, much information can be gathered from a study of their present-day fabrics. Even more stimulating, however, are the mantles, shawls, and shirts of forty or fifty years ago. At that time, as in the Southwest, commercialization had not spoiled the craft, and whatever the Indian made was still very largely a product of his own fantasy-world. Although European motifs were often used, the old manner prevailed in the technical approach, the feeling for color, and the significance of the decoration. Alien elements changed in the hands of the natives, and pagan symbols were blended among them into a splendid whole. Today, however, with the hordes of erratic souvenir-hungry tourists, the former folk art is rapidly becoming a dull and routine occupation. The white man's sense of time and money is penetrating into remote regions, and, as is only natural, merchandise destined for the market is made to suit the taste of the buyer.

On the other hand, his own costume is still very much a part of the Indian's life. Lilly deJongh Osborne, who came close to the soul of the native during the years she collected old Guatemalan textiles, told us about the Indian's habit of kissing a garment in parting from it after a deal. She also related an instance of a husband striking an old blouse, sold by his wife, to drive out any part of her spirit that might cling to it.[59]

The much worn *huipil* in *fig. c* was purchased a few years ago at San Antonio Aguas Calientes, Guatemala, from the girl who was wearing it. The name is derived from the Aztec word *huipili,* "my covering," and designates a woman's blouse. The colorful piece is woven in two strips, each about 12½ inches wide, and contains a number of medieval motifs worked on a dark blue ground. The two stripes that first strike the eye with their bold zigzag lines have six color combinations before a repeat, varying lavender and olive-green, deep red and green, and red and sky-blue. Lavender is the predominant note in the bottom stripes, and the two broad diamond bands are in a soft green set off with yellow and white. These tones are remarkably pastel, and the general effect is quiet, despite the great variety of color and pattern.

In *fig. a,* another scene taken from life, a woman of Santiago Atitlán is pictured working on her hand loom. The photograph shows how simple the apparatus is even today. This condition, however, is rapidly changing, and the standing foot loom is taking its place. The modern outfit offers new possibilities and will radically alter an art that has changed little since the Conquest, the last to succumb.

ANDEAN AREA

The Andean Area is the most fortunate of all pre-Columbian regions in possessing a climate and customs which preserved a vast number of its extraordinary textiles. The dead were often interred in a sitting position, dressed in elaborate clothing and bound with a simple white cloth. At Paracas one strip of a winding sheet measured over 37 feet in length. On top of some of the bundles an artificial head was attached, made of cloth and stuffed. Features were added, sometimes cut out of metal, sometimes in the form of a mask (see *Pls. 203* and *208, fig. b*). The effect was much like that of a child's rag doll. Pottery and personal possessions went into the bundle, and food for the journey to the afterworld accompanied it. Some mummies were so well outfitted that they measured more than 6 feet in diameter. They were placed in caverns scooped out of the sand or within a wattled-wall inclosure, but especially honored persons were set among the gods in the temples, for the people believed the spirit of the deceased ruler or high priest remained to help them.[30] Although artificial mummification seems to have been occasionally practiced in Peru, generally it is the arid climate, especially along the coastal region, which has desiccated and preserved the mummy bundles. Though sometimes stained and rotted, they have proved a treasure-trove for the study of pre-Columbian weaving.

From the earliest recognized culture on the North Coast, the Mochica, only one important specimen has been authenticated, while on the Paracas Peninsula, about one hundred miles south of Lima, a single cemetery site yielded more than three hundred such burials. These contained—to mention only the textiles— magnificent mantles, tunics, headbands, loincloths, sashes, and bags.

In color, the tendency is toward strong contrast rather than delicate harmonies. From seven to thirteen hues occur. Red, yellow, and dark brown predominate, but blue, purple, green, white, and black are also used. In the more elaborate specimens, different shades of the same color enrich the scheme.[83] With the patina of the centuries on them, the fabrics present today a considerably more mellowed impression than originally.

In general it can be said that all techniques were known in all periods, although each period shows decided preferences. Thus, embroidery is characteristic of the Nazca and Paracas periods and tapestry, of the Coast Tiahuanaco. Also, different periods feature different color combinations.[8]

The deep-seated artistic sense inherent in the ancient peoples of the Andean Area is neatly documented in the selection of bobbins and spindles shown on *Pl. 174, fig. b.* Such a little tool, so insignificant in the eyes of modern man, who sees in it only a means to a goal, was for them a medium of self-expression. We have seen hundreds of such instruments in various museums but never two alike.

Made of very hard wood and painted at least in two colors, sometimes even in-cised with exquisite miniature work, they have in them the naïve charm of an unpretentious but balanced civilization.

Above them the hand loom from the Ica culture (*fig. a*) still has a partly woven bit of double cloth on it, showing how the work was set up. After seeing this crude outfit, we admire even more their refined patterns and technically mature fabrics.

A finished piece of double cloth (*fig. c*), found among the ruins of La Centinela in the Chincha Valley on the southern coast of Peru, shows this weave more clearly. Conventionalized fish and bird motifs, large and small, are ranged in an orderly fashion, with the elements alternating in natural light and dark tones. Interlocking frets form the borders.

From the earliest times that we know, various kinds of embroidery were practiced in the Andean Area, some of which are difficult to differentiate from brocade. Needles of thorn and copper have been found. The running pattern in *Pl. 175, fig. b,* a Nazca shawl, is an illustration of this type. It is done in wool on cotton. Conventionalized reptilian or fish motifs, their wedge-shaped heads clearly distinguishable, make up a fret pattern without any pretense to natural-ism, which has an advancing rhythm.

Fig. a shows a fragment of a wool mantle from the site of Paracas. In the manufacture of such pieces, the sections to be filled with embroidery were some-times woven in gauze technique so that the finished product would not be bulky. In both the square medallions and the border the embroidery stitch can be traced, following the contours of the body and face. In this respect embroidery as a medium is more liberated than weaving, for it allows a freer use of curves. The distortion of the human figure into a twisting attitude produces a lively pat-tern, and streaming hair represented by long light lines contributes to the feeling of motion and connects one motif with another. Each medallion is about 1½ by 1¾ inches. The thick heavy fringe attached to the mantle should be mentioned.

Whether Paracas fabrics antedate the Nazca or should be classed as contem-porary is a question not yet settled. It should be noted that Paracas was identi-fied as a site only about 1925. Therefore, many earlier pieces in collections, which probably came from Paracas, were classified as Nazca on the basis of their designs, familiar from Nazca pottery.[8]

Each set of steps in the right half of *fig. c* must have been woven and tie-dyed separately, then joined. In the left half, interlocking warp technique can be seen. The "patchwork" figures are loom-woven together on one edge and sewed on the other in a singularly modern pattern.

In the fragment of a garment illustrated on *Pl. 176, fig. a,* of wool and cotton, a subtle pattern is woven in supplementary weft technique which has the effect of tapestry. The figures with their angular lines are similar in style to those carved on the Gateway of the Sun at Tiahuanaco and place the textile in the Coast Tiahuanaco Period, about A.D. 800. Eight rich colors are used in the fragment, which is slightly more than 19 inches wide. Although the same figure is repeated in each horizontal row, the repetition is disguised through a varied color scheme.

Feline figures, 6¾ inches high, stand out from the light background of the Paracas mantle in *fig. b.* Countless diamond shapes embroidered in various colors make up each animal, producing a Paisley effect. The large creatures, alternately inverted, are arranged in horizontal rows, but the vertical line of the heads and the diagonal line of the bodies greatly diversify the design. The rich border shows a condensation of animal and geometric motifs.

Fig. c is a sample of polychrome embroidery, also from the Paracas Peninsula. A plain dark ground serves to set off the embroidered figures of the warriors. They are very much alike in costume, each wearing a fringed tunic and a serpent headdress and carrying two trophy heads on a staff. Reared snake heads curving like feathers from the headdress recall the metal masks of Chavín (see *Pl. 195*). The arrangement of the figures is worth studying for its subtle avoidance of wallpaper monotony: in each row every other one holds his trophies in his right hand, and a repeat of colors does not appear until the fifth. The oblique rows alternate in light and dark, but even here great variety in color and expression serves to offset the regularity of pattern.

The whole of an embroidered Paracas mantle, almost 10 feet long and over 5 wide, is presented on *Pl. 177, fig. a.* What strikes the eye first is the vitality of its pattern continuity and, in the actual piece, the contrast in colors. Only after a moment of sheer delight do we turn to the individual motifs and find two fish, generally one light and one dark, that seem to revolve with a deftly contrived centripetal effect. There is no regular repeat in the center field. The use of the same motif on the border against a different colored ground is far from monotonous; rather it augments the turbulence of the whole. It will be noted that the border does not run all the way around but that a patch containing one element rounds out each corner. Since the main field is not circumscribed, the whole composition is given more breathing space. The fish are worked in shades of blue, green, and yellow on a black ground in the center and a red one in the border.

In the section of the Paracas mantle (*fig. b*), the demon motif that makes up the entire decoration is dictated by the same imagination that embellished the pottery of the Nazca region, conditioned by the technique of the loom (see *Pl. 161, fig. b*). The bright colored figures, each about 7 inches high, stand out all the more sharply for being embroidered in wool on the blue-black cotton base. The square head is turned sidewise, and a fantastically tripartite tongue curves above it. One hand holds a staff upraised and the other, a device resting on the ground that resembles a stem with lima beans attached. In every other row the figure is upside down, which adds to the confusion of the pattern. The line of small vegetable shapes that is noticeable down the center of the photograph seems to run the length of the piece. A running stitch skillfully used makes the mantle reversible. It is a characteristic example of Paracas textiles and dates from about A.D. 400 to 600.

Although tapestry was used in the early periods of the Andean cultures, it occurs more frequently in the middle and late.[105] The two plates that follow illustrate fabrics woven in this technique.

The poncho, or shirt, in *Pl. 178, fig. a* is from the Nazca region in Coast Tiahuanaco style. It measures 45 inches wide and 41 long, and was made by sewing two lengths of cloth together, with slits left for the neck and arms. Plain stripes set off the densely patterned sections. The geometric designs and abstractions of animal and plant origin that form the individual elements derive from the Tiahuanaco, though loosened and stereotyped.

A detail from a tapestry band, which measures in its entirety 46½ inches long by 5½ wide, is reproduced in *fig. b*. It also is identified as belonging to Coast Tiahuanaco from the Nazca region. The field is red, and the body and legs of the animal are orange. A white limning closes the slits. The creature, 6½ inches long and probably a textile version of the puma, shows how ingeniously a figure taken from nature was translated into a woven design of remarkable power and integrity. We even accept without question the exchange of a paw for the tail. In the band, the individual figure loses somewhat its identity and becomes part of a flowing and colorful pattern.

The Late Coast Tiahuanaco tapestry with woven fringe (*fig. c*) is thought to have come from the Central or North Coast and could be dated around the beginning of the 11th century. It is done in Kelim technique in wool on a cotton warp and was probably part of a garment. (Compare the fringed ponchos on *Pl. 190.*) Colored birds, staggered in a step design, are woven in white, dark brown, pink, red, and tan on an orange ground and blend in mellow color harmony with the plain fields of soft red.

If tapestry weaving of simple rectangles and bands requires great technical skill, how much more is displayed in the complicated design of the fish on *Pl. 179, fig. a,* from the Central Coast. It is 21 inches long by 9 wide, in late style of Pachacámac, and is woven in Kelim technique. Its shape is well defined by the white outline, and stylized parts of it, such as the gills, fins, and tail, contribute a certain naturalism. But the weaver was not content with these additions alone; the backbone is added as a decorative feature, and extraneous designs and abstractions are used to enliven the entire surface. All these additional elements are kept in balance and proportion without endangering the primary effect. The colors are tones of brown and cream with touches of green.

In *fig. b* we have a square of wool tapestry, roughly 18 inches on a side, that is classified as Ica Period from the Nazca Valley. The simplification of every element shows how weaving, during the centuries, shed its involved patterns. The complicated techniques, however, remained, and Kelim, eccentric, and figure-8 weaves may be found in this piece. The human figure is used merely as a decorative unit and repeated unchanged. From an artistic point of view, the most praiseworthy feature is the narrow border of marching birds, representing stylistically a different tradition.

The square medallion in *fig. c* is done in tapestry technique, wool on cotton, with needle-knitted borders. A stylized condor is spread on the light field, while the two borders are decorated with conventionalized two-headed lizards, creating a moving pattern above and below the static figure in the center. Compared with the other two designs on the plate, the bird is executed with more detail than the little men just seen but it is far less animated than the fish. This piece is said to have come from the South Coast of Peru and was seemingly made after highland influence from Tiahuanaco had stiffened and formalized the fantasy-world of the weavers there.

Peoples who possessed such a penchant for traveling as the pre-Columbian population of the Andean Area needed bags for various purposes—from the simple cloth of the agriculturist to the Gobelin-like tapestry materials that were part of the apparel of a high functionary. In the three examples illustrated on *Pl. 180,* one finds embroidery, tapestry, and rep.

The tapestry bag with plaited cord top *(fig. c)* is probably the earliest in the group, and is identified as Coast Tiahuanaco in style. A spotted catlike animal serves as main motif in a design that is not only more intricate than the others pictured here but covers the entire surface of the bag. Even without the secondary and tertiary elements that are ingeniously placed to fill up the space, this figure alone would produce an animated and continuous pattern. In it something of the droll quality of the Nazca animals is evident, filtered and toned down through the centuries—to appear here at its best. The piece, with its gathered top, is subtle and sophisticated enough to serve as a modern theater bag.

Fig. b, a bag with embroidered decoration and needle-knitted edges and tassels, is in the same style but later in date. The design consists of a fantastically involved animal shape from Nazca weaving, frozen through highland influence into a rigid fretlike motif, its formerly vibrant rhythm exchanged for cold geometric exactitude. The plain section at the top as balanced against the fringe at the bottom reveals deliberate artistic sense.

Fig. a, 7 by 8½ inches, is a simple bag of loom-pattern or warp-pattern rep. It comes from the Central Coast of Peru and is said to be Inca in style, dated about 1400. The dominant color is deep red, and yellow, blue, and green are used in the design. This late piece has nothing of the involved convolutions of *fig. b,* nor does it show the suavity of *fig. c;* rather one finds in it evidence that even the artistic imagination of the Chimú people, usually so fresh and charming, dwindled during the high-powered Inca administration.

Brocade came to Europe from the Orient, and fabrics woven in this technique, whether imported or domestic, were always among those most highly prized there. The pre-Columbian dignitary also had his brocaded garments, some of them made perhaps before Europe knew of this complicated weave.

One fragment with a pleasing tapestry border and woven fringe is shown on *Pl. 181, fig. a.* The brocaded top comes out in an oblique series of interlocking feline heads, woven in mauve-pink wool on yellow cotton cloth. The border, with its interlocking frets in three shades of brown with cream, is executed with amazing clarity, and the combination of these two diagonal patterns with the narrow horizontal stripes is highly effective. The piece is dated after 900 and probably belongs to the beginning of the Ica Period.

The other example (*fig. b*), 39 inches by 28, is a single-faced wool brocade on cotton crêpe. While the provenience of the first is somewhat in doubt, the second was excavated in the Nazca region and belongs to the Ica Period, about 1100 to 1300. There is a distinct stylistic difference in the two, a difference of artistic concept. In the first, the whole gains life through the striking combination of its patterns and colors, while in the second, a realistic figure loses life through its repetitious treatment. Peculiar charm is added by the tiny light-colored birds in the border, one of the favorite motifs of the coastal region. Birds of all sorts appear in Andean art, from the little humming birds, depicted on Nazca bowls, to the ducklike creatures on bands of tapestry and the conventionalized figures hammered into metal-work.

Flat and cylindrical molds are good evidence that block printing, or the stamping of a design by means of a cliché of clay, wood, or, eventually, metal, was widely practiced among the pre-Columbian peoples (*Pl. 182*). Even though many of them may have been used for body painting and some for pottery decoration, we have textiles from the Andean Area that prove that they were also applied to fabrics. In some instances painting and printing appear in combination; others seem to have been painted to imitate block designs. Cut-out stencils of silver also have been found.

A complete poncho, probably Chimú, between 1100 and 1400, is illustrated in *fig. a.* It is in plain weave and decorated with painted figures that were outlined before they were filled in (especially noticeable in the lower four birds). The unevenness of the squares arranged in a V at the neck would point to freehand painting; however, it must not be forgotten that since stamping was by hand and the amount of paint not accurately regulated, certain divergences might easily appear even in stamped units of the same motif. Sophistication is manifest in the placing of light birds on a dark ground in the yoke and dark birds on a light ground in the lower half.

As a design, the work is interesting, although the execution seems somewhat careless. Note the inverted bird in the upper right. The painting must have been done after the two strips of material were joined, for the bird in the center is split in two. Had the fabric been woven, this would have entailed fashioning half a figure on each strip, a procedure that would not have occurred under any circumstances.

Fig. b shows a painted detail from a band of coarse plain-weave cotton, said to have come from the Central Coast. In spite of the high degree of stylization, the beguiling playfulness and softness of the spotted kittens can be enjoyed. Each is about 4 inches high. They are executed in tones of tan, brown, and white on a pinkish-tan field.

In *fig. c* we have a portion of a cotton cloth, also in plain weave, covered with an extravagant variety of decoration that involves four separate pattern themes repeated in diagonal arrangement. Considering the small size of the squares—they are less than an inch high—the clarity of the composition is remarkable. It must have been extremely difficult to keep so many little motifs in line and to fill in the solid colors without smearing. The excellent dye should also receive mention, for the colors are still bright. Stylistic elements of the Coast Tiahuanaco are evident, although the piece probably belongs toward the end of that period. Stamped or painted designs would seem more susceptible to outside influences than those that are loomed, for in a woven pattern tradition and technical principles are more deeply involved.

The production of delicate fabrics brought forth correspondingly delicate patterns. In *Pl. 183, fig. a* a fragment of a painted cotton cloth from Trancas, a Nazca Period site, is shown, the sheerness of which can be perceived in the photograph. The tiny birds, each about 1½ inches long, moving in opposite directions in alternate rows, must have been painted by hand. An absence of all rigidity of line, the usual corollary of mechanical devices, gives the piece especial charm. There is a healthy naïveté and play of fantasy in the design that make it the equal of many Oriental fabrics featured in art museums.

A net for the hair (*fig. b*), woven of plant fiber, introduces us to the most fragile weaves, under which fall the laces, voiles, and gauzes. It is made in square-meshed netting with the design embroidered in double-knotted cross-stitch. The piece is identified as coming from the Central Coast and shows Chimú stylistic features. Nets such as this have been found on the heads of mummies *in situ,* and one has to admit that in few civilizations were the dead buried with such exquisite covering for their hair.

In *fig. c* a detail from a square-meshed lacelike fabric is reproduced that also comes from the Central Coast and is presumably Chimú. The designs are outlined and filled in with cross-stitch. Besides the human figure seen here, about 4½ inches high, animals enliven the decorative scheme. Airy fabrics such as these were manufactured for various purposes, ranging from fastidious hair covering to fish nets and from small bags attached to scale beams (see *Pl. 299, fig. a*) to veils.[84]

In *Pl. 184, fig. a* the familiar step-and-fret design is woven in gauze weave of cotton, giving the impression of drawn-work. The faultless transition from the plain section into the openwork pattern can be easily followed.[105] The piece is identified as Nazca.

The second example (*fig. b*) is probably Chimú and shows a combination of gauze with bands of plain weave and openwork. It is dated about 1300. The variation of tightly woven, fine-meshed, and openwork stripes is highly successful and so universally appealing that we can easily imagine the piece as a Sunday table cover in one of our own Victorian households.

The fragment of a poncho (*fig. c*) shows an unusual type of openwork which enhances the plain cloth through the lacy contrast of its squares. The border above the fringe is worked in tapestry weave in several colors and features the much stereotyped bird of Ica style, here almost lost in an interlocking-fret design.

It is not surprising that modern textile experts stand dumfounded before the manifold variety found in medieval Peruvian weaving. It seems as if technical hindrances did not exist for these people, nor any limit to their inventiveness.

The poncho in *Pl. 185, fig. a* displays the weft-loop weave, a technique used in our Turkish towels and terry cloth. In this photograph the fringe is parted to show the plain cloth between the rows of loops, but when worn the entire surface of the poncho presented a shaggy appearance. The slit at the top is the opening for the neck. A shirt of this type in such a good state of preservation is a rarity. What a striking garment it must have been when new, worn with accessories of metal, shell, or turquoise.

The foundation fabric in *fig. b* is woven with a cotton warp and wool weft in tapestry with spaced warps, giving an openwork effect. The tassels are of polychrome wool and are sewed on in groups.

Still more extraordinary is the complicated piece illustrated in *fig. c*. Here we have a closely woven tapestry in red, yellow, and brown, ornamented with a five-toothed motif in white and interspersed with openwork squares, over which are sewed tasseled rosettes of wool, fashioned separately—a prodigious task even for our machine age. The tassel colors are yellow, blue, and white; the rosettes, red and violet. These pieces probably come from the Central Coast and are Chimú in style. Contemporary Europe imported its choice textiles from the Orient, but they were less varied than those worn by the native chiefs in Peru.

Pl. 186 presents two caps, 5⅕ to 6 inches high, stylistically Coast Tiahua-

WEAVING

naco. Both are made of wool with a knitted base (see top), into which the silky strands are knotted and then clipped in a manner not unlike our plush or velvet technique.

In the first (*fig. a*), a meandering geometric pattern characteristic of the highlands appears, while in the second (*fig. b*), conventionalized birds stand out clearly against the varicolored ground. The pointed knitted ends of the one and the four fuzzy pompons of the other, as well as their distinctive patterns, demonstrate that even where tradition dictated the shape, material, and motifs, a piece could still be individualized. The photographs show not only the evenness of execution and the fine texture of the wool, but give a fair idea of the many colors involved. One of these trig and colorful hats above an elaborate, loosely fitting poncho must have added considerably to the picturesqueness of the costume.

Although the Paracas textiles are among the earliest of pre-Columbian finds, they show some of the greatest finesse of execution. *Pl. 187* presents a detail of a superb mantle in soft henna wool of gauzy quality. The cloth is 46 inches long and 20 wide. A solidly embroidered border in rich polychrome with fringe is sewed completely around the edge, and the sheer body of the piece is covered with a pattern of mythical figures worked in a delicate running stitch in cocoa-brown. The design is made up of a series of double-headed monsters forming converging V's, covered with masks and other elements, all connected with one another. They leave diamond-shaped fields of equal size, in which the single main figure—the many-tongued creature seen in *Pl. 177, fig. b*—is placed without crowding. The line of heads at the edge should not be missed, especially the central one, like a heraldic motif. The angular build-up of the units has something of an incised carving about it, and the separate demon figure is slightly reminiscent of the Sechín stone (see *Pl. 99, fig. a*). The iconography of this early piece contains many of those fantastically stylized elements which were used throughout later centuries with little change.

Older than many of the textiles already seen is the justly celebrated ceremonial mantle from Paracas reproduced on *Pl. 188*. It is 54 inches long and 21 wide, including the border, and was found in a tomb with other fabrics and some gold objects as part of the funeral raiment of a chief or priest. The gossamer material, woven of cotton and vicuña wool, carries a design of puma heads and frets exquisitely woven into a continuous pattern. Delicate tones are combined in a never-repeating scheme: maroon, rose, and peach-pink with turquoise and azure-blue, green, yellow, and gold.

The real sensation of the piece, however, is the amazingly decorative wool border that contains an endless procession of ninety figures in twelve colors. It is about 3½ inches wide and wrought in a technique resembling embroidery and knitting—a lost skill that is known as three-dimensional knitting. The legs appear against a dark solid background, but above the waist the figures rise free. Their definitely plastic effect is achieved by a core of stuffing that varies in thickness. In its marvelous state of preservation, the border serves as a fascinating inventory of the elaborate costumes, headdresses, and jewels worn and the weapons used in that early day. The llama appears, haltered and laden with ears of maize; other cultivated plants are represented, and the puma and numerous mythological creatures, whose significance can only be guessed at today, crowd together in an overwhelming display.[84] The section chosen for enlargement is shown between the two arrows. In the detail (*fig. b*), the many-tongued demon of the preceding plate can be distinguished on the right, with the figure beside him turned under to provide more background. The looped rosettes that join the border to the mantle are also clearly visible here. This piece is said to be contemporary with the Nazca culture, which would date it around 500, or even earlier. It exhibits a perfection in technique and a fantastic richness in the conception of its design which in all the centuries that have followed have never been surpassed.

Because of their familiar shape, the ponchos on the next three plates are easier for us to understand than the many fragments we have seen. By their tangible presence they attest to the civilized apparel of this area.

The first (*Pl. 189, fig. a*) shows Ica traits in technique and design, although it comes from Ancón, a site on the Central Coast. This piece, as well as those that follow, is full size for an adult Indian. It is a very rare and an excellently preserved specimen of openwork, woven in a variant of Kelim technique with spaced warp,[105] already seen in the tasseled fragment on *Pl. 185, fig. b*. The bold painted diagonals are remarkably effective. Note that the weaving in the vertical bars is straight and tight, while in the horizontals the thread is loose, producing a wavy line that gives variety and softness to the cross-bar pattern. Only the tapestry border with its small moving animal motifs is solid. The cuffs have a quadruple fringe that repeats the colors in the shirt—dark blue, beige, red, and white.

Fig. b comes from Pachacámac, an immediate neighbor of Ancón to the south. Cotton cloth in plain weave, very thin, serves as base for the appliquéd designs. The condensed symbolism in the figure is characteristic of the coastal cultures, and it is presumable that these finely woven Chimú tapestry medallions were taken off an older material and applied on another in a later century, just as old laces are used on clothing today.

The poncho in *fig. c* comes from farther north, the Chimú site of Huaco. Rosettes and tassels add a characteristic colorful touch with their tones of red, tan, and brown. Below the decoration, the plain weave changes to openwork, fourteen double rows of it, and a tapestry border with a cleverly contrived interlocking-fret pattern completes the exquisitely finished garment.

Some time ago Peruvian archaeologists discovered in shallow walled-in graves at Paracas four hundred twenty-nine mummies.[145] In the bundles there were some rather plain funeral ornaments cut out of hammered gold, but the textiles found were of greater value. Mantles and shawls of delicate weave and stunning color combinations were unearthed, many of them in an amazing state of preservation when we consider the fifteen hundred years that have elapsed since their manufacture.

Extraordinarily well preserved is the poncho on *Pl. 190, fig. b* from this cemetery. It is a very large garment, measuring 50 by 38 inches, with a braided fringe 28 inches long at each shoulder and a 20-inch woven fringe along the border. Sometimes these shirts are so large that one suspects clothing was worn under them or that they were woven especially for the mummies. Figural and geometric motifs, easily distinguishable, are skillfully handled to produce a rich and mobile decoration. Note the difference in the interpretation of the same figure in the embroidered and the woven bands. The contrasts of the plain dark material with the colored and the smooth fabric with the rough fringe make the piece outstanding even among Paracas textiles.

The sleeveless poncho in *fig. a* comes from farther south and shows a pattern that marks the transition from Coast Tiahuanaco to late Nazca. It is made of wool in a cloth weave, with borders embroidered in wool. The motif edging the monotone fabric is probably a stark conventionalization of a former cat pattern. (Compare with the bag on *Pl. 180, fig. b.*) It is now so condensed and unified, however, and so decorative that it does not occur to us to inquire into its origin. This piece also makes effective use of tassels and fringe, even if they are not so lavishly applied as in the other below it.

The four ponchos on *Pl. 191,* our last examples of pre-Columbian weaving, are especially noteworthy because they come from the highlands, where few textiles have survived the climate. All but *fig. a* are from Lake Titicaca, and two (*figs. b* and *c*) were found in a tightly covered stone box, which accounts for their excellent condition. All are made of vicuña wool in tapestry technique, with V-shaped yokes, and all feature in one way or another the checkerboard— as if this exact and organized pattern had become subconsciously the symbol for the tightly coördinated life under Inca rule.

It is possible that some of them were manufactured just after the Conquest; *fig. b* has a silver thread in the border, probably a Spanish innovation. But they possess generally stylistic features outspokenly Inca. We no longer meet the large mythological or symbolic figures of Nazca culture or involved geometric stylization. The application of the small square, the fret, and the step, among others, has become by now fluent and accomplished. The units are systematized, and there is no meandering of motifs. From the designs in *fig. b,* however, it is clear that ancient pattern elements of the Tiahuanaco culture persisted into later centuries, even into the Inca Period and beyond, as if a counterpoint in weaving threaded itself through all phases of the highland weaver's art. Here they too have become well-regimented decorative elements on a chessboard structure.

As a new motif of high rank the diamond appears (*fig. d*), executed with precision and somewhat suggestive of blanket designs in our own Southwest. Another new element is the suave arrangement of feathers on the same piece. Note also the human figures on its yoke, each wearing a shirt with checkerboard decoration and holding up a sketch of another. Figures are used in a different presentation on the lower border of *fig. b.* Their inclusion in such a design is considered by some also a mark of Spanish influence.

To appreciate the work fully, one must take into consideration the beautiful color modulations: the soft reds, vivid blues, and the olive-greens that are especially dominant in *fig. d.* In *fig. a* delicately conventionalized butterflies in rose and olive-green on a brilliant turquoise field enliven the rigidity of the pattern and individualize the piece.

An art so highly perfected and so vital to life in medieval America as was weaving could not cease to exist with the Conquest. The technical skill and feeling for design received new stimulus with the introduction of silk, linen, and sheep's wool from the Eastern Hemisphere. This meeting of two civilizations that had developed independently produced a blend, in weaving particularly, that has the fascinating quality of a fairy tale. The Spaniards, who embodied in their art influences from China, Persia, and other lands of the Near East, and the native American weavers, who achieved mastery by a very different road, turned out, especially in Peru in the 16th, 17th, and 18th centuries, tapestries which are today the cherished possessions of museums and collectors.

In style, some are strongly reminiscent of the Late Coptic. The human figure, so rigidly expressed or completely omitted in most pre-Columbian pieces, is now used more freely. New animals, such as horses and cows, and a new approach that encouraged the use of fruit and flowers in naturalistic form stimulated the talent of the native. Besides elements of European provenience, Levantine and Oriental motifs are sometimes blended into a beguiling potpourri. During these centuries an Hispano-American art flourished which surpasses all modern attempts at the neo-primitive, for here it was a true and spontaneous expression, not an artificial stumbling and stuttering in a highly technical age.

A post-Columbian tapestry poncho from the Lake Titicaca district in Bolivia is reproduced in *Pl. 192, fig. b.* In shape and general lay-out of design, it differs little from those we have already seen—even the V-shaped yoke outlined with squares appears. But the pattern in the yoke presents a stylized mixture of fantasy animals, flowers, and plants never met before. Even more striking are the dark stripes on the light base. The delicate motif woven into them actually has elements of a bird design, but it is organized into a floral effect with a continuity characteristic of European taste.

Much farther removed from the pre-Columbian atmosphere, both in shape and pattern, is the tapestry panel in *fig. a.* It measures nearly 8 feet by 6 and is all wool. Like an Oriental rug, it features as center a riot of flowers, with framing bands, each of which is made up of a different floral motif. Only the two lighter ones recall in their twining and winding elements pre-Conquest times; the others are well-digested decorative units such as appear frequently in Spanish colonial work.

Since there were no religious bans against using shapes of nature, as was the case in Islamic countries, all the European and Oriental motifs were at the disposal of the Peruvian weaver, and the result was especially rich and varied. Human figures, gesticulating dramatically, are introduced in the four small medallions. The couple on the left wear Spanish costumes of the 18th century—cocked hats, big boots, and pistols in their belts—while the other two seem to be Indians. Urns and baskets, infrequent in Peruvian weaving, show rococo influence. The Indian weaver's disinclination to repeat is manifest in the changes in the urns and birds and in the general color variations that disguise the inevitable recurrence. Pink, dark blue, yellow, and olive-green are the chief colors, each in several tones.[83]

A story-telling atmosphere pervades this exquisite and rare work of art, bringing to us the viceregal period of Peru. We can easily imagine this tapestry on the wall or floor of a proud and aristocratic palace of the 18th century there.

The textiles of the Andean Area reveal that the product can be highly complicated in pattern and intricate in technique even though the tool is primitive. The advance in this isolated civilization from the animal skins of the first hunting tribes to the Paracas mantle represents an achievement that is tremendous. The distance from this high grade of technical and artistic skill to our present-day production is far less. Not a single new type of weaving can be shown by modern industry. The hand-spun thread of the pre-Columbian natives was superior to ours in tensile strength, fineness, and evenness of quality. Furthermore, for durability of material and fastness of color, our production fails to show a great advance. We do not know how much would remain of our average wools and cottons after more than a thousand years in the earth.

VII

Metal–Work

WHEN Columbus pleaded at the Court of Spain for support of his expedition, he evoked the treasures of the East. The Admiral crossed and re-crossed the unknown ocean four times and touched upon the eastern shores of Central and South America, as well as the West Indies, but even the red-skinned population of these regions did not shake his belief that he was somewhere on the shores of fabulous Asia. As a token of the success of his undertaking, he brought back jewelry and small objects of gold and silver. By the time that Cortés's first shipments reached Europe, however, it was clear that it was a new world which lay beyond the seas.

The *conquistadores* could see on their first contacts with the natives that gold and silver had not the same value in the eyes of the Indians as in their own. It was not a medium of exchange for them but a resplendent material to be fashioned into articles for ceremonial and decorative use. Although the gold which Cortés collected consisted partly of raw metal, a great portion was already made up into objects—jewelry, statuettes, and utensils executed with artistic finesse. Even the unsentimental soldiers who took part in the Conquest were impressed by their beauty. All articles, however, had to be melted down into a more convenient form for shipping, and, at Montezuma's order, a group of the goldsmiths who had wrought many of the delicate pieces worked for three days casting the heaped-up gold into ingots and bars which were stamped with the royal arms of Spain. The more cautious of the soldiers ordered their share of the booty made into chains and other articles that could be carried on the person. Cortés had a small cannon made of gold and silver alloy. Upon seeing the greed of the Spaniards for the metal, Montezuma is said to have remarked, "The Christians must have a strange disease which can be cured only with gold."

But the thirst was insatiable. The lure of gold enticed other adventurers, and it was Pizarro who came upon the real El Dorado with its riches beyond the wildest dreams. In the realm of the Incas, gold and silver were used functionally. Besides "goblets, ewers, salvers, vases of every shape and size, ornaments and utensils for the temples and palaces," sheets of gold covered some of the buildings, dazzling as a mirage.[110] A fountain that sent up a sparkling jet of gold is described in one account, with birds and animals of the same material playing at its base, and mention is made of a golden ear of corn, sheathed in broad leaves of silver, with a rich tassel of silver threads. In some of the more northerly regions of South America, gold fishing hooks, tweezers, nails, spoons, and pins—even safety-pins—have been found.[9] So abundant was the metal that Pizarro, on his march into the interior of the country, ordered golden shoes for his horse as the iron was worn away. The picture of a small band of ragged Spaniards, marching in a hostile unknown land, their horses shod with precious metal, shows an illuminating paradox of the Conquest. Here, too, gold and silver were melted down and cast into solid bars of uniform standard. So great was the treasure that the Peruvian goldsmiths had to work at the task for a full month, ten times as long as was needed in Mexico.

By the middle of the 16th century, the importation of gold from the New World to Spain was so heavy that in the maintenance of her navy England reckoned with the booty seized from the Spanish fleet. In Spain itself, the enormous wealth proved unfruitful and transitory, and melted away in the hands of a corrupt administration.

Of the millions of dollars' worth of gold and silver that reached Europe in the Spanish centuries, we cannot trace a single object as an absolutely authentic survival of the Conquest.[71] Some of the extant pieces come from old collections, some from excavations, and many more circulate without data on their provenience. Even today, if worked gold and silver articles from pre-Columbian times are found by the ignorant population, they are apt to be looked upon only as a source of a few dollars, and it is fortunate if they are not melted down. A few of the specimens photographed for this survey have since disappeared, stolen and wantonly destroyed for the metal they contained. The "strange disease" still holds us in its grip.

The consensus of authorities gives credit for the early development of pre-Columbian metallurgy to South America. Indeed, according to some opinions many high cultural trends originated there and then worked north. This theory, challenging that of Maya precedence in antiquity, has many arguments in its favor. The Mochica, Chavín, Nazca, and Early Tiahuanaco cultures date at least within the first centuries of our era, and the earliest specimens shown in this chapter are believed to fall within this time. Most pre-Columbian metal-work, however, is generally placed after the turn of the first millennium.

"The golden land" of the Spaniards, the Inca Empire, comprised not only Peru and Ecuador but parts of Chile and Bolivia, and the art of metal-working extended beyond, into the regions of Colombia, Venezuela, Panama, and Costa Rica, where styles show local characteristics. Metallurgy is not believed to have reached the Maya and Mexican cultures before the 9th century—the 12th is more likely.

In both the Andean and the Interlying areas the mines were so situated that they could be worked by primitive methods. Gold was obtained principally by panning, while silver was extracted from surface mines. Besides these metals, copper, tin, mercury, platinum, lead, and iron in natural alloys are found in pre-Columbian objects.[71] The medieval Peruvians regarded their mines as living spirits and performed certain ceremonies in their honor. Those who worked them worshiped the hills that contained the minerals, and feasts were held with dancing and drinking to assure the benevolence of the spirits.[28]

Hammering, embossing, casting, plating and gilding, inlaying, sheathing, engraving, alloying, soldering, and welding were all processes known to the Peruvian goldsmiths around the 10th century. For these operations the use of hammers, anvils, furnaces, crucibles (probably made of pottery), and blowpipes was necessary.[70] It is interesting to note that comparatively few implements for such specialized techniques have been unearthed, probably because the excavated material up to now comes from grave sites rather than work sites.

Hammering, embossing, and engraving might be considered as belonging to the simpler methods, but the existence of cast and plated articles, of those with the design in an alloy of different color, or with inlaid lapidary material, shows real grasp of the medium and the achievement of highly specialized skills.

The *cire perdue,* or "lost wax," process of casting was widely employed. This method was essentially the same as that used for our bronzes today. It was known also in ancient Egypt and the Near East, then apparently lost to Europe in the first centuries of Christianity to be re-invented for the Renaissance shortly before Benvenuto Cellini. The perfection of this process in pre-Columbian America serves as a striking example of parallel development, when similar conditions produce similar results.

By this method the desired object was modeled first in wax or resin, sometimes over a core of clay, and covered with a clay mixture. When this was fired, the wax melted and ran out of vents provided for the purpose, leaving a mold corresponding exactly to the wax positive. Molten metal then poured into the mold took on the desired shape, and after it solidified the covering was broken away. The rough castings were often hammered and burnished for smoother finish and sometimes welded together to form a larger object. The nature of the procedure invited the use of fine and intricate detail, accurately reproduced in the soft wax. The fact that only one object could be made from each mold would not appear as a drawback to the craftsman of medieval America, who apparently shared with the modern Navaho the conviction that the gods would destroy his talent if he servilely duplicated a piece.

MOUND BUILDER REGION

The objects in the first two plates were produced outside the bounds of our five areas, but are included to show the wide distribution of metal-working on an outspokenly artistic level. They come doubtless from a late period in Mound Builder culture but are presented at the beginning of this chapter rather than at the end, where they might appear as an anticlimax after the metal-work of the more civilized areas.

The ornaments on *Pl. 193, fig. a,* found at Hopewell Mounds, Ohio, were cut out of a hammered copper sheet with bone or horn tools. A surprising neatness of finish can be observed in them. Their geometric design is not only decorative but intricate in composition. The swastika in the upper right documents an instance of the independent invention of this form.

Fig. b shows shapes cut out of mica. They were excavated from graves of dignitaries of the Hopewell people and appear to have been used as ornaments on clothing. The material is a laminated substance, one that requires considerable skill to work, and was brought into the region by trade from Virginia and North Carolina.[31] Both pieces show amazing certainty in linear conduct. The eagle foot with its translucent silvery tone is unique—highly sophisticated in its stylization.

Fig. a on *Pl. 194* is part of a headdress fashioned of copper and, although damaged, is impressive because of its shape and symmetry. It comes from Nashville, Tennessee, and is 11⅝ inches long. The type appears fastened at the nape of the neck of a figure on one of the shell gorgets, also from Tennessee (see *Pl. 280, fig. a*).

The two copper sheets embossed with faces (*figs. b* and *c*) are from Spiro

Mound, Oklahoma. On the larger, 9½ inches high (*fig. c*), plastic effects were attempted, and every detail is sharply executed. Eyes and hair in particular are skillfully drawn, the eyes showing a manner of delineation quite different from the Mexican or Maya. The face in *fig. b,* with its half-open mouth, teeth, elaborate earrings, and the thin lines suggesting hair, bears a certain similarity to the early prints of Indian chiefs.

Fig. d, 10½ inches high and also from Spiro Mound, is cut away from the background, producing a sharp silhouette. Especially well executed is the section between the nose and chin. Technical superiority is evident in the feather headdress, with its harmonious line; although almost detached it is nevertheless an integral part of the composition.

ANDEAN AREA

The name "Chavín," as was already discussed in sculpture, is applied to an ancient culture that apparently once dominated the upper interior of Peru and in places reached into the coastal valleys. All four pieces on *Pl. 195,* classified as Chavín in style, came from the department of Lambayeque on the coast. This section, which lies some two hundred seventy miles northwest of the site of Chavín, received its name from the river flowing through it and was in ancient times a part of the Chimú Kingdom.

All specimens shown on this plate present variations of the same theme. Not only is the central subject recurrent, but the manner of delineation is definitely of the same iconography.

The plaque (*fig. a*) is 8½ inches high and was probably fastened to a headband. The standing main figure, holding a staff in either hand, is a jaguar or puma demon with tusks and a wrinkled muzzle. Its body seems made up of masks and intertwining serpent bodies. Secondary designs of puma and serpent heads fill all available space and make the effect of the whole confusing.

The same technique—a pattern pressed out in relief on a thin gold sheet—was applied in *fig. b.* It is 9¼ inches high and was part of a crown. Here again the main figure is an anthropomorphic creature with a staff in either hand. In the surrounding pattern we find the same elements as in the preceding piece, presented, however, with considerably more clarity. The human element is brought out in the smooth surfaces of the face, shoulders, and legs—a trick which sets off especially well the fine mask on the torso.

In *fig. c,* nearly 5 inches high, the main motif is transferred from the cylindrical shape to a plaque with cut-out outlines. The sixteen serpents about the head have not changed their position too much, and the mask in the center has all the details necessary to identify it as the same theme, crystallized by tradition and clarified by good workmanship. Here, however, with the edges cut out, a certain live and plastic impression is achieved that is not apparent in the other two. The deep corrugated embossing, extremely telling in the medium of gold, is especially well applied.

In *fig. d,* a gold ornament 6½ inches high from the same region, appears the quintessence of the type. The main motif is loosened, and a remarkable lightness has been gained by cutting out the background. This mask has lost its fangs, otherwise the features are the same, perhaps the most clearly expressed of all. Entwined serpent bodies serving as frame for the head produce a highly decorative effect.

The transplantation of the same theme into different media by different cultures is illustrated in *Pl. 196.* The plaque (*fig. a*), said to have come from Pachacámac, shows influence of the Coast Tiahuanaco and Chavín styles. A thin silver sheet was cut out to the desired shape, then lightly embossed. It contrasts interestingly with the jaguar masks of the preceding plate. Hollow eye sockets and an open slit for the mouth line are effective in their negative emphasis.

The silver stirrup jar (*fig. b*), perhaps from the Mochica culture but with strong Chavín influence, presents an anthropomorphic jaguar god in the round. About 13 inches high and hammered of high-grade metal, it was made in several parts and soldered together. Characteristic features of the jaguar demon seen on the preceding plate appear: the eyes outlined in heavy loops, the curving eyebrows that flare at the ends into cat's ears, the bared teeth with four huge tusks which stand out even more prominently through plastic presentation. The snakes, however, do not appear, and more anthropomorphic elements are brought into the composition. The two rows of teeth are clearly defined as human, although stereotyped, and appendages are attached suggestive of human ears. That which in the other examples was a lively play with lines, producing a vibrant whole, has become in the silver piece merely the expression of a remote idea. Little feeling for the material is apparent. The shallow corrugated lines on the top suggest pottery, while the deep groove above the eyes would be more effective in stone.

In *fig. c* we have the same subject carved in the round from wood—a staff or paddle head probably of Late Coast Tiahuanaco style. Much similarity to the silver jug can be detected. The channel below the eyes, which shows up clearly at the right in the photograph, is deep and particularly expressive in the softer material. The headdress, only suggested in *fig. b* and simplified in *fig. a,* is here worked out into an animal-mask. Shell or bone inlay gives good emphasis to all the carving by the introduction of a contrasting material. The four fangs should be mentioned as a feature consistently present.

In medieval America earrings were a distinction allowed only certain ranks, and the piercing of the ears was a ceremonial occasion. As the wearer grew older and the lobes stretched, his ear ornaments became larger and larger. The derisive Spanish name for the Incas was "long ears."

The four earrings shown on *Pl. 197, fig. a,* were found at Chongoyape in Lambayeque, the same site where some of the other pieces of Chavín style (*Pl. 195*) were discovered. They are all of gold, with the largest slightly over 5 inches in diameter. In each case the design was pressed into the metal, then cut out and soldered to the tubelike cylindrical section, which was inserted into the lobe. In two of them the decoration consists of rectangular serpent heads made up largely of straight lines; the other two, representing bird heads and beaks, have more convulsive contours.

Fig. b presents another object of personal adornment, a necklace identified as belonging to the Mochica. In its present arrangement it is about 16 inches long and composed of thirty graduated heads, the largest about 1½ inches in length. The features are slightly diversified, but each wears a puma headdress, and all are hollow behind and perforated along the edges for attachment to cloth. A chief with such a golden string sewed to his colorful poncho must have presented a picturesque appearance. The Scythians of prehistoric Asia—known as the best metal workers of their time and the diffusers of many metallurgical inventions into Europe—also combined textiles and metal in the same sophisticated manner, ornamenting their tunics with small golden objects.

The magnificent ceremonial knife illustrated on *Pl. 198, figs. a* and *c,* was found with other remarkable gold and silver objects quite recently at Illimo, near Lambayeque, on the northern coast of Peru. The treasure came from funerary tumuli in which several Chimú dignitaries were interred. Their graves contained, besides this piece, gold cups, some with repoussé figural decoration and others with turquoise incrustation (see *Pl. 201*), as well as gold funerary masks, simple beakers of gold, spoons, bead necklaces, earrings, pins, bells, timbrels, and personal ornaments of gold and silver. This sensational hoard, which apparently had escaped the busy digging of intruders and robbers for centuries, constitutes both in value and artistic importance the greatest single recorded find made in South America since the *conquistadores* laid hands on the metallic wealth of the Inca Empire.[164] It is fortunate that this and that other all-important treasure from Tomb 7 at Monte Albán in the Mexican Area, remained undisturbed until scientific handling could be assured.

The Chimú people, like their predecessors, the Mochica, were characterized by a cruel and warlike spirit. According to some sources, they practiced human sacrifice, a custom with which this knife might be associated. Its elaboration points to ceremonial use. It is about 17 inches long. The figure above the half-moon-shaped blade has been identified as the Chimú demigod, Naymlap, and shows him with an ornate headdress, the two outer bands of which, wrought in filigree, give the effect of an aureole. Eight pieces of green turquoise stud the arc and two more, his earplugs; these, together with the two wings that extend from behind the arms, are legendary characteristics of this mythical figure. The beaded edge, remarkably well preserved, is carried into the smallest detail, appearing even on the minute exquisite birds suspended from either end of the aureole. The semicircular outlines of the headdress and the blade form parentheses which seem to inclose this perturbing symbol.

Even more decorative detail appears on the back of the statue (*fig. c*). The bell shapes in the fringe along the edge of the shirt and apron, as well as the eight dangling pendants outlined with rows of globular beads, are all intact. With his wings and the birds hanging from his headdress, he might be an Icarus of the Chimú people. According to legend, he gave himself wings with which to fly to heaven.

In *fig. b* further evidence of the settled iconography of this region is discernible. It is part of a gold ear ornament, 2½ inches in diameter, from Jayanga, near Lambayeque, in the heart of the Chimú Kingdom. The main characteristics of the former image are present, and doubtless the same personage is represented.

Superb craftsmanship produced the piece in *Pl. 199, fig. a,* a gold cup, 5 inches high, also Chimú. The embossing of the figure is very shallow, but a bolder pattern was applied in the shell-shaped ornament just below the rim. These two kinds of relief effects—protruding shells and flatter figure—add to the

artistic value and interest of the piece. Although the pose of the figure is somewhat different, the wing-shaped eyes seen in the Illimo knife reappear here.
This cup, as well as those on the following plate, is of an unexpected thinness,
yet faultlessly made. A number of them have been unearthed in a relatively
excellent condition.

Fig. b shows another hero-god with outstretched arms and elaborate garments, repeated on the divided surface of a gold plaque. This Chimú ornament
comes from the vicinity of Chan-Chan and is about 3½ inches high. Here again
the shallow repoussé of the figures is well contrasted with the more pronounced
dots that ornament the frame.

The figural decoration of a large earplug (*fig. c*) demonstrates the same
ideology and technique, with the additional interest of cut-out outline and per-
foration. Three of the four figures wear a modified aureole headdress, not so
elaborate as in the Illimo knife. The central personage holds in his left hand a
cup shaped in the round and in his right a bag with dangling pendants. Other
disks are attached as ornaments elsewhere. Note the long bar, with a monster-
head at either end on which the chief character seems to ride. Originally the
plaque was mounted on the front of a very large earplug and surrounded by an
exquisite frame of beaded gold (see *fig. b* on the preceding plate). Behind it
was the tubular section, also of metal, that was inserted through the lobe of
the ear.

Cups were common all over the Andean Area. Their decoration varied,
however, according to district, and silver and gold, or even wood, were used as
material. The shape is characterized by a flawless dignity of line. *Fig. a* on
Pl. 200 is of gold, about 5 inches high, and is said to have come from the highlands, while *fig. b* is of silver and from the coastal district around Ancón. The
silver beaker flares gracefully from the base and is covered with repoussé designs of cats and other patterns. The gold cup is broader, has straighter sides,
and a single protruding band is its only ornament; its simplicity of style is typical
of Classic Tiahuanaco.

In *fig. c* two gold beakers and cup-shaped earplugs demonstrate a variety of
patterns. The two larger pieces are 5¼ inches high, and were fashioned of gold
hammered over clichés, with the bottoms soldered on. They come from the
Chimú Period of the Lambayeque region. In the cup on the right, only a frieze
is used above an embossed double band, which employs, inverted, the bird figures common in the decoration of Chimú pottery, textiles, and stucco work. The

fact that the birds are in a natural position when the piece is turned upside down gives reason to believe that some cups may have been kept inverted. The more elaborate ornamentation of the piece on the left shows the familiar stunted figure with semicircular sunburst headdress, placed within a geometric border of frets and other elements which have some suggestion of masks.

The ear ornaments, 2¾ inches high, have a pleasant curving form and are very finely incised or engraved with an oblique spiral design that leaves only a narrow ribbon-like strip undecorated. Again we find a squat human, this time in profile, repeated at measured intervals within a border of frets. The design is lucidly carried out within the limited space allotted it. Extraordinary feeling for the medium is shown in the use of plain bands to relieve the incised design as well as in the cast beads along the edge, soldered together and applied with unerring precision.

In the gold and silver cups on *Pl. 201,* still more variety is displayed, not so much in shape, which seems to have been more or less standardized, as in decoration.

The main interest in the two gold pieces from the Illimo treasure (*fig. a*) lies in their incrustation with turquoise. In spite of a certain divergence, very slight, in the border patterns, it is clear that both were manufactured on identical principles; even the soldered sections added at the bottom are similar. The beaded setting which incases each stone is a graceful artistic solution, as it not only holds firm the colorful material but brings plastic variety into the composition.

The silver cup (*fig. b*) is said to have come from the Piura Valley in the realm of the Chimú. Motifs characteristic of this culture embellish the piece, applied with a fine feeling for pattern. Human figures are blended into the oblique band of birds, fish, and symbolical objects as in a tapestry, where all elements are subordinated to the general scheme. It was much more difficult to execute the pattern within these winding mounting ribbons than in the horizontal line more frequently seen. The damaged edge, like crumpled paper in appearance, gives an excellent idea of the thinness of the metal.

In *fig. c* the tall gold ceremonial cup, 12⅔ inches high, comes from the northern coastal region of Peru. Its narrow chimney-like cylinder flares slightly toward the top and is finished with a fine beveled lip. The sharp protruding line of the jaw gives the feeling of a goblet and marks off the elongated neck below, which offers a good grip. Such faces always show the angular U around the mouth, indicated by a single downward-curving line, and the nose is always aquiline and sharply modeled. Cups of this type are found quite frequently in excavations even today, after four hundred years of treasure hunting.

In *Pl. 202* three different interpretations of the human figure from districts near one another are offered for comparative study. In the first illustration (*fig. a*), it is embossed on a gold cuff, about 5¾ inches high. Seemingly each figure was hammered from the same cliché. The heads are large, with the main features of the face clearly indicated, while the body, arms, and feet are small in comparison and sketchily done. No framing motif or additional decoration is combined with this puritanical trio, but their placement with ample breathing space shows artistic deliberation. Stylistically this piece might belong to the Mochica culture; however, such cuffs were also found in graves in the Ica Valley south of this region.

The small gold statuette, 2½ inches high (*fig. b*), is from the Chimú culture. Except for the two hammered gold disks in his hands, it is cast in one piece. The nose is pierced for an ornament that has disappeared. As on the cuff, the head is disproportionately large, a common characteristic throughout pre-Columbian art, and some details, such as the navel, are so sharply brought out that we may assume for them, too, especial significance. Despite its static build-up, the figure has life and in its communicative appeal will stand comparison with the turquoise and silver statuettes on *Pl. 258*. There is a hook in the back of the head, probably for suspension.

Still more ingratiating is the Chimú doll of silver (*fig. c*), which was put together of several sections of hammered metal and is, therefore, hollow. In his hands he holds a cup with a face design like that discussed in the preceding plate. The act of drinking is well conveyed to the onlooker through his movable arms. There is a toylike quality in the piece that is sensed immediately, which gives us a new angle on the mechanical versatility of these people and the scope of their imagination.

Masks were composed of semiprecious stones in the Mexican Area; in the Andean, something on a similar order was fashioned out of metal. As mentioned under weaving, the use of masks on mummy bundles seems to have been quite general here, but we find outspoken plastic differences in pieces from different regions.

Both specimens on *Pl. 203* appear to have come from the North Coast and are characterized as Chimú in style. In such work the Chimú people show an advanced and articulate artistic expression, frequently superior to that of their southern neighbors. A mature—we might also say aristocratic—mannerism is evident when these masks with their sure lines are compared with some of the pieces from the Ica Valley, for instance. The plastically composed and positive expression is there flattened into a geometric design and the arrogant mouth, generally closed in Chimú pieces, is opened to show teeth that are primitively embossed.

The mask in *fig. a,* 6 inches high, is hammered out of very thin gold, while that in *fig. b* is made of base silver. The latter, found among the unpublished treasures of the British Museum, is extraordinary, not only in design but because its accompanying materials are still intact. It is made up on quite different lines from the piece beside it. The eyes represent monkey heads, lending it especial interest. Feathers denoting a beard offer proof of the importance of the personage, for beards were allowed only rulers, high priests, and chiefs. A brocaded or embroidered band frames the mask and once served to bind it to the mummy pack.

Veritable statuary is presented on *Pl. 204,* shaped with a beguiling blend of naïveté and realism. *Fig. a* is a silver alpaca of Inca style, 12 inches high. Plain surfaces are used for the head, but the rest of the animal is fashioned from a sheet of metal hammered in corduroy welts to convey the impression of its long woolly coat and even the contours of its body beneath. Its pose is natural and quiet; its realism, accentuated by the disdainful expression of its face, one of the beast's characteristics.

The small figures in the group (*fig. b*) come from the Titicaca region. The man and woman are cast in solid silver and decorated with inlaid golden bands and eyeballs. Their postures are uniform, with only the heads showing a slight difference. He wears earplugs and a high headdress; she is distinguished by long hair that is parted in the middle and falls over the back. The silver llama, about 9 inches high, is cast in several pieces and soldered together. In some cases, as many as ten to thirteen separate parts were used to make up such a figure. The tips of the cleft hoof and the scalloped edging of the blanket are of gold, while the blanket itself was inlaid, probably with turquoise or some other semiprecious stones to give the ground tone.

In *fig. c,* a copper statuette 4¼ inches high from near Cuzco, the humorous element is introduced, more frequent in Andean art than in Middle American.

A little hunchback figure is depicted, clinging to the back of a llama who seems to endure him with reluctance. The animal's legs, caught in slow motion, add to the realism of the portrayal.

An alpaca or guanaco, about 4½ inches high, is presented in *fig. d.* The piece would seem to have been cast by a worker of considerable experience, for the silver alloy of the body and the gold of the head are beautifully joined. In contrast to the animal above it, the pose is lively, with its turned neck, bent knees, and raised forefoot all suggesting motion.

The medieval peoples of the Andean Area had such a highly developed sense of decoration that they ornamented even their tools with human and animal figures in a way which would not occur to us with our utilitarian approach. These pieces radiate the same charm that marks some of the pottery and also show the enjoyment of these peoples in their implements, partners in their craft.

A bronze knife is pictured on *Pl. 205, fig. a,* with a golden bird, probably a flamingo, perched on one end and a serpent crawling along the back of the blade, its reared head especially clear. The total length of the piece is 5½ inches. The blade is very thin along the cutting edge and at the point and must once have been quite sharp. Both serpent and bird were cast separately, the snake being welded to the blade, while the bird, of high-grade gold, was set into a socket in the end of the handle. It is believed that the working of bronze originated in the Classic Tiahuanaco Period and was introduced to the coast with the spread of that culture. In some cases the natural material appears to have been used, in others there is evidence of alloying.[10] In this connection, it is interesting to note that a large sheet of tin was discovered at Machu Picchu.

Close to the first piece in idea and execution is another unusual knife (*fig. c*), only 5 inches long, which was found by Dr. Bingham on his expedition to Machu Picchu. Humor and keen observation are manifest in the attitude of the boy as he lies on his stomach in his peaked cap and short tunic, waving his legs and dangling a large fish on the end of a thick rope.

The same qualities are apparent in the bronze chopper with a man and llama on the top of the handle (*fig. b*). Although corrosion has blurred the details, the piece gives a good idea of the originality used in the decoration of these implements.

It will be noted that some little figures on these bronzes have a practical application: the pointed ends could be used as awls for boring; the flattened surfaces, as adzes; the rounded parts perhaps for burnishing. All are probably Inca and late in date.

The bronze knife in *Pl. 206, fig. a* may have been used for cutting, scraping, and chopping. The shape of the blade recalls the Illimo ceremonial knife (see *Pl. 198*)—a form which is said to have persisted long after the Conquest. It has been compared to the Eskimo woman's knife. A llama head with a long neck forms the handle, 4½ inches high. Delicate inlay work, admirable from point of view of design as well as technique, decorates the piece, with the laconic drawing of the llama in the second square particularly worthy of mention.

Inlay work on a larger scale is seen in *fig. e,* a staff head of bronze, 3⅝ inches high, representing a bird. Fashioned in the shape of an adze and decorated with stripes of copper and silver, it presents a skillful blending of the practical and ornamental. The parallel strips of metal by no means give a naturalistic representation of a cormorant's feathers, but the idea of the colorful creature is nevertheless well conveyed. Its legs are executed in high relief. A handle, probably of wood, was attached.

Fig. b is a small bronze spoon, pictured here in its actual size. It may have been designed for handling valuable powder or medicine, or as a ceremonial gift. The chewing of coca leaves mixed with lime was a habit long-established in the Andean Area and the little implement may have been used for measuring a dose of this. The pointed beak and tail, however, suggest its association with a craft.

Fig. c is of special interest because it is said to have been found in El Salvador, although it is typical of the Andean Area. It may have traveled all this distance by trade, or it may be an imitation or copy of an Andean piece made somewhere along the route. As small as they are (the whole tool is only 2¾ inches long) and even in their corroded state, the figures of a parrot and monkey are clear.

The copper awl, or pin, with a rattle handle (*fig. d*) is about 5 inches long and might be of Chimú provenience. In the openwork all around the domed top small human figures are wrought in an ingenious pattern—an unusually fine bit of casting.

In *Pl. 207* we reach a high point in the metal-work of this area. With technical problems no longer a matter of concern and with totemistic representations stylized to a high degree, the objects approach very closely what we term *objets d'art.*

In *fig. a* is pictured a group of small gold articles of unknown provenience but Chavín in style. Superior workmanship is manifest in all of them. Each bead in the necklace is composed of one solid and one openwork band, which, in turning one against the other, brings an unusual play into the design. The two objects at the top of the plate are identified as scrapers of cosmetic oils. The left one, 3½ inches long, is decorated with a human figure seated on an openwork base and blowing a shell trumpet; the right one has a tiny bird on top. Both are hollow and are composed of several pieces.

Condor heads in good Chavín style (see *Pl. 197, fig. a*) are embossed on the disk on the right. Even more fluent, however, is the decoration on the other dishlike ornament with its bulging center. Here the sinuous and interlacing ribbons resolve themselves into a feline mask in the medallion (inverted in the photograph). Note the two snake heads that make up the lower jaw.

The group is the product of a civilized people; there is nothing vacillating about the work. Material, shapes, patterns, and figural ornaments are homogeneous, all of one culture that had the power and the time to digest everything here expressed into one artistic language.

The two shallow plates and the pitcher with a stirrup handle (*fig. b*) come from Huarmey Valley on the coast of Peru and are made of an alloy of 64 per cent gold, 30 per cent silver, and 6 per cent copper. The pitcher was fashioned from two semispherical parts and the stirrup section. It is decorated with an interlocking fish pattern, one favored in Chimú pottery and textiles and well adapted to a rounded surface. The eye dot is the only globular detail in an angular composition. The two plates, about 8 inches in diameter, are simple in shape and ideal in proportion. The slanting-Z element, interspersed with dots, suggests a writhing serpent body and attains staccato rhythm. But here, as in the case of the pitcher, the totemistic significance of the motifs has lost its vehemence and become primarily decorative in character. Probably made between 1300 and 1400, the forms are the result of the refinement of centuries.

As stated at the beginning of this chapter, it would appear that metal-working was first developed in or around the Andean Area. From here, certain pieces may have found their way into very distant regions where they fructified the local arts.

In *Pl. 208, fig. a* the golden breastplate, 5¼ inches in diameter, is said to have come from the highlands of Peru, although disks like these are actually more common in Ecuador and even farther north.[123] Stylistically it is classified as belonging to pre-Inca times, because of the resemblances to both Chavín and Tiahuanaco styles. The plaque, with its involved decoration, is not of high artistic quality, but the organization of its symbols into an apparent scheme gives good reason to argue that some kind of a system is involved in the piece. According to certain interpretations, the large face in the center represents the sun and the intricate characters on the rim stand for the various months of the year.[96] This is particularly noteworthy since the Andean Area is not known to have had any calendar comparable to the Maya or Mexican.

Interesting discussion centers about the gold disk in *fig. c.* It is said to have been found in a vaulted tomb near Zacualpa in the highlands of Guatemala under circumstances that would date the burial around the 10th century.[69] It can be seen that it bears some similarity to the foregoing piece, although in its crushed condition details are indistinct. Its style has been analyzed as combining elements of Chavín and Middle Chimú.[60] However, it has also been pointed out that it contains features of the Mexican Tlaloc, a circumstance that would suggest its manufacture nearer the place where it was found. It is 5 inches in diameter and shows another face when inverted. The eyes in the center are easily distinguished and the hanging tongues and the mouths, one wide with fangs and the other narrower with teeth, can be recognized after a moment's study. The rim is narrow and plain. Little calendrical content can be read into this second piece. The first plaque with its series of involved symbols would appear to antedate it.

Fig. b shows embossed silver ornaments from Cuzco, which may have been applied to mummy heads. The round one is considered an ear ornament; the almond-shaped one, 4⅞ inches in length, was perhaps for the eye. They are crudely executed with not too interesting patterns. On the second, two animals are roughly drawn in repoussé. Both are probably Inca, examples of a late and mass-producing culture.

More artistic deliberation can be discovered in the fragment in *fig. d,* taken from the same tomb at Zacualpa mentioned above. It is a piece of a small gold plaque, 3¼ inches in diameter, featuring a bird framed by a composite border design. The center and the rim seem to have been beaten out separately in two pieces, then welded together; the break follows the line of fusion. The design is very unusual. Dotted lines on metal-work are primarily a characteristic of the Chimú or their neighbors. The delineation of the bird, however, has no stylistic affiliation with any known culture; Dr. Lothrop recalls only designs on Managua-ware pottery from Nicaragua that might be said to resemble it.[69]

Animal representations of late cultures of the Andean Area are shown in *Pl. 209*. The gold beard-tongs, or tweezers (*fig. a*), is about 2½ inches high and from the Central Coast of Peru. In the droll and well-executed scene on top of the instrument, two monkeys sit nibbling, as if perched there only for a moment.

The gold disk (*fig. b*), perhaps an earplug, is about 2 inches in diameter and identified as Chimú. It shows a flock of monkeys encircling a central figure portrayed in the round. The intermingling arms and legs and the curling tails are used to the best advantage to create a decorative design.

A pair of humming birds decorates the gold ear ornament from the Ica region of southern Peru (*fig. c*). The piece is 1¾ inches in diameter and presents the subject in perfect three-dimensional plasticity. All the grace and volatility of these colorful creatures have been transmitted in this diminutive representation.

Fig. d, slightly enlarged as shown, doubtless had symbolic content. Its provenience is unknown. The condor head with its static strength of a totem is reminiscent of Tiahuanaco or Coast Tiahuanaco. But the realistic creeping attitude of the little amphibian suggests cultures north of the Inca realm. Birds, amphibians, and reptiles attracted generally great interest because of their affiliations with the sky and water. The ability to fly or to live under water always has had a fascination for the human. Its association with supernatural power is still more evident in the cultures of Ecuador, Colombia, and the Isthmus.

INTERLYING AREA

Although certain similarities in technique and ideology were spread over the Andean and Interlying areas, outspoken stylistic characteristics can be found in the different cultural regions that are clearly indicative of their locality.

An example of this is seen in the Bat-god (*Pl. 210, fig. a*), a figure strange to the iconography of Peru. The piece came from the Tola Islands in Esmeraldas, in the northwest corner of Ecuador. Quito, the capital city of this once independent nation, fell under the domination of the Incas for a time, and it is known that certain of its districts thereafter produced chiefly bronze tools for the Empire. There was no time for Inca influence to go deep, however, as the Conquest soon put an end to it. The culture of Ecuador seems to have been allied more closely with the north; the figure of the Bat-god extends from here through the Isthmian region and into lower Middle America (El Salvador and Honduras), where we have already seen it on pottery.

This piece records, in a cruder edition, the same technical achievement that we saw in the Andean Area. It is 9½ inches across and cut in the shape of the deity out of one piece of medium-thick sheet gold, with the details embossed. The outline of the wings is irregular, the rows of dots unevenly applied, and the sides unsymmetrical. The body is compressed and the legs are only indicated, doubtless deliberately, so as to throw full emphasis on the head. This part is executed with a definite feeling for the use of various planes. It was made separately and joined by soldering. A new manner of representation is revealed in the treatment of the eyes and nose. Although the face of the god is stiff and inarticulate, the plaque has the compactness and vigor of all true primitives.

The mask (*fig. b*), also from Esmeraldas, is made of bronze with a low tin content and is about 7½ inches long. The hollow eyes and mouth are unusual and add a fantastic touch. Two tusks protruding from the lower lip offset the human features. In impression, the piece recalls masks of modern Latin America.

Fig. c is a bronze disk, 13½ inches in diameter, from the Manabí district of Ecuador. In contrast to the plain bowl-shaped rim, the center carries an embossed face, hammered over a mold. The dotted lines seen in *fig. a* appear here in the headdress as a more organic part of the composition. Such pieces were probably used as breast ornaments, although it has been suggested that they were gongs.[54] While the material from Esmeraldas (see also *Pl. 151*) is stylistically quite distinct from the Peruvian, showing relationship with the north, that from Manabí has been linked with Peru. Both sites are presumably pre-Inca.[8]

The breastplate on *Pl. 211* offers a much riper example of the Bat-god concept. It is 13½ inches across and came from Esmeraldas. The bat head, thrust savagely toward the onlooker, was hammered out separately and joined to the beaten plate. Although the noseplug seems to pass through the septum, it was in reality two separate pieces soldered on either side. Embossed patterns, the meaning of which is unclear, ornament the background of the middle field. Four uniform human figures are placed on the sides, their large headdresses worked out with crude but decorative detail while embossed legs suggest their bodies.

A human face surmounted by a helmet-like headdress appears on the small gold plaque from Ecuador (*fig. b*), about 4 inches in diameter. The composite animal frieze on the rim is made up of bird and monkey elements, very decorative in their stylization.

While the Bat-god was represented in the two preceding plates, first with the contours of a body, then surrounded by a stylized abstract pattern, the head of the deity on *Pl. 212* seems almost subordinated to the elaborate independent decoration that surrounds it. This golden ornament is 14 inches across. The head in the center, even though somewhat modified, shows enough similarity to the other two to be identifiable. The strong plastic effect still prevails. It also was fashioned separately by hammering and stands out 1½ inches from the background, to which it was joined by a fine bit of soldering. Highly interesting is the middle section where four double-headed alligators—very animated, with their upturned snouts—appear in faultless repoussé. Dots and triangles represent the scales.[34] The embossed lines are attractive in themselves, with their alternating courses and lively changing shapes. The design has the appearance of quilted work of remarkably even quality. The outer edge of the breastplate is slit to represent feathers. Their plain surface, vibrating and shimmering, adds a new decorative variation, which makes the piece most striking in its artistic balance.

With Ecuador we leave the territory which could have received first-hand artistic impulses from the center of the Andean Area. In Colombia we shall notice not only the ideological change, perceptible in certain Ecuador pieces, but also utter differences in technique and construction, involving primarily cast objects, the manufacture of which was undoubtedly a later achievement than cold hammering and soldering.

A semicivilized concept is manifest in the gold ornaments in human shapes (*Pl. 213, fig. a*) from the region of the Chibcha people. This powerful tribe resided in the highlands of the Cordillera Oriente, one of the rich gold districts of Colombia, and resisted the Spaniards valiantly at the time of the Conquest. Isolated not only from attack but also from many outside cultural influences, they were inferior to the Incas in their social and artistic development. Their gold work and other minor arts reveal a mixture of individual traits with peripheral designs borrowed from neighboring cultures.

The five pieces in the middle of *fig. a,* which were probably fastened to robes, show a uniform technique. The center figure is about 5 inches high. The gold background cast in one flat piece was intended to represent the outlines of a human body considerably simplified; features and other elements were applied in gold wire where a suggestion of detail was deemed necessary and separate dangling ear pendants were attached by links. By comparing the posture of the three central figures with *Pl. 218, fig. c*, an obvious similarity will be noticed. This Chibcha type will appeal to the neo-primitives of our own day. The two flanking figures are solidly cast in an axe-shape, the blade section serving as lower half of the body and the heads and arms forming the top. This form could derive from earlier similar shapes in stone, which, indeed, might have served as the first positives for molds. (Compare *Pl. 237, fig. a.*)

The pre-Columbian peoples had a predilection for bells of various sorts, sometimes without clappers, sometimes with pebbles or pellets of clay inside them. Tinkling ornaments of shell or metal were frequently attached as a fringe to garments, as pendants on jewelry, or to the legs. The two gold bells in *fig. b,* the taller 2½ inches high, come from Colombia. They were cast, with the exception of certain wire decorations which may have been soldered to them. In the smaller, a tiny figure is seated on top of the bell; in the larger, the body of the animal serves as the bell-jar. The contrast of plain surface with twisted and composite wire decoration shows an advance over the Chibcha figures. Both are inarticulately crude in style, however, when compared with other Colombian ornaments.

A rare piece of gold work, said to have come from La Guaira, Venezuela, is pictured in *fig. c.* Although this region is outside our five areas and the archaeology of the country is only now beginning to be organized, this striking image should be included here as evidence of the widespread metallurgical knowledge below the Isthmus and as an example of still another style. The figurine stands about 5½ inches high. Cast parts are fused with hammered surfaces, and some of the lighter decorative elements, made up of coiled wire and nail-head shapes, may have been soldered on, while others were doubtless cast with the main body. The subject of the piece is an anthropomorphic figure with ferocious tusks and button-like eyes (discernible in the diamond sector directly over the teeth). An extravagant headdress is featured, with frondlike plumes and two stylized animal profiles on either side. Two solid beaks jut forward over the creature's forehead. It may be presumed that local stylistic elements mingle here with foreign motifs, already stereotyped when taken over.

All the flasks on *Pl. 214* are of gold and come from Colombia. The largest (*fig. a*), about 7½ inches high, shows a male figure embossed on one side and a female on the other. The shape of the vessel is pleasing, with the curving lines of the sides well balanced by the bulging bottom and heavier shoulders. No hesitancy is apparent in the execution of the neck, although it too was difficult to fashion. The form is living; the most static element is, perhaps, the fetish-like image in the center which changes the mood of the piece. We shall meet this rigid figure stepping out into the three dimensional (see *Pl. 218*); even then its ineloquence does not disappear.

The flask in *fig. b* is a variant of the one beside it. Instead of the concave line that serves to lighten the latter, this piece has convex sides, adding corresponding bulk, and an onion-shaped neck that harmonizes with the curves of the body. The composition of the human figure is more or less identical.

The two smaller flasks in *fig. c* likewise seem to have presented no problems to their makers. Even to our eyes they are perfect in their proportion, the shapes are civilized, and the execution is faultless. The piece at the left, about 4 inches high and in the form of a gourd, has a jovial rotundity suggesting the flesh of a living plant. It could have been suspended on a ribbon by the two loops on the sides. The flask on the right has absolutely no decoration and its surface is smoothed and burnished. Shaped with consideration, its contours bring to mind an almond or some delicate exotic fruit.

The Quimbaya people, who inhabited the region of Antioquia on the Cauca River in the northwestern part of Colombia, were among the most skillful gold workers of medieval America. Pure gold or gold alloyed with copper was used, and broad polished surfaces, enlivened by intricate relief work of coiled wire and neat braided bands, characterize their art.[70] It is noteworthy that no air bubbles are present in any of this cast work and that there is no evidence of a period of experimentation.

Pl. 215 and those following take us into a strange fantasy-world where human elements are blended with animal shapes and decorated with what appear to us abstract or geometric motifs.

The pendant (*fig. a*) is a rare specimen of craftsmanship, even among the works of the Quimbaya culture. The main part is only about 3 inches high, but the piece appears much larger because the bird heads extend for an inch and a half. The principal elements are strongly plastic, with all minor detail abbreviated. A human head and shoulders are easily distinguished, but all human likeness is dispensed with below, where the figure blends into twin bird bodies with sharply delineated heads and beaks. The elaborate headdress with its two bell-shaped ornaments and the winglike wire spirals on either side will be seen again on the next plate. There was apparently no intention even to suggest arms, and the hole in the chest is impossible to interpret realistically, although it is of value in balancing and lightening the design. A realistic tendency is again evident in the compact bodies of the birds, with which the human figure merges so smoothly that the point of fusion cannot be defined. Although the eyes protrude too far and no bird ever wore such a plaited "harness," it is just this part of the faultlessly cast pendant that needs no interpreter; so expressive is it that we accept it without question.

The same type of semicircular nose ring as that worn by the figure is shown in *figs. b* and *c,* 4 and 4¼ inches wide respectively. These come from Antioquia, where they seem to have been quite common. The rows of openwork, fashioned in a highly complicated technique, look as airy as if made in crochet but are quite solid to the touch. Remarkable continuity is observed in the composition. On comparing the two pieces, it is interesting to note that the creature on the top edge of the first has degenerated in the second to a mere zigzag.

A diminutive idol, 2½ inches high, with a head composed of stylized animal elements placed on a human body, is the subject of *Pl. 216, fig. a.* It was cast of gold in several pieces and reveals full command of the technique. The emphasis is laid on the ornamentation of the upper part and the face is almost submerged. However, a wedge-shaped alligator-like head is discernible with a grinning pointed mouth, on top of which, at the apex, is a tiny rounded snout and perhaps eyes close to either side. The two bell shapes noted on the preceding plate are still more prominent here, and similar wire coils sweep upward as if in an elongation of the mouth. The hands of the idol, the five fingers well defined, grasp ceremonial bars. Below the belt, plain flat sections are used to signify the legs, and a complete departure from realism is reached in the feet with their eight toes. The small piece shows unexpected deliberation in its composition. From the point of view of design, the smooth lower part with its flaring base counterbalances the bell-shaped ornaments on the top, and the broken elements are concentrated between them.

Further disintegration of the human figure is shown in *fig. b,* about 10 inches high, another Quimbaya gold breast ornament. The leg sections are now merely two vertical sheets of metal, and the feet, with no suggestion of stance, have become a single finlike appendage, with the toes a series of numerous incisions. Five birds are ranged across the breast on a gold scaffold, producing a second plane. On both ends of this support, conventionalized "flowers" of wire form a motif that appears also in *Pl. 218, fig. d.* The bell-shaped elements at the top are more pointed than in the idol beside it, and the two slender winglike compositions at either side narrow as they mount, thus augmenting the vertical effect. Their lines remind us of those in medieval European manuscripts where the Gothic tendency saturates even the angels' wings.

The transmutation of the central anthropomorphic figure into an abstraction is fully realized in the three pendants of Quimbaya type shown in *fig. c.* The tallest is about 10½ inches. Such ornaments must have been manufactured frequently, for a number of them have been found showing very slight deviations. This would help explain the high degree of formalism involved in them. All three examples illustrated here show to an identical degree the boiling down of naturalistic elements into flat, round, and coiling units. The headdress "bells" are no longer laid horizontally, but are tipped forward; the mounting "wings" have become tight cautious coils, and the wire elements are multiplied, with the topmost spiral the largest. Instead of arms with ceremonial bars as in *fig. a,* we find here only two sticks, like elephants' tusks, issuing from the center, and the fingers that grasp them are denoted with wires, sometimes five, sometimes only three to a side. Nose and eyes can be inferred in the thimble-shaped protrusion beneath the bells and the two screw-head shapes at either side of it. A zigzag pattern decorates the base in complete disregard of its derivation. The nose piece with its four spirals is a new element, as is also the double whorl below it, but all their number does not bring new charm to the whole.

The circle of conventionalization that started with the first figure on the plate is closed with these ornaments. Both *figs. b* and *c* branched out from the same idea, and which of them has more conventionalization depends on the evaluation accorded certain elements. Only by looking at *fig. a* can we trace faintly the impulses which fathered such pieces. It is worth noting that this type of ornament is conceivable only in metal, proof of the deep-rooted feeling these artisans had for the medium.

Fig. a on *Pl. 217* shows a knife-shaped pendant about 11 inches high from Popayán, Colombia, south of the Quimbaya region. It is made of an alloy base of gold, silver, and copper, with a thin plating of fine gold, the process of which is still problematic. The central anthropomorphic figure and the four small beaked creatures were cast by the lost-wax process and are hollow behind, while the thin knife blade below was probably hammered from cold metal. The variously executed sections were joined by soldering. A circular nose pendant and three bead necklaces decorate the main figure, whose body is outlined and divided by delicate beading. Its legs are short and out of proportion, the knees encircled by tight bands frequently met with in Colombian work (see next plate); the screwhead eyes are already familiar. The hanging mass of feathers on the headdress counterbalances the upward sweep of the knife blade, and the approaching finger tips of the main figure contrast with the outward-turned palms of the smaller ones. Tactile variation is furnished by the flat "bird-monkeys" and the finely executed geometrical pattern of the openwork nimbus. A heavy loop is soldered to the back for attachment.

This piece shows influence from both the north and south. The general idea of the figure above a curving knife blade recalls the Illimo knife of Peru (see *Pl. 198*), while the divided crest and the multiple fingers and toes—perhaps symbolizing supernatural power, as do the many arms of Hindu deities—suggest the work of Panama and Costa Rica. Its date would probably fall between the 11th and early 15th centuries.[16] In its general aspect the ornament is unique and presents a crystallization of the "primitive" that is exemplified in the more familiar African wood carvings. Nothing in this piece is completely realistic; elements of life, of fantasy, and abstractions combine in frozen flamboyancy.

In *figs. b* and *c* we have variants of the same theme, also from Colombia but on a lower artistic level in both composition and decorative effect. *Fig. b* introduces an amphibian element that we shall encounter more and more frequently as we proceed toward the north. In this piece the human face is square when compared with the V shape of *fig. a,* and the eyes and mouth are represented by depressions on the surface in contrast to the protruding elements of the larger piece. Wings replace the arms or forelegs, and the "knife" section is tapered down until it resembles a tail. The nose rings are identical, and the headdresses, especially in the inner geometric arc, show similar design.

In *fig. c* human characteristics again predominate, although the face or mask is strongly reminiscent of bird features. The openwork in the headdresses just seen has here been transferred to the blade, and the feathers are again more realistically portrayed than in the conventionalized presentation in *fig. b*.

Besides the general idea, all three pieces have in common the beaded trim which ornaments the body of each central figure. It conveys the most realistic suggestion on that one with amphibian qualities (*fig. b*). On the plate just preceding, we can trace the stylization of an anthropomorphic figure into abstraction; on this, we may be confronted with steps toward the personification of an idea, perhaps of the Crocodile-god.

The golden plaque on *Pl. 218, fig. a* bears a subtle relationship to the pendant from Popayán in the curving outline of the upper section and in the bird heads and tails with their perforations at the sides. It is well proportioned, with the broad base line successfully carrying the weight of the whole. The seven embossed figures, with headdresses little more than suggested by beaded aureoles, are uniform, but the central personage—who is leaning forward as if from a balcony—and the two just below him are represented in different attire. He wears a three-dimensional headdress somewhat similar to that of *fig. c* on this plate. There is a ring in his nose for an ornament that has disappeared, which, from the general design, may have extended into the blank space below. The two figures at either side wear headdresses in the form of birds that show marked similarity to the next piece. Cautious craftsmanship is seen in the small supporting sections, which, nearly unnoticed, strengthen the most fragile side parts. The hooks at the bottom may have served to affix it to another material or have held dangling pendants. Mention should be made of the plaited edging, outlining the entire plaque.

Interest is due the gold breastplate in *fig. b* for its rare subject matter—a tower with four birds of prey sitting on the top. It is about 6 inches high and is identified as coming from the Quimbaya region. A kind of artistic shorthand is employed to record the birds. Only the heads received real emphasis; the bodies are practically non-existent, and the claws are depicted in relief, artistically less powerful, although there would have been space for bringing in more details if desired. In this respect, the composition recalls the bird figures of *Pl. 215, fig. a.*

Fig. c is a gold figurine from Antioquia, done in the lost-wax technique of which the people in the Quimbaya region were such masters. It is 6 inches high and presents a female figure. She wears the tight knee and ankle bands that have been noted elsewhere and a crownlike headdress with two beak blades and wire spirals at either side. A large lunate pendant hangs by two rings from the nose, covering the lower part of her face, and two others, circular in shape, are affixed to the hands.

There is considerable resemblance between this figure and one 9 inches high shown in *fig. d.* This statuette wears a conical headdress, and the hands, which are in the same position, hold spirals of gold wire suggestive of flowers. The nose is pierced and doubtless once carried an ornament. Even if the proportions are not in accordance with our ideals of beauty, the body is young and vibrant; the shoulders and knees have the static elasticity of the prehistoric sculptures of other great early civilizations, and the slim waist would satisfy the fashion designer of our own day. As in so many South American representations, the legs are short.

Both pieces have the same tapering base which might have been attached to a staff or other similar object. Both have the qualities of an idol, emphasized by the presentation of a figure completely nude, with jewelry and ornaments. A discussion of the reasons why so many idols of prehistory are thus represented would require too great a digression here; however, it may be pointed out that their symbolism is connected with fertility rites and goes back to the earliest times of mankind.

The technique and artistry of the Quimbaya region reach their peak, perhaps, in such pieces as those reproduced on *Pl. 219*. The modesty of subject, the immediacy of the representation make them not only easily understood and enjoyed, but give an insight into the more relaxed moods of this people when they were not weighed down by a mystic-totemistic sorcery. Nothing conveys their inherent talent and keen nature observation so simply and with so much naïve charm as these pieces. Despite a certain stylization, which is apparent, all embody the spirit of life.

The gold staff head representing a pelican (*fig. a*) manifests lively realism and technical assurance. It is 5 inches high and was cast in several pieces, then soldered together. Eyes, beak, claws, and tail are fashioned skillfully and simply; neck and legs are static. As in all good sculpture, not all the elements have the same quality of motion. The openwork of the breast contrasts with the solid surfaces and makes the piece appear lighter in weight. Even the unevennesses of tone due to soldering seem to enhance its animation.

Fig. b is a golden staff head, about 8 inches long, from Montería, Colombia. The five birds standing in a row on a latticed bar are humorously appealing. Heavy, weighing more than one pound, the piece nevertheless gives the impression of lightness: the birds are alert, as if about to take flight from a riddled crumbling log. The use of a lattice pattern for the base prevents this subordinate element from distracting from the focus of interest. From the technical as well as the plastic point of view the work is outstanding. It was made by the lost-wax process; the base and the lower lines of the bird on the extreme left show best the great skill essential to its execution. Both birds and base are hollow, yet so solidly cast that not one beak or section of the bar can be bent.

Two more staff heads are seen in *fig. c,* executed in the same technique. In the diminutive dog, shown in actual size, there is a broader use of openwork.

The animal has a toylike charm, and its expression is droll and humorous. Still more humor is discernible in the human figure beside it. The little man is seated on a low chair, blowing on a trumpet—a common musical instrument throughout medieval America—and shaking a rattle with his right hand. His left arm is realistically modeled; it is part of a living body engaged in making music. The sense of tone is rarely present in representations of musicians of any age or region, but this little man seems surrounded by the din he is creating. The decorative bands around the crown and on the edge of the brim of his broad hat are clearly marked, corroborating the description of the earliest Spanish writers regarding the picturesque headgear of the natives.

These are some of the rare pieces of pre-Columbian metal-work completely plastic in radiation, released from any remnant of two-dimensional tradition which cut its shapes from sheets of metal.

The jewelry and metal trappings of chiefs included far more impressive objects than the golden staff heads just shown; headgear, more ornamental than protective, was also made of the precious metal. The crown from Antioquia (*Pl. 220, fig. a*), 6 inches high, was cut from a sheet of beaten gold. It is rare, not only because of its perfect state of preservation, but also because it has more decoration than most of the extant crowns. An embossed geometric pattern covers much of the surface, but the feature of the piece is the concise cut-out representation of a soaring condor. Little scrolls moving upward from the outspread wings add to the feeling of height.

Headgear of considerably greater weight (over twelve ounces) is pictured in the massive gold helmet from the Quimbaya culture (*fig. b*). It was fashioned in semispherical form, full-size and shaped for a human head, with repoussé decorations hammered in afterwards. Such gold helmets from pre-Columbian America are infrequent and most of them bear convulsive animal or geometric patterns. This casque is a rarity on account of the single female figure embossed upon one side. It is a crude representation to our eyes, but there is no denying that it is well placed within the space accorded it and the design shows vigor. The hammered dots and lines curving away from the head may be the conventionalization of a great headdress extending across the upper field and ending on the opposite side of the piece. This conjecture is supported by the position of the hands, which appear to be clasping the edges of the huge ornament. (Compare *Pl. 148, fig. e*.)

Headbands, crowns, and helmets of solid gold have been found in Peru,

Ecuador, Colombia, and Panama; north of this, there is no record of this type of headgear. In Mexico, the inventories of the loot at the time of the Conquest mention wooden helmets, gilt-edged or sheathed in gold and combined with feather-work and stone mosaic.[70]

Another gold helmet, about 4¾ inches high and weighing eleven ounces, is pictured on *Pl. 221, fig. a.* It comes from Darién, Panama. The surface of beaten gold is divided into four equal fields, each embossed with a double-headed crocodile. So precisely is the subject pattern repeated that we may presume its application by the use of a cliché. The realistic impression of the amphibians is offset by a second head where the tail should be.

That there was no intention of producing a record true to life in these helmets is doubly clear in the next piece (*fig. b*), from Coclé, Panama. It is made of thin beaten gold and weighs slightly less than eight ounces. Here the entire surface is covered with a highly stylized pattern of similar ideological content, showing repetitions of the double-headed Crocodile-god, one in the center of the photograph and two others on the sides. The tendency was to cover all available space. Human, reptile, and geometric elements are condensed, and in the restless crowded texture we discern mainly the vibration of a positive decorative talent. Note the perforations around the edge for sewing in a lining.[70]

Panama and Costa Rica used techniques similar to those of Colombia, but their art shows definite local motifs. In studying stylistic divergences, however, it should not be forgotten that until 1903 the territory known today as Panama formed a part of Colombia. Throughout the Isthmian region, the same veneration was bestowed on crocodiles and alligators that rattlesnakes received in the Maya and Mexican areas. The aborigines fought them and made use of their bodies according to the traditions of the land; but they also incorporated them into their fantasy-world, elevating them to the symbol of a god. We find them partly realistic, partly stylized, embossed in relief in curious patterns, or, as they appear on this plate, cast in three dimensions. Other reptiles, such as frogs, lizards, and turtles also occur frequently.

Pl. 222, fig. a, about 4¼ inches long, is now in the Museo Nacional at San José, Costa Rica. It is made of eighteen-carat gold and weighs about two ounces.[65] In style it appears to be an offshoot of the Chiriquí culture. The alligator or crocodile is pictured here quite realistically, with human prey; the man's head with earplugs, his body, arms, and legs are clearly depicted. As will be seen, this rare presentation may furnish a clue to problematic elements in many of these pendants.

The gold alligator from Coclé (*fig. c*) is 7 inches long and quite massive. It was cast in one piece with an open channel underneath that held the core around which the molten metal was poured. Small eyes on the under side show that, heavy as it is, it was attached to another material. The body of the creature, with its bulging eyes and creeping posture, is quite naturalistically observed; there are even certain suggestions of muscular build-up. On the other hand, the tail, with its divided curling flukes and the bars and rings on either side, is completely unrealistic. The same is true of the object carried in the reptile's mouth, which is probably a highly conventionalized human body. Upon comparing it with the piece above, we can discern the great loops of the earplugs; the element beside them may represent a waving arm, and the toothed edge in front, the feet, with the pattern then doubled in mirror fashion for the sake of symmetry.

The twin reptiles in *fig. d,* about 3½ inches long, are of gold and also come from Coclé. The protruding eyes, sharp bared teeth, springy elastic legs require no explanation; they testify to the talent of the goldsmith who wrought the piece. Cuneiform depressions along the bodies represent the markings of the reptiles. Their curling tails have decorative effect, although the position is not natural.

We should compare the objects in their mouths with those in *figs. a* and *c* to see how much change could occur in one motif within the frame of a single idea. Considerable difference can also be noted in the treatment of the tails and scaly surfaces of their bodies. Such a combination of good naturalism with strange symbolism is one of the main characteristics of medieval American art and complicates not only the problem of interpretation but the analysis of style as well.

The shark pendant (*fig. b*) comes from Chiriquí, Panama. It is about 4 inches long and was cast in one piece. Of brilliant yellow gold, it reveals a smoothness and elegance that are extraordinary, even among the many other faultless pieces from this region. In the lively representation of the body even the glutinous quality of the skin can be felt. The rings at the ends are for suspension.

The two embossed gold plaques from Coclé on *Pl. 223* show a mastery in technique and stylization such as we have not met since certain early cultures of the Andean Area.

In *fig. a,* about 8 inches in diameter, there is a similarity in build-up—even though the decorative effect is different—to gold work from Chavín, Lambayeque, and, to some extent, Tiahuanaco. These older pieces are perhaps quieter in their stylization, more suave in linear conduct—more civilized, one might say; in the specimens from Coclé, the expression is brought out with brutality, a cruder plasticity, but certainly with primeval vigor. It is interesting to find the same ground idea depicted in *fig. a* as in the Gateway of the Sun at Tiahuanaco (see *Pl. 46*), the Chavín stone (see *Pl. 99, fig. b*), or the gold plaques of Lambayeque (see *Pl. 195*). The figure in the Coclé piece has the same frontal pose, with arms outstretched, each holding a staff; the elaborateness of the headdress, the emphasis on the belt which resolves into a fantastic animal on either side, the exaggerated teeth, and the decorative presentation of the feet all register a certain relationship. Technical aptitude is shown in the extraneous elements added for decoration, in the palms, the feet, and the grooved bodies of the monsters, for instance. All contours are sharp and angular in contrast to the rounded corduroy effect of Lambayeque work.

Still more enjoyment in the command over the material is visible in the other gold disk (*fig. b*). This one is slightly larger and shows two identically gesticulating figures with bodies more or less human and heads like birds. The extravagant belts that sweep to the edge of the piece are suggestive of the flowing plumes of a tail and an instance of the exuberance in technique, for the same idea could have been conveyed much more simply. In spite of a certain crudeness in the delineation, the power and movement in the design are immediately sensed.

Both culturally and artistically, much is unbalanced in the Interlying Area, but for this very reason these examples are especially important to our survey as artistic milestones on the way up from the south. Because their language is so sharply minted, it is easier for us to approach through them the works of other cultures whose expression is less articulate.

The same vigor and the same enjoyment in ever-changing plastic surfaces, already met in larger specimens of Panama, are even more apparent in the jewelry shown on *Pl. 224,* all from Coclé.

The first gold pendant (*fig. a*), 2 inches long, is fashioned in the shape of an insect. Its head and thorax are cast in gold; the abdominal part is made up of light translucent quartz. Two hooks for suspension are at the tip. The casting and handling of such small and delicate details may be regarded as one of the triumphs of the lost-wax process.

Fig. b is a gold cuff that was found on the arm of a skeleton in one of the richer graves at Sitio Conte in the Coclé region. It is of thin sheet metal, and the pattern, hammered in over a cliché, shows two crocodiles, each with a bird perched on its tail. The hind legs of the amphibians are omitted, but the fore-feet recall in their gesture the second gold plaque on the preceding plate. The headdress, too, and the sharp contours and decorative depressions of the general pattern show similarity. Cuffs of gold, silver, and copper are not common in medieval America but they have a widespread distribution.[70]

The gold pendant with four curly-tailed animals (*fig. c*)—probably alligator cubs—measures only about 2½ inches in length. Miniature animals with elongated and curling tails were quite common in Panama and have been found made of agate also. Here the alert little creatures are placed side by side, coalesced in such a way that they stand on a total of only ten legs, the front five of which are clearly visible in the photograph. The pendant was cast as a unit, and part of the clay mold still adheres to the under side.

The combination of two or more different materials in one piece is always a sign of superior workmanship—when skill has leisure to play with its medium. In Renaissance Europe ivory, rock crystal, and mother-of-pearl were framed with metal by Benvenuto Cellini and his followers. The combination of metal and semiprecious stones, such as serpentine and opal, besides the quartz and agate already mentioned, appears frequently in the jewelry and other small objects of the Interlying Area. *Fig. d* shows an impressive pendant of solid gold, 4¼ inches long, representing a fantasy animal whose body is a fine dark emerald. In this unusual and fascinating piece, the same skill already observed is apparent, perhaps to an even higher degree. Stylized elements, like the bifurcated tongue, are combined with such expressive naturalistic details as the springy legs, and virtuoso embellishments—products of pure fancy—are added, such as the "cog-wheel" at the end of the tail and the dangling pendants at the back.

Of the four objects on this plate, three were cast, one was hammered, and two of them were fashioned in combination with precious stones—no mean achievement for a semicivilized people.

Casting reached such perfection and routine on the Isthmus that metal-work complicated in both structure and decoration was turned out as a matter of course. And if these products are not especially appealing to our eye, the reason should be sought in the obscurity of the concept rather than in any technical ineptitude.

Pl. 225, fig. a is not only interesting as a piece but also because of its material. It was made of an alloy of gold and much copper, a mixture now generally called *tumbaga* (from the Malay word for copper) and easier to handle than gold alone. As gold was more plentiful than copper in these regions, the combination must have resulted from considerable experience in working with the metals and observing their durability. The gilded *tumbaga* pendant shown here is about 5 inches wide and 3½ high. After seeing animals in groups of two and four, we now have two warriors, mirror images, one of the other, standing with bowed heads side by side, their toes clinging to a thin metal rod. They wear conical caps upon their heads and over their chests hang necklaces of several strands. Across the body of each runs a braided "bandoleer," which supports at the hip a tiny bird. One hand grasps a paddle-shaped club; the other, a bundle of spears. The twin figures are joined at the shoulders by three small knobs, from which, suspended by a braided cord, hangs a human head. Originally two other heads (the left one is broken off) hung from the lower ends of their weapons. The statuette evidently depicts the return of victorious warriors, carrying their battle trophies. There is doubt as to whether this type of work originated in this area; compare it with the stone carving of the "dual officiants" (see *Pl. 97, fig. d*).

The next illustration (*fig. b*) shows a somewhat similar gold pendant that is said to have come from Colombia. It is about 4 inches wide and presents an octette of flageolet players—twin major figures and six smaller editions of the same type. Whether they are human or animal cannot be determined; their posture is that of men, but their faces and clumsy feet are rather animal-like. Considering the many open spaces between the constituent elements, the whole piece is remarkably compact.

Fig. c, from Costa Rica, is an interesting parallel to the first piece. Here the twin figures walk hand in hand. There is a suggestion of the war clubs in the bars at the sides; on the other hand, the wire coils that decorate the heads and form the hands connect them also with *fig. b.*

The east coast of Costa Rica was first discovered by Christopher Columbus on his fourth and last voyage. Port Limón lies today on the bay in which the Admiral's exhausted men rested and repaired their ships in 1502. The Indians were not hostile toward the newcomers, but rather were disposed to barter their goods; they even made presents to the Spaniards of fruit, animals, and gold ornaments. The name "rich coast" was thus given to Costa Rica with reason, for, when compared with those first touched by the Spanish ships, it was a country with an abundance of metal objects. The inhabitants are reported to have known the arts of weaving and casting gold. They were clever wood and stone carvers and no mean potters.

An interesting compositeness is evident in the next specimen from this region (*Pl. 226, fig. a*), a gold pendant about 4 inches high that undoubtedly shows a blend of local and imported ideas. At least three different creatures are incorporated in this symbolic piece: the main motif is a condor with flattened wings and tail; two grinning reptilian heads branch to right and left, and a heavy bovine animal gazes out from the breast. The use of smooth cast surfaces is striking, revealing a sure feeling for the medium and a grasp of the technique.

Beside this pendant we show one typical of the Quimbaya district of Colombia (*fig. b*) to indicate how far the threads of influence stretched. Some affinity to the Bat-god (see *Pl. 210, fig. a*) is evident in the squat body with drawn-up legs posed between the outspread wings, and a certain relationship with the plaque in *Pl. 218, fig. a* can be discerned in the rounded sections at the top, the broad flat base, and the cut-out bird heads at the sides. At the same time a similarity of idea between the two figures on this plate will be noticed, even though they come from widely separated regions. This likeness extends not only to the form but also to the build-up of the central bird head, presented in the round with profile silhouettes on either side. Each, however, speaks its own language. The fine stylization and superior workmanship in the second let us forget for the moment to delve for the complex idea behind it, while in the first, a less-refined execution and bolder delineation emphasize its puzzling qualities.

The cast gold figurine, 2¾ inches high and from Panama (*fig. c*), shows a little man carrying a pipe or blowgun in his left hand and in his right an object as yet undefined. Reptile heads seem to be represented in the protruding elements of his headdress. Flattened surfaces, such as those in the arms and feet, appear frequently also in Costa Rican work, but it is undecided where this manner originated. It contrasts effectively with the rounded body and head, bringing out the sheen of the metal. The braided headband and twisted belt likewise add variety to the composition. The hands are interestingly stylized.

The gold rattle or bell in the shape of a seated man (*fig. d*), shown in actual size, comes from Costa Rica. Its utilitarian purpose prescribed the bulky shape. One feels, nevertheless, more life in this figure than in the little man just described; even a touch of humor is apparent. The piece was cast in several parts and one line of fusion is visible at the belt.

MAYA AND MEXICAN AREAS

Nicaragua, Honduras, El Salvador, and Guatemala are poorer in metal objects than the areas just discussed. The gold figurines and ornaments that have been taken from graves here, particularly those dated from the 13th century on, bear, for the most part, characteristics of Costa Rica, Panama, and Colombia.

Figs. b and *c* on *Pl. 227* are cast copper bells found in the Maya Area. Both have a fine definite tone, proof of good clean casting. *Fig. b,* a little over 3 inches high, comes from Honduras. It has a grotesque face as decoration, with the slit of the bell serving as a mouth, through which the clapper, a pebble or clay pellet, may be seen. Excellent use was made of the available surface. The same drollness pervades the turkey bell (*fig. c*). This piece was found in British Honduras, near the border of Guatemala, and is also about 3 inches high. There is a naturalistic quality about the representation that can be universally understood, although the details are not carried out all over the piece.

The copper mask in *fig. a,* about 5½ inches high, was identified as belonging to the Tarascan culture of Mexico. Note the vast difference between this and the one of bronze from Ecuador (see *Pl. 210, fig. b*). In the latter, the expression is rather grotesque, the work bold and rough; here a symbol of death is cast with such finesse that it appears modeled. The subject is Xipe-Totec, God of the Flayed. His closed eyes and sagging mouth, the two braided lines running down the face to hold up the skin of the cheeks produce a remarkable intensity. The piece has something in its plastic make-up of an early Romanesque sculpture.

The Codex Mendoza (see *Pl. 269*) offers pictorial evidence that gold formed a part of the yearly tribute paid by the southern provinces of medieval Mexico to the Aztec kings. Names of the towns levied and the quantities exacted are recorded in glyphic signs, a list which was of great assistance to the progress of Cortés during the Conquest. The gold was delivered in gourds or cane tubes, or cast into bars. Manufactured articles in the Codex Mendoza include diadems, headbands, bells, breast ornaments, earplugs, labrets, and round beads.[121] Díaz records that gold, silver, and other metals, as well as precious stones and jewelry, were sold daily in the great market at Tenochtitlán. The Aztec goldsmiths' center was a town not far from the capital and the artisans were famed throughout Mexico. One might say that the intervening goldless region between Mexico and the south served as an insulator and a refining filter as far as stylistic influences are concerned. More problematic is the acquirement of the technical knowledge that enabled these people to produce autochthonous shapes in metal on a par with their other arts that were developed over a far longer period.

It is in the region around Oaxaca that the most elaborate pieces of jewelry in the Western Hemisphere have been excavated. Nearly a thousand miles by air-line from the nearest archaeologically established metal-working center (Costa Rica), the Zapotec and Mixtec inhabitants of this section made use of all the techniques known to the southern areas, applying them in a vigorous and individual manner, and invented new forms.

The gold ring from Oaxaca (*Pl. 228, fig. a*) is an example not only of virtuosity in casting but also of increasing refinement in artistic taste. At its greatest length it is about 2½ inches, slightly less than pictured. In the body of the ring, whorls and beading have been combined against a solid background. The ornament on the shield, expertly cast in separate parts and soldered to the base, represents a descending eagle, symbol of the setting sun, bearing in its beak the glyph meaning "precious" or "jade." Five minute drop-shaped bells, which tinkle as they strike one another, hang from the pendant and two more dangle from the bird's outspread wings, making the piece sprightly. The cast wire work of the wings and feathers above the head has been individualized and brought to a higher artistic level than we have met before. When compared to the much cruder specimen that follows, this work shows obvious development.

The copper ring, about 1¼ inches high (*fig. b*), is said to have been found near the border of El Salvador and Guatemala. It was made by the same technique as *fig. a,* but there is little comparison. The difference may be accounted for in part in the 500-odd miles that stretch between the places where the two pieces were found. The cruder material is also partly responsible, and the layout of the features would indicate a lower level of craftsmanship. Its chief interest lies in its material and in the unique design.

A gold ring from Oaxaca (*fig. c*), about 1 inch high, shows the most delicate execution in this group. The narrow lacelike band is composed of two double wires that frame a series of the ∽ motif. A design of the feathered serpent, daringly unconfined by a rim, replaces the shield, and a tortuous movement pervades the entire piece.

The ring in *fig. d,* only seven-tenths of an inch in diameter, is of a type quite usual in Oaxaca. It imitates filigree but was produced by the lost-wax process. The fashioning of the model in wax gave opportunity for inventive play with curving threads and globules. In the tiara-like construction a series of double loops, very characteristic of Mexican gold work, is used to form a glyph, and another symbol is applied directly below it.

Fig. e, the last of the rings, is among the most exquisite examples of this technique. It is about 1 inch high and belongs to the Oaxaca type. In the illustration it is shown in a horizontal position to bring out the design more clearly. After a moment of observation, we recognize the contours of a human profile at the right edge. The large nose and mouth and the eye appear first, then the earplug and headdress. After that, it is easy to find two hands nearer the center of the ring, one extended in a normal position as if in a gesture, the other placed above the head for the sake of symmetry. Four fingers are clearly executed, with even the nails suggested by small globules, and the thumbs, widely separated from the rest of the hand, hold the central panel. Dots are also used to delineate ornaments on both wrists, as frame for the headdress, and on purely decorative sections of the ring. The various framing motifs are distributed in such a way that they strengthen the center.

Our approach to the crowns, helmets, and rings of medieval America is made easier by the fact that we are accustomed to these shapes in our own civilization. But when it comes to earplugs, lipplugs, and noseplugs, we are hindered in our appreciation by unfamiliarity with their use. Nevertheless, many of these pieces are works of art and excellently contrived from a technical point of view.

The labret, or lipplug, from Oaxaca (*Pl. 229, fig. a*) measures about 2½ inches, including the tongue. It represents a serpent head, at the base of which is a plain section that was inserted into a slit in the under lip. Smooth solid surfaces have been well used. Twisted wire and series of globules, characteristics of Zapotec-Mixtec work, ornament the top of the head.

The smaller lipplug below it (*fig. c*) also comes from the Oaxaca region. Here again appears a serpent with outlashing tongue. There are less broken surfaces than in the first example. Each detail is outlined with a fine ridge. This ensemble play of wavy lines gives not only a higher artistic touch to the piece, but removes it deeper into the world of fantasy. Delicate perforated work adorns the outer edge of the plug proper.

Fig. b shows a plain headband and a feather of gold from Oaxaca. The diadem is oval in shape, with the rim wider in front than in the back. The feather, a little more than 13 inches long, carries a loose design in repoussé. Both objects were found together and the feather may have been worn affixed to the headband. The simplicity which permeates these pieces is not without subtlety. It would seem to be more characteristic of Chimú culture than of the area in which the articles were found.[60]

In *fig. d* a piece from the famous treasure is shown that was discovered in 1932 in the Mixtec burial of Tomb 7 at Monte Albán. This sepulchre contained nine skeletons decked in all the pomp and riches due kings or high priests and yielded over five hundred objects. The bracelet is of normal size and executed, like so many of those here considered, in repoussé. Two endlessly intertwining serpentine lines make up the pattern, with less protruding dots, doubtless eyes, between the convolutions. These are the same decorative elements that appear in the Chimú "plates" (see *Pl. 207, fig. b*), but are used here with greater force and assurance. The gold is of an amazing thinness and shows neither breaks nor cracks, proof of excellent workmanship.

Every one who enjoys jewelry will immediately grasp the beauty of the necklaces shown on *Pl. 230*. The first (*fig. a*) is of gold and from Tomb 7. Each section is about 2½ inches long. Jaguar teeth are represented in the corrugated units at the top,[23] and a moment's consideration of the entire row of thirty-nine will demonstrate how well the grinding jaw is suggested. It will be recalled that in the art of this area especially a warrior's head usually protrudes from the gaping jaws of an animal headdress. The loops and rings are precisely executed and divide with their faultless line the smooth surfaces. Each bell is slit and tinkles softly when it strikes its neighbor.

Fig. b shows a necklace of Toltec workmanship found near Texcoco. Fashioned of an alloy of silver and copper, it is much corroded and appears dull beside the shining gold of the others. However, the beautiful graduation of the beads justifies its presentation here. They run from about the size of a pea to that of a hickory nut, more than an inch in diameter, with the largest cast in two halves, then soldered together. All are hollow and astonishingly thin.

Another of the treasures from Tomb 7 is the gold necklace in *fig. c*. It is designed on the same general plan as the first but has enough individuality to be included beside it. Instead of the flat tier of golden jaguar teeth, here there is a row of plain round beads, between which pear-shaped drops are strung. From these, without an intervening element, hangs a smaller bell. Twenty-eight of the pendants are uniform, while in the three in the center the lower bells are smaller. In comparing the two necklaces, both a consistency in type and a divergence in detail will be noted, evidence again of the nuances the goldsmith was capable of creating.

The gold pectoral on *Pl. 231, fig. a* also comes from Tomb 7. It measures 4½ inches in height and weighs a little more than three ounces. While it looks as if it were fashioned with wires in filigree technique, it was actually produced by the lost-wax process. The piece is usually called the "Jaguar-Knight." He probably represents the Death-god, wearing a buccal mask in the form of a jawbone, held in place by a double cord that passes under his nose. Above the forehead is a helmet, formed by a blend of jaguar and serpent heads and surmounted by feathers and round medallions which were of plaited paper. Two serpent heads protrude from his large earplugs. Bells are attached to the lowest strand of the necklace, and a pendant features an eagle swooping downward with outspread wings. In connection with this motif, it is interesting to remember that the descending eagle symbolized the west, the point of the setting sun, or the end of life.

The neck of the deity rises out of a flat plaque instead of a body, on which glyphs are outlined in the same technique that is used in the headdress. These are far from symmetrical in their linear distribution, but nevertheless fulfill a decorative purpose. Dr. Caso believes that the piece commemorates an important mythological or historical event.[25] The whole portrayal of the god attacks us immediately through its expressive presentation of the power of death.

A pectoral from Costa Rica is shown in way of comparison in *fig. c.* Though here the human element is practically non-existent, certain details of the two bear relationship, while others, namely, the crescent "bird heads" at either side of the head and feet of the main figure, as well as its numerous toes, hark back to the south of Panama.

The gold statuette (*fig. b*) is supposedly a portrait of Tizoc, who stood at the head of the Aztecs from 1481 to 1486. It was claimed to have been a gift from him to a contemporary lord at Texcoco, where the piece was found. The figure is 3½ inches high, and its gold content is said to be over twenty carats.[128]

For a portrait, we certainly do not discover many individual characteristics in it. The stocky figure sits in a tight pose. This position would simplify the shape for casting; but the same squatness occurs also in pictorial representations of the king where such technical considerations would not influence the delineation. He wears the royal crown decorated with plumes. A slender tubular object adorns his nose and a lipplug (see *Pl. 229*) protrudes from his chin. A string of large beads arranged on his chest ends in a circular disk, similar to the one shown on *Pl. 234, fig. a,* but with a top piece added. Studded bracelets and anklets decorate the arms and legs, and in his right hand he holds a baton of command.

In the back, extending over the hair, crown, and feather headdress, is the symbol of a wounded or bleeding leg. This is Tizoc's glyphic identification and always accompanies his figure in the several codices and stone carvings where he appears. His name is a combination of *zoc,* "bled," with the prefix *ti,* signifying "the bled one." Interwoven in a wire-work design on the back, which gives the impression of a mantle, is the date glyph for 1481, conforming with the year of the election and elevation of the ruler. He was the seventh in line of the Aztec dynasty, of which Montezuma II, ruler at the time of Cortés's arrival, was the ninth.

From an artistic point of view, the piece has not the exuberance characteristic of Zapotec-Mixtec work, although it is approximately correct in iconography. Within the past few years, technological investigation of the material and technique have enabled the specialist to declare it less than a hundred years old—a revealing glimpse at how carefully copies and fraudulent and combined pieces are fabricated.

With the gold pendant on *Pl. 232,* also discovered in fabulous Tomb 7, we reach the highest achievement of the goldsmith's art in medieval America. It is 8½ inches long and was probably used as a pectoral. Several pendants exist, discovered earlier than this one, that might be regarded as forerunners or provincial examples of the same idea; one of these has a plaque with figural content at the top and three simple loops holding bells. However, they contain fewer elements than the piece illustrated and are far inferior to it in execution. All of them are said to have come from the Tehuantepec region, more than one hundred fifty miles south of Monte Albán, and are allegedly of Zapotec manufacture,[121] while this one, from Tomb 7, is of Mixtec origin according to Dr. Caso's classification.

This masterpiece, produced by the primitive implements of the pre-Columbian goldsmiths, could not be surpassed, either in design or in technique, by the use of modern equipment. It is built up of seven units, each different in shape and content, loosely connected by links and separated far enough so that each element is accorded the emphasis due it. There is no repetition—rather a sequence, planned with unparalleled artistic deliberation. The angular plaque at the top, massive in background and largest of all the sections, is followed by a disk, also with a massive back. The third part is openwork in a squarish frame, and the fourth is made with the same technique within a narrower space. Next come four "cockades" with very little openwork, followed by four hollow balls. Bells in elongated drop form constitute the seventh element, providing an effective contrast to the solid top piece.

In spite of the general horizontal trend in the design of each of the first four sections, there are always connecting lines that direct the eye on to the next. The progressive loosening of the respective parts, from the angular plaque to the dangling bells, is so subtle that the vibrancy of the piece can be felt, even though it is fastened to the black velvet holder in the museum.

The pectoral embodies an indigenous cosmic representation.[25] The rather macabre ball game of the gods across a grinning skull at the top is the glyphic presentation of the nocturnal heaven with stars. On the second section is the sun disk, and below it is the moon, symbolized by the "flint knife." Finally, the earth-monster is shown, with open jaws, fangs, and a forked tongue. Feathers—ceremonial ornamentation—are represented by the cockades, and the bells at the bottom are symbols of the music of life.

The gold mask of the god Xipe-Totec (*fig. b*) is also one of the finds from Tomb 7. It measures nearly 3 inches in height and weighs slightly more than three ounces. Its precise use is uncertain; it may have served as a belt buckle or a clasp to fasten the hair, or even as an ornament on a necklace. Xipe-Totec, as has been mentioned under sculpture, is the God of the Spring. But, since the skin he wears is also similar to the thin sheet of gold which jewelers used to cover wooden objects, he was also regarded as God of the Jewelers. Drooping eyelids and a sagging mouth, shapeless without indication of lips, express the flabbiness of the flayed skin. The four cords on each side of the head that served to hold the skin in place are executed with such skill that they seem as pliant as twisted cotton. Stepped and V-shaped lines applied around the eyes denote face painting, and a dangling nose ring, earplug disks, and a band which fastens the hair complete the adornment. The band seems higher on one side, indicating that the wearer is a warrior, and has the characteristic tuft of the military class.[25] The chimney-like opening at the top was for additional ornament, probably feathers.

It was inevitable that the often bloody ceremonies of these people should be expressed in their art, and this mask, with its terrifying and complex associations, so utterly strange to us, conveys much of the atmosphere of pre-Columbian Mexico. We are forced to ponder the spiritual world that inspired it, so un-Christian yet so expressive in its art that even we can grasp something of its significance.

Realism is blended with symbolism in such a masterly way that we cannot define where one begins and the other ends.

Our last gold necklace (*Pl. 233, fig. a*), another gem of the Oaxaca type, is 20 inches long, with cast beads featuring turtles as the main element. The delicate wire loops and bell pendants, one hundred twenty in all, are similar to those seen on *Pl. 230,* yet produce a different effect, with three of the pear-shaped pendants hanging from each bead. Of all the necklaces shown, this one gives the smoothest and most solid impression and is actually the heaviest in weight. All the Oaxaca necklaces attest to a long road of civilization—from the shiny colored pebble-stone string to *colliers* such as these, highly sophisticated and technically impeccable.

Although the Tribute Roll of Montezuma and the contemporary writers of the Conquest mention towns in what is today Vera Cruz as paying tribute in gold objects, few examples from this region have as yet come to the fore. It was probably customary here also to bury with kings, priests, and chiefs, their jewelry and other personal effects, but so much movement has passed across this territory since the landing of Cortés that the ground must have been pretty thoroughly combed over at an early date. However, little surveying has been done archaeologically, and no one knows what still remains in these "hot lands." The few gold plaques that are known lean in composition toward the Oaxaca style, showing generally a more or less plastic head, sometimes with shoulders and arms, that flattens down into a plain sheet with a raised rim.

Among the newer acquisitions of the Museo Nacional in Mexico, however, is a red-gold plaque from Vera Cruz (*fig. b*), about 2 inches high, which offers a contrast to the type just described. A seated figure with elaborate headdress is represented, holding an object with both hands. Legs and feet are depicted with the same clarity and emphasis as the head and shoulders. This is the only case known to the writer in which a plaque of any pre-Columbian area contains the entire human figure cast in relief. The head is part and parcel of the piece, emphasized by its uneven upper rim but firmly tied into the framework of the plaque by delicate reeding edged with diminutive circles. The bird-mask, with its solid and irregular line, and the two rosettes on the corners retain their customary shape. A row of teeth that marks the animal jaw of the headdress and the beads of the necklace effectively frame the face of the man. Note the cape that falls in folds behind the figure. The lower third of the plaque is devoted to a glyphic representation, in which a segment of a circle—suggestive of a shield

—irregular step-frets, and five dots are discernible. Judging from the concavity in the object the dignitary is holding, it may have been inlaid, and it is possible that the background also contained either inlay work or enamel.

The figure does not show great individuality in its features. There is nothing ferocious in the expression; rather it seems somewhat contemplative. The only reminders of the more familiar type lie in the filigree wire elements and in the raised edge that frames the composition. To execute this small and difficult subject represents an achievement in casting; but still more important for us, from an artistic point of view, is the sympathetic air of the piece. Saville illustrates a 4½-inch gold ornament which shows stylistic affinities to our plaque. It was found at El Tajín and had Nahua glyphs on the back.

Pl. 234, fig. a takes us about one hundred twenty miles northwest of Oaxaca into the neighboring state of Guerrero, where at Texmilincan this solar disk of beaten gold, 6 inches in diameter, was found in an ancient sepulchre. Classified as a product of the Mixtec culture,[3] it is important not only as evidence of the wide influence of these people but also because of its complete dissimilarity with Tomb 7 specimens said to belong to the same culture. The fact that it was discovered near the border where the Aztec language meets the Mixtec may explain somewhat the great stylistic and technical differences between it and the Oaxaca pieces. Besides the gold disk, the grave contained earrings, bells and blades of copper, small onyx vases, fragments of jade, and a small turquoise mask.[98]

The disk is ornamented with the intertwining bodies of two feathered serpents in a design similar to that on the well-known stone ring in the Ball Court at Chichén Itzá. It is divided into two sections, and a narrow embossed edge marks the inner and outer margins. The more important elements—the heads, from which two human figures emerge, and the rattles bound with plumes —occupy the outer circle; the inner half contains the finely laid and artistically stylized serpent bodies, the scalelike markings forming an unbroken rhythmic circle. The crossing of the two bodies is smoothly and effectively solved. Slight differences in the two reptiles indicate that a full cliché was prepared for the embossing of the disk. The fret-scrolls resemble the main pattern of the Ulúa vases. Caso designates the piece as pre-Aztec because of the *atlatls* wielded by the small human figures, a weapon which antedates the bow and arrow supposedly introduced by the Aztecs. Its disk form and the suave and undulating lines of the serpents recall certain admired Chinese jades.

A suggestion as to the use of this disk is offered by the ornament seen in the Tizoc statuette (*Pl. 231, fig. b*). Gold figures have also been found in the

Totonac region wearing a disk-shaped jewel hanging from a necklace, and the large pottery statue from Mexico (*Pl. 119, fig. b*) is depicted with a circular ornament framed by carefully plaited paper. It would seem that thin gold sheets were often combined with other materials, such as feathers, paper, wood, semiprecious stones, or woven stuff.

The three pieces in *fig. b* are spectacular examples of such a combination. They are the frames for eyes and mouth of a life-size mask, probably originally mounted on a base of wood, and were dredged from the bottom of the Sacred Well at Chichén Itzá. As has been described, boys and girls, ceremoniously adorned, were sacrificed here to the Rain-god, and pilgrims cast valuables into the water to secure the benevolence of the deities. An inventory of objects brought up through the operations of the late E. H. Thompson lists other masks, one of which is given as of solid gold and 7 inches in diameter. (Compare the Chimú mummy masks on *Pl. 203.*)

The embossing is unusually shallow, little more than faint ripples, yet clear enough to define the theme. Two ovals in a zoömorphic pattern ornament the mouth, edged with a series of blunt hooks suggestive of plumes. Each of the eye frames is decorated with a cut-out stylized figure of the feathered serpent, facing toward the center. The open mouth with fangs and an exaggerated forked tongue are clearly visible, particularly over the one on the right. Four rings mark the rattles at the opposite ends. The great loops formed by the sinuous writhing bodies, furiously waving plumes, and lashing tails lend superb fluency to the composition. Both clarity and a feeling of motion are gained by the spacing of the various elements and the lacy arrangement of the openings.

Like the preceding disk, the piece technically is not complicated; its remarkable feature lies in the conception of the design. Here the feathered serpent, an ever-recurrent theme in medieval American art, comes to its most flamboyant expression. So powerful is the purely decorative effect that without attempting to fathom its symbolism, we recognize in it the hallmark of genius.

In the transformation of Late Romanesque into Gothic in different regions of medieval Europe, art-history is presented with a spiritual as well as a stylistic problem, which is still to a certain degree unsolved. With incomparably less data at its disposal, pre-Columbian archaeology is confronted with a problem even more obscure. Although valuable contributions on the subject of metallurgy in medieval America have been made within the field of general survey and analysis as well as in specialized laboratory investigations, too few pieces of metal-work have been excavated under scientific conditions to establish a sequence of styles such as has been built up for pottery in a number of our regions.

The evolution of design as revealed in these pottery sequences is of uneven value as far as gold is concerned. In the first place, some prolific metal-working centers produced no top-rank pottery; in the second, one of the highest cultures, the Maya, had practically no gold until its late and final period. In the Andean and, to a certain extent, the Interlying areas, metal-work developed technically and stylistically in pace with the other applied arts. In the Mexican and Maya, however, it came as a new and attractive medium into the dexterous hands of an already artistically conscious people who made use of it in their own way. Their iconography was already articulate and well developed; the craft did not have to grope its way through primary processes.

Much of the surviving material comes from the so-called middle and late epochs of various cultures, which had their periods of flourishing and of decline. The influence of their art traveled far, at times to sections where technically the people had not advanced to as high a level. This resulted in peripheral versions. Also, stylistic trends were sometimes better preserved in geographically pocketed districts than in those that lay along the main arteries of travel, producing a shift or lag in chronology.

The tribal talent of the various pre-Columbian regions was so strongly individual that the application of the same techniques yielded very different effects, and, as paradoxical as it may seem, the mastery of the most complicated technical processes did not always produce the most highly artistic results. The first Lambayeque plaque (*Pl. 195, fig. a*) and the mask from Chichén Itzá (*Pl. 234, fig. b*) were both worked from thin sheet gold in repoussé; but while in the former the symbolic content is rigidly held down by spiritual inhibitions, the Late Maya piece shows amazing maturity and facility of expression. The disk form was used for both the ear ornaments (*Pl. 197, fig. a*) and the solar disk from Texmilincan (*Pl. 234, fig. a*); the scroll designs of the Lambayeque pieces are balanced and pleasing, but brief study will show the far superior and more subtle values of the Mixtec specimen, in spite of its more regular form. The Chibcha figures (*Pl. 213, fig. a*) have the same build-up as the mask from Monte Albán (*Pl. 231, fig. a*) yet show technical infancy and a helplessness in expression when compared with this masterpiece of international esthetic worth.

Of the two main problems presented by a study of the metal craft of medieval America, the technical will be solved much before the stylistic, for technological analysis in our age has advanced far more rapidly than our ability to penetrate the spiritual complexities of a vanished and alien world.

VIII

Jade and Other Semiprecious Stones

THE attachment of man to stones of unusual color and shape is as wide as the world and as old as civilization. Amulets, bracelets, beads, and ceremonial objects made of some kind of lustrous stone occur generally among prehistoric peoples, and the popular costume jewelry in our department stores, vying with expensive jewels, shows that even our enlightened era still feels the fascination. We are familiar with the ornaments shaped by the early artisans of the Near and Far East, but have had little opportunity to appreciate the skill and artistry of the lapidary of medieval America, although here, after pottery sherds, semiprecious stones are the tokens most commonly found in excavations from the higher cultures.

Among the stones used in medieval America were jade, turquoise, rock crystal, and serpentine, as well as amber, onyx, jasper, and agate. Of these, the jade work stands first in quantity and in its artistic quality. The finest carving, however, is confined to the Mexican and Maya areas, where the styles are frequently so interrelated that they will be presented here as if from one vast region.

The Southwest and the Andean Area had no jade but used turquoise, a material also esteemed in the other areas of high culture, as will be seen in the chapter on applied arts. In the Southwest, the worked shapes are more or less simple, generally with little or no elaboration, and do not represent as high an artistic invention as the craft in the other areas. However, the stones are put together in a tasteful and appealing way and show inimitable color sense, whether in the working of single pieces or the juxtaposition in a string of beads. In the Andean Area, turquoise was delicately carved into figurines and vessels and was used also in inlay and mosaic-work. It is comparatively rare, probably because gold held more meaning for the Children of the Sun. The absence of carved jade in both of these regions is an argument against any intensive intercourse between them and the Mexican or Maya areas in the first half of the Middle Ages; otherwise, some traces of the jade cult would surely have found its way hither, just as metal from the Interlying Area reached the land of the Maya as civilization spread.

Besides its rarity and beauty, jade had a deep symbolic meaning for the Maya and the Mexicans. The Maya word for it was *tun*. The Nahua name *chalchihuitl,* or "green stone," carries an association with "grass" or "herb," emphasizing the color which is the symbol of life itself. It is known how Montezuma, on seeing the great delight with which his gifts of gold were received by the Spaniards, promised them more valuable presents for the following day, and how disappointed Cortés was when "some green stones" were proffered on this occasion. Although the offering was an anticlimax to the Spaniards, to the Aztecs it really comprised their most choice possessions.

The word "jade" is of Spanish origin and, contrary to general belief, is closely connected with the discovery of America. The Chinese names (*yü* for white jade and *pi yü* for the green type) clearly have nothing to do with our term.[88] In European literature the first mention of the stone occurs in the work of Monardes, a physician of Seville, in 1565.[147] He calls it "piedra de hi*jada*," the hypochondriac or colic stone, from the Spanish *hijada,* meaning "loin." The Indians believed it efficacious for certain disorders and passed on their tradition to their conquerors, together with other exotic remedies, drugs, and foods of more actual value. Medieval Europe, even prior to the Conquest, was wont to prescribe pulverized stones mixed with animal or plant extracts for certain illnesses—a practice handed down since the times of Babylon and ancient Egypt. *Piedra de hijada* included carved or shaped stones varying in shade from a very pale to a blackish green. The mineral content was of no importance; the stones were selected on the ground of their appearance, color, and tactile qualities.

Although known in Europe since the Conquest, jade may be said to have first impressed itself on public consciousness after the sack of the Summer Palace in Peking in 1861. Before that time, all worked green stones with a luster were popularly put under the general heading of jade. It was only after Chinese jade objects began to appear in greater quantity in the European art market that the necessity arose for a more exact differentiation between the different types of stone, and the classification was undertaken on a chemical basis.

While the word "jade" was coined by a Spaniard to designate a pre-Columbian importation, the term "jadeite" was invented by the French chemist and mineralogist, Augustin Alexis Damour, after the opening of China. With the aid of chemical analysis, two separate types were distinguished; both have a high silicate content, which makes it possible to mistake one for the other. The first, nephrite, sometimes called "true jade," is a lime magnesia iron silicate. It has a wide range of colors and a waxy sheen. To the second category belong jadeite and the subgroup, chloromelanite, silicates with alumina and soda content. Jadeite is often pale, but it may run to brilliant greens with a vitreous luster; chloromelanite is a darker shade, frequently almost black. Thus, the much misused term "jade" covers two types of stone; it is a cumulative expression and will be used in this survey to denote all those stones of high silica content which were called *tun* by the Maya and *chalchihuitl* by the Aztecs.

Recent investigations with the spectroscope show a definite mineralogical divergence between the jades of America and those of the Orient. The American jadeite contains always a large amount of diopside, not found in the jadeite of Burma and China. Phosphorus, nearly always present in Oriental nephrite, was entirely lacking in all the thirty-odd pieces of American origin examined.[101] These modern scientific tests should finally put to rest the false and fantastic ideas that jade is not native to America and must have been imported from Asia.

Substantial evidence of the autochthonous origin of jade in America existed along several lines long before scientific investigations began. The Tribute Roll of Montezuma, which served Cortés so effectively in locating regions where gold was produced, contains place names in which the Aztec glyph for *chalchihuitl* occurs, suggesting that the green stone was to be found there. The quantity of pre-Columbian jade extant, either undocumented in circulation or found by excavators, testifies further that the stone was fairly common, though the finer types seem to have been rare and may have been traded from one district to another, even occasionally reworked. In the Museo Arqueológico in Guatemala there is a magnificent block of it, weighing about two hundred pounds, that was excavated from the pre-Columbian site of Kaminaljuyú by the Carnegie Institution of Washington in 1937. Sawed and chipped at various points, it shows the marks of the lapidary, made apparently to determine the color grain and to remove smaller pieces for working.[165] Pre-Columbian jade objects which have turned up in Honduras, El Salvador, and Costa Rica frequently vary enough in color and quality to make one suspect different local deposits. Jade has been reported from several Mexican states, chiefly in the form of nodules in the beds of some of the rivers, notably in Hidalgo, Guerrero, Puebla, Oaxaca, Chiapas and Vera Cruz.[86] Furthermore, jade has been found as far north as Alaska and as far south as Brazil; and, what is known by very few, true nephrite has been discovered in our western mountain states, in California and Wyoming.[51]

Thus, archaeological, historic, and mineralogical evidences combine to prove beyond doubt that the jade of medieval American art is as indigenous as the limestone used for Maya temples. Contrary statements may be considered as misconceptions, smuggled into general opinion. Before any serious research was conducted, fanciful theories were already widely circulated, particularly by those fantasts of archaeology (all too frequently Teutonic) who persist in trying to link Babylonian astronomy and Greek mythology with the past of medieval America. Little has been known about jade in America simply because no systematic investigations were begun until very recently.

The stone was esteemed in the Maya and Mexican areas as a mark of rank and was worn by the hierarchy. Most of the pre-Columbian objects fashioned of jade were personal ornaments, amulets, masks, and figurines; in the Early and Great Maya periods we find cuffs and anklets also represented. Its masterly carving and polishing is one of the amazing accomplishments of these people. How such delicate lines and fine contours could have been executed without the use of metal chisels and drills is difficult to imagine. The work was done with primitive implements, probably of hard stone. Indeed, by the time they had succeeded in shaping their tools, they were well on their way toward mastery in the carving of any subject.

As jade was very precious, the smaller pieces were often used in their natural shapes to insure as little waste as possible. The larger stones were split along the grain or sawed into units with at least one flat surface, probably by means of cords and abrasive powder. For boring and cutting both solid and hollow drills of bone, stone, or other hard material were used, revolved in the manner of a primitive fire-making tool. The limitations of these drills were overcome in ingenious ways. To form depressions, the lapidary might bore several holes side by side and then rub the cavity smooth. The hollow drill held at a slant would produce the segment of a circle. Straight lines were often achieved by sawing with cords or rubbing with wooden or stone implements. The work was polished with abrasive powder or wood. It required great patience and skill to smooth the carved surface and rough edges without injuring the shape or blurring the sculptured details. The time element, however, was never a consideration in medieval American art, and pre-Columbian craftsmanship can scarcely be understood without keeping this in mind.

The development of several distinct methods in handling jade can be observed, just as in the sculpturing of stone or stucco, and local preferences and styles suggest themselves. The color and shape of the material often gave inspiration for the subject and design to be followed. We shall see pieces where the natural form of the stone was used without change as sculptural frame. Again, usually in later times, the edges were chiseled and polished off to form a basic outline, before sculptural embellishment began. Fetish-like three-dimensional subjects are found, and figures composed in relief; some designs flow to the very edge of the irregular stone, while others are placed within the restricting frame of a medallion. Oftentimes the color grain was used to good effect to highlight the plastic contours, and admirable efficiency developed in combining and calculating defects to sculptural advantage.

The great importance of carved jade in setting and transmitting style should be stressed. So deep-rooted was the veneration for the green stones that even after the late introduction of metal, it persisted, as we have seen, until the Conquest. Thus the working of jade covers the time-span of the civilization discussed in this survey. Styles in carving and changes in technique were exchanged from one region to another by means of the prized and easily handled jades, and stylistic influences can be noticed in distant and peripheral districts, much as one hat from Paris has been known to change the fashion in many a provincial town. In view of this complicated exchange, no attempt has been made here to try to classify the various types presented into a tightly knit series for the sake of chronology. Nor would a precise mineralogical differentiation be productive from our point of view.

The associations connected with jade in the culture of medieval America go far back, beyond the time on which we have any adequate archaeological data. The artistic impulse of peoples of prehistory manifested itself much earlier and in a more articulate manner than most of us would expect. Jade beads are found in the earliest graves. The custom of putting a piece of jade in the mouth of the deceased—it stood for the heart and was supposed to help him on his way to after life [151]—shows that symbolic meaning was attached to it. In China also, carved jade was placed in the mouth of the dead as a tongue piece. This does not imply any connection with the American practice, but points only to the very old use of this stone in both civilizations and to the fact that the formative periods of each go back into a distant age when no metal was known.

MAYA AND MEXICAN AREAS

The Leyden plaque and the Tuxtla statuette (*Pl. 235, figs. a* and *d*), bearing glyphs interpreted as belonging to Cycle 8 of Maya chronology or about the 4th century of our era, have been considered two of the earliest dated objects found on this continent. It is quite probable that both pieces were moved not once but a number of times hither and yon before they came to rest in the spots where they were discovered.[91]

The Leyden plaque (*fig. a*) was unearthed near Puerto Barrios, Guatemala, during the digging of a canal in 1864, and is now in the Rijksmuseum at Leyden, Holland. It is of a very pale jade of fine quality and about 8 inches high. On one side of the smooth celt-shaped plaque is a column of hieroglyphics, characteristic of the archaic or early period of Maya art and not yet identical with Maya codex technique. On the other, a dignitary is shown, standing on another human whose uplifted and backward-turned head and upswung feet are clearly incised. The delicate tracery of the balls, tassels, and curlicues in the elaborate ceremonial costume is fluently drawn. Horizontal lines in the belt and the flaring jaws of the serpent headdress divide and clarify the design. The three-quarters pose seems natural and is delineated with assurance. Dr. Morley reads the date as A.D. 320 and from the position of the figure associates the piece with early Tikal.[90]

The Tuxtla statuette (*fig. d*) was plowed up in a field near San Andrés Tuxtla, in Vera Cruz, Mexico, about 1907, and is now in the National Museum at Washington, D.C. This jade, 6 inches high, is of a darker tone. Here the outer layers of the stone have been shaved down to a somewhat clumsy but definite shape, and plastic expression has been attempted. The eyes and nose are human, the eyes achieving an alert penetrating look, which is one of the statue's powers, by the simple means of bored holes. The jowl line is brought down deep and broad and shaped as if in a grin. Fantastic elements appear in the lower part of the face where the mouth or mouth mask is shaped like a duck's bill, with incised marks on either side of the center line in realistic representation of the bird's nostrils. The lines starting at the shoulder level and curving down each side are suggestive of folded wings or of arms covered with a cloak. Clawlike hands emerge from them toward the bottom of the piece. (Compare with *Pl. 68, fig. b* and *Pl. 132, fig. b.*) Recently doubt has been cast on the interpretation of the glyphs as Maya; it has been suggested rather that they are Olmec—as yet undeciphered.[154] This, however, in no way detracts from the intrinsic strength of the figure. Regardless of its origin, it carries within itself the concentrated energy of truly primitive art. Its remarkable tactile quality—that appeal to the hand to grasp and fondle it—is naturally more apparent in the statue itself than in the photograph.

These two specimens of pre-Columbian lapidary work exemplify the same two tendencies noted in sculpture: in the first, the stone serves as a background for the delineation; in the second, it is shaped in the round, into a three-dimensional object. It is noteworthy that in pre-Columbian jades the manner of delineation, that is, the convention of representing the eyes, ears, nose, and the like, never became restricted to a single style. The eyes, for instance, seldom show the double-rimmed lids and convex eyeballs of realistic Greek interpretation; the nose is sometimes wedge-shaped, sometimes "hammer head" like an inverted T, sometimes bulbous; ears may jut out into handles or be reduced to an incised spiral.

The next three pieces show, primarily, subtly worked shapes. The first (*fig. b*), 5¾ inches long, is probably a pectoral. It bears a lozenge of Maya glyphs, identified as quite early in type, incised in a frame at either end of a fine light green jade bar. It is highly polished and evidently was finished with great care.

In *fig. c,* a recumbent human figure is scratched on the surface of the stone. In his outstretched right hand he carries a torch or perhaps a weapon, while the left grasps some object. His headdress is subdued and apparently is not Maya. The square mouth also bears out the impression that we are dealing here with a different regional tradition. The even rim around the entire piece suggests that it may have been a palette.

Fig. e, a small idol from Uaxactún, takes us again into the field of the three dimensional. Here a seated human figure is represented with a disproportionately large head and bulging eye. As we have noticed in other categories of pre-Columbian art, the head and upper part of the body are often emphasized and more realistically treated than the lower half of the figure, which may be dwarfed or barely suggested.

Pl. 236, fig. a presents a sculptured stone slab, Stela I from Copán, dated 677, and shows an early style, often considered related to wood-carving. Note the hieratic position of the hands holding an ornate ceremonial bar. An interesting resemblance is found in *fig. d,* a jade plaque of fine quality which was unearthed during the building of a railroad near the city of San Salvador. The hands are placed back to back, as in the stela—though here they support nothing —and the headdress is an animal-mask. The feet, however, are not pointed outward in the traditional Maya pose. The subject covers the entire face of the stone—only in the beading on the top is the even outline broken. High and low planes, smooth and broken surfaces are well utilized for clear delineation.

The head is square, the mouth thick and widened, the nose and eyebrows carved in one with simplified lines. A necklace and the edges of a tunic are emphasized, and drapery reaching to the feet is suggested behind. (Compare with *Pl. 69, fig. c* and *Pl. 82, fig. c.*) Despite the fact that there is a suggested level beneath the feet, the figure does not seem to stand but gives the impression of being suspended.

The two pieces in *figs. b* and *c* show more plastic consideration; even though the right edge is a straight and static line, on the left, use has been made of a more defined language of sculpture. In the first, a human figure is depicted, arms crossed, head turned to profile; along and above his forehead rests the snout of a water monster that lies folded over on itself. (Compare with *Pl. 139, fig. b.*) The piece is 6½ inches long and comes from Kaminaljuyú. The jade is very fine and its tactile quality here comes forward. It is pierced at both ends so as to hang face downwards.

A somewhat similar figure is presented in the whitish bar from Quiriguá (*fig. c*). Its arms are also crossed and the legs are represented in the same dangling position. But with its simpler headdress, the whole piece is easier to grasp.

The universal appeal of charm stones is exemplified in the large breast bars from Venezuela, approximately 12 inches long (*Pl. 237, fig. b*). In this case the carefully shaped and smoothly polished pieces of slatelike texture—said to be symbolic of the Bat-god—were apparently worn as ornaments. They are light in color and weight and are extremely pleasant to handle. The shape in itself has dignity and accents the beauty of the stone. Very early Chinese jades were treated in the same manner, the lack of any embellishment serving to enhance their significant form and fine color. Here might be mentioned also the bird and banner stones of Mound Builder culture which show real feeling toward balance in form.

Fig. a is a bluish jade from Costa Rica, about 7 inches high. On the upper half a masked figure is carved, terminating in an undecorated blade which, perhaps because of the contrast, makes the whole into a shapely and pleasing piece. The deep eyes may have been inlaid. The crossed hands are depicted in an abbreviated manner. Two stylized intertwined serpents, the heads of which can be seen on the sides, make up the headdress. This same type appears on two jades found in El Salvador, as well as on a piece dated mid-7th century from Copán (not shown here), and is very clearly represented in *Pl. 247, fig. a.* The tonguelike affix before the mouth and the lines suggesting a shoulder remind us of the

Tuxtla statuette. Several similar jades are known to have come from the Nicoya Peninsula, a district that produced also a high grade of pottery (see *Pl. 145, fig. a*).

Fig. c is unusual because of its modeling. The heavy rounded section at the top flattens out into a shape like a police whistle. How important this section is in maintaining the subtle balance of the piece can be seen by blocking it off with the hand. The plastic contours of cheeks, eyes, and nose are brought out with assurance and simplicity. Mouth and jaws broaden into the same duck's bill seen in the Tuxtla statuette, with a contrast as effective as that in the blade at the left of it. Perforations to suspend it as a pendant or attach it to another material were bored in each edge just below the eyes.

Realism and the humor of a caricature are manifest in the carving from Oaxaca (*fig. f.*), about 3 inches high. Here once more the stone was the medium for only an engraving and even the unused sections before the face and behind the head were not carved away. The lower half of the body has been neglected to emphasize the sharp and clear-cut profile of an elderly smiling man, who appears to be seated with his forearm laid along a horizontal rest. Features, headdress, and earplugs are well defined and remind us of the Monte Albán *danzante* type seen in *Pls. 57* and *91*.

Fig. e, 3¼ inches high, is actually more akin to the Monte Albán slabs in manner of carving. Mouth and nose are depicted in a kind of sculptural shorthand and lean toward the Olmec in type. The piece shows a full figure sitting cross-legged. At the bottom center can be seen a miniature hand resting on a knee that depends largely on the contour of the stone for its shape. The necklace and tulip-like earplug were apparently considered of greater importance than the realistic representation of the body. The face has expression and is the *raison d'être* of the whole piece.

Fig. d shows a much more settled manner of depiction. Here also main consideration is given to the face, but the composition of the whole figure is more distinct. A careful study of the stone before carving is evident in the placement of the subject and in the clever use of the light streak in the jade to emphasize the shoulders and the lower part of the face. The lines of the forehead, eyes, nose, and mouth are executed with a sure and routined hand. This piece has a compact robust appearance, multiplying several times the effect one might expect to find in such a small space. The brain that conceived it had a definite idea of what it wished to represent and was able to impart the inspiration to the simple tool.

The serpentine plaque in *Pl. 238, fig. a,* about 6 inches high, may be considered as late in style. It shows Tlaloc, Rain-god of the Aztecs, as an older man with heavy headdress and earplugs with pendants, holding a serpent in his left hand and in his right, a symbolic object. In contrast to the earlier figures, he stands firmly on the ground. The background is filled in with explanatory symbols such as usually surround Aztec figures in the codices—appendages which are decorative, though they make the piece more difficult for us to understand.

Fig. b, somewhat over 5 inches high, was found at Teotihuacán. It presents a seated chief in full regalia attended by a smaller figure in the lower left. In the upper left is a demon in the jaws of a serpent. The central figure, with its elaborate feather headdress, is a hieratic representation, very detailed but less liberated as a sculpture than a number of other less pretentious pieces here shown. Note the bar-bead pectoral and the jade mask on his belt. Considerably greater sculptural vivacity appears in the subordinate characters. Dots, circles, and curving lines are evidence of ingenious work with round drills. T. A. Joyce connects this carving with the style of the "celebrated site of Copan," [56] but stylistically it is nearer the reliefs of Piedras Negras and Yaxchilán. The speech scroll that appears before his face is associated with the Toltecs.

The plaque in *fig. c,* shown in actual size, is carved from a stone of good quality and high luster. Here the face is presented in full front. Almond eyes, beaklike nose, and grim mouth identify it as typically Maya. The body is facilely and economically done, and the placement of the figure within its allotted space is perfect. For the first time in this chapter a raised carved frame appears, well within the margin of the stone itself, with the flowing plumes of the monster-headdress effectively utilized for the upper part.

A comparison of the two pieces (*figs. b* and *c*), both Maya, demonstrates the considerable stylistic divergences which existed in various regions of the same folk, not necessarily widely separated in time. The gestures are similar but reversed. Facial differences could be analyzed, going deep into detail, but here it will suffice to call attention to the different execution of the eyes and mouths. In relief, a profile lends itself to sharper characterization than a full face, but even aside from this, each piece speaks its own language. The technique of the one might be called pointillistic and of the other, impressionistic.

In *fig. d,* nearly 4 inches high, costume and gesture derive from another tradition and another region. The round heavy-lidded or half-closed eyes, apparent also in the mask, are characteristics of Oaxaca. The broad necklace is well brought out and the monster-mask headdress that frames the face shows real virtuosity in the carving of complicated scrolls, curves, and undulating lines. The nostrils of the animal, conventionalized, can be discerned in the swirls just above the forehead. By adding the small feather sections at either side, the carver has skillfully suggested a full swaying feather ornament.

One of the several sculptural directions taken by jade carving seems to have placed more and more emphasis on the head. In all the pendants on *Pl. 239,* the head was given the main consideration, although in *figs. a* and *b* a body, dwarfed and out of proportion, is also indicated.

Fig. b, about 5 inches high, is composed largely of curving lines. The introduction of the horizontal in the "coffee-bean" eyes and mouth and in the arms brings the face out of the swirling ornament and rim of suggested plumes. The round knees and tab of the belt are so executed as to complement the pattern formed by the eyes and open jaw of the monster-mask.

The face in *fig. a* is definitely framed by double and triple parallel lines which indicate the headdress and show the arms in ceremonial gesture, a pose, as in *fig. b,* that is physically impossible but has decorative value in the design. Circular earplugs and a "choker" necklace of large beads cut the rectangular surface and harmonize with the scrolls in the headdress and the eyes of the monster-mask. A new feature appears in the two "concealed" profiles at the upper corners of the stone. Such faces occur in jades from the Guatemala highlands and from El Salvador, as well as the Olmec region. Maler mentions superimposed heads on stelae and other sculptures at Tikal,[75] and Means speaks of "hidden faces" in monumental stone carving from the Andean Area.[84]

The work in *fig. c* shows much more virtuosity in the deeper carving and deliberate contrasting of high lights. This piece is less than 1½ inches high. The face is the bulbous-nosed, heavy-lidded Oaxaca type, with even the eyes of the monster on the mask half-veiled. The use of round and curving lines throughout results in the absence of real "center" in the design; the effect is that of a delightful arabesque. In Copán, beneath Stela 3, dated mid-7th century, some jade pieces were found which show a certain similarity to this in build-up.[143] It would seem that in many early jades the lapidaries were content if they could place a face in the middle of the stone—then whatever surface remained was filled in with condensed symbols.

Fig. d is carved on a thin brownish slatelike stone. Here the idea has flattened down or thinned out to a degenerate and simplified expression. A monster-mask with especially ferocious fangs is recognizable just above the forehead of the human face. Little of the power and skill which created its numerous fore-runners is apparent in the carving.

Fig. e, only 2 inches wide, shows a head in profile, emphatic in facial lines but with the headdress less clearly worked out. The intertwining elements may be a conventionalized representation of a sinuous serpent body and a serpent's vertical jaw is visible behind the head. Center is given to the design by the earplug, the sharpest element in the whole. Details in this piece bear little relation to others on this plate and may indicate a different region of origin.

The profile in *fig. f* is liberated from all its wrappings. Although the natural shape of the jade was evidently the starting point for this design, it has been completely subordinated to the composition. The subject fills the entire stone and all irrelevant material has been pared away. The face, with its hooked nose and curling lips, is the feature of the piece. As there was apparently no space above the forehead for the headdress, it sweeps behind. Only a tuft of feathers remains of the familiar trappings; mask and round earplug are here absent. The material is good crystalline green jade, and the streak of lighter coloring, which extends from the forehead in front of the eye, beside the nose, and down the cheek, has been well utilized for plastic effect. The expression of the eye, which is bored through the stone, is greatly enhanced by the wing-shaped groove under it. A flamboyant rhythm permeates this piece, particularly noticeable when it is compared with the others.

The first two pieces on *Pl. 240* show persons engaged in activities not clearly definable. In *fig. a,* slightly over 4 inches high, an old man is seated with knees up and fingers outstretched, evidently concentrating his attention on one point. The edge of the stone is cut to conform with the elaborate carving which surrounds him, the lower part of which seems to represent a serpent in profile.

The figure on the whitish jade (*fig. b*) has Oaxaca-type features. He holds in his right hand an implement that resembles a stylus or quill, and in his lap, a good-sized jar, perhaps of paint. There is tension in the half-raised hand, and the gesture of the whole figure shows real working activity. A large monster-mask appears above him, perhaps part of his headdress. The original edge of the stone seems to have been left to a certain degree, though shaped to symmetry in the lower portion. Note the similarity of action in the top figure on the page from the Dresden Codex, *Pl. 266.*

In the four pieces that follow, the definite placing of a figural composition within a frame is evident. All the faces are typically Maya, though far from stereotyped. In the first three, the feather headdress overflows the frame, each in its own manner. The feathers in *fig. c* are horizontally placed; in *fig. d,* the edge of the stone is utilized as outline for the headdress which flows backward and down. The inner rim of the frame here is interestingly interrupted on a level with the thighs. Although the warrior in *fig. e* is confined within his frame, it is clear that he was only a part of a larger carving, for a fragment of a grotesque mask can be made out on the right. This pendant is 2¾ inches high in its present state and of a brilliant true "jade green." Note the pectoral that the warrior wears, like the piece shown in *Pl. 241, fig. h.* In each of these jades the pose of the hands is individual, but all show ceremonial gestures.

In the last pendant (*fig. f*), about 5 inches at its greatest height, a fine springy rhythm enlivens the figure who is apparently making an offering. The glyph before his mouth is as yet undeciphered. He wears an antlered headdress, unique in the jade carvings illustrated in this survey. The style has been identi-fied as Ocosingo, or Tonina, from central Chiapas. The piece is a perfect medal-lion, with the subject placed, unbroken and uncrowded, within the given space and framed by an even rim, bearing its own subordinate decoration.

These last two pendants, though clearly in the style of the Old Empire—par-ticularly reminiscent of Palenque—were dredged from the Sacred Well at Chichén Itzá. Possibly they had been handed down through generations before they were cast into the water as offerings to the Rain-god. We have a somewhat similar custom in passing on the amulets, lockets, and crosses of our forebears.

The Sacred Well at Chichén Itzá has proved a repository of objects from widely diverse regions and times, providing invaluable information on the inter-relation of cultures in Middle America since the 12th or 13th centuries.[150] Re-cently some amazing finds of jade were made in southern Vera Cruz and vicin-ity, where a great number of worked pieces were discovered, representing sev-eral styles and types.

The emphasis on the head with the subordination of every decorative motif is unmistakably evident in *Pl. 241. Fig. a,* about actual size as shown, illustrates very well the use of the round drill. The human head, which is carved here in low relief and placed within a triangular-shaped stone, steps out into three di-mensions in *fig. b,* and the unrelated or medallion rim of the first has been fash-ioned in the second into ears and a thick neck. A head of the same tradition appears in the thumb-nail sketch from the Guatemala highlands (*fig. c*), about 1½ inches high. The jade is a clear limpid green, but the carving is weak and unclear in detail, perhaps because it is so minute. These three pendants all show similar features: the almond eyes, rounded nose, and drooping mouth are Maya; the tall headdress with curling ends suggestive of maize leaves and, in *fig. b,* the arrangement of the hair in pompadour fashion are not only Maya but Maize-god attributes as well. *Fig. f,* although said to have been found at Monte Albán, possesses a number of the same characteristics. Here the rim has entirely disappeared and the face has a full expression, the result of a routined sculptural interpretation.

The fragment in *fig. e* shows an advanced technique in its use of sharper relief. The face itself is framed by the open mouth of the animal on the mask. Above is a considerable headdress. Although Mayoid in style, the features show another manner of carving.

Fig. d, 3 inches high and found in the Sacred Well at Chichén Itzá, is carved from an unusually fine apple-green jade. Here the head was sculptured out of an oval stone into a three-dimensional representation. The monster-mask, which appears foreshortened and is treated plastically, extending toward the back, is rather less defined than the clear-cut face with its somewhat vacant expression. Typically Maya is the receding chin, more readily seen here than in the first three specimens. Glyphs adorn the edges and even the back, which is flat.

In *fig. g* the stone again becomes the medium for a relief, with the edges trimmed to produce a symmetrical shape. The monster-mask here takes the form of a casque and the rim below the chin is worked out into an evenly executed collar, which, with the emphasized earplugs, helps balance the composition. The prominent jaw contrasts sharply with the almost chinless figure beside it. A similar type, though more uncertain in execution, was found in El Salvador.

A square shape and a predominance of straight lines lend a stern expression to *fig. h.* Compare it with the preceding head—a similar shape in which curved lines are the rule. The expression is quite conventionalized. He may be wearing a stylized headdress or the lines at the top may indicate hair. This pendant is 1⅔ inches high and was found at Zacualpa.

Pl. 242 presents larger pieces of carved stone. *Figs. a* and *b* come from Copán, Honduras, a Maya site that produced several styles during its existence. Some stylistic differences are manifest in these two statuettes, though the oblong shape and ceremonial posture, by now familiar, show a uniform idea. The first (*fig. a*), 7¾ inches high, is rounded and more squat in form, and the face is set off from the body, masklike, by sharp contours. There was apparently no attempt to adjust the shape to the imperfection in the stone (left) and the bent leg is merely carved across it. In general effect the piece is reminiscent of the stone carvings called *tortugas* or "turtles," at Quiriguá.

Fig. b is more elongated and angular, with the stone apparently cut to the contours of the figure. The carving is more simplified and the details are generalized. The man wears another type of headdress, with the wide-open jaw of the serpent extending above his forehead. It may be remarked that neither of these Maya jades shows the strongly almond-shaped eye. The designated pupils in *fig. b* are unusual.

Fig. c is another of the remarkable finds made by A. Ledyard Smith at Uaxactún. The figure, 10½ inches high and devoid of all decoration, is seated in somewhat the same pose as those above it, but with the hands crossed over one another. The same stereotyped expression is evident as in the other two, but here more clearly perceived, perhaps, because of the clear green of the material. This piece, however, is not a mere lump of stone fashioned in the semblance of a human, but a real three-dimensional statuette. The eyes may have been inlaid and there are traces of red in the eye sockets and mouth. Noteworthy are the incised fingers and the "eyebrows," associated with Olmec traits (see the next plate), and the numerous piercings, apparently for added ornament. The absence of a headdress is another non-Maya feature.

A kneeling woman is represented in *fig. d*. The shape, the dark-toned material (a green diorite), and the economy of detail are typical of Aztec work. In this small piece, about 3 inches high, the head has received all concentration to the detriment of the body, which is little more than a rounded base with arms suggested at the sides and small feet extending to the rear. The static effect of the carving, created primarily by its solid shape, is augmented by the empty eye sockets, which were probably once inlaid, as was the medallion on the breast.

The statuette in *Pl. 243, fig. a,* 4¼ inches high and said to have come from Vera Cruz, is of an agreeable pale grayish-green color. The little figure has tattoo marks over his body. His ears are pierced for ornaments but he does not wear a headdress. The pose is more relaxed than in the pieces on the opposite plate and he appears to be blowing on some instrument, perhaps an ocarina. A hole is bored up through the center of the stone, possibly for mounting it on a staff.

We now come to that puzzling manifestation of medieval Mexican art, known as the "baby face" or "tiger mouth" type. It is a characteristic tentatively assigned to the mysterious Olmec people, who are believed to have inhabited a part of the state of Vera Cruz, south of the city of that name, as well as the contiguous areas of Tabasco, Chiapas, and parts of Oaxaca. Olmec is said to mean "dwellers where rubber grows." They exerted an influence on the Maya art of Cycle 9 (A.D. 435 to 830) and again, in the New Empire, on the art of Yucatan with its strong Toltec infusion. This art and culture are now called La Venta, after one of the sites where it occurs in most characteristic form.

"Most typical of Olmec art," as J. Eric S. Thompson writes, "are the treatment of the muzzle and mouth in anthropomorphized representations of the jaguar and the blending of these feline features with those of a youthful deity. The characteristics . . . are: the flaring nostrils at the base of a narrow nose, the muzzle shaped like a croquet hoop, the triangular or square appendage from the upper lip, the uptwist of the lower lip to follow the line of the upper lip and muzzle, the nick in the forehead." [154]

The tiger-mouth deity (*fig. b*) has an interesting mixture of human and animal features. As fantastic a creation as it is, it was, nevertheless, like other representations of medieval American iconography, clearly defined in the imagination of the carver. The headdress with its hanging ear-flaps is skillfully worked over the head with a facile touch, and not only patience but very mature technical skill are shown in the execution of the minute details in the face. Ferocity in the general impression is neutralized by the childish roundness of the forelegs that end in human hands, the ribbons tied at the neck and wrists, and the tassels flaring at the back. Note the medallion with a cross on the breast, similar to that on *Pl. 235, fig. c.* This photograph brings out the brilliant luster of the stone.

Fig. c shows a representation a little more on the human side. At first glance, it might be taken for a child, with its soft square face and hanging jowls. The over-developed mouth, however, with its moustache-like addition, and the stumpy nose are rather elements of fantasy or symbolism. A band around the forehead and ear-flaps are the only ornaments. From the shoulders down, the body is condensed into a cubical shape which, with hands tip to tip and the stubby feet only indicated, is in sharp contrast to the clearly developed and alive expression of the face.

The same idea prevails in the last piece (*fig. d*). The face has the same exaggerated features and the body is even more out of proportion. The only real carving in the figure was in the shaping of the chin, mouth, and nose—the symbolic elements; the rest that was plastic in *fig. c* is here only incised. It has slanting eyes that are distinctly crossed and "cockscomb eyebrows" that are somewhat similar to those in the little naked idol on the opposite plate. Here the forehead shows the deep V-shaped nick, a characteristic of the Olmec.

Pl. 244 presents two necklaces fashioned by the medieval American lapidary. Beads, especially from Oaxaca and Guerrero, were much in demand as objects of trade over a wide area. The first (*fig. a*) is of graduated translucent quartz and comes from Chichén Itzá. Rock crystal is recognized as one of the hardest stones and the beauty of the shaping and the polish, as well as the skillful uniform boring, are admirable, particularly so when it is remembered that the pre-Columbian worker had only simple tools at his disposal.

In the jade necklace (*fig. c*), the beads are neither so even nor so regular but the quality of the stones is very good. The color ranges from a marbleized dark gray to a light greenish crayon gray. Some of the very different shapes may have been added later, as the arrangement with the pendant—upon which a face is suggested with a few essential lines—is recent.

The broken circular disk in *fig. b* is of an unusually fine jade color and demonstrates great technical ability, both in the carving and in polishing off the undesired sections to produce such a difficult form. It would have been task enough to cut down the stone into a circle, but to bore the hole in the center was a still more risky matter. The thin flat body and the ring shape are responsible for our having only a fragment, but even this shows the delicacy of the work. An off-color cement used in restoration makes the seated figure at the edge rather unclear in the photograph. Nevertheless, it is apparent that only a gifted and experienced craftsman could have conceived and produced the design. A staccato rhythm is created by the interspersing of figural and decorative motifs.

The following plates unfold before us a variety of shapes and color, techniques and expression, a range in region and time, but all show clear envisaging of the subject and command over technicalities.

All examples on *Pl. 245* measure from 2½ to 3½ inches in height. *Figs. a* and *b* are conceived on the same general plan: an idealized elongated head shape, executed without any decoration but highly plastic. Their ears are conventionalized to the simplicity of handles, and the slightly opened lips have a greater or lesser tendency toward the Olmec tiger mouth. The first piece has more life than the others; there are no eyeballs, but it has a live and penetrating look. The upward lines between the eyes are carved deep with considered sculptural effect. To us the cheeks appear swollen. The thickened nose combines with the upper lip and probably carried a nose ornament.

The two figures below these (*e* and *f*) are related to them. Both show artificial deformation of the skull to an even greater degree. Both have a narrow rim under the chin. *Fig. e,* however, has a quieter facial expression and more realism, while *f* is made uncouth for us by exaggeration in the eyes and mouth.

The rounder shapes in *figs.* *c* and *d* reveal grotesque humor. Whether they represent a crying baby face or a mask of some fantasy-world, the force of expression in these small pieces cannot be denied. Pronounced angles in the upper lips give them both outspoken tiger mouths. Note the incision work around the eyes in *fig. c* that may have denoted tattoo or paint. The mouth is hollow; in *fig. d* it is only deepened. Here luglike ears occur, similar to those in the group just described.

It should be pointed out that where a human face with Olmec features appears the dome of the head is bald and without headdress. This observation holds for the great number of jade pieces which we have studied.

Fig. h presents a profile view of a pendant with characteristic Maya ornamentation around and above the face. It is carved from a light jade of better quality than most of the others on this plate and is executed in a very different manner—much more decorative and flamboyant.

Fig. g has the same hanging lower lip, half-closed eyes, and rounded nose. The straight lines above the forehead are similar to those in *fig. d,* but while the piece in the upper row has an articulate expression, this one is stoically uncommunicative. It is a mask in shape, quite deeply hollowed out in the back. Acquired in El Salvador, it is a mottled light green flecked with gold, a material seen so frequently in jades thereabouts that we may speculate on its local origin, perhaps around the region of San Miguel.

The pectoral in *Pl. 246, fig. a* is 3¼ inches high and of the finest quality jade, a deep rich green in tone. From several points of view it is unique. The unusually plastic head does not occupy the entire stone and flat surfaces extend on both sides. Again the skull is dome-shaped, but the arrangement of the hair in locks, incised in turn with fine lines, does not occur in any other known pre-Columbian work. There are masks in the Museo Regional of Mérida, Yucatan, and in the Musée de l'Homme in Paris, on which locks of hair are indicated, and there are also stucco reliefs where the same detail is implied, executed, however, with incomparably less artistry. Especially remarkable is the treatment of the eyes with their slight cast, revealing deliberate use of the effects of light and shade. Flattened circles in the iris catch a luminous reflection and deep incisions above the eyeballs serve to intensify the gaze. The tiger mouth is so discreet that it is little more than a disdainful droop. A finely chiseled nose with a pierced septum is evidence that the carver could be realistic when he chose. The ears are delicately sculptured, and decorated with earplugs. On the left the two glyphs, as yet undeciphered, appear to be Olmec; Joyce reports traces of two others, one on each side where the stone is broken off, and estimates the piece therefore as having been originally at least 6½ inches wide. Because of its technical and artistic superiority, he places it at the highest period of Copán. However, the non-Maya glyphs and Olmec features would remove it rather to that region where Maya and Olmec art meet. The face has real spiritual content. Its penetrating forcefulness and mysterious beauty combine to make it a *chef-d'œuvre* among pre-Columbian jades.

Strong kinship in ideology and appearance can be discerned in the companion piece (*fig. b*), a profile carved in relief on a shield-shaped stone, one corner of which has been broken off. Here also the subject does not take up all the available surface. On the upper edge and again under the chin smooth sections are left that emphasize the passive frame into which the head has been placed, balanced. The carving is very shallow. In front of the sculptured forehead, a second head appears, lightly incised in the margin, and a third is found facing out of the top line of the shield, with the forehead of the main head forming its chin. On the cheek of the main face are outlined two minor profiles, facing each other—from their design and position possibly representing tattoo. These faces all show strongly Olmec features. It is possible that some of these subordinate profiles were cut into the stone later. The hollowed-out eye and the vertical lines in front of and behind the ear in the large head may have been inlaid.

Each of the four small heads shown on *Pl. 247* differs in style as well as in the quality and color of its material. Three different ways of carving the eyes are evident. In *fig. a* the stone is alabaster-like. The most distinguishing features of the piece are the serpent headdress and the execution of the eyes and mouth. Eye sockets and lids are lifted out of the stone and a channel carved all around them, giving the coffee-bean effect familiar from pottery. The two condensed intertwined serpents are a rare decorative addition as headdress, on which incision is utilized in contrast to the strongly plastic face. (Compare with the headdress on *Pl. 237, fig. a.*) Ears are indicated by a coil, and the distended lobes are bored with large perforations.

Fig. b breathes a martial air. A singularly hard-bitten expression is given the face by the deeply cut crescents that outline the nose and suggest eyebrows. The nose is broadened and flattened into a triangle and nostrils are indicated by shallow round depressions at the base, produced by the same method that bored the iris in *fig. a* on the opposite plate. The mouth, represented by a broad curved band, tending downward like a drooping moustache, and the lug-shaped ears lean toward the Olmec. A helmet rather than a headdress is suggested by the lines that divide the head into three sections. Compact, succinct, and vigorous, this little piece, not 2 inches high, has the vehemence of a portrait.

Fig. c presents a more realistic head. It is about 2½ inches high and cut from pale jade in an acorn shape that must have been difficult to carve. The face has considerable plastic detail, and, in comparison with the straight lines of the others, its peaked outline is striking. A unique feature is the pointed helmet, fashioned in perfect symmetry and counterbalanced by the natural almond shape of the face. The deep-cut rim of the headdress produces a pleasing shadow.

Fig. d can be regarded as the product of a lateral development, with similarities to the Olmec heads on *Pl. 245* and to the square baby faces of *Pl. 243*. No headdress, no hair, no helmet, no ears even are indicated; the nose is only half-heartedly three dimensional, and two holes are drilled through the upper lip for nostrils. This conventionalized face has, however, an indisputable mystic radiation. Here we approach the complex idea of the fetish, in which not the simplified sculptural representation was of importance but the magic power which was attached to it and lay behind it. The piece was bought at Chichén Itzá but may have traveled a considerable distance from its place of origin.

In the next three plates larger masks are presented. *Pl. 248, fig. a* is a pale sea-green jade about 4½ inches high. It represents Coyolaxhqui, sister of the Mexican War-god, Huitzilipochtli. The image, in itself far from sympathetic, seems to be weighed down by the bulk of the stone. The face proper is nearly square and appears stretched between the earplugs. An inert headdress and cumbrous ornament increase the heavy impression. The milky color, the expressionless slit eyes, and swollen lips all combine to give a feeling of deadness to the subject.

Fig. c below it, 7⅛ inches high, shows technically a new approach. The use of several planes in the execution of the mouth and forehead creates sharp contours, utilizing the effect of light and shade. Incision underlines certain sculptured details. Deep bored holes used in the eyes and nose intensify the fierce and demoniac expression.

Fig. d is rounder but has similar features in its build-up. The protruding forehead and mouth are evident, but the general surface is smoother. The drooping mouth is simplified into two bands, and the headdress, fully executed in the piece beside it, is here only suggested by the flamelike middle section. Slight markings denote ears that are not represented on the other at all. The eye sockets may have been inlaid with another material, as cavities for affixing it are visible in the inner corners.

Fig. b, about 4½ inches high, is the quietest among the four on this plate and the most human. The stone is agreeably rounded and polished. All features are in proportion. The mouth and nose have not the unnatural emphasis seen in the masks below it and only the raised upper lip with its suggestion of the tiger line shows relationship to them. Here the decoration on the forehead—plastic in the other pieces—is only incised, a deterioration of the same motif, probably indicating, with the other lines about the face, tattoo or paint.

Pl. 249 demonstrates how powerful artistic concepts of certain pre-Columbian periods were stereotyped into formulae through frequent repetition. The mystic quality of the work diminishes as the lapidary approaches naturalism.

Figs. a, b, and *d,* all Toltec in style, range from 6 to 10 inches high and are variations of the same theme with few divergences. The heraldic shape of the masks is similar, and a complete absence of decoration is common to them all. The eyes in general suggest the coffee-bean type, but the slits are widened and shaped to resemble more nearly an eye socket. Particularly good workmanship is manifest in the first.

Fig. c, about 9 inches high, is executed in a different sculptural manner. Eyes and nose are less pronounced and even the protruding mouth does not show the sharp contours of the companion pieces. A rim above the forehead—which will be met again on the next plate—points to another provenience.

Fig. a on *Pl. 250* is a round mask and, as such, is quite rare. It is a Xipe-Totec representation, seen also in sculpture and metal, executed here in a very dark stone with a high polish. An unusual feature is the hair, divided in the middle and stylized with even strokes. The piece is 4¼ inches high.

Fig. b may be an unfinished carving. Better than any of the other illustrations it shows the technical approach of the lapidary. Marks left by hollow drills of various sizes can be seen in the eye sockets, and a print of a "reverse" is still visible on the left, below the nose. Nostrils are indicated by segments of a circle; the mouth is but a sawed line. The headdress is only outlined, and the circles drilled at the sides may be the beginnings of earplugs. After comparison with the piece beside it, it becomes evident how much contour and expression could be given by further working; note especially the similarity of the noses.

Fig. c, 4¾ inches high, also has the rim above the forehead. The mouth is somewhat open. The vaguer expression is the result of the standardization of a sculptural manner.

The mask in *fig. d* is very large, 18 inches high, and of bright green serpentine. It probably represents a dead warrior. An unusual feature is the lolling tongue, which is sometimes suggested but seldom executed with such realism. The depiction of the row of upper teeth is also unusual. Otherwise in sculptural build-up the mask is quite similar to the Toltec type.

The small objects on *Pl. 251* exemplify the broad skill of the lapidary in many regions. In *fig. a* we find the jaguar head that has appeared on so many headdresses with symbolic intent carved in a more natural form. It is not surprising that the little piece, about 3 inches high, exhibits such good workmanship and realism in expression, for it comes from Piedras Negras, a site which had the ripest plastic talent. The jade is a mottled apple-green and of finest quality. There are glyphs carved on the back.

The beguiling monkey head in *fig. b,* about 4 inches high, is said to have come from the state of Puebla, Mexico. It was here that influences from the distant tributary states met the inner circle of Aztec iconography. The piece is made of obsidian. This material was commonly used for sacrificial knives, daggers, and other sharp-edged implements, which the pre-Columbian lapidary split off from "cores" with great dexterity. But the shaping and polishing of this figure with its many rounded surfaces must have required especial skill and patience. It has fine tactile quality. Although the eyes have lost their original inlay, they still have a live expression even with rough blank sockets.

Fig. c is simpler in its carving but telling in its effect. This is one of the rare cases in which the inlay has survived. The white shell in the eyes, with red dots for pupils, augments the bizarre effect of the whole little mask. Compare the grotesque nose with that of the large pottery figure at Oaxaca (see *Pl. 124, fig. c*).

In *fig. d* only the main contours of the amphibian are plastically executed;

all surface representation is done by shallow incised lines. This example, better than many others, demonstrates that the pre-Columbian carver saw nature in his own way and did not hesitate to apply incision, relief, and even three-dimensional sculpture on one and the same piece. What merits special attention in this carving is the contented expression in the face, achieved obviously with intent.

The serpent fan handle in *fig. e,* about 5 inches long, is another of the gems found among the treasures of Tomb 7 at Monte Albán. The jade is very fine, both in luster and color. Not only is the sleek creeping quality of a reptile well caught, but excellent skill is shown in the cutting: to chisel out, shape, and polish so perfectly the slender cylinder required great deftness. Here is proof that the Zapotec-Mixtec region, so different in its stylistic language from the Maya, was also master in the technical field.

The jade hand (*fig. f*), perhaps a votive offering, comes from the Ulúa Valley in Honduras, a region which held several strong Maya characteristics, as in a pocket, when they had disappeared elsewhere. The quality of the stone, milky in tone, is fine. An amazing command of technique is displayed in the living gesture in all the fingers, whether opened or closed. The piece is truly three dimensional; even the knuckles are worked out on the back.

Full standing figures carved in jade are rare in medieval American art. Of the three on *Pl. 252,* the first to our eyes seems somewhat ponderous, the second, rather grotesque, while the third is the most perfect in expression. Certain features of the Olmec type can be discerned in all of them; not one has any head-dress and the luglike ears and bald dome prevail. A truly Olmec mouth, however, appears only in the last.

Fig. a, about 20 inches high, is one of the largest pre-Columbian jades ever found. Hands and legs are stiff in execution but the contours of the chest and cheeks are ably worked out. The neck is not so deeply defined as in the others, perhaps for fear the head might break off, but it nevertheless sits naturally on the massive shoulders. Glyphs are inscribed on the belt and the edge of the kilt. The eyes may have been inlaid, as there are depressions in the inner corners. Here we must admire the skill which was able to carve a statue of such dimensions without breaking the stone.

Fig. b is only about 5 inches high and stands in a more vivacious pose. The elongated head is by now familiar but the pointed beard and prominent teeth are unusual.

The statuette shown from the side in *fig. c* and from the front in *fig. d* is 9½ inches high. Of the three, this one is made of the best jade and, as carving, it is the most articulate. The contours are smoothly rounded and agreeably plastic. He stands without support, with slightly bent knees, a posture that gives the figure more elasticity. The hands seem to have held a separate object.

After seeing the standing figures, it is interesting to observe that the seated pose offered more opportunity for variation. All the statuettes on *Pl. 253* have more life in pose and expression. The position of the man in *fig. a* recalls that of the jade from Uaxactún (see *Pl. 242, fig. c*), but here the limbs are freed from the mass of the stone. A close cap is suggested, the only indication of headdress among the seven figures in this display. The face has strength and authority; tattoo or paint may be indicated by the incision work, which intensifies its severity.

The material of *fig. b* is pyrite, an iron ore with a metallic luster, very difficult to work. There is some similarity here to the baby faces of *Pl. 245,* but the eyes slant downward and the face does not show the same plasticity. The tiger line in the upper lip is pronounced—note the depressions made by the round drill in the angles of the mouth. Stumpy arms and legs add to the amusing impression.

A completely different language of expression is manifest in *fig. c,* about actual size as shown, which comes from the Ulúa Valley; evidence that the people of this region had excellent plastic feeling and a correspondingly able technique has already been seen in the marble vases. This figure is bearded, with a fringe of moustache at the corners of his mouth—a rarity in Middle American sculpture—and shows relationship to *fig. b* on the opposite page, the only other bearded one in this group. The forward thrust of the elongated head and the wide shoulders dominate the impression. Different planes of the face are sharply contrasted and add to the power of attack on the onlooker, despite the relatively small size of the piece. His hands are well worked out, but the feet are only incised.

In *fig. d,* the statuette, 4¼ inches high, is sculptured from the finest green jade. The pose is the freest represented here and harks back to Maya statuary (see *Pl. 81, fig. b*). In his right hand, the figure holds a plant, in his left, an unidentified object. The head shape and many of the other features are quite similar to those of the standing statue in *figs. c* and *d* on the opposite page. Again, in this example, the Olmec mouth has no repelling effect.

Besides their different poses, these four little figures also manifest diverse spiritual content. The first is intent and has poise; the second is droll and restrained; *fig. c* has an aggressive, almost ferocious air throughout, while *fig. d*, the masterpiece, displays an aristocratic refinement, imparted with grace and subtlety.

The heavy jade vessel on *Pl. 254, fig. a* is carved in the likeness of the Rain-god, Tlaloc.[25] A little under 9 inches high, it weighs ten pounds and three ounces—a compact piece of rather dark, pleasantly green stone. As the verdure brought by the rain was symbolized by the color, one can readily understand why this beautiful block of precious material was used for an image of the Rain-god. The deity's upper lip has the tiger line, and his fantastic tongue may represent falling water. A hole bored just behind the tongue is visible in this picture. His bulging eyes and knoblike nose are fierce and powerful enough to match the heavy sculpturing of the lower features. The ears, with their straightened lines and the convolutions indicated by an incised S, serve as handles. Below the prominent head, a body, hands, and legs are suggested. The hands can be seen on either side under the ears, holding upright some object. Other details of figure and dress are reduced to geometric patterns. A finely rounded rim finishes the vase effectively.

This piece shows a transmutation of a utilitarian shape into the likeness of a mythological being, such as was also seen in pottery. Much in the composition was dictated by ritualistic iconography, but it required remarkable talent to realize it in such balanced form.

The unique statue in *fig. b,* 7½ inches high, was cut from a rather pale mottled jade of fine color (called wernerite) and is unbelievably smooth over the entire surface.[44] The figure has been identified as Toci, Mother of the Gods, from whom the deities sprang full grown. The goddess is shown clasping her buttocks in the typical crouching position of Indian women in childbirth. Her labor is conveyed by the cramped expression, the prominent collar bone, and straining lips. The face of the small figure is mature and the animal paws give to the birth a symbolic significance.

On every side the piece is equally worked out. Straight hair, only partly visible in this illustration, hangs halfway down her back. The ears are unusually realistic. Holes are drilled not only in the earlobes to hold jewelry, but in the feet, body, under the chin, and into the hair, indicating the application of other materials for ornament. When photographed, the statue was tilted forward to stand the figure in a natural position which was probably achieved in pre-Columbian times by additional props, since then disappeared. A monumental quality is embodied in the small piece; despite its harrowing theme, it has dignity and austerity.

Two objects cut from rock crystal, a hard yet easily cracked stone, are presented on *Pl. 255*. The goblet in *fig. a* was found in the celebrated Tomb 7 at Monte Albán. It is about 4½ inches high and 3 in diameter and is carved from a single piece. Its shape is pleasingly proportioned, the polish fine and smooth, and the edges are perfectly rounded. The base was hollowed out to about a third of its height, enhancing the delicacy of the whole, and the translucent material was worked up into a frosty tone. The piece gains dignity by the omission of decoration; there is life enough in the undisturbed play of changing light caught and reflected through the rounded surface.

The life-size skull (*fig. b*) is realistic in detail. Crystal, here polished to a glassy finish, is remarkably effective for this gruesome subject.

Pl. 256 offers other examples of a most remarkable technical skill in working hard and brittle materials. The life-size representation of a frog cut from rock crystal (*fig. a*) speaks for itself. Its naïveté and humor are so eloquent that we have only to enjoy it, unhindered by strange ideology. Reflections are subtly utilized to give it life. Even though unnaturalistic in many details, it appeals to us through the universal language of straight-forward sculpture, the language of toys.

The crystal man in the moon (*fig. b*) is so sophisticated that one may question whether it is a product of pre-Columbian times. According to some writers, the theme was not strange to medieval America: a jade representation, found in a tomb near Quiotepec, Mexico, was reported in 1916.[53] Seler points out that similar figures are found in Zapotec codices, and de Rosny described a sign of the month as "a crescent to which is attached a face in profile." [116] Even if the carving was made after the Conquest, this should not lessen our enjoyment; the illustrations in this chapter have already demonstrated that the pre-Columbian artist possessed the ability to execute such a piece before contact with the white man's civilization.

The model of a temple-base, 8 inches high (*fig. c*), was carved from one flawless piece of obsidian. The evenness of detail is particularly worthy of mention; note the stability gained by cutting the lowest terrace on a slight slant, while the sides of the other four are more nearly vertical. On the top is a depression which suggests additional decoration.

Fig. d is an eccentric flint, a type of object generally found in the region of the Maya Old Empire, frequently in votive caches. Creatures such as the dog, snake, bird, and scorpion are represented, but some pieces defy interpretation. They must have had some ceremonial significance, since no practical use can be divined for such fragile and irregularly shaped objects. The piece here illustrated is said to have come from near the border of Guatemala and Honduras. It is about 7½ inches long and less than one-quarter of an inch thick. To chip off the stone to this bizarre outline, depicting profiles, headdresses, and ceremonial paraphernalia, must have involved expert craftsmanship.

Fig. a on *Pl. 257* is a tripod vase from Tomb 7, Monte Albán, made of a kind of onyx which the Mexicans call *tecali.* This material is well adapted to carving and, like alabaster, can be reduced to sheets so thin that light shines through them; after the Conquest, windowpanes for churches were sometimes made of it. Like the crystal goblet from the same tomb on *Pl. 255,* this vessel has no decoration of any kind; both depend on their pure shape and unadorned surface for artistic effect. The whole interior is hollow and the walls are extremely thin. When the photograph was taken, an electric light was placed inside (the wires were painted out in the print) to give an idea of its translucent quality.

The miniature vase of grayish-green jade from El Salvador (*fig. b*) is only about 2 inches high, but considering the much harder material from which it was carved, the accomplishment is considerable. Its fine spherical shape would in itself excite admiration. In contrast to the onyx vase, the surface is covered with a meandering pattern, probably a stylized serpent body, with the characteristic lattice-and-bar motif of the Maya. The rim is very symmetrical and well rounded.

The remaining specimens are again of Mexican onyx and are said to have come from the Isla de los Sacrificios, situated just outside the modern seaport of Vera Cruz. This region was inhabited by the Totonacs, skillful stone carvers, as other plates in other chapters have already shown. The first of the two (*fig. c*), about 13½ inches high, is carved from a creamy-colored stone, with brown and yellowish veins that accent its vertical lines. Especially noteworthy are the fine line of the fluting on the body, ending in scallops, and the perfect execution of the double rings above them. The combination of incised symbols on the neck—the circles for "jade" or "precious," the fret-scrolls for "liquid"—occur often in

Teotihuacán and Aztec glyphs and has been interpreted as signifying sacrificial blood.[25]

The vase with the lizard (*fig. d*) is about 9 inches high. While the fluted vessel, with its glyphs and mystic associations, is composed and uncommunicative, this piece has an outspoken naturalistic accent. The little creature, its head raised inquiringly over the edge, introduces a comic touch. There is excellent balance in its position, even when viewed from another angle. The bases of each, as well as the use made of the veining in the stone, are completely different.

ANDEAN AREA

This chapter would not be complete without some contribution from the Andean Area. The little Mochica masterpiece on *Pl. 258, fig. a* is of mottled greenish turquoise and only 2¼ inches high. The head and headdress appropriate nearly two-thirds of the piece, but it is this disproportionate presentation that gives to the figure the charm of a good fairy-tale illustration. His face has the preoccupied expression and composure of some one doing something important, and his outstretched hands holding the offering have the gesture of willing and friendly giving. The gift in his right hand appears to be two shells sealed together, a contrivance often used to hold a treasure. As a visible sign of his ceremonial occupation, he is wearing a puma pelt, the head of which serves as headdress—its forepaws hang at the side of the ears and the hind feet and tail are worked out on the back of the statuette.

How standardized were certain plastic features, regardless of material, is demonstrated once more in the panpipe player of cast silver, 6¾ inches high, also from the Mochica culture. Here the headdress is more elaborate, the costume more detailed, and the fingers of the little man are more clearly defined. His carriage, however, the length of dress, the feet, and especially the delineation of the features are identical. Even such a small detail as the eyes is expressed with the same lines and convexities, whether in stone or metal.

Below it (*fig. c*) is a small cylindrical vase of turquoise. The stone has a good even color, and the matt surface gives it tactile charm. Its decoration appears abstract and geometrical, although a symbolic serpent body and monster-heads of Chavín style can be discovered in it. Balance appears in the decorative elements, but beyond that the piece makes no great appeal to us. The ingratiating little Mochica gift bearer and this small impersonal vase show the difference in artistic temperament between two early cultures, in regions not far from each other, both in the north of Peru.

The tools of the pre-Columbian lapidary were less advanced than those of the Chinese. Nevertheless, numerous pieces of medieval American jades can compete in beauty and interest with those of the Orient. Amazingly varying styles will have been observed in these pre-Columbian pieces, although a relatively small range is discernible in technical development. Modulations in taste seem to have influenced the styles over wide regions from period to period. As documents that would help reconstruct the sunken cultures, these small pieces are not of primary importance; their artistic appeal, however, is so obvious that they can be enjoyed *per se*.

Jade was singularly adapted to cult purposes here. Even while still unworked, it presented with its frequently mottled tones the broken surfaces which the Maya deliberately created in their sculpture and pottery. Its extremely pleasant tactile quality, the great variety in color, the suggestive shapes in the raw material all inspired the lapidary not only to bring forth objects of high craftsmanship but to imbue them with a mystic content.

IX

Murals and Manuscripts

PRIMEVAL man scratched and painted on cave walls pictures of the animals upon which he depended, probably as a magic ritual to assure success in the hunt. Here began the art of recording on a two-dimensional surface, a form of expression which has passed through more changes than architecture, sculpture, or any of the applied arts.

· As long as the walls of caves served as medium for the animal and human contours, this art had a universal quality. Later, the picture was drawn on animal skins or sheets of plant composition and each civilization created its own pictorial language. In the beginning, each symbol stood for one concept, such as sun, moon, rain, death. Gradually, characters taken together developed into hieroglyphic writing. As the culture became more complicated, the ideas broadened in their association to cover the needs of a growing perception and the writing became more and more fluent, often achieving the state of cursive script.

For this reason it might be said that the recording symbols of a people reveal the grammar of its mind, the whole process of thinking, as fundamental as speech construction. The sequence of the symbols—their arrangement to express a thought—is also peculiarly individual with different civilizations, a revelation of the manner of their approach to an idea. This is a difficult point for us to grasp, for, as most of the languages with which we are familiar are basically related, we seldom have to deal with an absolutely different ideology.

In some civilizations writing developed on the flat surface of the sheet, scroll, or folder, while in others it was inscribed on stone tablets, clay, wax, or metal. Egypt recorded on pages made of papyrus reeds, and young Christianity used animal skins for the scrolls which passed on to posterity the words of the Gospels. Paper, as we know, is a Chinese invention. Ancient as is the practice of writing, the present shape of the book is relatively young. We do not find pages bound into book form until the 11th century, and at that time the written word was at least four thousand years old.

In pre-Columbian America the origins of writing cannot be traced so far back. We do not even know the circumstances of its creation, although it may safely be stated that it was more recent than in the Eastern Hemisphere. In the Southwest, there was some method of communication before the Conquest, but little is known of it beyond the fact that crude signs were cut on the bark of trees to register the time-count.[169] In the Andean Area, counting, records, and communications were effected with the help of the *quipu,* an ingenious invention of cords of varying colors, thickness, and length, in which knots were tied at certain intervals (see *Pl. 299, fig. b*). It is possible that these people might have developed writing in time, as China also had a method of knot-recording before written characters appeared. The scope of the *quipu* is still a matter of conjecture; in the Inca dramatic legend "Ollantaytambo" it is read as a message.

Only the Maya and the Mexicans had developed systems of writing. These were idea-associative in mental structure and pictographic in appearance. Like the early European codices, which treat most frequently of dogma, legends, history, and astronomy, the writings of medieval America pertain chiefly to calendrical, religious, and historic matters. The gods intimately connected with agriculture and fertility were of great importance—as is generally the case among people whose existence depends upon the size and quality of an incalculable harvest—and the pictorial representations of these deities always retained certain attributes from nature. In addition to those gods who grew out of the life of the common people, there was another group embodying the more esoteric ideology of the priestly caste. Gods ruled each day or period, as indeed they once dominated our own, judging from the names of our days and months, and the figures of many of them came to stand for the time-span over which they presided.

It is believed that after A.D. 889, when the Maya custom of erecting dated stelae was abandoned, the records were kept on the more easily handled codices, or manuscripts. The material used for these was deer hide or a "paper" made from the maguey; the surface was covered with a very thin lime wash to receive the text. In Mexico, glyphs were painted in red, blue, green, black, white, yellow, orange, brown, and purple.[169] Most of the primary colors appear in different shades, a sign of refinement in color appreciation. All figures and designs were outlined in black, which bound the different pictorial elements into one composition. A fine brushlike implement was necessary to make the slender contours of this writing and the work could have been executed in hardly less time than was required for the miniatures of medieval Europe.

The extant codices consist of a single long sheet, folded like an accordion, or *leporello*. Each page is 6 or 7 inches from top to bottom, and the unfolded manuscript has been known to measure as much as 34 feet. At each end were covers of wood or hide to protect the contents. In one instance—the Codex Vaticanus B in the Vatican Library (see *Pl. 267, fig. a*)—jade set into the wooden back reminds us of the decorated bindings studded with semiprecious stones of Europe's Middle Ages. As in early European manuscripts, the pre-Columbian codex did not tend to individualize the human figure. The identity of a person was expressed by a name-sign, or glyph, and the gods were differentiated also by costume and their own special attributes. Since the entire life of the community was highly hieratic, little importance was attached to the individual. There are, however, a few codices in which lives of personages are related, such as Codex Colombino, which gives an account of the Zapotec or Mixtec warrior, "Eight Deer," to be discussed later in this chapter.[26]

The Maya, outstanding in their other arts, excelled also in the calligraphic work of codex illumination. It may be supposed that a great number of codices existed at the time of the Conquest. However, Diego de Landa, one of the first bishops of Yucatan, in his religious zeal ordered an *auto-da-fé* of all these works of the devil. Only three survive. Later in his life, he assembled a mass of material on the ancient culture of the Maya, which constitutes the main source of information from Conquest times. But the harm done was irreparable; the deciphering of Maya writing is greatly hampered by the scarcity of comparative material. To date less than one-third of the total glyphs known have been interpreted, including numerical symbols and those with astronomical significance.[92]

The numerals are expressed in two ways: by dots and bars and by characteristic heads. A bar-and-dot system for numbers was used also by the Zapotecs, but these were placed below, not above or beside, their glyphs.

After the Conquest several of the Maya-speaking tribes, among them the Quiché who dwelt near the shores of Lake Atitlán in Guatemala, wrote down the legends, mythology, and history of their people in their own dialect, inscribed phonetically in Latin characters. These books, the best known of which is called the *Popul-Vuh,* meaning "Book of the Community," have been translated into Spanish and reveal valuable details of the ancient beliefs and customs. However, since they do not contain pictorial and glyphic material, they furnish no clue to the hieroglyphs of pre-Columbian times.

Aztec writing had a more direct pictographic approach than the abstruse symbolism of the Maya. For example, the conquest of a town was indicated by a spear driven through a temple, above which the name-glyph was inscribed. The name-signs of personages developed into decorative appendages.

As fourteen medieval Mexican codices survive, a larger field is disclosed by the writings of these people. Besides religious and astronomical subjects, there are lists of the tribute exacted from vassal tribes, certain legal documents, and polychrome maps (see *Pl. 267, fig. c*). When Cortés landed on the coast of Mexico, Aztec scribes immediately painted pictures of the Spaniards, their horses, ships, equipment, and other novelties seen in their entourage to supplement the verbal report carried to Montezuma (see *Pl. 270*). Historical codices also exist, telling of the Aztec migrations and giving the general outline of their history. In these, tribal movements are shown by a line of painted footsteps passing from the glyph of one town to that of another, together with the date-signs. The codices were used in the schools of instruction and in the training of initiates for the priesthood. The number of persons, however, who could interpret the text was probably always quite small.[151]

In some civilizations, a symbol came to indicate a sound, and from there on writing and painting separated. Whether the pre-Columbian systems were standing on the brink of phonetics at the time of the Conquest is still a matter of discussion.

The fresco of medieval Europe was frequently a symbolical scene enlarged from manuscripts which the friars had illuminated. On walls, however, the condensed character of the compositions disappeared; the large surfaces called for and absorbed more and more decorative elements, until the spiritual content of the fresco tended to become of secondary importance and the main purpose came to lie in its decorative quality. Later the panel was placed on an easel and finally abandoned for canvas. Thus the manner which had been adapted to the static wall went through a great transformation and received at the same time considerable stimulus to further development. If a parallel could be drawn in medieval America, it might be found in the painted pottery vases of the Maya, where perhaps traditions of both mural and manuscript meet.

The mural in pre-Columbian America did not have the broad educational purpose as in medieval Europe, but rather was reserved for the initiate. It decorated the temple sanctuary and the palace, far from the walks of humble folk. The painter must have been a distinguished member of the artisan group, like the scribe who illuminated the codices, or the carver of jade, or the "jeweler," but it was apparently not the intention of any of these craftsmen to create art for art's sake, for the mere practice of virtuosity and the production of "beautiful" objects. The primary purpose of their work seems to have been to record or to invoke the power of magic, and the art never completely lost its symbolism to become purely decorative.

Pre-Columbian painting told its stories on the flat surface of a wall with the same pictorial language used on the page of a codex. Although on the walls, the figures were often enlarged, and the animal, plant, and building details frequently carried more minutiae, the modern eye will notice in both pictorial manifestations an absence of perspective. The lowest section of the picture is used to present that part of the scene nearest the spectator. Each level above it represents growing distance, although the figures are not necessarily reduced in size.

This manner of composing may appear strange to us, but we must not forget that in Europe, too, early painting denoted different distances by using different levels; with the exception of our western civilization, even today many cultures tell their stories without our studied use of perspective. The modern Russian icon does not employ it. Chinese scrolls, Japanese woodcuts, Persian miniatures all indicate it by working from the lower edge toward the top. The contrast of light and shade, one of the tricks of suggesting perspective, is not practiced by any of them. Figures are evenly lighted, without shadows; trees stand in the same tone of color in the foreground as in the background, and movements are conveyed mainly through the expressiveness of the lines. The surface to be painted is, as a rule, fully used—too crowded and too decorated for our eye. Yet, our own age shows the same symptoms, and our own illustrations, advertisements, moving pictures, and even more pretentious paintings are often crammed with people and detail.

If we keep all this in mind, the wall-paintings of pre-Columbian America may seem perhaps a little less strange. Unfortunately, far too few of them remain to allow a comprehensive study either of methods or development. The friable stucco wall of a temple or palace was the first part to disintegrate. Exposure to dampness, the growth of the jungle, whose rootlets spread like a web over the surfaces, have raised havoc among those wall-paintings that have survived the hands of man. Many must have been ruined in pre-Columbian times through the practice of filling in the lower rooms with rubble when a new building was superimposed. The ingenuity of the archaeologists, however, has rescued some buried murals. One at Chichén Itzá, revealed inch by inch on the crumbling plaster, was copied piecemeal by the artists, who did not perceive the full content until their work was fitted together.[94] Other paintings that did not disintegrate at the time of their discovery have since faded so badly that they are practically indecipherable; only the immediate copying in water color has saved their subject matter from being lost.

For this reason, most of the illustrations of murals shown here are necessarily copies, conscientiously executed, which give at least an impression even if lacking the weight of the original.

THE SOUTHWEST

The Indian in the Southwest carved human and animal figures on the rock walls of canyons and painted murals on the walls of his kiva. In some cases, the pictographs can be related to the wall-paintings and also, through certain ancient symbolic paraphernalia still surviving, to Indian designs of the present day. Some primitively painted figures in certain Southwestern sites have been known for a long time, but the recent excavations at Awatovi, in northeastern Arizona, and Kuaua, New Mexico, have considerably changed our ideas of the standard attained in this medium.

The section of wall-painting from Awatovi, reproduced on *Pl. 259, fig. a,* features human figures engaged in a ceremony. The geometrical shape at the extreme left doubtless has some symbolic significance. Note that the frontal figures are not full length: the central one is cut off below the waist and the second seems to stand elevated, with only the upper part of the body detailed. The two men in profile, on the other hand, are drawn in full, with the feet carefully executed. This may indicate that the first two are standing in the background, while the others are dancing in front of them, an impression borne out by their bended knees. The signs before their mouths may signify chanting. An elaborate object appears above the head of each—in the case of the largest figure, a bowl decorated with the step design, a favorite even today among the potters of the Southwest. Their ceremonial make-up shows great variety; even the patterns on the kilts of the two "dancers" are dissimilar. The lunar ornament at the throat of the chief celebrant shows not only excellent drawing but gives the impression that the piece itself must have been of delicate construction.

Fig. b shows another mural, 10 feet long and 4 feet 2 inches high, painted on a kiva wall at the same site. It presents an abstract design, highly complex and symbolic; but even though ignorant of its meaning, we are impressed with its stunning decorative character, the vigor in the layout, its play of line and color. Although the composition itself has complete equilibrium, the individual units are far from symmetrical, and it is this which gives the mural much of its interest and life. The birds on the upper edge differ in kind and color and few details are repeated in the right and left halves. Besides the white bands, which seem to embrace and connect the whole composition against its coral-red background, the color scheme includes blue, green, yellow, brown, and black. In contrast to the impression received from the abstraction of some modern paintings—which epitomize not so much an idea as a bid for attention and the will to be "different" —one is struck here with the integrity of purpose.

Another group of mural fragments was found on ancient kiva walls at a site called Kuaua, near Albuquerque, New Mexico. The preservation and removal of the crumbling adobe surfaces was a remarkable technical achievement for the University of New Mexico. In the painting (*fig. c*) a human figure is depicted holding a long slender staff bound with a tuft of feathers. The body is stylized into a long rectangular shape without proportion, but care is bestowed on the details of the skirt and the pendants or tassels on the belt. Execution of the face, especially the eyes, shows individual treatment when compared with the fragment in *fig. a,* although the painted design on the chin and the long hanging about the head make the expression remote for us.

The Indians in the Southwest never lost their talent for painting. Scenes picturing Spanish horsemen in a Christian procession were found on a cave wall, delineated in a style very similar to these kiva murals. The sand paintings of the present-day Navaho preserve many pre-Columbian characteristics, among them the angular elongated treatment of the human body. Even the splendid storytelling or decorative paintings of the young Indian artists at the United States School at Santa Fé display this atavistic trend.

MEXICAN AND MAYA AREAS

In medieval America the painter apparently had no intention of decorating a surface for the mere sake of beauty. His purpose was to commemorate an event, or, by applying magic symbols, to state an esoteric truth, or assure the benevolence of gods in whose honor a particular building had been erected. Therefore, if we, with our conscious esthetic approach, find our standards applicable to his work, it is purely fortuitous.

‹ 318 ›

The fragment on *Pl. 260, fig. b* was painted on the base wall of a large altar in the Temple of Agriculture at Teotihuacán. This composition is among the very few in which accurate symmetry between the right and left halves can be observed. Even conceding a certain amount of simplification by the hand of the draughtsman who made this copy, we cannot escape the marks of intention in the use of two central units of glyphic significance—a stylized mask with feather headdress and a serpent scroll with stones and shells—as an axis from which wavelike motifs flow. These are chiefly floral and plant forms, rare in pre-Columbian art. In between, simple scalloped bands run across the surface, holding together the entire design.

In contrast to the horizontal linear conduct of this mural, there is in the second detail from this temple (*fig. a*) an outspoken tendency toward verticality. This results from an attempt to depict a complicated scene that for our eyes would demand a knowledge of perspective. Since the idea of foreshortening and the other devices for denoting distance were unknown to these people, the problem was solved by placing the figures on different levels. The picture supposedly represents a Toltec ceremony. The buildings at the right and left might be temples; their decorated character seems to support this impression. In front of each a fire is burning, the tall flame of it highly stylized. Men and women are making offerings—the symbols before their mouths denote speech or chanting. Care has been taken to differentiate the personages by costume and gesture. Particularly appealing is the figure seated at the right in the first row, holding a bird in his hands. On the third level, a man in dark raiment, his hand upraised, gives an idea of Toltec dress unlike any we have met before. The headdress also differs considerably from the elaborate ceremonial style with which we have become familiar. His necklace is emphasized, and his decorated shawl is an indication of an advanced textile art, even in that early period.

As in numerous early civilizations, the arts in medieval America were closely allied. Color was lavishly applied on masonry surfaces. Sculptured slabs, also painted, constituted structural parts in some of the temples and palaces. In certain cases a decorative effect similar to that of the mural was achieved by sculpturing the stone blocks of the walls themselves with a very shallow relief and painting the carving.

Pl. 261, fig. a shows a section of such a wall found in the small building at the base of the Temple of the Tigers in Chichén Itzá, called the Temple of the Bas-Relief. It pictures a ceremonial procession of priests and warriors moving toward an altar to do honor to their god Kukulcán. At the risk of seeming repetitious, we must call attention again to the fact that there is not the slightest sign of serializing the units which form the whole; no two of the elaborately dressed dignitaries, with their spears and spear-throwers, are exactly alike in attire or pose. Great differentiation in certain details is not evident; nevertheless the scene has none of the monotony of an Assyrian stone relief, though it may seem more remote to us because of its less familiar ideology. In other late structures of the same site the same technique is applied to square piers at entrances and in colonnades.

A comparison of the two illustrations on this plate shows the contrast in both composition and figure delineation between even the late Maya art and that of the Mexican high plateau. *Fig. b* presents a section from a mural painted on the sacrificial altar in Tizatlán near Tlaxcala. The Tlaxcalan people were kindred of the Aztecs and their name in Nahua means "land of maize." This tribe was the first to ally itself with the Spaniards and thus aided in the downfall of the whole pre-Columbian civilization.

In the fresco fragment here pictured, two figures face each other. The left, with a skull as head, represents the Death-god. Opposite him stands Tezcatlipoca, the God of Youth, who was believed invisible, omnipresent, and all-powerful.[151] Both were gods of primary importance, occurring frequently in codices. Death seems even more ferocious in his attack than the God of Youth, who shows a certain deliberation in his attitude. Both are dressed and ornamented with such a profusion of trappings that the outlines of their figures proper are virtually concealed. Their characteristic features, such as the open-mouthed skull and tufted headdress of the Death-god or the forward-thrust, clawlike right foot of Tezcatlipoca and the two painted streaks across his face, appear in every representation of them.[97] The skull of the Death-god is painted in white and his feet are white, otherwise the chief colors used in his costume are blue, red, and yellow. A darker scheme was employed for the God of Youth, with black and deep red predominating.

In technique and delineation, the frescoes were not far removed from the illumination of manuscripts. The ignorance of perspective or scale is noticeable whether the scene was painted on an immovable wall or a fragile sheet of animal or vegetable material. The medium did not affect to any great extent the composition or linear conduct; a closely related stylistic manner will be observed in either case.

The Maya offer an exception also in this field. They were so highly developed in their artistic sensitivity that they "felt" differently for a mural than a manuscript. This will be especially evident in the two plates that follow.

The ruins of Uaxactún in Guatemala have revealed the spectacular achievement of the early Maya people in architecture, pottery, and jade. Recently A. Ledyard Smith of Carnegie Institution of Washington uncovered a mural fragment which raises considerably the already high opinion held of their remarkable talent (*Pl. 262, fig. a*). A comparison of it with the murals of any other culture here presented will make clear why the art of the Maya has received the keenest interest and most favorable comment from outsiders.

The Teotihuacán painting (see *Pl. 260, fig. a*) is composed of small wooden units, and, while each figure has a certain animation in itself, the picture as a whole is flat and static. In contrast, the people in the Uaxactún scene are not detached from one another, as if introduced one after the other into the composition, but are blended into a rhythmic free-flowing procession. While in the Teotihuacán piece the figures are placed above each other, apparently as space afforded, in the Uaxactún mural use is made of two divided levels, exactly defined. Superior effectiveness must also be granted the delineation of dark figures on a light ground.

An evaluation of the drawing will also reveal the greater artistic talent of the Maya in the portrayal of such a diverse group of persons, no two quite alike in dress or deportment. The eye falls first on the three sitting inside a house; especially noteworthy is the one in white, admirably drawn. Outside, on the left, two elaborately dressed figures face each other, one in a commanding attitude, the other with his right hand on his left shoulder in sign of submission. At the right, taller and shorter persons are assembled in animated groups. Near the door, two are engaged in conversation, as are the two above them, but with what contrast in mood and appearance and how ingeniously spaced to bring out the difference in feeling. Above, one member is detaching himself from a loose group of four, apparently to join the others on the left—a clever connective in the composition. Below, a line of followers is massed behind a small seated figure with a scroll or drum. The variations in height, the uneven spacing of the feet express perfectly the shifting and straining as they await the result of their leader's discussion. It is difficult to realize that there is little overlapping of the figures, only the two on the extreme right being actually superimposed. There is no shading whatever; the highly differentiated poses and complicated drapery are communicated by outline alone. One more factor should be pointed out among the many real pictorial values of the piece, and that is the individual pose of all the feet. The clear fine glyphs may identify the event as well as the participants.

That the high standard of artistry shown here is not an isolated case is manifest from the free designs and rhythmic compositions painted on the extant polychrome vases discussed under pottery. But in this mural a more human atmosphere prevails when compared with the hieratic air usually dominant. A freedom from restriction is noticeable, perhaps resulting from an innate feeling for the broader surface.

Fig. b is a water color of a fragment found on a wall of Edifice 3 in Chacmultun, Yucatan. Although doubtless a less exact copy than the one above, enough of the composition is caught to give a good idea of the original. Its story takes place on one level. The ceremonial character of the scene is evident. In the upper half of the surface the lavish headdresses, standards, and canopies are distributed with considerable decorative feeling. Even if this mural has not the artistic finesse of the one from Uaxactún, it is still a whole world removed from the frozen friezes of Egyptian tomb frescoes and has nothing of the stiffness of early Christian mosaics and wall-paintings. The figures are light and varied, as they stand poised, step onto the platform, lean forward, or rest the hand on the hip; an adroit execution of details proves that the abundant artistic tradition of the Maya prevailed to a high degree also in the New Empire. In accordance with Dr. Spinden, we find the Maya spirit still predominant here.[137] When these illustrations are compared with those on the following plate, which seem to be of a later date, the transformation in Maya art due to Mexican influence becomes evident. The highly decorative pageant-like representation gives way to a less refined drawing with more agitation—one might say the key of the composition changes from minor to major.

A mural that originally covered a space 9 feet high and 12½ feet wide on one of the inner walls of the Temple of the Warriors at Chichén Itzá is reproduced from a water color on *Pl. 263, fig. a*. It was found in fragments in the débris of the temple. A scene of every-day life in a seacoast village of Yucatan is depicted. In the upper two-thirds of the picture land is represented, upon which stands the same type of whitewashed hut with a thatched roof that is built in that country today. The building on the right, with its greater size, more elaborate execution, and the serpent poised above it seems to be a palace or temple. The settlement is full of activity. A woman is seated by a cooking pot that stands over an open fire outside a door; men are starting off on a journey with staffs in their hands and burdens on their backs, held in place by straps around their foreheads. There are trees with spreading tops. A crane wings across the scene, and the fisherman's catch lies in a little heap on the shore. At the left, a figure is kneeling at the water's edge.[94]

The lower part of the painting is gray-blue water. Three canoes in a row move across it, each paddled by a standing rower and carrying two Indians in warrior's dress with shield and arrows. Fish and reptiles of various sizes, shapes, and colors swim through the waves.

The earth is painted a reddish brown, the color of the soil of Yucatan, the flying crane is a natural pearly gray, and the trees show variations of green. In the water large reddish crabs, white shells, and a turtle with brown head and legs and green striped back are recognizable. Here the same pictorial manner is applied as in the Teotihuacán mural, but with much more dash. The strange but appealing atmosphere conjures up something of the mood of Gauguin's Tahitian paintings, bringing with it an association that may help us come nearer to the vanished world depicted here.

Fig. b is a detail of the mural from the east wall of the inner chamber of the Temple of the Tigers at Chichén Itzá. Although not from the same building as the preceding illustration, it seems, nevertheless, to complement it. Stylistically both murals are related, although a comparison of the trees will show differences. Representations of plant and animal life predominate in the scene, with a jaguar pictured in the foreground, another clinging to a tree, three serpents, each differently posed, and a bird. The warrior at the lower edge and the figure at the right introduce the human element.

A detail of a wall-painting copied in water color from the west wall of the Temple of the Tigers at Chichén Itzá is shown in *fig. c,* depicting a battle in and around a town. The difference between this mural and the others lies not so much in its technical execution as in the subtle combination of figures in repose with those in highly agitated attitudes. Each of the four men seated in the center foreground is differently dressed and is drawn in a different posture. They might represent a war council; some have speech scrolls before their mouths. Note the woman in a relaxed position in the lower left corner, a figure that would not be out of place in any of the other scenes on this plate. The seated warrior in the opposite corner with his leg pulled up seems to be working on a weapon, while the five fighting men in the second plane are wielding darts or spear-throwers. Their costumes are worth study. Not only are all individually outfitted, but each reveals another fighting pose. Considering the crowded space, the variety and turbulence in the scene, the picture is beautifully composed. The presentation of the action is especially ingeniously solved: the quiet happenings take place on a horizontal line, while the vehemence of the fighting group is augmented by the oblique, upward trend of their movement.

The inclination of the Maya of the Great Period for calligraphy, apparent also in their other arts, is markedly present in the Uaxactún mural. It is noteworthy that, while here the figural composition is interspersed in several places with columns of glyphs, no writing appears in the later murals. On the other hand, the speech scroll, associated with Mexican cultures, is seen in *figs. b* and *c*. The Uaxactún fresco and, to a certain degree, that from Chacmultun represent an early and pure Maya art and the battle scene, with its companion pieces, a late period, permeated with alien influences. However, all radiate strong storytelling atmosphere. We can enrich ourselves with this pictorial symphony, from the *andante maestoso* of Uaxactún to the *allegro vivace* of this last illustration from Chichén Itzá.

Mural painting at Chichén Itzá does not seem to have been practiced continuously during the life of the city. At any rate, of the one hundred thirty-one coats of whitewash in the Temple of the Warriors, only one, the twenty-second from the wall, was so decorated. The pictures were sometimes executed ". . . on freshly applied stucco, still soft enough to groove beneath the stylus, with which, in such cases, the preliminary sketches were drawn, but more commonly upon hardened plaster where the sketch lines were done in red. After being outlined, the figures were filled in with the desired colors, then re-outlined in black. . . . Often there is marked divergence between the sketch and the finished painting. Sometimes the pose of a limb is changed, or the proportions of any feature may have been altered in size or relation, as revealed by the faint sketch lines to be found upon scrutiny beneath the later applied pigments.

"The nature of the colors that have so successfully resisted time is a matter of interest. The early colonists . . . enumerate various dyes of permanent color to be obtained from native trees and plants, and the Maya today affirm that the colors of the old paintings can be duplicated with vegetable dyes which could be made from growths in the neighboring bush. However, samples of every color found in the frescoes in the Warriors complex have been examined in the Geophysical Laboratory of Carnegie Institution and found without exception to be of mineral origin. Red clay, composed principally of iron oxide, is plentiful beneath the surface soil in depressions in the limestone everywhere about Chichen, but most of the greens, blues and yellows must have been drawn from far sources.

"Of the medium or media in which the pigments are mixed, nothing of a positive nature can be said. Commonly the wall paintings have the flat surface and clear transparency of water colors, but in some cases, notably on the benches in the buried temple, the different pigments, when applied, had a viscosity as of oil paint. Indubitably the medium used there was of syrupy consistence. Presumably it was some sap or other organic liquid, the dried residue of which has been so broken down by time that it is not recognizable to the chemists." [94]

Pl. 264 presents yet another style of wall-painting. Many of the tomb chambers explored recently at Monte Albán disclosed finds of gold, pearls, jade, turquoise, bone, and pottery, but Tomb 104 had something quite different to offer, though of equal importance. In this subterranean chamber the painted walls were in such a good state of preservation that they give a rare opportunity to study the original mural. The entrance to this tomb is now reconstructed so that the chamber proper can be closed off from the outside, thus preventing damage from exposure or defacement. The pottery figure above the outer doorway was seen on *Pl. 15, fig. d.*

In *fig. b,* a photograph taken from the door of the tomb is reproduced, showing the two side walls and the farther end. The general decorative effect of the mural is sensed at once. Pottery and offerings were found in the five niches in the walls and personal ornaments on the one skeleton—apparently that of a high priest—that lay outstretched on the floor.

As in some of the paintings at Chichén Itzá, the figures were first drawn on the smooth plaster in red, then the details filled in with red, blue, yellow, black, and gray. The white of the wall itself was also used in the design. A final touch was given by framing each detail with a black outline. An occasional divergence is noticeable between the original as sketched and its final execution. Dr. Caso remarks on the haste with which these walls were painted, caused apparently by the urgency of the interment. As a result, the red used in the two side figures is darker than that in the end wall, where the color seems to have been thinned to eke it out. Investigations show that all the pigments were derived from minerals.[24]

The figure on the left (*fig. a*) is supposed to represent Xipe-Totec, the God of the Spring and of the Flayed. On the end wall the great mask with ornaments extending at the sides and on top is a Zapotec god, not definitely identified, whose body seems part of the center niche. The figure on the right (*fig. c*) appears from its make-up to be a local version of the Maize-god. Smaller pictorial elements, such as the parrot on the left, the masks, and numerical glyphs, form connectives that bind the mural into one continuous unit (*fig. d*). The ceremonial attire of the two deities, quite specific in each case, can be studied on the unrolled aquarelle. Headdress, necklace, breechcloth, sandals are all executed in detail. Both figures hold a pouch in the hand nearer the spectator, while the other is extended. What orthodoxy governed this iconography is manifest in the different execution of the eyes: in the C-shaped eye of Xipe-Totec, the Mongol cut of the center mask, and the almond shape of the Maize-god. Note the use of jaguar tails in the costume of the last.

Such frescoed tombs seem to have been fairly common in Monte Albán, as others of the type have since then been discovered there. However, none so far has contained such well-preserved paintings.

The murals on this plate have a completely different pictorial atmosphere than those previously discussed. In the first place, they are not story-telling. In considering the design, it is noteworthy that it has elements of both wall-painting and the manuscript—neither realized to its full possibilities. A certain connection could perhaps be traced with the fragments of murals in Mitla (shown on the following plate), particularly in the glyphic units, but no similarity at all can be found to those of Teotihuacán. The great differences between the two cultures are apparent in this field also.

The same dual nature—with qualities of both mural and manuscript—is discernible in *Pl. 265, fig. a,* a section of a painted lintel at Mitla. Here, however, the leaning is more toward the manuscript, in which gods and other supernatural elements are presented with a condensation approaching glyphs. The total effect is that of a miniature, done in negative painting and applied on a large scale in combination with architecture. This same manner of decoration is also recognizable on pottery in the Mexican Area (see *Pl. 111, figs. d* and *f,* and *Pl. 116, fig. c*).

Fig. b is a detail of a painting on the Temple of the Frescoes at Tulum (see *Pl. 30*). The use of stylized serpent bodies to divide the surface recalls the painted relief at Chichén Itzá (see *Pl. 261, fig. a*). The Old Empire tradition of the manikin scepter is manifest in the figure in the lower right corner. In many of the figures, however, Mexican mythology seems to dominate; trends from as far as the Pacific coast of Nicaragua and northern Costa Rica have been recognized in certain details.[67] The condensed quality seen in the Mitla murals can be sensed also here.

While in Mexico, manuscript and mural remained close in their general aspect and pictorial quintessence, in a certain period of Maya art these two branches of painting found expression in divergent visual terms. A section of a page of the Maya Codex Dresdensis, or the Dresden Codex, presented in *fig. c,* will show the manuscript style. The fluent drawing that was apparent in the Maya murals and which is characteristic of all Maya art, here is raised to the quality of tinted copper engraving. Two rows of seated individuals are pictured, each of whom—with the exception of one raised on a dais—is apparently holding a smaller person in front of him or carrying one on his back. Some of the major figures are strikingly alike in appearance, even to pose, headdress, and ornament, and it is believed that they are different representations of the Moon-goddess.[155] Above each row a series of glyphs is drawn, which at a glance may seem fairly uniform but on closer inspection will reveal more individual differences than our Latin characters. When we consider that the section reproduced is less than 5 inches long, we can appreciate the skill required to execute so much design in such a small space.

Fig. d is a page from an Aztec codex (Borbonicus) which depicts the renewal of the sacred fire at the beginning of a 52-year cycle, a solemn ceremony in the Mexican Area. The year is indicated in a small square at the top of the page (left center). To the right of it, the tribal god of the Aztecs descends from his temple, above him the blue and white flag of the month. In the extreme right corner is the glyph of the place (Hill of the Star) where the new fire was lighted. A road, designated by footprints, leads down from the hill, passing in front of the houses, to the temple which the priests approach with their torches. Other dignitaries will be seen coming from the left carrying large fagots in their arms. The men, armed, await the result of the ceremony. In the houses of the village all the inhabitants, even the children, have their faces covered with masks made of maguey leaves, and, shut in a granary, a pregnant woman is guarded by a warrior, for according to their belief she may at this particular time turn into a beast.[21]

With this slight explanation, we find the page telling more of a story than is gathered at first glance, giving us a taste of the strange psychology of these people. It will be noted that in the frescoes the tendency was to fill up the surface with decoration or color, while in the manuscripts much of the background was left empty, in the natural color of the paper.

A full page of the Maya Dresden Codex is reproduced on *Pl. 266,* somewhat enlarged to show the miniature-like quality in the execution of the three figures. Interesting differences in the individual poses also led to the choice of this particular page for reproduction. The first two are believed to represent two manifestations of the god of the planet Venus, while below lies a prostrate victim.[155]

The seated figure at the top is strongly reminiscent of two jade pendants, both in costume and pose (compare *Pl. 240, figs. a* and *b*). He wears the same elaborate headdress, with the eye of the mask emphasized; his right hand holds a stylus-like tool, and the left lies unoccupied. This similarity between an early manuscript and jade pieces of rather late date—in all probability not even from the same region—offers further proof that the pantheon of the pre-Columbian peoples was settled and that a certain god had always certain irremissible iconographic paraphernalia.

The kneeling figure in the middle is the clearest; his whole attitude is that of a young and powerful warrior. His costume is minutely delineated, even to the fringe and tassels of his breechcloth and the ornaments which he had to wear on legs and wrists. The violent gesture of the right hand with the darts is so convincing that one fails to notice at first that the fingers are reversed. (In a naturalistic representation, the back of the hand would be seen.)

The recumbent figure at the bottom of the page wears a monster-mask. His position seems natural, if somewhat uncomfortable. Both feet are shown, giving the impression that one is looking at him from above. Particular finesse is evident in the drawing of the right arm, which appears actually to bear the body's weight. In its linear facility and the compactness of its execution, this figure recalls to a certain degree the great Initial Series glyphs carved in stone at Quiriguá (see *Pl. 71, fig. b*).

The combination of glyphs with such exquisite miniatures reminds us of the illuminated manuscripts of medieval Europe, with their finely painted initial letters always related in subject matter to the text. The writing here is fluent, almost cursive, with "air" provided by the numerical dot-and-bar symbols. Lively coloring is used in these three vignettes, and the outlines are brought out in dark brown which may originally have been black.

From the subtle and flowing delineation in the Maya codices, we turn to the more angular and static work of illumination found among the cultures of the Mexican high plateau.

On *Pl. 267, fig. a,* a section of an Aztec manuscript from pre-Conquest times, the Codex Vaticanus B, is opened to show the screenlike folding of the pages. Each carries a main figure supplemented with a number of subordinate details and is framed on the top and right sides with glyphs. Some of the codices were read horizontally from left to right across two pages, then down and back from right to left, the two pages in this way forming the unit. In other cases, the text follows a horizontal and vertical route, across and down, and still others are read by unfolding the screen, turning it in a vertical position, and following the glyphs from top to bottom in serpentine curves—a veritable puzzle to which only the initiate had the clue.

Although most of the pre-Columbian manuscripts are concerned with rituals and astrology, a few are devoted to genealogies and historical matters. In a scene from the Codex Colombino (*fig. b*) an individual, identified as Eight Deer, is pictured kindling the sacred fire in the presence of a high priest. The story of this hero seems to have been recorded in several codices. It is thought that he was a Zapotec or Mixtec king, named, as was usual, for the day of his birth.[26] Both figures are dressed in ceremonial garb. Beside the fire drill, flames are drawn. The temple at the left is ornate in its decoration, with the alternate stairs painted red and green. On the entrance platform is an altar with offerings.

A comprehensive idea of the type of map made by the Aztecs is given in *fig. c.* It shows a section of rather mountainous land, on which roads are marked by two parallel lines with footprints in between. Rivers (lower right corner and top left) are painted blue and designated by three parallel lines between wavy ones; the interspersed circles are abbreviations of the glyph for *atl,* meaning "water."[116] Towns are represented by cartouches with their name symbols, placed to show their relative positions to the road—different in every instance, just as the lay of the settlements doubtless differed. A glyph similar to the character in the lower left center—an open animal jaw—appears also as the name of a town in Montezuma's Tribute Roll (see *Pl. 269,* the center of the page). Mountains are painted dark green, representing the vegetation which covered them. On the left, a temple is found, drawn upside down, possibly to show that its entrance faced the crossroads. It is worth while to compare the trees in this map with those of the murals from Chichén Itzá. Maps of quite recent date from the Far East show a naïveté in cartography similar to this ancient example, perhaps as much as four hundred years old.

On *Pl. 268* drawings from pre-Columbian and post-Columbian times that use the same manner of delineation are placed side by side.

Fig. a was executed by a Mexican after the Conquest but retains much of the pre-Columbian spirit. It comes from the Codex Magliabecchiano, a pictorial series illustrating ancient Mexican feasts and deities. Judging from the bird-mask, the god Xochipilli is depicted here, taking part in a ceremony that occurred every seventh month of the Mexican year.[102] He is borne by two attendants and preceded by a musician blowing on a conch, whose dress is much more elaborate than that of the carriers. The three scrolls above the instrument denote the sound (compare *Pl. 294, fig. f*).

The Codex Mendoza, from which our next illustration is taken, was painted after the Conquest on the order of Don Antonio de Mendoza, the first and greatest of all Spanish viceroys of Mexico. He instigated the recording of the pre-Columbian history of the country. This manuscript, made on European paper and completed before 1550, incorporated a copy of an old Mexican chronicle, the original of which has since been lost, recounting the history from year to year of the kings of Tenochtitlán and their conquests, beginning with 1325 and ending with 1521. A copy of the Tribute Roll of Montezuma (see the following plate) was also included. The last portion, compiled by a Mexican scribe, is devoted to "life from year to year," and gives vignettes of the country as it was before the arrival of the Spaniards.

The adventures of this codex are typical of the century which produced it. The ship on which it was sent was captured, and the book was taken to Paris. Thirty years later, it was purchased by Richard Hakluyt, chaplain to the English ambassador, and brought to England, where an English translation was made soon after at the instance of Sir Walter Raleigh. It now rests in the Bodleian Library at Oxford.[27]

The drawing in *fig. b* shows a group of Aztec warriors in full regalia. All have a certain uniformity of make-up, but the feather ornaments fastened behind the neck show variety in execution, as do also the garments, necklaces, and spears. Note the insets, which were usually of obsidian, in their lances. The shields especially have individual patterns.

Fig. c, from the pre-Columbian Codex Borbonicus, pictures a fiesta of youths who have not yet graduated as warriors. They dance around a gaily decorated pole to the music of a drum (compare *Pl. 292*). In the lower right stands Otontecutli, the Otomi God of Fire, at the foot of his own temple stairs.[155] The celebration reminds us of the games of pole-climbing still to be seen in Mexico on certain feast days or of our own Maypole.

Pl. 269 shows one page of the original medieval Tribute Roll of Montezuma II, preserved in the Museo Nacional, Mexico. The reports of the *conquistadores* attest to the well-knit organization of the Aztec confederacy; this page, drawn in colors on maguey paper, is tangible evidence of it.

The Tribute Roll contains a list of more than four hundred tributary cities of the Empire, together with information on taxes in kind exacted from each. On the page illustrated, the names of the towns levied—in this instance, those of the "hot countries" or tropics—are placed in the bottom row and up the right side of the sheet. It is interesting to note the individuality that characterizes the glyph of each. The cone and flag-shaped designs above the articles listed denote the quantities required. Beginning in the upper left corner and moving right, the items are, row by row: varnished yellow gourd bowls, little pots of bees' honey; a large wooden pack full of grain (maize, sage, beans, and various seeds), baskets of white copal; balls of unrefined copal wrapped in palm leaves, five strings of jade beads; war dress—note the long legs, visible also in the preceding plate—in sets of yellow, blue, and green, respectively, with matching shields (the center type is reproduced on *Pl. 287, fig. a*); below these, white mantles of a specified size, and, next to them on the right, a number of copper axes; finally, quilted, striped, and richly embellished mantles and women's garments.[107]

Other pages list gold dust, small turquoises, diadems, and earplugs of gold, bags of cochineal, reams of maguey paper, salt in molds (for use of the nobility alone), loads of chocolate and small pottery vessels out of which it was drunk, cotton, scarlet feathers, and jaguar skins.[27]

Among the historians of the Conquest and of the pre-Columbian culture in Mexico, Bernardino Sahagún ranks as one of the greatest. This young Franciscan arrived in Mexico in 1529, before the cultural and artistic traditions of the country were completely shattered. He acted as Superior in several monasteries and finally settled in a college in the Mexican capital. Wherever he was, he tried to establish contact with the Indians, and later, after his research had received official sanction, he frequently assembled the most intelligent and best educated of the older natives who had grown up before the Conquest. He questioned them in friendly conversation about their ancient customs and beliefs and had the answers given him in the form of Aztec picture-writings. In this way, he compiled a manuscript of twelve books, containing, besides records of the religion, history, and social life of the Aztecs, a grammar and dictionary of the Nahua language.[57]

Sahagún wrote his volumes in this tongue and then translated parts of them into Spanish. The pictures which illustrate his work show a high degree of skill, combining the old Aztec tradition in picture-writing with much learned from the Europeans (*Pl. 270*). The evenly laid brick walls, for instance, the foreshortening attempted in the interior (*fig. a*), and the landscape (*fig. f*) demonstrate familiarity with Spanish pictures, while certain primary forms, such as the mountains (*fig. h*) and the Indians themselves, retain their glyphic outlines. Their keen observation embraced all phases of life. *Figs. c, d,* and *e* are examples of their accurate depiction of animals.

Their botanical knowledge was no less thorough. In 1552, two Indians compiled an "Herbal" from Aztec lore, with illustrations and descriptions of one hundred eighty-five plants as well as their medicinal value. They divided the plants into classes, orders, families, and genera and presented them in color with remarkable clarity, showing leaves, flowers, and even roots.[37]

ANDEAN AREA

In the Andean Area, especially in the coastal region, walls were finished with plastered surfaces on which paintings were applied. The subject matter was generally similar to the stucco relief decoration of the walls (see *Pl. 43*) or reproductions of arabesque or animal patterns from their weaving and pottery. Fragments have been uncovered at Chan-Chan, Paramonga, Pachacámac, and elsewhere, but unfortunately none of these is well enough preserved to furnish any satisfactory impression.

There were no manuscripts in this area. Markham mentions pictures of past events painted on boards, but not a single such tablet has survived.[78] Various scenes appear on pottery, as has been shown. This type, however, becomes less frequent after the spread of the Inca Empire. Seemingly the subsequent stepping-up of production resulted in the abandonment of this naïve, sometimes virtuoso, but always delightful manner of recording.

X

Miscellaneous Applied Arts

IN THE dark ages of Europe, when the continent was one vast battlefield of invading barbarians, applied arts, such as the fashioning of jewelry and horse trappings, weaving, and wood-carving, throve, laying the groundwork for stylistically independent national schools of later centuries.

If only the so-called "fine arts"—architecture, sculpture, and painting—are contemplated in medieval American civilization, the picture lacks the depth and color that the textiles, metal-work, pottery, and jades provide. But these people reached out even farther for raw materials and developed amazingly skillful techniques in carving wood, bone, and shell and in making mosaic and featherwork.

WOOD-CARVING

As common as stone and more easily worked, wood, next to clay, is the most obedient medium for the use of temple and palace. As it is more perishable than most other materials, little has survived unfortunately, even from less remote periods. Without question, the budding cultures of the Western Hemisphere used wood widely for articles of daily life as well as for the more obvious purposes of building. It is believed by some that the earliest glyphic writing was inscribed on it. Wood was generally a staple article of trade. Bernal Díaz, chronicler of the Conquest, describes a special precinct in the Aztec capital where boards, cradles, beams, blocks, and benches were sold, each commodity arranged separately. Even some of the tribute paid to Aztec rulers was in firewood, beams, and planks. Chairs, benches, thrones, and other furniture were made of wood. Montezuma is said to have had a wooden screen, brilliantly colored and gilded, which was set before him when he dined, for it was regarded as improper to see the ruler eat.

That there were objects of wood among the gifts which Cortés sent to Seville in 1519 is documented by the inventory that accompanied them. Among other things, suits of wooden armor, helmets, shields, bows, and *atlatls,* or spear-throwers, are mentioned.[126]   Some of the *atlatls* now in European museums may date from that occasion.   Besides the spear-thrower and wooden helmet, later discussed in more detail, the most unusual device is, perhaps, the slat armor, which was used in the Pacific section of the United States, also in the Southeast and possibly in the Mexican Area.   Constructed of small ribs of wood held together with cords, it gave adequate protection against arrows and stone missiles, although not against bullets.   Scarcely less important than the weapons were the images of the gods.   Wooden statuary was common over a wide area at the time of the Conquest.   Utilitarian objects were frequently made of wood. In the ruins of the Southwest, crutches were found which utilized the V-shaped crotch of a branch as arm support.   Although household utensils for holding liquids and storing corn and seeds were generally fashioned of clay, they were also made of wood.

Even the simplest article nearly always carried on it some embellishment, if only a medallion.   Wooden spoons or scoops, boxes, trays, and such small objects were decorated with carving in low relief or were sometimes painted, sometimes inlaid with turquoise, shell, and bone.   Techniques related to lacquer were also applied.   The artistic talent of the pre-Columbian Indian and his love for his craft are documented in these unimportant pieces as surely as in the more spectacular ones.

Mention should be made of the great trading boats, or *canoas,* sometimes capable of holding twenty-five to thirty passengers.   The prow and, less frequently, the stern were ornamented with symbolic designs and human and animal shapes.

The great untapped forests of medieval America furnished in abundance the raw material.   In Central America the chief wood for building was the extremely hard and durable *chico-sapote,* well adapted for structural purposes. Other woods commonly in use were cedar, cypress, pine, spruce, oak, laurel, mahogany, and other hard varieties peculiar to tropical and semitropical regions.[126]

The tools used in working the wood ranged from the primitive stone axe to —at late last—the copper hatchet and axes and adzes with copper blades.   Large trees were probably felled by burning.   Although the technique acquired in wood-carving may later have been applied to stone, it should be pointed out that finer and sharper implements are needed to sculpture wood without splintering it or raveling the long cross fibers.   For this, the craftsman probably employed sharpened shells, bone, and obsidian.

The use of animal masks in ceremonies or for totemistic purposes was a widespread practice in medieval America. Two wooden masks from states outside our areas are presented on *Pl. 271* because of their remarkable workmanship. The first (*fig. a*) is about 11½ inches high and represents an antlered human head. Shell is set into the eyes and mouth, and it may have decorated the earplugs. The carving comes from the Spiro Mound in Oklahoma, which also yielded the embossed copper plaques shown on *Pl. 194,* as well as a large and important collection of stone pipes.

It is interesting to note how differently the same idea was expressed in a different culture. The masquette in *fig. b,* 10¾ inches over all, does not blend the human with animal features. It is the pure and beautifully naturalistic representation of a doe, executed with sculptural command. An amazing maturity, rare north of the Mexican Area, is manifest in this piece, unequaled in the delicacy of its linear conduct and full-blooded plasticity. It was found at Key Marcos in southern Florida and is said to have been carved about the 15th century by the Calusa Indians, a tribe now extinct. Besides the work illustrated, a number of masks, representing among other animals the deer, alligator, and wolf, were dug up from deposits of wet muck. All retain traces of paint and the eyes show inlay of shell. Parts of some, like the deer's ears in *fig. b,* had leather hinges so that they could be moved with strings.[31] Early Spanish reports mention a monumental art in wood in that region, all evidence of which is now lost.

The spear- or dart-thrower, called *atlatl* in Nahua, was for centuries the most effective weapon of pre-Columbian America. It was common to all areas here discussed and can still be found in use in remote districts. In certain regions the blowgun also was employed. The bow and arrow did not appear until late in medieval American history.

The butt of the spear or long dart rested against a peg or hook near the tip of the spear-thrower, which furnished, as it were, an extension of the throwing arm. With the aid of this contrivance the projectile was sped farther and with greater force than by hand alone. The sling, one of the earliest weapons of mankind, and one widely used in the Old World, is based on a similar principle.

Pl. 272 shows spear-throwers from three areas. The first (*fig. a*), a plain well-balanced piece, comes from the Southwest. Clearly visible at the top is the hollowed-out section with the hook to hold the spear; the grip at the other end resembles a saber hilt.

Fig. b is an elaborate specimen from the Mixtec region in Mexico. The length of the carved section is 13¾ inches and of the whole piece, 21⅜. The accompanying drawing (*fig. c*) gives the decoration in clearer detail. Four figures are depicted in various poses: the top one diving downward facing the left, the second standing with upturned face, the third facing right, and the fourth, like the second, looking upward. At the bottom is a finely executed mask with a glyph. The wood is very hard and highly polished. On the other side the groove, 19½ inches long, which held the spear, is bordered by a pattern of intertwining serpents.

The three weapons in *figs. d* and *e* come from the Andean Area and seem to be Ica in style. The first two, rounded and without a groove, have bone handles carved to represent heads, one animal and one human. The third carries a complete figure, also carved of bone, a little seated man only 3⅓ inches high playing a panpipe. Despite his oversize head and certain undeveloped details, the piece is as expressive in its modeling as the statuettes on *Pl. 258*.

The elaboration of the *atlatl* resulted in such magnificently carved pieces as those presented on *Pl. 273*. The very rare specimen covered with gold leaf (*fig. a*) was undoubtedly made for ceremonial use. Nine figural elements, one above the other, embellish it. As in *fig. b* on the opposite plate, a diving figure is at the top, here in frontal view. The carving is exquisitely wrought and would bear considerable enlargement to show the fine relief work employed—the same sculptural language as that used in stone on a much larger scale. The bone grip with its precise binding is additional evidence of remarkable workmanship.

The two *atlatls* in *fig. c,* also in a perfect state of preservation, were included to show that the decorative scheme was not always divided into small sections with mythological figures. In the one on the left the undulating body of a feathered serpent fills most of the ornamented space. At the top a human head can be discerned, emerging from the reptile's jaws—a motif often found in the late art of the Mexican Area (see *Pl. 234, fig. a*). The grooved face of the piece on the right carries two condensed motifs, geometric in effect. Both specimens bear traces of red and green paint.

In *fig. b* a part of a wooden ceremonial staff is shown. It is 11¼ inches long and was recovered from the Sacred Well at Chichén Itzá during the dredging operations there. The larger figure wears a tall headdress, while the smaller head below is sculptured within a serpent's jaws. In both cases, tiny arms and legs on the sides, more clearly seen in the lower figure, suggest a condensed body in a diving attitude. The character of the carving differs completely from that on the *atlatls*.

Some authorities believe that the forerunners of the Maya stone stelae were of wood. At any rate, a number of the early monuments show a shallow rounded style better adapted to the softer material than to stone (see *Pl. 236, fig. a*, dated 677). Later the art of wood-carving attained such heights as that reproduced on *Pl. 274*.

As a composition, this piece, taken from Temple IV at Tikal, Guatemala, and dated 741, is completely in harmony with the severe and awe-inspiring style of this religious center. The precision of outline and the softly rounded surfaces show complete mastery over the medium. The lintel measures about 5 by 7 feet. Its central theme is a standing dignitary and the feeling of ceremonial pomp is well conveyed. His face, turned toward the left, is typically Maya in feature. The spreading headdress is a study in small elements of decoration, pressed one beside the other. Shoulders and chest are also covered with dense ornament. His apron-like hanging in front and the befeathered shield and staff which he carries should be noted.

He stands within a loop formed by a great feathered serpent (compare *Pl. 9*), one head of which, with half a masked figure emerging from the jaws, can be seen at the left in the photograph. The stylized elements of a second head, discernible on the extreme right, are similar in line to the fret-scrolls on the marble vases from the Ulúa Valley (see *Pls. 94* and *95*).

This relief is not only the largest extant wood-carving of the Maya, but it embodies the essence of their greatest period in art. The fine differentiation between the larger motifs that make up the serpent body, flowing and less dense in arrangement, and the compact smaller elements of the main figure successfully throws the emphasis on the human, despite the wealth of detail. It required great skill to separate such ornate units, practically superimposed, in such shallow relief. The Serpent Bird at the top center, which also appears at Palenque, Piedras Negras, and Copán, should be mentioned. Tablets of glyphs fill the upper corners.

This flamboyant manner of presentation—almost overornate for our taste—is evident also in Chinese, Hindu, and Tibetan art, where there is so much detail that the main subject often seems submerged in the surrounding embellishment. Although the Maya's preference for extravagant decoration remained a characteristic until the Conquest, in later centuries it lost its exuberance to give way to a more loosely composed and more conventionalized style.

The great thickness of the walls at Tikal accounts for the large size of the lintel. Several of this type were removed by Dr. Gustave Bernoulli in 1877 and are now in the Museum für Völkerkunde at Basle, Switzerland. Maler's account explains in great measure their damaged condition. The problem of dismantling them was a difficult one, as Indians do not use the saw. Consequently, the natives frequently resorted to burning off the beams at both ends to save the cutting edges of their *machetes*. As this was a slow process, they often left the fire to go for their meals or a drink, heedless of the damage done to "a pair of sacerdotal feet, the plume of a helmet, or some interesting hieroglyphs." Furthermore, unless watched, they were apt to throw away one piece or another of the heavy wood to lighten their loads on the long journey back through the jungle.[75]

The arid climate that prevailed along the coastal strip in the Andean Area preserved in excellent condition wooden objects that escaped vandalism. *Fig. a* on *Pl. 275* shows the decorated top of a long pole which has a flattened section at the opposite end. In the rows of lacy carving below the sextette of stiff little wooden men, one feels the influence of woven patterns. Even the human figures are pattern-like in their uniformity. This type of work seems to have been practiced in the Ica Valley and its vicinity. The purpose of such pieces is unclear. According to some they served as tomb markers, while others would have them steering paddles.

Fig. b is allegedly the decorative pendant which hung from a woven cocabag and is also Ica in style. Coca leaves, from which we derive cocaine, were mixed with lime and chewed, especially on long journeys, to provide extraordinary endurance. On the wooden section alternating rows of two motifs are carved in low relief, the top one similar to the perforated "star" pattern in *fig. a*. The center of each unit was inlaid with shell, and four rows of silver bands ornamented the heavy strands of the fringe. This piece was probably not of great importance, nevertheless the good taste and skill shown in combining the materials reflect the high quality of this culture.

In *fig. c* are four wooden spoons with figures on the handles. The larger two are about 4 inches high. There is a flat two-dimensional quality in the carving. In the third from the left the material below the design was not even cut away. Nevertheless, the figures, even though sketchy, have considerable liveliness when compared with *fig. a.* The pattern build-up and technique of execution are characteristically Coast Tiahuanaco, and the figures are reminiscent of Viracocha's two types of attendants on the Gateway of the Sun. All show the kneeling or running posture seen on this monument and "starred" heels which appear on the pottery. Note the ceremonial staff with a human head carried by the one on the right and the small bent figure at the feet of the one beside him.

The art of applying a lacquer-like finish to wood or calabash was known in the Andean as well as the Mexican Area. This pre-Columbian accomplishment is one of the few that continued into post-Conquest times. On *Pl. 276* a group of wooden cups is shown treated in this manner, called by the Quechua name, *kero*. All date from late Inca, some even from post-Columbian times, and many have been handed down in families. The wood was first covered with a clear varnish, then the surface to be colored was lightly engraved, and finally the pigments were applied.

The decoration on *fig. a* is especially delightful because of its spacing, with widely separated human figures in the upper section and, in the center, a tight geometric pattern recalling textile motifs (see *Pl. 191*). Flowers at the base, harmonizing with those just below the rim, serve to unify and balance the composition.

Fig. b shows a goblet, about 7 inches high, decorated with encircling bands of geometric and stylized bird elements. (Compare *Pl. 192, fig. b.*) Variety is furnished by the vertical incised lines on the body of the vessel and the striking zigzag on the rim against a cross-hatched background.

Nearest to our esthetic standards is the beaker in *fig. c,* 6½ inches high, with its pleasing row of birds carved in low relief. A plastic band, suggestive of a snake, encircles it like a cord, and is, with its series of mushroom-shaped ornaments, a rare feature; unusual skill was necessary to execute it on the curving side of the vessel.

In *fig. d* an interesting division of figural and geometric themes is again apparent. The handles here are particularly noteworthy, carved in the shape of animals—probably pumas—holding tenaciously to the edge of the beaker. Although the creatures are not too naturalistic, the clinging position, especially of the forepaws, is distinctly conveyed.

The *kero* in *fig. e* is shaped like a puma head. Flat story-telling pictures in brilliant hues cover the plastic representation—an example of the composite language of decoration in the Andean Area.

Fig. f presents an unusual shape: a shallow bowl standing on three curving legs set on a rounded base. In this piece the inlay-like appearance of the finish is particularly clear. The geometric patterns, the serpent on one leg, and the other motifs taken from nature on the base furnish indeed a miscellany of designs. The "fortress" with banners carries a cross at the top—an indication probably of post-Conquest inspiration.

In the coloring of these *keros,* glowing red predominates; buff and yellow, blue-green, brown, olive, black, and salmon also occur. It is believed that the cups were used for the native beer.

A wooden seat from late Inca times is illustrated on *Pl. 277, fig. a.* Compare it with the Late Maya jaguar throne on *Pl. 92.* The piece is over 11 inches high, 14 long, and 11 wide. The two animals, each on its own oblong base, face in opposite directions, connected only by the hollowed-out seat which they support. They are painted a greenish black with yellow spots and have scarlet tongues and grass-green eyes. The use of much cream and white lightens the general effect. Note the elaborate designs everywhere along the edge.

Fig. b shows a wooden beam of a scale, 7 inches long and probably Chimú in style (see *Pl. 299, fig a*). In the balanced combination of human, animal, and geometric designs the characteristic charm of Chimú art is perceptible.

TURQUOISE MOSAIC

An original and very skillfully handled technique was that of mosaic-work, by means of which objects of various sizes and shapes were incrusted with turquoise and other semiprecious stones. Just as jade was revered in the Maya and Mexican areas, turquoise was highly prized in many regions for its symbolic meaning. In the soft blue of the stone was envisioned the spirit of the vaulted heavens or of an expanse of life-giving water.

Examples of mosaic-work have been found in the Southwest, the Mexican, Maya, and Andean areas. The Incas, however, although expert lapidary workers, do not appear to have engaged in this craft; at any rate, no specimens are known. It would seem that not only the greatest number but the greatest variety has been found in the Mexican Area, but even here they are comparatively rare, with less than fifty known at the present time. Seventeen were uncovered in one cave in the Puebla region, where they had been treasured by the natives for years after the Conquest, probably revered as precious relics of a lost but not forgotten epoch.[125]   Still more recently in the Maya Area at Chichén Itzá a number of objects incrusted with mosaic were dredged from the bottom of the Sacred Well, among them, staff heads and masks.   During the reconstruction of the Temple of the Warriors, a beautiful mosaic plaque was uncovered, composed of more than three thousand bits of stone,[93] and another was found in the throne buried in the Castillo (see *Pl. 92, fig. b*), embedded in the back of the jaguar.

Unworked turquoise as well as finished mosaics was exacted in the annual tribute of the Aztecs; on the Tribute Roll eleven towns were assessed for it and five more for *piedras ricas de azul*.   According to the description of Cortés, in the great market of Tenochtitlán the merchants who sold gold and the venders of precious stones displayed their wares side by side.

One of the earliest expeditions from Cuba toward the mainland, made in 1518 under Grijalva, received presents of mosaic-work with stones resembling turquoise, and between 1519 and 1525 Cortés obtained on various occasions, either as gifts or loot, a number of articles mentioned in his letters or in the writings of early chroniclers.   A glance at a partial list of these will reveal not only the wide application made of this art, but its importance as decoration.   The stone was used with feathers in a very original combination.   According to one description, there was a large feather-work box "lined with leather and ornamented with a large disk of gold and a design in blue stones; a sceptre with inlaid stone mosaic with two golden rings and feather decoration; an armlet of stone inlaid with mosaic; a mirror placed in a piece of blue and red stone mosaic with feather-work stuck to it; sixteen shields of stone mosaic with colored feathers hanging from the edge; a piece of colored feather-work which the lords of the land wore on their heads and from which dangled two ear ornaments of stone mosaic work with bells and golden beads; a bracelet of gold with ten pieces of blue and two of green stone; a butterfly of gold with wings of scallop shell and body and head of green stone." [125]

The development of the art of the lapidaries and mosaic workers in Mexico, like that of the goldsmiths, is attributed by Sahagún to the Toltecs.   He describes the elaborate technique of preparing the turquoise, mentioning also the working of pearls, amber, and amethyst and their incorporation into jewelry.   Walter Lehmann, however, believes that the art became known to the Aztecs by way of the Zapotec culture.[64]

The materials most commonly used in mosaics were turquoise, jade, malachite, quartz, beryl, garnet, obsidian, pyrites, and shell.   Wood generally constituted the base, but stone, bone, gold, silver, and perhaps even vegetable paper were also used. Turquoise of good quality is not very hard and can be easily worked. In Sahagún's description of the technique, it was shaped by an instrument of tempered copper and scraped with sharpened flints. Facets were cut and the piece polished with great care, sometimes with bamboo, which gave it a special luster. Stones were carefully sorted for color and shade. The inlay was built up, bit by bit, often into a highly complicated pattern, and glued to the foundation by a vegetable pitch or gum.

The principle of mosaic-work may be said to appear also in the composite stone ornaments on buildings. The ruins at Mitla (*Pls. 16 to 18*) show the idea, enlarged on a grand scale. Also, according to tradition, the inner walls of certain edifices at Tula, on the Mexican high plateau, were ornamented with colored jasper and shell set off by plaques of gold and silver.

The turquoise mosaic mask in *Pl. 278, fig. a*, 6½ inches high, is one of the best preserved pieces extant. The base is of cedar and painted red on the inside. The turquoise used in the incrustation is rather pale, except for the minute particles which rim the eyes with brilliant hue. Cabochon stones stud the face, ingeniously breaking the monotony of the even surface. Eyes, nostrils, and mouth are pierced through, and the eyeballs are designated by pieces of iridescent pearl shell with holes bored in the centers for iris. Shell teeth are inserted between the parted lips, and the gum which holds the shell in place is gilded.[125] The rows of small stones are tellingly placed to bring out the lines of the features. A black-and-white photograph can only slightly convey the vibrant color scheme of any of these mosaics.

Fig. b is a sacrificial knife about a foot long, the blade of which is fashioned of light-colored waxy chalcedony chipped to a leaf shape. Its carved wooden handle, overlaid with mosaic, represents a crouching human wearing an eagle headdress and a feather cloak falling over his shoulders and back (compare *Pl. 286*). The figure, grasping the blade in both hands, is so firmly bound to it with cord that he seems to be pushing it with his whole body—a conception singularly appropriate to an instrument of a savage rite.

The large double-headed serpent of mosaic in *fig. c*—interpreted as the monster that carries the sun [153]—was probably a breast ornament. It is 17½ inches long and 8 high, with the foundation again of wood, hollowed out at the back and painted red. The teeth and fangs are of white shell, while the gums are indicated by a strip of pink shell. A raised band of turquoise and deep red shell is laid across each nose. The sparing contrast of coral-pink and rich red on the heads gives a dazzling effect. Turquoise of the finest quality was used throughout, shading deepest toward the edges to bring out the rounded body.

The helmet, 7½ inches high (*Pl. 279, fig. a*), is hollowed out to fit the head and painted green inside. In spite of whole sections of missing inlay, the composition is striking, both in color and shape. Two gaping serpent heads can be distinguished at the base of the two crests, picked out in iridescent shell. It is possible that the main surface of the helmet was covered with a design denoting their intertwining bodies.

Because of its decoration and its almost perfect state of preservation, the shield shown in *fig. b* is one of the most important examples of aboriginal American mosaic. It is 12¾ inches in diameter with an average thickness of ¾ of an inch. The holes in the margin indicate that it was either applied to another piece or was rimmed with another material, perhaps an edging of feathers. The wood of its base is probably cedar. For the most part, this splendid mosaic consists of minute circular pieces of sky-blue turquoise, and the pattern is brought out by the fine gradations of color as well as by the use of larger pieces in outlining. It has been estimated that nearly fourteen thousand stones went into the composition.

A sun disk is represented, with eight points extending across the wide outer circle. In the upper center the sun appears again, inclosed by the "celestial band," with a female figure, probably a goddess, plunging head downward from it. Two other persons stand holding objects somewhat similar to those borne by the deity. An irregular shape, probably a speech scroll, emerges from their mouths. All these figures are composed of larger pieces of turquoise shaped and often incised to represent details of features and costume. The earplugs protrude above the surface of the piece, as do a number of other rounded elements, somewhat in the manner of the cabochons of *Pl. 278, fig. a*. At the bottom of the inner circle, very distinct against the darker background, is the glyph for Colhuacan, an important town in the Valley of Mexico in medieval times. The string of four dots at either side of this is believed to have calendrical meaning. Saville is of the opinion that the scene relates to the worship of the planet Venus and reads the date as 1461 or 1513.[125]

Two types of shields were in use by the Aztecs: one for war, the other ceremonial. The shield of the common soldier was probably plain, that of a man of rank was often painted. Shields used on festive occasions were very ornate.

< 343 >

Most of the hundred and fifty listed among the booty of Cortés carried feather-work, twenty-five were ornamented with mosaic, and some were adorned with gold (see *Pl. 287*).

In addition to the examples illustrated here, earplugs, idols, and animal figures studded with mosaic-work or inlaid with stones and shell should also be mentioned. The artistry in this work was appreciated quite soon in Europe, and as early as the middle of the 17th century a book was published in Italy, describing and illustrating this Mexican craft.[125]

SHELL-WORK

To the pre-Columbian peoples, who put their hand to all the gifts of nature in their arts, shells offered still another medium. Sea shells, naturally highly prized in the interior, were valued as ornaments and for inlay also by the inhabitants of coastal regions.

As in numerous early cultures, shell played a multiple rôle in the Western Hemisphere. In Alaska, among certain tribes of California, and widely among the aborigines of eastern and central United States, it constituted a medium of exchange. Its most general use, however, was as jewelry, either in combination or alone. Quetzalcóatl, the tribal god of the Toltecs—Kukulcán in Maya mythology—is traditionally depicted with a section of conch as breast ornament. Small shells were used as pendants on the mantles of young men of the military school in several highland tribes of Mexico,[151] and among the coastal people of the Andean Area the material was cut into shapes of small animals, birds, and fish and sewed onto garments.

Although five of the shell ornaments illustrated on the next two plates do not belong to the areas presented in this survey, they are included because of certain technical and iconographic affinities they have to late works from the Mexican Area.

On *Pl. 280, fig. a,* a shell gorget from Tennessee is pictured, nearly 4 inches in diameter. A human figure is incised on it in a half-kneeling or leaping pose. In his right hand he holds a human head or mask, in the left, a short club or ceremonial staff. His head is drawn in sharp profile, turned right. Noteworthy are the copper head ornament, which is like a double-bladed axe (see *Pl. 194, fig. a*), and the leaf-shaped "apron" or breechcloth that also appears in the next illustration, a piece from a distant region. The thick necklace may be a twisted rope of shell beads, such as has been found in many burials. Concentric incised circles form both frame and background, serving almost as a lens to focus attention on the figure.

Fig. b presents an incised conch, 13 inches long, from Spiro Mound, Oklahoma. The unrolled pattern appears beside it, showing more clearly the mythological bird-man with outspread wings and tail. As ingeniously as the design is arranged, the shape of the shell itself is not utilized to bring out any plastic effect of the subject.

The gorget with the scalloped edge (*fig. c*), 5 inches in diameter, comes from the same site in Oklahoma. The attitude of the figure is quite similar to that in *fig. a,* but has more dash; the static quality of design in the Tennessee piece is here replaced by vigorous drawing, which gives the figure a rushing, leaping, almost flying appearance. A certain emancipation is also shown in the liberty with which the incised right hand and both feet trespass into the plastic border, and a more articulate artistry is manifest in the combination of incised design with a raised and evenly "beaded" frame. Note the eyes on the elbows.

From the subject matter of these pieces contact with Mexico is hypothesized, believed to date after the 15th century, probably in the spread of a cult.[108]

The examples on *Pl. 281* show a certain development in that the background is cut away, producing an openwork effect. The gorgets in *figs. a* and *c* also belong to the Mound Builder culture and were excavated from the Etowah Group in Georgia. A motif common among the Etowah people, the pileated woodpecker, is featured in the first (*fig. a*). The two birds, standing on a perfect cross (inverted) are as pleasing in their stylization as a Byzantine design. There is a certain heraldic and outspokenly decorative quality in the ornament that reaches beyond the culture group which produced it.

In contrast, *fig. c* is characteristically pre-Columbian. It shows a warrior-like figure wearing a headdress of deer antlers and a breechcloth tied with a large loop. Except that the profile is turned to the left instead of the right, the subject is in linear conduct quite like that of *fig. a* on the opposite page. At the same time, there is an interesting similarity of design to the bird-man on that plate: the barred section at the right resolves itself into a wing resembling those incised on the conch. Both figures have an aquiline nose and paint around the mouth; even the necklaces appear to be of the same type. The clawlike right hand of the Georgia piece supports the idea that an eagle-man is represented.

Fig. b speaks a different language. This pendant, highly articulate in both concept and execution, comes from the Huaxtec region of the Mexican Area. It is about 7 inches high. The subject seems to be of a sacrificial character. On the left, leaning forward, a male deity is shown holding a tube which leads down to a broad shallow vessel in the center of the piece. At the right is seated a female deity who carries two darts or arrows bound together. Both figures rest on the open jaws of two feathered serpents, whose intertwined bodies support the bowl mentioned above. The lozenge-shaped section below the group signifies water. Although the lower frame is lacking, a recumbent figure with upraised knee and arm can be discerned at the bottom.[11]

An interpretation of this mythical scene would lead too far afield and is unnecessary for an appreciation of the art in the piece. The general impression is highly decorative. Openwork alternates with solid surfaces in perfect balance, and the graceful loop in the center breaks any monotony that may be felt in the build-up. Various incised elements are introduced, not only in the execution of the two main figures, their jewelry, teeth, even fingernails, but also in the free-flowing lines of the snake heads and plumes. The serpents themselves are differentiated and the shift of their individual markings can easily be followed.

The small finger ring (*Pl. 282, fig. a*), scarcely three-quarters of an inch in diameter, comes from a Hohokam village in the Gila Valley in southern Arizona. The material is glycimeris shell, common in the region but originating in the Gulf of California, a distance of nine days' journey on foot. The perforations appear to have been made by deepening an incision with a sharp-edged sandstone tool until the core could be broken out by tapping, for the use of a drill would doubtless have shattered the brittle material. Piles of such cores have been found in the district. This technique is similar to that employed by the Alaskan and British Columbian natives in the manufacture of jade implements.[170]

The enlargement in the photograph shows the details—considerably more than one would expect to find in such a diminutive piece and in a material so fragile. Two birds perched back to back constitute the face of the ring, each holding the head of a serpent in its beak and clutching the rattles in its claws. The twined bodies of the reptiles form the hoop of the piece. We may assume that the eye-holes were originally inlaid, and paint may have contributed to the effect. Within these lilliputian dimensions, material and composition are brought together in a solution that would have never occurred to the white man.

The miniature head in *fig. b*, 2½ inches high, is fashioned in the round from a solid ball of yellowish-red shell. Objects made of reddish shell are listed among the treasures which Cortés received from Montezuma. The general absence of contours in the features and the double mouth show this to be another representation of Xipe-Totec, the God of the Flayed. So realistic is the execution that we can sense the god's eyes and nose beneath the sagging skin. Remarkable detail work is noticeable in the headdress, earplugs, the hair pulled back toward the side, and the collar that frames the face. Here a round drill must have been extensively used, a highly difficult operation in this medium.

The beautifully opalescent mother-of-pearl, 3¾ inches high (*fig. c*), was allegedly found at Tula, Hidalgo, a site fifty miles north of Mexico, D.F., and believed to be one of the earliest cities on the Mexican high plateau. Toltecs, Chichimecas, and Aztecs occupied it in turn and left the marks of their respective cultures there. Certain similarities between sculptures at Tula and those of Maya sites would indicate an exchange of cultural ideas, and trade might account for this piece turning up here, for its stylistic characteristics are strongly Maya.

The use of this medium for such a representation is very rare. A chief is shown, seated cross-legged, wearing an elaborate headdress. His placement and posture remind us of figures on jade pendants; but, though the subject is handled in the manner of a jade carving, the softness of the shell and the high lights bring out more sensuous qualities in the figure, well caught in the photograph. His headdress has received much attention, with the extraneous material at the side cut away. The left hand with its closed fingers is a particularly fine detail that deserves mention. The ornament is quiet in atmosphere and superb in execution. It has four glyphs on the back, and was bored for suspension.

On this plate, three areas with markedly different styles are represented, as well as three different ways of working the same material: openwork technique, three-dimensional carving, and relief—a variety which should be noted.

Three examples of the skillful and appealing work in shell from the Andean Area are presented on *Pl. 283*. The two earplugs (*figs. a* and *c*) are about 2½ inches in diameter, and both show human figures pieced together out of many small colored bits of shell. The task of fitting and setting the small units, one beside the other, required much dexterity, and the effect is naïve and toylike. In *fig. c,* the little man stands in a static pose, with feet turned outward and arms outstretched, holding objects in both hands. In the other (*fig. a*), movement may be expressed; the feet, both pointing to the right, and the floating line of the mantle suggest motion. The rim in each case is of iridescent shell and the background a deep lavender; tones of orange-tan and jade-green are used, and the inlaid eyes of the figure on the right seem to be turquoise. From their style, the earplugs are thought to belong to the Chimú culture.

Still greater patience, as well as a marvelous color sense, was required to produce the central piece (*fig. b*), a shell cup with an inlaid base, fashioned in an interesting hour-glass effect. It is nearly 9½ inches high, Chimú in style, and comes from Lambayeque. The cup is admirably proportioned and sophisticated in conception. Unfortunately in a black and white reproduction the refinement of the color combination is lost. The cup proper consists of four slightly curving sections of translucent white shell, evenly cut and polished, which are ingeniously held together with metal clasps concealed by four inlaid panels. It blends smoothly into the main body of the piece, which is made of wood and inlaid with shell. The bulk of the fish in the center is eased by the tapering lines of its head and the brilliant pink stripes of the fins and tail. Its head is a solid piece of the same bright tone. Inlay of milky color in the body also serves to lighten the effect and makes a good connection with the translucent white above it. Inlaid fish motifs of pearl and darker iridescent shell enliven the dark brown of the wooden stem.

BONE-CARVING

In early medieval times, ivory—rather neglected today—was much valued in the Eastern Hemisphere. The pre-Columbian carver of our areas did not have this material at his disposal but utilized to good advantage the bones and teeth of smaller trophies of the hunt, among them peccary, jaguar, deer, and mountain sheep.

The skull of a wild boar was used for the carving, or rather engraving, shown on *Pl. 284, figs. a* and *d,* a piece found in a tomb at Copán. The main subject, incised on the top of the skull (*fig. a*), depicts two men seated within a quatrefoil medallion, facing each other in a conversational attitude. More unusual is a detail from the side (*fig. d*), where a group of running boars is pictured with considerable verve. Animal representation in such a realistic manner as this is quite rare in Maya art. The problem of superimposing one body on the other seemingly did not hamper the carver. Smaller animated figures of a jaguar, monkey, deer, and a flying bird appear on the same piece. It is interesting that peccaries are drawn on peccary bone.

In addition to its treasures of gold, jade, and rock crystal, Tomb 7 at Monte

Albán yielded more than thirty pieces of carved jaguar and deer bones similar to those shown in *figs. b* and *c,* some studded with turquoise. They range between 6 and 8½ inches in length and their use has yet to be definitely settled. It has been suggested that they were nose ornaments, knife handles, or ceremonial daggers.

In the compositions, gods are represented in human and animal form, some of which have been described as having calendrical significance. A discussion of the glyphic meanings of the carvings is not necessary, however, to enjoy the full extent of the carver's mastery, especially when we consider the limited surface upon which the complicated and condensed subjects had to be placed. The diversity of the design arrangements—now horizontal, now vertical in tendency, and in others, separated by oblique bands—makes an interesting study under a magnifying glass.

A small tool, only about 2 inches high, from the Hohokam culture of the Southwest is presented on *Pl. 285, fig. a.* It was made from the leg bone of a mountain sheep or a deer and used as the handle of a bone awl. Its relationship to the bird ring cut from shell (see *Pl. 282, fig. a*) can be sensed. The piece was calcined in a crematory fire, but was saved after excavation by ingenious chemical treatment. A mountain sheep stands above entwined rattlesnakes, combining favorite motifs of the region. The carving is simple but cleanly executed and somewhat reminiscent of early Near Eastern statuary. The tubular formation of the bone was utilized for the shaft of the implement and the natural contour of the end, for the sheep's horn.[171] Although it expresses a totally different and much simpler artistic concept than the companion figure on this plate, it holds its own beside it through its power and sincerity.

Among the masterpieces of Maya art—perhaps the smallest in size but by no means the least in importance—is the diminutive figure, 2¾ inches high, carved from the femur of a jaguar (*fig. b*). Its provenience is unknown. It has been suggested that it was used as ornament for the top of a scepter or ceremonial staff; holes in the base would indicate some such application.

As the figure carries no weapons, it is thought that he represents a priest.[25] His unbending and stoic expression is emphasized by the arms akimbo. He is clothed in the skin of a jaguar and the large fan-shaped headdress doubtless was made of quetzal feathers. Its lines are carved with such variety that it avoids ungainliness. The hole above the forehead was very likely for a jade or turquoise inlay, and a carved pendant in the shape of a monkey head hangs on the breast. Remnants of red paint are visible, which may have caused the roughened surface noticeable in the front. Maya glyphs, probably of chronological significance, are carved both on the front and rear of the narrow pedestal.

In *fig. c* is seen the back of the statuette. The jaguar pelt wrapped about the hips shows clearly, with its spots and hanging tail. The back of the headdress was worked into an inverted jaguar mask. Another stone was doubtless set in the depression at the waist as ornament for the broad belt.

Even were bone sculptures from the Maya Area less rare than they are, this little piece would demand especial attention for the monumental qualities embodied within its small dimensions.

FEATHER-WORK

Mankind on all continents has been fascinated by the birds. Their secret of flight, their gorgeous plumage have made them the subject of many stories and legends, from Daedalus and Icarus of Greek mythology to the naïve couple, Papageno and Papagena, in Mozart's *Magic Flute*. All civilizations have appreciated the decorative value of their feathers and perhaps even attributed some symbolic significance to them, as is shown by the ostrich-plumed helmets of knights and warriors, the colorful regalia of savage dancers, and the splendid standards which appear at a festival Papal Mass. But no one has used them more ingeniously than the peoples of medieval America.

Before advancing modern civilization disturbed the belt extending from the southern border of Mexico to Colombia, this region abounded in birds of real paradisiacal appearance, and even today in the more remote sections some of them survive, a delight to the traveler and a reward for all the discomfort and fatigue endured on his journey.

The most renowned, and justly so, is the quetzal, a bird about the size of a turtle dove. Its feathers are a deep iridescent green, turning at an angle to midnight blue, above a flaming scarlet breast. The tail of the male develops three plumes, which measure about three and a half feet long, emerald-green in color with a golden shimmer. The bird is further remarkable for the absence of down and the large size of its contour feathers, which are extremely soft and so loose that they come off easily in the hand. Before the Conquest, the gorgeous plumage of the quetzal was reserved for the chiefs alone, a symbol of their rank. Eagle and turkey feathers were also used in the Indian's regalia.

Among numerous other birds resplendent in color were the various humming birds of different hues, one species of which had a brilliant turquoise breast that was used with exquisite effect. Throughout pre-Columbian America the parrot also plays a rôle in some form; its likeness is found in Mound Builder remains as well as in the carvings of Copán. Members of this family were quite common as far north as Lake Erie and Lake Ontario and as far south as the Strait of Magellan. In the Andean Area, feathers of the duck and hen were used, as well as those of the rhea, or American ostrich, which was domesticated not only for its meat but also for its plumage. Father Cobo, the chronicler, writes of a humming bird upon whose breast was a tiny gold-green spot, highly prized for decoration.

Birds were hunted with bird lime, traps, or slings, and were not necessarily killed when robbed of their feathers. According to the early writers, Montezuma had an aviary where richly colored birds were plucked once a year and their feathers carefully classified as to shade and texture.

The plumage was used to embellish headdresses, shields, standards, garments, bands, and other accessories. The technique of applying feather beside feather —called, rather inaccurately, "feather mosaic"—was developed to a fine art. A few specimens from the Mexican Area and many from the Andean survive. The elaborate plumed headdresses of the Maya dignitaries depicted on stelae, pottery, and carved medallions, as well as the occasional fans of honor (see *Pl. 129, fig. c*), attest to the skill of these people, too, in feather-work, although probably due to the unfavorable climate, no examples survive.

For pieces intended as wearing apparel, a fine woolen or cotton cloth was first woven, then feathers were laid on a row at a time, each quill hooked over a thread and secured by a knot in a second thread running parallel to the first. The subsequent rows were completed in like manner, one after another, each sewed to the cloth in such a way as to conceal the quills of the row below, leaving only the colored portions visible. Thus row by row the design was built up. In the arrangement of a pattern the position of the feathers of each tint had to be carefully calculated beforehand. When fixed in place, the tips were clipped to give a sharper contour to the design.[84]

For headdresses, standards, and similar articles, an ingenious light-weight construction of reeds and small sticks held the showy parts together. After the pattern arrangement was made, the colorful material was glued to a base of hide or dried plant fiber with a sticky juice. When the piece was completely dry, it achieved considerable durability—as is proved by the specimens which were sent to Europe at the time of the Conquest and are still on display, showing even today not only a veritable kaleidoscope of color but a fairly well-preserved and sound inner structure.

Pl. 286 features the feather headdress traditionally presented by Montezuma to Cortés as a gift to his sovereign. It first appears in an inventory from the late sixteenth century in the Habsburg castle at Ambras, Austria, where it was discovered toward the end of the last century and transferred to the Museum für Völkerkunde, Vienna.

The feather-work symbolizes a gigantic settling bird, and as such once had a golden head and beak, probably a casque, which was mentioned in the early inventories of the collection at Ambras but disappeared during the 18th century. Well over 4 feet high, the piece is divided roughly into three zones. Four different kinds of feathers are used. The gathered furry section at the bottom is of brilliant turquoise-blue, decorated with twenty-eight crescents and fifteen step-shaped plaques of gold. A fluffy band of crimson separates this from the second zone, where a few short uneven quetzal plumes are laid against a ground of rich cocoa-brown feathers, so placed that their white tips form an edge for the band. Three rows of small gold disks, one hundred eighty-seven in all, decorate its border. Beyond spread the iridescent tail feathers of the quetzal, shimmering gold and emerald-green. The protruding center is built up on a similar scheme.

The number of gold disks, crescents, and plaques has been explained as of calendrical significance. The blue, brown, and white of the composition are said to symbolize the sky, earth, and water, and thus the wearer of the headdress may have personified the power of these three elements of nature.[115]

The sketch at the right (*fig. b*) is another illustration from the Sahagún Codex, showing craftsmen engaged in making a large piece of feather-work, while at the left a merchant brings in the raw material from the "hot lands."

For the Aztec shield in *Pl. 287, fig. a,* about 2 feet in diameter, feathers were mounted on an animal pelt, apparently from a jaguar, stretched over a wooden frame. Long tufted plumes trailed from the lower edge like a fringe. A shield of this pattern is specified on the Tribute Roll (see *Pl. 269*) and also appears in the Codex Mendoza (see *Pl. 268, fig. b*), carried by one of the warriors.

In better condition and displaying a far more impressive pattern is the feather shield in *fig. b,* which has the same history as the headdress. On it is emblazoned the figure of a coyote rampant in turquoise-blue with a purple belly against a background of mottled red feathers. A weblike frame of thin narrow strips of pure gold marks the outline of the animal and delineates its claws, teeth, eye, and fur. The coyote is one version of the Fire-god of the Aztecs, and its lashing tongue, as well as the tufts of yellow and red shaded feathers around the rim, signifies flame. Mouth, claws, eye, and the ragged back and tail display excellent observation and sprightly talent for the decorative. The technical execution in such an unusual medium is astonishingly inventive.

Fig. c shows a princely standard which was worn on the back, rising like a colored aureole behind the head. The standard proper is about 18 inches in diameter and made up of a ten-spoked wheel with an outer rim of stiff feathers radiating in a fanlike fashion. In the center of this side the "fire-flower" is represented; the "fire-butterfly" is depicted on the reverse. A band of twenty-eight chevrons, worked in various colors, encircles the medallion, giving a rotating effect to the pattern. Note that this design moves from left to right, a convention observed in the chevron bands seen in Maya Chamá pottery (see *Pls. 130* and *131*). This is inclosed and set off by a frame of purple, beyond which come the unclipped feathers of the rim. The handle is of a light reedlike wood with a finely woven scaly cover.

It is interesting to speculate whether Mozart's librettist had not seen some of these pre-Columbian garments and objects of feather-work when he clothed his Papageno and Papagena in the unprecedented feathered raiment frequently commented upon by both contemporary and later critics. In mid-18th century such pieces probably existed in greater number than today, for, as we know, the art of feather working was not abandoned immediately after the Conquest. Mitres, stoles, and holy pictures were made of feathers during the Spanish vice-regal period, some of which are still preserved.

The mitre and infula illustrated (*Pl. 288*) were made in the first decades of Spanish dominance and present an achievement well worth consideration—a proof of the Indian artist's remarkable ability in this medium, even though the subject was alien to him. Steeped in the concepts of his own religion and art, which had been formulated for centuries, he was confronted almost overnight with a specialized technical civilization and a religious iconography completely different from his own. These pieces also show the far greater talent of the Indian in reproducing a Christian scene than that of the contemporary Spaniard when depicting the Indian.

The details of minor scenes, such as the Last Supper at the bottom of the mitre or the Resurrection on the infula (left), as well as the main subject, are well worth study under a magnifying glass for their story-telling quality. They reflect unmistakably the ecstatic pictorial mannerism of the 16th-century Spanish paintings that were placed before the workers to be copied. Scrutiny will reveal that the same method was applied here that went into the construction of medieval American feather-work. The technique of outlining seen on the coyote shield in the preceding plate was used, not only on the figures but also for the floral garland which meanders between the individual scenes.

The general background is a deep iridescent purplish blue, against which the fiery dots scattered here and there seem actually luminous. All the colors are rich in tone. The figure of Christ is executed in every instance with especial care—even the eyelashes are depicted with an infinitesimal feather tip, shimmering gold.

Only a few colonial specimens of this unique art remain. Besides churchly objects of the sort illustrated, holy pictures have been seen in Vienna, London, and Madrid. In the last city there is an arresting feather-work shield, fashioned for Philip II. It carries four complete battle scenes on its surface, showing the greatest triumphs of the Spaniards over the Moslems.[33]

With *Pl. 289* we return to medieval times and enter the Andean Area. The fan or headdress in *fig. a,* about 10 inches high, probably came from the Central Coast of Peru. A woven framework holds the feathers firmly in the arc. White tips are most effectively used as edging. The depth of color, the richness and density of the plumage are remarkable after so many centuries.

A pair of earplugs, a little more than 2½ inches in diameter, are shown in *fig. b.* These are Ica in style, and bear the ∽ motif already familiar from the pottery of the region. Even on such small pieces, contrasting colors and a divided pattern were applied, rendering them lively and appealing.

The fondness for striking colors and designs observed in the textile art of this area expresses itself with increasing brilliance when woven materials were covered with feathers. The poncho in *fig. c* came from a Chimú grave. A rich canary-yellow is the color of the body of the piece; the two bands are brown. In between them flows a scroll in black, a sharp and well applied contrast.

A different build-up of design is seen in the Ica poncho with animals (*Pl. 290, fig. a*), showing strong affiliation to the textiles of this culture. Here the dark subjects stand free against a white background. Neat clipping of the feathers makes the figural and geometric decoration clear and precise.

The large feather poncho in *fig. b,* 51 inches long by 42 wide, is Chimú in style. The body is a yellowish red, and yellow and black alternate in the small circles, the centers of which are turquoise-blue. This brilliant hue is repeated in the yoke at the neck and the bands on the lower edge. The fantasy play of shades is most subtle and effective.

Such gorgeous pieces of ingenious craftsmanship—feather mantles, ponchos, and ornaments—help one to visualize the pomp that dazzled the Spaniards when they first met the dignitaries of medieval America. The high standard of this civilization is confirmed by those small pieces of the applied arts which belonged to and beautified the life of its people. In addition to objects for ceremonial use, we have seen articles of lesser importance—all bearing the stamp of artistic talent.

XI

Facets of Daily Life

PEOPLE who had such varied and ingenious impulses in the arts as the natives of medieval America could not help but manifest their talent in the ordinary walk of life. There are a number of accurate and colorful books describing their customs in detail and, therefore, we shall give in the following plates only random aspects of the field, which may be pursued further by any one who takes an interest in one or another. The illustrations bring up material that falls outside a rigorous interpretation of the arts, showing either some lesser known or spectacular facet of their daily life. In the broader picture thus presented we gain a deeper appreciation of their achievement.

AGRICULTURE

Medieval America never knew the plow. The chief implement was the planting stick, and, as corn is planted a few kernels at a time—not sown broadcast like wheat—it served its purpose very well. In some regions ancient agricultural methods are still in operation, each adapted to a specific climate.

Pl. 291, fig. b shows Sahagún's illustration of the planting stick from the Codex Florentino. A remarkable parallel appears in the picture beside it (*fig. c*), taken after the turn of the century in our Southwest, where the Indian methods of dry-farming still prevail.

Remnants of irrigation canals have been found in all our areas, and the use of fertilizers seems also to have been fairly general. Frequently a small fish was deposited with the seed, and in certain parts of the Andean Area guano was used. In the Maya and Mexican areas land was prepared for cultivation by burning it over—a wasteful method, producing a steadily diminishing crop, as is often pointed out.

Agriculture in the Andean Area, also pursued under especially great handicaps, shows marvelous organization. In the coastal regions, systems of aqueducts made the arid valleys bloom, while in the highlands, terraces were laid out with arduous labor along the precipitous shoulders of their mountains. The magnitude of this task can be judged from the photograph reproduced in *fig. a,* showing a site recently excavated in southeastern Peru. The terraces average from 20 to 24 feet in height.[35] Note the almost endless system of stairways, cutting directly across them or leading from one level to the next. The expert contour farming of these people is also evident in the terraces seen on *Pl. 51, fig. a,* and *Pl. 56, fig. b.* The irrigation water was guided in at the top and flowed from one section to the other.

It might be of interest to mention here that the metabolism of the corn-eating Indians of the lowlands in Yucatan differs from that of those living in the extremely high altitudes of the Andean highlands and both are found to be quite different from ours.

In many ways the fare of the aboriginal American was superior to that of his European contemporary, although he did not use milk or its products. We have only to list the food and medicinal plants of American origin that have been adopted into our civilization to make this clear. The most important are maize, potatoes, sweet potatoes, tomatoes, pumpkins, squash, beans (lima, kidney, and others), peppers, cocoa, pineapples, and peanuts as foods; quinine and cocaine as drugs; henequen (sisal) as fiber, and rubber and chicle as gums.

MUSICAL INSTRUMENTS

No one who has ever witnessed an Indian dance can doubt the remarkable sense of rhythm of these people. They have subtle changes, variations, and crescendi, which we distinctly feel but try to analyze without satisfaction.

In medieval times, their instruments were drums, rattles, whistles, trumpets, panpipes, and flutes. All of these point to a very early stage of musical development. We should not forget, however, that music as we know it came late even to Western Europe. The lack of fixed tonality and any system of musical notation made the medieval festivals even of that continent noisy and unmelodious affairs.

A detail from the Codex Florentino (*Pl. 292, fig. c*) pictures a festival scene in medieval Mexico. Two drums are shown in use, the smaller, a slit one tapped with sticks, the larger, covered with stretched jaguar skin, beaten with the hands. The other participants in the ceremony are apparently chanters carrying rattles.

An example of the larger type of drum—carved of wood and remarkably fine in its detail—is reproduced in *fig. b.* An eagle, the symbolic bird of the Aztecs, stands probably on the double-bodied serpent of Aztec mythology. The sign near the beak has been interpreted as the glyph of the war cry it utters.

The Aztec slit drum (*fig. a*), called *teponaztli,* is about 28 inches long and made of basaltic rock. It has a clear bell-like tone. The figure Macuilxochitl, or Five Flower, is represented, his own weird features spelling out his name. Note the effective expressionistic manner of denoting the eyes. Jaguar skin is carved on the ends of the drum.

The *teponaztli* had two tones of different pitch. It varied in size from the larger type set on a stand, seen in the Sahagún sketch, to those about 12 inches in length which were suspended on a cord around the neck. These are said to have been used to tap out signals on the battlefield.[126]

Two pottery flutes from Mexico, each with four finger holes, are seen in *fig. d,* the longer about 7 inches. A gaping monster or a snake mouth forms the end of the smaller instrument. Both have a fine red polish, very well preserved.

Fig. e shows a group of pottery figurines from Monte Albán Period III. Three of the little men in front, each about 4½ inches tall, are blowing trumpets, while the fourth, on the left, appears to direct them. Small as they are, one feels they fill the air with their blasts, and the dignitaries arranged behind them seem to swell to the sound.

Pl. 293 presents examples of drums which are masterpieces of the wood carver's art. The composition of ornately costumed figures in the lower piece of *fig. a* is carried out with deep precise incisions, but the bland surfaces and shallow carving of the single figure on the one above it is far more fluent and effective, seeming almost winged with its smooth contours and plain background. The drumsticks were padded or tipped with rubber.

Different styles are pictured in *figs. b* and *c,* one carved in human and the other in animal form. *Fig. b* is unusually plastic and has inlaid eyes and teeth of shell. The arms and legs, awkwardly placed, add a certain strangeness to the piece, but the carving is concise and shows assurance. Far more decorative is the drum shaped into an animal body (*fig. c*), which was also further embellished with inlay. The curling motifs are excellently applied and the treatment of the fringed legs and plumed tail is highly ornamental.

More melodic possibilities are offered by the instruments of the Andean Area (*Pl. 294*). The various lengths in the panpipes—which were made of reed and stone (*figs. a* and *c*) and even of clay—produced a variety of notes. Their music has a melancholy pastoral quality, and the five-tone scale is used. (See also *Pl. 258, fig. b,* and *Pl. 272, fig. e.*) The panpipe is still played in the region, as is evidenced by the scene in *fig. b,* taken on Lake Titicaca, which shows a group of Indians in a *balsa,* or reed boat, with a sail of the same material.

The bulbous clay flute, or ocarina (*fig. e*), fashioned in the semblance of an animal, came from Costa Rica, but the type was widespread, and human as well as various animal figures are found. The instrument has a dull hollow note, not shrill. It is interesting to note that in Europe the ocarina cannot be traced farther back than mid-19th century.[119]

The Mochica, excellent observers of details in other phases of their daily life, also left records of musicians in their pottery. The two in *fig. d* are playing flute and drum. Mention also should be made of the whistle jars of the area. These were double vessels that, when half full of liquid, made a whistling sound if blown into at one end.

In *fig. f* a conch trumpet, wooden flute, and clay trumpet are shown, all from the coast of Peru. Together, these instruments were capable of producing a considerable range of sound because of the variety in their materials.

The recitation of dramatic legends and the many types of dances and festive performances cannot be taken up here. There is too little authentic information concerning them to form a definite picture, but there is no doubt that such performances occurred everywhere and were elaborate affairs. The text used was polished and flowery; it would seem that it resembled in style more the poetry of a Li T'ai-po or a Rabindranath Tagore than the classics of Europe. There was no rhyming in the composition, but it was held together by an inner rhythm of thought and cadence.

There were even puppet shows. Sahagún describes one presented by a "necromancer" who made a tiny figure dance on the palm of his hand. There is evidence that medieval America had string-operated marionettes, used by the medicine men.[62] A suggestion of this art is found in the deer mask with movable ears (see *Pl. 271, fig. b*) as well as the silver doll from Peru with hinged arms (see *Pl. 202, fig. c*).

PIPES

On the next three plates, pipes from the Mound Builder culture and the Mexican Area are illustrated. Because of their plastic qualities, they could have been included under sculpture and pottery, but since they add to the picture of daily life, they are shown here instead of among the more imposing works of stone carving or modeling. As is known, tobacco is a plant indigenous to America and smoking was a ceremonial act. The stem apparently was not held between the teeth but only between the lips and the pipe puffed through a reed.

On *Pl. 295, fig. a,* we see the most universal type, undecorated—except for the one in the upper right, with its charming little squirrel—and absolutely modern. The two smaller ones are made of stone and come from Georgia, while the larger piece, 9½ inches long, is of pottery shaped like a corncob and was found in Mexico.

In *fig. b* the human figure appears. This example, 8 inches high, comes from a Mound Builder site in Ohio, but has plastic characteristics that recall the art of the Mexican Area. Note the large circular earplugs. The mouthpiece of the pipe is in the top of the head.

Although the pipes of the Mound Builders were sometimes carved in human shape, they were generally fashioned into animals, chosen with amazing variety. *Fig. c* shows an owl effigy from Illinois, 7 inches high. The eyes were inlaid. Here attention should be called to a certain sculptural relationship to Totonac work (see *Pl. 65, fig. a*). Influence from Mexico can be discerned also in *fig. e,* a limestone carving from Carthage, Alabama. However, considerable originality is embodied in the piece. The duck figure with an owl's head on its tail (*fig. f*) comes from Virginia. It is 10 inches long, and the dark mottled stone is polished to a high degree. The realistic portrayal of the duck is not in the least influenced by the unexpected addition of the other bird's head. As a sculpture, the composition is singularly well knit. In *fig. d,* from the Tremper Mound, Ohio, a squirrel stands on a curving base, 3¼ inches long. Gray with red marbling, its color adds to the naturalness of its appearance.

Three examples on *Pl. 296* (*figs. a, b,* and *d*) were found at the same site as the squirrel, Tremper Mound, Ohio. All have the same curving base, and are made of local pipestone, an indurated material much valued by the Indians for pipes. Its wide variety of colors was used to advantage for realistic effects. *Fig. a* is the only dog effigy found in the many Ohio mounds, although bones of dogs have been excavated.[130] Compare his pose with that of the mythical animal from Puebla (see *Pl. 60, fig. c*). *Fig. b* represents an otter carrying a fish. In *fig. d* a hawk is carved in greater detail. The claws especially are faithfully portrayed. Its eyes are inlaid with copper.

In *fig. c* a duck is strikingly caught in the movement of swimming. Its placement on the tubular pipe shows admirable balance. The pipe in *fig. f,* from Ohio, showing a spoonbill duck on the back of a fish or amphibian, is a more elaborate variation of a similar theme. Despite the fantastic coupling of the two creatures, it gives a highly realistic impression. Note the shiny uniform quality of the stone.

Perhaps the greatest artistic courage is manifest in the crane effigy (*fig. e*), a red clay pipe, 5½ inches long, also from Ohio. The daring line of the long neck produces an unusually beautiful effect. Besides the reaching head of the bird, the terse but expressive outline of the wing and leg is noteworthy.

The portrayal of the various animals on Mound Builder pipes is generally so naturalistic that they can be identified by species within the genus.

The pottery pipe on *Pl. 297, fig. a,* a little over 5 inches long, comes from Mexico. The human figure is excellently employed and the elongation of the left leg to serve as the pipe stem is resourceful and original. Especially noteworthy are the elaborate headdress with its flower-like decoration and the large round ornament on the chin. The bow at the belt is executed with the ease typical of this area.

Fashioned in a somewhat similar attitude is the figure on the effigy pipe from Oaxaca (*fig. c*), about 6½ inches long. The face, here half turned away, seems to have a beardlike appendage, and the small pellets of clay covering the head are unusual. Glyphs characteristic of the region appear on the back and around the bowl of the pipe. (Compare *Pl. 125, fig. a.*)

Glyphs also ornament the tripod incense burner from Oaxaca (*fig. b*), a little over 12 inches long, which is included for the sake of comparison. Here the human figure is used only for decoration on a utilitarian vessel; he lies along the handle in a comfortable pose, while a snake is shown crawling toward him from the opposite end. The facial features have definite Oaxaca traits (see *Pl. 123*).

MIRRORS

Before the mirror with mercury was invented, it was a universal custom to use the polished surface of metals and hard shining stones. On *Pl. 298, fig. a,* we find a rounded slab of obsidian employed, placed within a carved and gilded wooden frame. It is said to come from Vera Cruz. How well it reflected is shown by the image of a small effigy vessel that was placed before it but which is not visible in the photograph (see *Pl. 118, fig. a*). The frame, similar on both sides, with its alternating elements of the double-headed serpent and a four-leaf-clover pattern, still retains enough of its gilding to form an excellent contrast to the black volcanic glass.

In the hand mirror from the Andean Area (*fig. b*), pyrite is used as the reflecting surface. Though broken and dulled today, it must have served its purpose well when new. The three alert heads on top of the wooden frame lend the piece a certain piquancy. It allegedly came from the coast of Peru and might be Chimú.

The wooden frame for a hand mirror, the back of which is shown in *fig. c,* is said to have come from Lambayeque. It is 9½ inches high, including the handle. The small figure standing under a roof is characteristically Chimú. This panel must have been carved separately and set in, for the grain of the wood differs from that in the frame. The upper rounded molding is well worked out and the section above it, now broken off, also probably carried some kind of decoration. Adorned with painted patterns in various colors, this small utilitarian object again bespeaks an originality and talent that left its mark on anything it touched.

COUNTING AND MEASURING

The markets of medieval America aroused the enthusiasm of the *conquistadores* wherever they saw them. They were held several times a month and surplus products of garden plots and labor were exchanged by barter, for there was no money as we know it. Controllers were present to check on weights and measures and the quality of the merchandise.

The balance scale with its beam of bone and finely netted bags (*Pl. 299, fig. a*) is an unpretentious but *éclatant* example of the great Chimú culture which produced it. Note the tiny birds carved on top.

Various ingenious methods of counting and recording were devised in the different regions. Grains of maize, beans, or pebbles were used, and still are, in calculating addition and subtraction. Among the highland Maya, accounts were kept by means of counted kernels set aside in separate boxes or bags. In certain regions of medieval America there are indications of the existence of a type of primitive abacus.

In the Andean Area private trade was confined within narrow limits. Commerce was in the hands of the state, which managed it according to its own rules. There was heavy traffic in the interchange of regional products. Into the highland warehouses flowed cotton, peppers, fruits, and fish from the coast, and wood, coca, feathers, and dye stuffs from the eastern forests. In return, wool, meat, potatoes, and metal were sent down from the mountains.[95]

Although the inhabitants of the Andean Area never developed the glyph, they had nevertheless a system of numeration and invented an ingenious device upon which they did their counting and kept certain records. This is the *quipu* (*fig. b*), a series of knotted strings of different colors and lengths, sometimes a yard long. The one illustrated here was found at Chancay, on the Central Coast of Peru. Each color referred to a separate subject or category. The knots denoted numbers and those designating the same number were tied in a horizontal line, the same distance from the top on all the strings. On the six strings tending upward from the heavy twined base in this illustration, units, tens, hundreds, and thousands are registered, while in the lower groups units, tens, and hundreds are shown.[82] Those who know the system give remarkably parallel readings.

By this means the complicated business of the great Empire was transacted, a census of the people and animals recorded, and an inventory made of grain, cloth, and other produce. The device is still in use today among the Peruvian shepherds. In China and Tibet, knot records are said to have preceded the invention of writing.

Among the Incas, the accounts were in charge of officials trained for the service. Youths were prepared for these positions in schools, where they learned the traditions, history, and even geography of their land. Relief maps, modeled in clay, were used to help them visualize certain topographical features. Traditions were preserved by memorizing past events. Here the *quipus* were of assistance, suggesting facts and figures, in the reconstruction of the great panorama of the past. As is known from other civilizations without written signs, those who do not write generally have prodigious memories.

ROADS

It is not surprising that the splendid cities of medieval America were joined by roads or that the highways were constructed with the same thoroughness that characterized other phases of this civilization, even though there were no carriages and wheeled vehicles, no beasts of burden, except the llama in the Andes, to make use of them. They were built for travelers and carriers on foot, for men bearing palanquins with chiefs and priests going from one city to another with pompous suites. So wide were they that four files of men with their loads could easily pass. Relay runners even carried sea fish alive in salt-water containers from the shore to the palaces of Aztec and Inca rulers.

Most of the roads, however, are now buried in jungle growth or obliterated by the shifting sands of the Pacific coast. A study of them has been undertaken. Flights over the jungle of northeastern Yucatan have resulted in such photographs as that reproduced on *Pl. 300, fig. a*. It shows the intersecting of two ancient Maya highways, now buried in the bush, on the outskirts of Cobá. One of them led to a village a short distance from Chichén Itzá, sixty-five miles away. The fresh-water lakes and ponds that dot the scene made living possible here in earlier times. Investigations by the Carnegie Institution of Washington reveal that a network of roads was laid out between the once-flourishing Maya cities.

Maya highways were constructed no less carefully than the causeways of medieval Europe. The ancient road builders began by digging down to hardpan and erecting on either side retaining walls of roughly dressed limestone set in mortar, sometimes to a height of eight feet. A foundation of heavy boulders was then laid and the spaces filled with smaller stones. The surface may have been leveled with stone rollers. One such stone, 13 feet long, 2¼ in diameter, and weighing about five tons, was discovered near the section shown here. It has been suggested that the roads were surfaced with cement; if so, they must have been dazzling in the tropical sunshine. From the material found in connection with them, they are believed to have been constructed between the 4th and 7th centuries.[19] A few years ago the writer saw the same method of road building in practice on the border of Guatemala and El Salvador.

To facilitate travel, bridges had to be erected and rest houses built for the traveler. Simple thatched-roof shelters stand today in the highlands of Central America, sometimes on passes from 12,000 to 14,000 feet above sea level, at a distance of one day's journey on foot. Here the tired Indian finds protection against the icy chill of the night and prepares his warm meal—a wise custom which he follows at least once a day even in his "hot country." In the morning a few fresh pieces of straw and the dying embers of a carefully covered fire are all the evidence left by the nightly visitor, already well on his road.

In the Andean Area under Inca rule these wayside stations, or *tambos,* grew into veritable hostelries, born as they were of the same need as the romantic caravanseries of the Orient. They were built of stone and had blankets, firewood, food, utensils, and, in many cases, a caretaker; in the absence of an attendant, it is recorded that the travelers showed considerable responsibility for the welfare of those who would come after them. One squadron of *conquistadores* lived for weeks on such supplies during a reconnoitering trip into remote parts of the Andes.

Many chroniclers consider the Inca roads the most outstanding achievement of this remarkable people. For the stretch that passes over the great mountain plateau from Cuzco to Quito, galleries were cut through solid rock, rivers spanned by swinging bridges, ravines filled up, and precipices scaled by steps cut into their sides.[82]

When a new land was conquered, part of the inhabitants were moved over these highways to other parts of the Empire, while loyal subjects were brought in to take their places, a precautionary measure taken against rebellion and for the dissemination of the Quechua tongue (the language of the Incas) over the subjugated territory.[29]

But even before the Inca organization stretched out its fingers after distant provinces, there were roads on the coastal plain. *Fig. b* shows one that led to Talara through the Chicama Valley, near the great Chimú center of Chan-Chan. As straight as if laid out by a surveyor, broad and comfortable, it still gives one a profound respect for the culture that flourished here before the Incas rose to power. The ruin with its walls and high fortress-like base was probably a station.

Equal to the roads as an achievement were the aqueducts which brought water from the mountains and distributed it over large tracts in the coastal districts that otherwise would have been uninhabitable desert. The very engineering skill of the people, however, contributed to their own overthrow. Many aqueducts were too long to be adequately defended, and as soon as the upper channels were in the hands of the enemy, the whole region was faced with starvation or surrender.[54] Now everything that man built here is going back to the sand from which it was made, but if desolation and decay can speak, these ruins are indeed eloquent.

CITY-PLANNING

The views on *Pls. 301* and *302* present different sites from the air, showing well-planned layouts that are little suspected from the ground.

The Southwest, frequently overshadowed by the other areas, furnishes brilliant examples of organized city-planning. One case in point is Pueblo Bonito, already shown on *Pl. 4;* another is Aztec Ruin in New Mexico (*Pl. 301, fig. a*).

This is a rectangular walled-in complex, with the largest kiva near the center, the interior of which was illustrated earlier (see *Pl. 5, fig. b*). Smaller kivas, recognizable by their circular outlines, can be singled out, set among the living quarters and storage rooms. It is a clearly conceived and evenly walled construction.

A bird's-eye view of Tulum (*fig. b*) gives a broad picture of the defense wall and the cliffs which protected this Maya town (see also *Pls. 29* and *30*). Though crumbling before the aggressive growth of the jungle, the barrier still has enough stones left in place to make an impression. At the corner the ruins of a watch tower are distinguishable. The grouping of the buildings is clear in the photograph, some concentrated around the center, others scattered farther away and now completely overgrown.

Teotihuacán and Chan-Chan stand among the most venerated of the numerous sites of medieval America. An airview of the former has already displayed to advantage the impressive layout of this early Toltec ceremonial center (see *Pl. 7, fig. b*). Here a more comprehensive view of the Citadel is presented (*Pl. 302, fig. a*). It faces the broad Avenue of the Dead (right) that leads directly to the Pyramid of the Moon and on that side a wide stair mounts the embankment. Within the square of the rampart rises the solid pile of the Temple of Quetzalcóatl, only partly reconstructed (see *Pl. 8*). The centuries have greatly changed the aspect of this place, but the regular lines of the square, the even level of the platforms still show a precision of workmanship that could not be improved upon today.

Chan-Chan also has been discussed under architecture. Its ruins as seen from the air (*fig. b*), showing the beautifully planned construction of the vast Chimú capital, need little elucidation. Approximately 250,000 people are estimated to have lived on the site amidst palaces, temples, and sunken gardens. Remnants of walls are evident everywhere—walls that once supported the roofs of dwellings, walls that separated one palace or one section of the city from another. Details of the splendid stucco decoration lavished on them were shown on *Pl. 43*. The dark oblong in the center of the photograph was probably a reservoir, overgrown with vegetation since the city was abandoned. Although Chan-Chan was overshadowed by Inca grandeur, the site even in ruins still remains a most impressive monument of one of those great cultures from which the Incas drew strength for an empire.

BATHS AND RESERVOIRS

The display of clear water in fountains, pools, and basins, as well as the use of hot and mineral springs for medicinal purposes, was revived in medieval Europe by the Moors and Turks. The people of pre-Columbian America made these discoveries for themselves.

Near Texcotzingo in the Mexican highlands, some thirty miles from the former Aztec capital, the king of Texcoco built a royal retreat. Here a large basin was hewn from the solid rock, with steps leading down into it, stone seats, and a fountain. The bath is still in relatively good condition.

Medicinal bathing was practiced in all areas, and even today ceremonial baths persist in many regions. Many Indians in the tropical and semitropical countries preserve their ancient tradition of cleanliness, bathing and changing their meager garments every evening upon returning to their thatched huts from work.

At Chichén Itzá a sweat bath of the Maya was excavated. The building (*Pl. 303, figs. a* and *b*) is in the late style of this site, plain except for flaring cornices. The vault of the spacious antechamber has not been fully reconstructed (*fig. a*), and reveals the built-in dais and a small square door opening into the bath proper. Here, within a low chamber, water was poured over heated stones, producing somewhat the same effect as our Turkish steam bath. The superfluous vapor passed out through a small round opening in the wall that can be seen in *fig. b*. It is interesting to note that another such sweat bath was discovered at Piedras Negras.

Mention has already been made of the involved irrigation works of various arid regions. In *fig. c* we see the remnants of a distributing plant at Sacsahuamán in the Andes. A section of narrow channel lined with massive stones (right foreground) gives an idea of the thoroughness that extended to even the smallest detail in the construction. The carefully plotted layout of the whole system is again an impressive example of Inca genius for organization.

STAIRWAYS

Stairways are among the most grandiose features of Maya, Mexican, and Andean architecture and deserve separate consideration. Inviting as the idea would be to present a series of them, only a few can be included here. It is noteworthy that they were generally in the open, like those of ancient cultures in the Eastern Hemisphere and early Christianity.

El Castillo at Chichén Itzá has already been described (see *Pl. 41*). The main stairway of the four that mount this symmetrical temple-base is shown on *Pl. 304, fig. a.* As was mentioned in an earlier chapter, it is two feet wider at the top, which exaggerates its monumentality. The sharp incline of the steps and the narrow treads are apparent at first glance.

In contrast, the Southwest made little use of stairs. People here employed ladders, which, in case of attack, could be pulled up into the building. These were of the same primitive type as seen in the inset—a tree trimmed of its branches with footholds hewn along its length. This particular example was found and photographed by us quite recently; it was in use by a road gang of Indians on the border of Guatemala and El Salvador. The two pictures, side by side, demonstrate the unbelievable contrasts in the civilization of medieval America. From what lowly beginning did the grand stairways spring.

On *Pl. 305, fig. a* we see the Temple of the Dwarf at Uxmal from the southeast, photographed before any preservation work was undertaken (see also *Pl. 35, fig. a*). The tapering artificial mound upon which the temple stood is imposing in itself, much more so if we try to visualize its whole great bulk covered with regularly laid stone facing broken with sculptural decoration. Up the side of this pile of masonry leads the stairway, steep and broad, crumbling from age so that in this photograph the single steps look like ripples on its surface. The climbing quality, however, is still in them and a certain detachment from the structure can be sensed.

Although some of the mounds in the coastal districts of the Andean Area reached two hundred feet in height, no stairways survive. The mass of sun-baked clay could not withstand the rare but devastating rain storms. In the highlands, however, many striking examples remain, made of stone. In the detail from Machu Picchu (*fig. b*) the completely different position they held in Inca architecture is evident. They are not dramatic decorative features. Neither so steep nor so thoroughly digested into the structure as in the Mexican and Maya areas, they are here purely functional.

The stairway of each people reflects the particular civilization which produced it. Pre-Columbian America developed its own, uninfluenced by the achievements of other continents. They have little in common with the broad steps of Egypt, the heroic lines of those of Greece, or the luxuriously sweeping stairs of Rome. They were adapted to the use of the ancient red man with his agile wildcat tread and his clinging sandals. How much so, we realized when we saw modern Maya waveringly making their way up the stairway of their ancestors.

ENVOI

The impressive site pictured on *Pl. 306* was discovered in southeastern Peru by the late Paul Fejös. It lies at an altitude of 12,000 feet about one day's distance by mule from Machu Picchu and was named by the natives Phuyu Pata Marka, "the city above the clouds." Approximately five and one-half acres were cleared and surveyed.[35]

In *fig. a* we see the northeastern part of the settlement. The masonry is of polygonal white granite blocks and the ground is squared off with characteristic precision into evenly laid terraces, cut through by two breath-taking flights of steps. The large white granite boulder in the foreground of the picture is carved with two couchlike depressions on the east side and two seats, like armchairs, on the west. Their similarity to the better-known Throne of the Inca at Sacsahuamán (see *Pl. 49, fig. b*) would point to some ceremonial use for such monuments.

Immediately above it is a row of five cubicles. These are water basins or baths, all connected by subterranean channels and fed from the main canal, visible at the left though not entirely excavated when the picture was taken. Apparently this aqueduct supplied the water for both household purposes and the irrigation of the terraces farther down the slope. A sixth cubicle can be seen to the left nearer the foreground. This outlying section is connected with the city by a monolithic bridge.

The other side of this site (*fig. b*) gives an even better idea of the immense and precipitous mountain slope to which it clings. The whole ground is shaped into rounded terraces, the outcroppings of ledge apparently taken into account and neatly skirted. Flights of steps, like flexible bands, follow the slope, slanting now mildly, now steeply. The houses, too, conform to the contours of the terrain. Nothing is incidental or casual; each building has a well-laid plan and even the bedrock was carved to receive the masonry. Seemingly constructional difficulties did not deter these ancient builders—witness the house at the left, poised so skillfully above the precipice; probably the tillable land was so precious that every bit of it had to be reserved for the terrace fields.

Phuyu Pata Marka, the City above the Clouds, is the last of our illustrations. After the dazzling array of the more famous sites in this survey—all generals— it lies, an unknown soldier, appealing through its very obscurity for more effort, greater understanding, deeper homage.

XII

Evolution or Influence

SINCE the discovery of America, the civilization of its aborigines has been the subject of fantastic conjectures. In the 16th, 17th, and 18th centuries, the study of human races was haphazard and weakly organized. The comparisons and allusions of travelers in the service of Spain concerning the American natives were accepted at their face value. Accurate information was almost impossible to obtain. The hardships of travel, the constant battle with diseases of a most deadly character, the despotism of local "little kings," as well as the overwhelming vastness and foreign aspect of the land, all weighed upon the visitors and made it difficult for them to form objective opinions. At the same time, most could not see beyond the conceptions of their day.

In addition, a strict control and censorship were exercised over the Spanish colonies of the New World until the movement for independence at the beginning of the 19th century. With the exception of a few cases—such as that of the English priest, Thomas Gage, who, after twelve years in Mexico and Central America, returned to his native land—all descriptions and reports had to pass the scrutiny of the Council of the Indies in Seville. Carloads of unpublished material on the colonial empire and its past lie even today in the stately Renaissance building there which was its headquarters. As late as the beginning of the 19th century, the scientist Alexander von Humboldt, sent to investigate the mineral resources of New Spain, with personal letters of recommendation from the king himself, met the barriers maintained by the Inquisition. He writes that in the Mexican capital he obtained permission to dig up and study a gigantic Aztec statue, buried since the Conquest in the patio of a monastery, on the express condition that it be re-interred before sundown of the same day.[50]

The study of man developed slowly in the early centuries of our age even with reference to the European nations and their immediate neighbors. The Turkish domination of a large part of Europe, the religious struggles among the

Christians themselves permitted little time or inclination for the study of savages on distant continents. However, with the Renaissance a certain interest in other great civilizations was aroused. The cultures of China, of ancient Egypt, and Mesopotamia began to be extolled and interpreted for the European and the arts and customs of these countries described and illustrated. By the early 19th century, a fairly well established basis of art appreciation already existed, and the framework of what later became art-history and archaeology was laid down. The humanistic writers of this post-revolutionary age consolidated certain principles of esthetics, guiding the taste and interest of the rising middle class. At that time, the cultures of the Near and Far East were looked upon as mere fore-runners of our European civilization, and whatever we had adopted from them —from gunpowder and printing to the making of porcelain—we took unto ourselves for our own glory, giving little credit to the country of its origin.

In such a set-up there was no place for pre-Columbian America. Although shortly after the Conquest it was conceded that the American Indian had a soul (which it behooved the white man to bring within the realm of Christ), he was too far from Europe to be considered seriously as a humanistic problem. America was for centuries only a land of the present: El Dorado for the Spaniard, the land of golden opportunity for the Anglo-Saxon settler and the other colonists. When its amazing early civilization, overgrown with the destructive tropical plants of the jungle or buried beneath the shifting sands of deserts, finally demanded attention, the science of the day made elaborate endeavors to file it in the pigeonholes already existing.

Thus, regardless of striking differences, the remnants of medieval American art were coupled with every possible culture of the Eastern Hemisphere by savants who had never visited the scene or studied any great number of pre-Columbian objects. Kinship with the lost tribes of Israel and the Egyptians of the Pharaohs was thrust upon the native American. Scientists in general had already built their structure of classifications and were unwilling to make any drastic change in it.

But with the opening of better transportation facilities and the consequent freedom of movement in Latin America, the accounts of these regions became more enlightened. As the 19th century neared its close, all America began to receive greater attention from the rest of the world, not only because of its industrial and social achievements but also for its scientific activities. In the short span of about seventy years, travelers and scientists, for the most part unknown to the general reader, have put together piece by piece the picture of pre-

Columbian America. Although still far from complete, the elements in general are assembled and, within the last fifteen to twenty years, many details have been worked out.

At the same time, research in early civilizations in the rest of the world has also advanced, so that the characteristics of both hemispheres are much more clearly defined and better differentiated than in the last century. Today we have a greater knowledge and a more efficient method of procedure to help us form conclusions on the origin and development of the pre-Columbian peoples.

Remnants of human skeletons have been found in America in proximity to extinct mammals, and arrowheads, fashioned by the hands of man, have been excavated alongside skeletal parts of the ground sloth and three-toed horse, animals which disappeared from the Western Hemisphere long ago.[114] Experts who reckon cautiously declare this era to be some fifteen to twenty thousand years ago. More and more support is being given the theory that as America had a developed plant and animal life in such early times, the presence of man also may be assumed. The abundance of fish, fowl, and wild game, the richness of the primeval forests and the plains with their edible plants, wild grains, and berries, and, toward the south, a climate well suited for the beginnings of agriculture, argue for this thesis.

For our purpose, however, the indisputable date of the earliest habitation of the Western Hemisphere is not of primary importance; our concern in this chapter is whether medieval American art is the result of autochthonous evolution or of influence from another continent. It has been noted that everything here of high artistic value, in a universal sense, is coincident in time with the appearance of Christianity in Europe and the centuries after. But it does not follow that this date marks the beginning of great art in the Western Hemisphere. While it is true that the earliest stelae of the Maya Area are contemporary with the first Christian centuries, they cannot be taken as products of a budding culture; they and the art surrounding them are too mature not to have a longer past behind them. However, the remnants of the beginning phases of pre-Columbian civilization are lost, just as children's clothing disappears from the wardrobe as a boy grows to a man; it is doubtful if they will ever be found to any great extent.

In examining the problem of evolution or influence, let us first consider the date and type of the earliest veritable arts in the Eastern Hemisphere. Investigations in China, in the Mohenjo-daro Valley in India, in the Ur Valley of

Mesopotamia, and in Egypt enable us to look back as far as 3800 to 4500 B.C., and, since the architectural or minor-art discoveries from that time show so much expression and skill in technique, we can assume that a formative period preceded them. Thus, considering the slow movement of prehistoric development, the so-called "horizon" of the cultures there can be pushed back well beyond the fourth millennium before Christ.

The prehistory of less civilized regions, on the other hand, is more uncertain. Various findings suggest movement of peoples and very early intercourse over long distances. As early as the Middle Stone Age, pottery types of the Danube Basin turned up in India. Nor was the spread of culture prevented by strips of water: as early as 7000 B.C. small geometric flint implements, known to have occurred previously only in eastern and northern Europe, had crossed over Gibraltar into North Africa.[106]

The greater migrations of some of the Mongolian peoples into Europe since the Christian era are familiar to us from history. The Huns, Avars, Magyars, Tatars all started in central Asia and in some cases reached as far as France. These waves, accelerated by the use of the horse and wheeled cart, brought numerous innovations from the nomad peoples that enriched European civilization—the stirrup, trousers, the cup with handles, among others.

It is possible, however, that even before the great migration took place in the direction of Europe, there were drifts toward the east into America. Most migrations seem to start from the need of new hunting and fishing grounds, or, with a pastoral people, for more adequate grazing land; the push of successful warlike tribes often drove before them a more peaceful population. These martial forces were doubtless at work also before history was recorded. Primitive peoples, as hunters and fishers, mobile and with few possessions, would follow first the forest and the water, and only later, as herders of domesticated cattle, more numerous and ponderous in movement, would they search the plains.

As such hunters and fishers, the early inhabitants of pre-Columbian America are believed to have crossed the Bering Strait. They came in bands, clad in animal skins, possibly over a land bridge or perhaps in boats, using the islands as stepping-stones. Probably they never amounted to any great number; this hemisphere was populated not by them but by their descendants. Certainly they were not conscious of the fact that they were treading the soil of another continent. The distance today from one mainland to the other is fifty-six miles. The stretch is broken by three islands, one of them four miles in length, so that the longest section of open water is twenty-five miles, across which one can see even in moderately clear weather. The embracing line of the Aleutian Islands marks off a sort of basin—the Bering Sea with its shores in both Siberia and Alaska. Even with crude water craft it would not require too much courage to cross to a land clearly visible with islands breaking the way. It has been pointed out that travel on foot would also have been possible during the time when the region was covered with ice.[134]

The case for the land bridge is also good. Where the two continents approach, like two animal profiles facing each other across the strait, the present depth of the water is less than one hundred eighty feet. This shallowness might indicate that a land bridge, now submerged, existed before cosmic upheavals produced the present topography. Excavations thirty feet below the present water level have revealed old beach deposits.

The Mongolian and the American Indian have some physical characteristics in common. Their head measurements are close. Both have scanty beard growth and little body hair in contrast to the Caucasian. Their hair is generally straight, while that of the white race is wavy and of the black, woolly.

Dr. Ewing, as quoted by Hans Zinsser in the following excerpt, introduces the head louse of the pre-Columbian peoples as evidence from another angle. "The scalps of hair samples from twenty prehistoric American Indian mummies were secured. It was found that the insects from Peruvian mummies were slightly different from those taken in the Southwestern United States, and that all the lice from prehistoric mummy scalps showed differences from some of the lice obtained from a living Indian. The louse adapts its color to that of the host, so that we have the black louse of Africa, the smoky louse of the Hindu, the yellowish brown of the Japanese, the dark brown one of the North American Indian, the pale brown one of the Eskimo, and the dirty gray one of the European. This prehistoric American louse has been described as quite similar to the Chinese head louse and to the lice found upon Aleutian Eskimos—another argument for the 'Migration' across the Bering Straits." [173]

Thus, there is evidence of relationship between the pre-Columbian American and the Mongolian or proto-Mongolian; but contact must have ceased early, as there are a number of basic Old World inventions and cultural achievements that are not found in the New. Early archaeological finds in Asia, dated approximately 4000 B.C., reveal an established and well-developed agriculture. On a cylinder seal of the fourth millennium B.C. from the Ur Valley in Mesopotamia the Sumerian type of plow is depicted, with a plowshare and two handles, a long curved pole, and two tackles for yokes over a pair of oxen.[172] The same subject, an animal-drawn plow, appears in a wall-painting from the 12th Dynasty in Egypt, about 2800 B.C. Terra-cotta models of chariots with disk wheels are also found in Mesopotamia from a very early Sumerian period. Certain Chinese ceramic pieces show the use of the potter's wheel before 1800 B.C.

On the other hand, the principle of the wheel, the use of the plow, and the domestication of beasts of burden (except the llama) were all unknown to pre-Columbian America. The agricultural implement here was the planting stick (see *Pl. 291, figs. b* and *c*). The only domesticated animals were the dog, the turkey, some other forms of poultry (ducks and hens) in certain regions, and, in addition, in the Andean Area, the llama and related groups. The case of the llama, herded locally for its wool and sometimes for its meat, serves to strengthen the argument for the early isolation of the continents, for this member of the camel family must itself have branched off at a very early period to have developed into an animal so unlike its Asiatic relatives.

The domesticated horse figures in the prehistoric civilizations of Asia from at least 3000 B.C.,[113] but the pre-Columbian peoples were overwhelmed at the sight of the horses ridden by the *conquistadores*. They thought at first that rider and horse were one, a superhuman creature. Even later, in one isolated stronghold of the Maya, an incapacitated animal left behind by the Spaniards was treated with reverence and awe, as if it were a living god; offerings of maize, flowers, and copal were made to it. At its death, a statue was erected to the new deity. A population so ignorant of the use of the horse could certainly not have had much intercourse with Asia, where for millennia the movement and migrations of nations had been based increasingly on that animal.

Rice, wheat, rye, and barley, the staple grains of the Near and Far East from prehistoric times were alien to the Western Hemisphere, while maize, beans, squash, tomatoes, potatoes, peanuts, and tobacco were New World discoveries to the Spaniards. The early Americans used the spear-thrower and blowgun, much more primitive weapons than the bow and arrow which appear late, relatively a short time before the Conquest and only in some sections. Bronze was unknown except in parts of South America. To all intents and purposes, the people remained within the neolithic phase. Furthermore, no satisfactory evidence has been found to identify a New World language with an Old World stock, except for the idiom of the Eskimos, who are a group by themselves.[169]

The great variety of Indian tongues indicates that numerous waves of different peoples, perhaps originating in diverse regions of the Old World, found habitation here. The difference in quality of the various pre-Columbian cultures, as well as the various burial customs, substantiates this theory. That the American Indians are, however, closely related to one another in racial stock is shown by the fact that a very high percentage (80 to 90) of pure-blooded Indians, whether from Peru, Yucatan, or Baffin Bay, belongs to the blood-group O.[173]

Musicology adds its own findings to the problem. It is interesting that all relatives of pre-Columbian musical instruments, aside from a few universal ones, are found exclusively in China, India, the Malay Archipelago, and the Pacific Islands. Outside of America, the notched flute is said to be confined to the Far East, including Mongolia. The absolute pitches and the scales of pre-Columbian, Melanesian, and eastern Asiatic panpipes have been found to be alike. Against these findings stands the complete absence of stringed instruments in the aboriginal cultures of America. In Asia as well as the Near East, the lute and lyre were known in legendary times. They were not only recorded on reliefs and in minor sculptures, but remnants of actual instruments have been excavated in several sites, in connection with cultures older than 3000 B.C. In China the long zither is mentioned in an ode written about 1100 B.C.; in due time it spread to the Malay Archipelago and most of the larger Pacific Islands. In pre-Columbian America all the instruments belonged to a groping stage of musical development. If those regions in the Old World had any influence on the cultures here, it must have been in very early prehistoric times.[119]

All this evidence would indicate that migrations of any importance must have ceased before the Old World achievements mentioned had been acquired or, at any rate, before they had reached that part of Asia from which the early Americans came. It does not, however, preclude a drift of Arctic tribes back and forth, relaying locally certain cultural traits. Bone and wood carvings of the northwest coast of British Columbia and Alaska point to this and are frequently referred to in discussion of similarities between the pre-Columbian and Asiatic arts. These cultures unquestionably profited from the rich and established form-world of the northeast coast of Asia. But in concept and execution their work is strongly differentiated from the art of the various pre-Columbian areas presented here. The specimens offered are mostly of post-Columbian date and prove only that local contacts had been made from Asiatic to American shores even before the Russians came with their ships as far as San Francisco Bay.

The thesis that there was also a prehistoric migration to America across the Pacific Ocean cannot be accepted so far. Accumulating facts point more and more to the relative lateness of the movement which populated Polynesia.[17] The early Maya and Andean cultures were already past their zenith when the Pacific Islands were being settled by the races who dwell there today. The migrations to the Polynesian Islands from the Asiatic mainland required considerable seamanship and knowledge of navigation, and the people of this region still retain their nautical skill. At the time of the Conquest, however, in America, there was not the slightest evidence of a seafaring tradition such as would surely have survived among a people able to cross the vast Pacific.

Today when the synthesis of Eurasian cultures has been achieved to a considerable extent, it is tempting to formulate conclusions in a similar vein for the pre-Columbian civilization. However, before our knowledge will be adequate for the task, much further investigation will first be necessary—not only in the Western Hemisphere but in the northeastern regions of Asia, where the Stone Age lasted longer than in what we know as China.

On the whole, the arts of most early cultures seem nearest alike when they first express their ideas unhesitatingly and, to our eyes, artistically, although without the sharp regional characteristics which later serve to separate them. We must not forget that in primitive art parallel solutions for parallel problems were often worked out with similar neolithic tools. On the other hand, we ourselves are doubtless frequently at fault in failing to see greater differences in the various manifestations. All of them have an alien radiation for us; we are deceived by their "primitiveness" and their strangeness and class them all together, unable to distinguish with finesse the unrealistic, the stylized, and the symbolic. Our eyes and minds are still inadequate for the full appraisal and we find ourselves trying to measure incommensurables.

There are some semblances between the mature arts of medieval America and the higher civilizations of the Eastern Hemisphere that have led to attempts to establish a definite connection between these, too. Careful cool-headed comparison of specimens from both regions, however, will show that such similarities are optical illusions.

The scholars indulging in such theorizing all too frequently are primarily Sinologists, Egyptologists, or others from remote fields, who would not venture into far-fetched deductions in dealing with early civilizations of the East. Their methods show from the start several defects. They have seldom been in any of the regions where pre-Columbian art originated. Their conclusions are based on second-hand reports and are the result of preconceived ideas, not of a careful and impersonal survey of the entire field. In the absence of the actual objects, they have hunted out illustrations to substantiate their theories that are too often retouched photographs or inaccurate drawings, thus betraying a lack of discrimination in a most important factor in any discussion of the arts. It requires great skill and thorough occupation with the pre-Columbian cultures to make adequate copies of their specimens. Pre-Columbian art was created and developed by a mentality totally alien to ours. An artist trained to our beauty ideals and technical mannerisms will unconsciously approach the pre-Columbian subject biased by his preconceptions. The writer was furnished startling proof of this during the preparation of this survey, when a friend, an anthropologist steeped in the study of primitive art, failed to identify a small sculpture from a new photograph, although he was familiar with a drawing of the same piece as published in an authoritative book. He admitted that the subject was identical but maintained that both spirit and linear conduct in the two reproductions were dissimilar.

Photography and the making of plaster casts are methods in which our function is purely administrative and not creative. A clear photograph, a precise cast, remaining neutral, at least will not guide us onto false trails, as sketches, retouched plates, and the like, unavoidably do. It is for this reason that we have included very few drawings and models, even though occasionally a photograph is not entirely satisfactory.

One of the comparisons most frequently presented to link medieval American and Oriental art places Ulúa marble vases (see *Pls. 94* and *95*) beside Chinese bronze vessels from the Shang or Chou dynasties. At first glance, even to one familiar with the two styles, a certain pattern will show a superficial similarity, but sober scrutiny will dispel this impression. The group which advocates direct Asiatic influence in this instance bases their argument on one particular element. This is the curving "dragon" motif of the Chinese vessels, which they consider to have influenced the fret-scroll pattern, the main decorative theme, of the Ulúa vases.

As we have seen in the chapter on sculpture, the Ulúa vases are a localized product from one valley in Honduras and are believed to date around the 10th century of our era, or later. They do not show great variety of form and are, upon inspection, quite simple—generally cylindrical, varying from deep to shallow, and almost without exception with handles in the shape of animals. The greater part of the surface is carved with fret-scrolls and with animal-masks made up of the same elements. Gnashing teeth are always features.

Compare these with the ceremonial bronzes of the Shang (1766–1122 B.C.) and Chou (1122–249 B.C.) dynasties. The many hundreds of these beautiful specimens of cast metal fall into twenty-eight general types, with complicated and often unsymmetrical shapes, many with deep spouts, movable handles, and especially fitted and ornamented covers. There are square canisters and gourd-shaped wine vessels. The horned animal—not the toothed—is featured and some are stamped with the Chinese character for "ox." The mask-panels of the Chinese pieces are executed in high relief and embellished with intricate ornament, while the backgrounds are filled with subordinate designs. Bernard Karlgren, who made an intensive study of the ancient Chinese vessels, proves that in the earliest examples every curve had a dragon head, and analyzes the permutations of the figure through the centuries until it became more and more a conventional coil.[111] A vertical tendency is apparent in the pieces.

In contrast, the decoration of the Ulúa vases presents a horizontal trend. Their relief is low, the design linear, the masks are unemphasized, and there is an absence of secondary pattern. It is evident that the fleeting similarity between the fret-scrolls of the Ulúa vases and the Chinese bronzes is most marked when the Chou design loses its realistic meaning and becomes a facile stylized pattern.

If there had been intercourse between China and pre-Columbian America, then the art of complicated bronze casting also should have reached the Western Hemisphere; as we know, it was only approximated here millennia later, within a limited area, and with small objects. One would expect writing in characters also to have been transmitted or the use of coins adopted—current in China since the third millennium B.C.—to take the place of the woven blankets, cocoa, and the like, which served as a medium of exchange among the Indians. In other words, China had many more important cultural advantages to pass on to the rising pre-Columbian peoples than a mere square-cornered spiral motif.

If, as has been suggested, contact was only sporadic, one asks why the precious vessel was not more accurately "copied." If nothing even approaching the shape or general design of the Chinese bronzes is visible in the Ulúa vases, why should we accept as an indication of influence the application of one reminiscent detail-motif of a scroll, used as a stereotyped "fill-in"—one of the least obtrusive features of the bronzes? How did it happen that a Shang or Chou vessel, dating from three hundred to eighteen hundred years before Christ, should have reached the Ulúa Valley, not one more nearly contemporary to the period of "copying," for instance, a vessel from the Han or T'ang dynasties, very different in character?

The greatest argument, however, for the independence of the Ulúa vases from Chinese influence lies in the fact that they are completely integrated with the artistic scheme of indigenous Middle American cultures. They show some relation to the Chorotegan pottery with animal handles from the south and to certain other pottery types of the neighborhood. The fret-scroll motif runs throughout Middle American art, from the early wood lintel at Tikal to the stone relief at Tajín. As individual and localized as the marble vases are, they nevertheless speak an autochthonous language to those who are familiar with it and do not require a far-fetched theory to explain their presence here.

Where similarity to the Oriental motif exists, it is in examples from both continents in which the pattern has become degenerate. Peru offers another case in point. Here the art became much more stylized and condensed than in Middle America and its geometric character lends itself still more easily to generalization.

There is and probably always will be a school of archaeologists and art-historians—"insectologists" of the humanities—who value the detail above the whole. For them, sections of a design will always carry more weight than the spirit of the entire piece. They start from a spiral, a step pattern, a repeated square, knowing already where they intend to arrive. The specimen is important for them only because it carries the motif upon which their theory is based. What does not fit their picture is disregarded. The ambition to bring parallels and to show influences becomes a working method, so that in the end not the essence of a civilization is taken into consideration but rather the best examples obtainable for a series of comparisons.

To pursue pattern details that are only superficially similar brings one to a dead end. The invention of patterns is technically limited and many of them are universal; the dash, circle, square, oblong, spiral, star or cross, swastika—all were invented and used by several civilizations independently during long centuries of development. The models for most of them can be found in nature. Even similarity in ideology is not necessarily to be explained by contact, for it may be the result of parallel development—very possible in races that branched from the same family tree in an early time, at present undeterminable.

The problems facing research in the civilization of medieval America are far from solved. Because of the mystery which surrounds most of its phases and because the approach can be made through different branches of the humanities —exploring new ground—the field is all the more fascinating. But its greatest attraction lies in its imposing body of art, unique in its psychological apartness. When finally, in decades to come, the chronology of pre-Columbian cultures has been established in greater detail and the various styles are more precisely defined, it will still remain for our perception to read from the reconstructed picture the living impulses that created on this continent in isolation the admirable material for a new chapter in the history of art.

Addenda to the Second Edition

THE area of present-day Mexico included the greatest variety of individual artistic cultures in the New World before Columbus. At the sites of La Venta, Tres Zapotes and San Lorenzo in southern Mexico, colossal stone heads of an ancient culture were excavated. The head in *Pl. 307, fig. b* was found lying on its side almost completely buried in the dense jungle of San Lorenzo, by the distinguished archaeologist Matthew W. Stirling, who is here pictured beside it. Measuring 5 feet 4 inches in height, it is in a perfect state of preservation. The face has powerful sculptural detail, an unparalleled achievement with tools of stone. Chin, mouth, nose, cheeks are admirably modeled. But most remarkable are the eyes, carved with a fine, sure line. Their gaze is focused; the iris even has the naturalistic, accomplished touch of a double margin framing it. The headgear is highly conventionalized; any protruding elements would have been out of keeping with the unyielding monumentality of the piece. Four horizontal bands with oblique grooving contrast with plain vertical ones that suggest drooping feathers or perhaps tassels. Ear-flaps complete the casque-like effect. Up to now, ten such colossal heads have been unearthed in this region, sometimes near stone altars of comparable dimensions. With their distinctive character, these heads are a great addition to the artistic picture of the Olmec culture. (For Olmec jade carving see *Pls. 243, 247, 252* and *253,* with corresponding text.)

Monumental stone figures of diverse styles have been found in northern Mexico, in Guatemala, Nicaragua, Costa Rica, Colombia, Peru, and Bolivia. In southern Colombia, several centuries before the Spanish Conquest, a culture flourished which left about 300 stone carvings within a comparatively small region. The statues among these usually combine human and animal traits and range as high as 14 feet (see p. 149). Traces of black, white, red, and yellow coloring are to be seen on them. Since many were found near the village of San Agustín (Department of Huila) that name was given to the culture. They

The material in this section originally appeared within the preface to the second (1956) edition at the place indicated on page xviii of the first volume of the present edition.

are thought to belong to an early period of Colombian archaeology, but on account of their diversity of manner they may have been produced over several centuries. The sculpture (*fig. d*), nearly 3½ feet high, re-erected on the site, presents a warrior brandishing a club with both hands. The carving is angular, the expression uncommunicative. The animal headdress, which was found broken off from the lower section, is given more plastic treatment. Animals as "totems" or symbols of the "alter ego" appear frequently in these works. In this case, the attitude suggests the Diving-god encountered also in other pre-Columbian cultures.

An entirely human representation, 4½ feet tall (*fig. e*), comes from Moscopán in a neighboring region and stands today in the courtyard of the University of Popayán. The manner of carving the body shows relationship with that of the statue of San Agustín, in the angularity of the legs, the stance with forward bent knees, and the overlarge head. The face is more communicative, the expression less grim. He wears a breastplate on a chain and his large earplugs are carefully depicted. The headdress is standardized into a block. On the bulging stone surface of the eyeballs no sculptural attempt was made to suggest the iris; perhaps this was done with color.

The Diving-god or a being descending from the sky occurs also in metal, on a gold mantle pin (*fig. a*) from the Quimbaya culture of Colombia. The pre-Columbian Indian generally wore untailored garments and such ornamental pins served to hold the textiles in place. This one is 12½ inches in total length, the figure 2⅛ inches high. It was manufactured by the "lost wax" process of casting (see p. 241). Here virtuosity in handling the medium is revealed in the highly stylized representation with its ceremonial feathers, extended arms and trailing legs. The zigzag decoration on top gives us the sense of propulsion by lightning.

The plumed and helmeted man on another gold mantle pin (*fig. c*) is related artistically to the three other Colombian examples on this plate. He carries a spear-thrower in his right hand and a ceremonial knife in his left (see *Pls. 217, 272*). His earrings, dangling free, add special animation. The little ram-like animal on his back may have symbolic meaning. A rich quilted pattern decorates his poncho, or shirt, which is repeated on the lower part of the socle. This figure proper measures 1¾ inches and is cast also by the lost wax process so skillfully that, from the front, his eyes can be seen shining through the slits of his helmet. Among San Agustín stone sculpture, one encounters a version of this helmeted man, simplified for the medium. The concept of the Diving-god ap-

< 383 >

pears over a wider territory. He is depicted in Late Maya art, in stucco, on the Temple of the Frescoes at Tulum (see p. 74). Flying or plunging figures are represented also on Peruvian textiles (see *Pls. 175, 177*). Further examples of iconographic parallels in different media or from different cultures will be found in the book.

Many exciting discoveries of Maya art have been made in southern Mexico, where the state of Chiapas meets Guatemala territory. Unfortunately this is a region of tropical rain forest which not only jealously guards the treasures within its boundaries but also destroys them with its climate. Some ruins along the Usumacinta River have long been known, such as Piedras Negras and Yaxchilán. About 20 miles south of the latter site, a ruined city was discovered which harbored the murals of Bonampak, "the painted walls." The building had been familiar to the Lacandón Indians for a long time and contained some of their incense burners. Taken to the temple by a member of the tribe, Giles G. Healy brought the first photographs out of the jungle. On the walls of three rooms of a single building, an epic tale is unfolded. In the first is seen a dance by impersonators of gods to the accompaniment of rattles, drums, and trumpets. In the second room, prisoners are taken in a raid and brought before high dignitaries. Finally, a ceremony of great pomp and a triumphal dance take place. Reproduced here (*Pl. 308, fig. a*) is a scene showing the arraignment of captives before a group of chieftains gathered on a platform to which broad steps lead. The ruler is distinguished by his swaying feather headdress and imperiously posed staff, which require twice as much space as the others; thus spatial emphasis brings out his importance. Including his plumes, the figure stands about 4 feet tall. A large jade mask adorns his chest (see *Pls. 89, 90*). His nearest companions carry clubs, distinctly different from the staffs that appear on the extreme left. Every one of the high-ranking personages wears an individual costume—their headdresses of jaguar, peccary, and deer heads, their clothing of feathers and textiles, as well as animal skins, can be noted. In the display of jaguar skins and heads analogy might be found to the lion skins worn by heroes of classical times and the lion masks on helmets and breastplates of Renaissance armor. At the extreme right, a woman—probably the wife of the ruler—appears in an off-shoulder white gown, with necklace of large jade beads, pendant earrings, and a fan. One prisoner cowers at the ruler's feet and others crouch on the steps below, naked except for loincloths, in amazingly differentiated attitudes of trepidation and despair. The prone figure in the center—

< 384 >

their leader perhaps—is unconscious or dead. The red on their fingers and the drops visible on the left have been interpreted as blood. The captives are represented as of lower intelligence than the victorious chiefs; their features are coarse, their hair is stringy and unkempt. This manifest contrasting of pomp and dignity with dejection and misery creates an artistic counterpoint of universal emotions.

Eye-witnesses of the Conquest of the Americas describe in detail the dazzling splendor, the colorful costumes and fantastic paraphernalia of the Indians with whom they dealt in their first meetings. In this mural, though it is not fully intelligible to us, we have a sample of such magnificence. Those who are shocked by the barbarism of the scene are referred to the innumerable acts of the Inquisition and courts of treason in Europe, when so-called civilized Christians tortured and burned their brothers and their neighbors, into the present century.

The murals were reconstructed in a water-color series, from sketches and measurements made at the site. In *fig. b,* the twisted figure of the prone captive is shown in the original photograph taken at Bonampak. While not as colorful as the larger scene above, the photograph shows the drawing as the mural painter executed it at the beginning of the 9th century. This detail is fragmentary, yet the impact of the figure is forceful and immediate. The admirably turned pose presages the invention of three-dimensional representation. The conduct of the brush can be intimately followed, suggesting in a single sweep the elasticity of the young body. Note the light shading under the chin, the softness of the hair in contrast to that of the other prisoners, the right hand with its curled fingers curving forward with full naturalism to rest on the thigh. The laxness of the hanging left arm is expressed with assurance. An engraving-like unbroken line frames the outstretched body. Although the mural is devoted to the depiction of victory, through the arrangement of the various compositional elements the prone captive becomes the vital center of action.

It would seem that, as with most wall-paintings in pre-Columbian America, the outlines of the composition were first drawn on the dry wall and the colors then filled in. The mastery of the Maya painter becomes evident in its full dimensions only when pottery and manuscripts, as well as the murals, are considered.

Not far from Bonampak, also in the state of Chiapas, is the great Maya site of Palenque, famous for many decades. Here a rich tomb was discovered beneath the massive pyramidal base of the Temple of the Inscriptions. The stucco head in *fig. c* was apparently broken from a statue. It is 17 inches high and

< 385 >

has been dated around the end of the 7th century. In elegance it rivals successfully the head of the ruler in the Bonampak mural. But while the mural painter had only to delineate a head in profile with its picturesque paraphernalia, on a wall surface, the Maya sculptor had to form it in three dimensions. The flattened forehead, the nose and chin, as well as the flat surfaces on the cheekbones, make up the classic Maya profile. An extremely fine, aristocratic ear is clearly modeled. The headdress with its flamboyant feathers reminds one of the Maya Maize-god (*Pl. 90*). Tassels with their grooving are arranged in a two-tiered build-up. A garland of lily buds introduces a different texture, with their well-caught waxy quality, and a new plastic element. (See also *Pl. 81*.) All this is crowned by a feather bush in truly lively flow. The soft material of the stucco lent itself excellently for such a depiction—from the technical point of view a delicate and difficult task but, as seen here, also a most grateful one. Lively colors most probably defined the various details. (For other stucco work, see *Pls. 80, 86*.)

< 386 >

Bibliography

The literature dealing with pre-Columbian civilization is extremely voluminous. Eyewitnesses and early chroniclers of the Conquest treated it mostly from a historical point of view, but their works are full of important observations which give a clue to the archaeology and ethnology of the various regions. During the viceregal period, a long line of commentators and historians, many of them influenced by preconceived theories or prejudices, occupied themselves with the past of the Indians. With the 19th century, the study of man began to be permeated with an enlightened spirit, and the literature of this period shows a tendency toward objective approach and accuracy. In the last thirty years, the field of research has divided itself more and more into particular branches of the subject.

Lack of space prevents us from giving a full list of these books as well as the names of various scientific and museum periodicals and publications in Europe, Latin America, and the United States, which are full of valuable notes and papers. Our modern and admirably organized libraries can furnish comprehensive bibliographies. Only those titles are included here which were used as source works or may be suggestive to the general reader for further pursuit of the subject. Books which have an extensive or valuable bibliography are marked with a dagger; the numbers denote text references.

Ackerman, Phyllis
   Tapestry, the Mirror of Civilization. London, 1933.
   [1] Handwoven Textiles. Pasadena, 1935.
Adam, L.
   Primitive Art. London, 1940.
Alexander, Herbert J., and Reiter, Paul
   [2] Report on the Excavations of Jemez Cave, N.M. Albuquerque, 1935.
Amsden, Charles Avery
   Navaho Weaving. Los Angeles, 1934.
Andrews, E. Wyllys
   A Group of Related Sculptures from Yucatan in *CIW Contrib. to Am. Anthro. and Hist.* Washington, 1939.
   Chronology and Astronomy in the Maya Area in "The Maya and their Neighbors," *q.v.*
[3] "Archeological Monuments of Mexico." 150 pages of illustrations. New York, 1933.

Baessler, Arthur
   Altperuanische Kunst. Berlin, 1902–03.

Baldwin, G. C.
Further Notes on Basket Maker III Sandals from Northeastern Arizona in *American Anthropologist,* 1939.

Baltimore Museum of Art
The Art of the Maya. Catalogue. Baltimore, 1937.

Bandelier, Adolph F.
The Islands of Titicaca and Koati. New York, 1910.

Bandelier, Adolph F., and Hewett, Edgar L.
[4] Indians of the Rio Grande Valley. Albuquerque, 1937.

Bartle, Ira B., San Luis Obispo, Calif.
[5] Correspondence on diseases of pre-Columbian times.

Basler, Adolphe, and Brummer, Ernest
L'Art Précolombien. Paris, 1928.

Bennett, Wendell C.
Peruvian Gold in *Natural History,* 1932.
Excavations at Tiahuanaco. New York, 1934.
[6] Machu Picchu in *Natural History,* 1935.
[7] Weaving in the Land of the Incas in *Natural History,* 1935.
Excavations at La Mata, Maracay, Venezuela. New York, 1937.
Chimu Archeology in *Scientific Monthly,* 1937.
Archaeology of the North Coast of Peru. New York, 1939.
Chavin Stone Carving. New Haven, 1942.
[8] Critical review and correspondence on this survey.

Bergsoe, Paul
[9] The Metallurgy and Technology of Gold and Platinum among the Pre-Columbian Indians. Copenhagen, 1937.
[10] The Gilding Process and the Metallurgy of Copper and Lead among the Pre-Columbian Indians. Copenhagen, 1938.

Bevan, Bernard
The Chinantec. Mexico, 1938.

Beyer, Hermann
The Stylistic History of the Maya Hieroglyphs. New Orleans, 1932.
[11] Shell Ornament Sets. New Orleans, 1933.

Bingham, Hiram
[12] The Discovery of Machu Picchu in *Harper's Magazine,* 1913.
[13] Inca Land. Boston, 1922.
Machu Picchu, a Citadel of the Incas. New Haven, 1930.

Blom, Frans
Commerce, Trade and Monetary Units of the Maya in *Middle American Papers.* New Orleans, 1932.
The Maya Ball-game in *Middle American Papers.* New Orleans, 1932.
L'Art Maya in *Gazette des Beaux-Arts,* 1933.
The Conquest of Yucatan. Boston, 1936.
[14] Unpublished manuscript on Maya pottery flasks (with H. Beyer).

< 388 >

BIBLIOGRAPHY

Blom, Frans, and La Farge, Oliver
[15] Tribes and Temples.   New Orleans, 1926.

Boas, Franz
Album de Colecciones Arqueológicas.   Mexico, 1911–12.
Primitive Art.   Oslo, 1927.   (Dover reprint)

Boyle, Mary E.
In Search of Our Ancestors.   London, 1927.

Brand, Donald D., and Harvey, Fred E. *Editors*
So Live the Works of Men.   Albuquerque, **1939.**

Braunholtz, H. J.
[16] A Gold Pendant from Ancient Colombia in *The British Museum Quarterly,*
1939.

Brenner, Anita
Idols behind Altars.   New York, 1929.

Brown, F. Martin
America's Yesterday.   Philadelphia, 1937.

Brummer, Ernest.   *See* Basler, Adolphe

Bryan, Kirk
Geologic Antiquity of Man in America in *Science,* 1941.

Buck, Peter H.
[17] †Vikings of the Sunrise.   New York, 1938.

Butler, Mary
A Pottery Sequence from the Alta Verapaz, Guatemala, in "The Maya and
their Neighbors," *q.v.*

Byers, D. S., and La Farge, Oliver
The Yearbearer's People.   New Orleans, 1931.

Cahill, Holger
American Sources of Modern Art.   Catalogue.   Museum of Modern Art, New
York, 1933.

Carbrera, Paul Felix
[18] Description of the Ruins near Palenque.   London, 1822.

Carnegie Institution of Washington
[19] The Great "White Ways" of the Maya in *News Service Bulletin,* Sept. 24, 1933.

Caso, Alfonso
[20] Las Estelas Zapotecas.   Mexico, 1928.
[21] The Use of Masks among the Ancient Mexicans in *Mexican Folkways,* 1929.
[22] Las Exploraciones en Monte Albán.   Mexico, 1932.
[23] Reading the Riddle of Ancient Jewels in *Natural History,* 1932.
The Religion of the Aztecs.   Mexico, 1937.
[24] Exploraciones en Oaxaca.   Mexico, 1938.
[25] Thirteen Masterpieces of Mexican Archaeology.   *Tr.* by Edith Mackie and
Jorge R. Acosta.   Mexico, 1938.

Pre-Spanish Art in "Twenty Centuries of Mexican Art," Museum of Modern Art (N.Y.) Catalogue. 1940.

Casson, Stanley
  Progress of Archaeology. London, 1934.

Catherwood, Frederick
  Views of Ancient Monuments in Central America, Chiapas and Yucatan. London, 1844.

"The Changing Indian." *Ed.* by Oliver La Farge. Norman, Okla., 1942.

Chapman, Kenneth M.
  Pueblo Indian Pottery. Nice, France, 1933 and 1936.
  The Pottery of Santo Domingo Pueblo. Santa Fé, 1939.

Charlot, Jean
  Mayan Art in *American Magazine of Art,* 1935.
  See also Morris, Earl H.

Charnay, Désiré, and Viollet-le-Duc, E. E.
  Cités et Ruines Américaines. Paris, 1863.

Clark, J. Cooper
  [26] The Story of "Eight Deer." London, 1912.
  [27] *Editor* and *translator,* Codex Mendoza, the Mexican Manuscript known as the Collection of Mendoza and preserved in the Bodleian Library, Oxford. London, 1938.

Cobo, Bernabé
  [28] Historia del Nuevo Mundo. Seville, 1890–93.

Colton, Harold Sellers
  Prehistoric Trade in the Southwest in *Scientific Monthly,* 1941.

Cordry, Donald B. and Dorothy M.
  Costumes and Textiles of the Aztec Indians of the Cuetzalán Region, Puebla, Mexico. Los Angeles, 1940.

Cortés, Hernando
  Five Letters. *Tr.* by J. Bayard Morris. London, 1928.

Cossío-Pijoán
  Summa Artis. Madrid, 1931.

Crawford, Morris De Camp
  Peruvian Textiles. New York, 1915.
  Peruvian Fabrics. New York, 1916.
  The Heritage of Cotton. New York, 1924.
  The Conquest of Culture. New York, 1938.

Cunow, Heinrich
  [29] Geschichte und Kultur des Inkareiches. Amsterdam, 1937.

Davis, Emily C.
  [30] Ancient Americans. New York, 1931.

Densmore, Frances
  Cheyenne and Arapaho Music. Los Angeles, 1936.

Díaz, Bernal, del Castillo
    The Discovery and Conquest of Mexico. *Tr.* by A. P. Maudslay. London, 1928.
Doering, Heinrich. *See* Lehmann, Walter
Dorsey, George
    Archaeological Investigations on the Islands of La Plata, Ecuador. Chicago, 1898.
Douglas, Frederic H.
    Numerous articles on Indian art in *Denver Art Museum Leaflets.*
Douglas, Frederic H., and d'Harnoncourt, René
    [31] †Indian Art of the United States. New York, 1941.
Douglass, A. E.
    [32] Dating Pueblo Bonito and Other Ruins of the Southwest. Washington, 1935.
Dupaix, Guillelmo
    Antiquités Mexicaines. Paris, 1834.

"Early Man." A compilation. *Ed.* by George Grant MacCurdy. Philadelphia, 1937.
Ekholm, Gordon F.
    The Archaeology of Northern and Western Mexico in "The Maya and their Neighbors," *q.v.*
Emmons, George T.
    Jade in British Columbia and Alaska. New York, 1923.
"Essays in Anthropology." A compilation. *Ed.* by Robert H. Lowie. Berkeley, 1936.
Estrada, Genaro
    [33] El Arte Mexicano en España. Mexico, 1937.
"Exposición de Escultura Mexicana Antigua." Catalogue. Mexico, 1934.

Farabee, W. C.
    Ancient American Gold in *The Museum Journal,* Philadelphia, 1920.
    [34] A Golden Hoard from Ecuador in *The Museum Journal,* 1921.
Fejös, Paul
    [35] Correspondence concerning excavations in Andean highlands.
Ferdon, Edwin N., Jr.
    Reconnaissance in Esmeraldas in *El Palacio,* 1940.
    Preliminary Notes on Artifacts from La Libertad, Ecuador, in *El Palacio,* 1941.
Fergusson, Harvey
    [36] Rio Grande. New York, 1933.
Fewkes, Jesse Walter
    Two Summers' Work in Pueblo Ruins. Washington, 1904.
    Antiquities of Mesa Verde National Park. Washington, 1911.
    Designs on Prehistoric Pottery from the Mimbres Valley, New Mexico. Washington, 1924.
Fleure, Herbert John. *See* Peake, Harold

< 391 >

Fogg Art Museum
  † An Exhibition of Pre-Columbian Art. Catalogue. Cambridge, 1940.
Fry, Roger
  Last Lectures. New York, 1939.

Gage, Thomas
  The English-American. A New Survey of the West Indies, 1648. *Ed.* by
    A. P. Newton. London, 1928.
Gallop, Rodney
  Mexican Mosaic. London, 1939.
Gamio, Manuel
  Las Excavaciones del Pedregal de San Angel y la Cultura Arcáica del Valle de
    México. Mexico, 1920.
  La Población del Valle de Teotihuacán. Mexico, 1922.
Gann, T.
  Mounds in Northern Honduras. Washington, 1900.
Gann, T., and Thompson, J. Eric
  The History of the Maya. New York, 1931.
Gates, William, *editor* and *translator*
  Yucatan by Friar Diego de Landa. Baltimore, 1937.
  [37] The de la Cruz—Badiano Aztec Herbal of 1552. Baltimore, 1939.
Gladwin, Harold S., and associates
  Excavations at Snaketown. Globe, Ariz., 1937.
Goddard, Pliny Earle
  [38] Indians of the Southwest. New York, 1931.
Golden Gate International Exposition
  Pacific Cultures. Catalogue. San Francisco, 1939.
  Aboriginal Cultures of the Western Hemisphere. Catalogue. San Francisco,
    1940.
Gordon, G. B.
  [39] Pre-Historic Ruins of Copan. Cambridge, 1896.
  [40] Caverns of Copan. Cambridge, 1898.
  [41] Researches in the Ulua Valley. Cambridge, 1898.
  Examples of Maya Pottery in the Museum and other Collections. *Ed.* by J. A.
    Mason. Philadelphia, 1925 and 1928.

Halle, Louis J., Jr.
  [42] River of Ruins. New York, 1941.
Hammond, Harriet
  [43] Maya Art in *Fogg Art Museum Notes*. Cambridge, 1930.
Hamy, E. T.
  Galérie Américaine du Musée d'Ethnographie du Trocadéro. Paris, 1897.
  [44] Note sur Une Statuette Mexicaine in *Journal de la Société des Américanistes,*
    1906.

d'Harcourt, Raoul
Les Textiles Anciens du Pérou et leurs Techniques. Paris, 1924.
L'Ocarina à Cinq Sons dans l'Amérique Préhispanique in *Journal de la Société des Américanistes,* 1930.

d'Harnoncourt, René
North American Indian Arts in *Magazine of Art,* 1939.
Living Arts of the Indians in *Magazine of Art,* 1941.
Indian Arts and Crafts and their Place in the Modern World in "The Changing Indian," *q.v.*
See also Douglas, Frederic H.

Harrington, M. R.
Certain Caddo Sites in Arkansas. New York, 1920.

Hartman, C. V.
Archaeological Researches in Costa-Rica. Stockholm, 1901.

Harvey, Fred E. *See* Brand, Donald D.

Haury, Emil W.
The Age of Lead Glaze Decorated Pottery in the Southwest in *American Anthropologist,* 1932.
The Mogollon Culture of Southwestern New Mexico. Gila Pueblo, 1936.

Hay, Clarence L.
[45] A Contribution to Maya Architecture in *Natural History,* 1935.

Hewett, Edgar Lee
[46] Ancient Life in the American Southwest. Indianapolis, 1930.
[47] The Chaco Canyon and its Monuments. Albuquerque, 1936.
[48] Ancient Andean Life. Indianapolis, 1939.

Hodge, Frederick Webb
Circular Kivas near Hawikuh, New Mexico. New York, 1923.
Co-editor, "Introduction to American Indian Art," *q.v.*

Hollenbach, Marion
Pre-Columbian Art. Catalogue. Los Angeles County Museum, 1940.

Holmes, William H.
The Use of Gold and Other Metals among the Ancient Inhabitants of Chiriquí, Isthmus of Darien. Washington, 1887.
[49] Archaeological Studies among the Ancient Cities of Mexico. Chicago, 1895 and 1897.

Hooton, Ernest A.
The Indians of Pecos Pueblo. Cambridge, 1930.

Humboldt, Alexander von
[50] Vue des Cordillères et Monuments des Peuples Indigènes de l'Amérique. Paris, 1810.
Essai Politique sur le Royaume de la Nouvelle-Espagne. Paris, 1811.

"Introduction to American Indian Art." *Ed.* by Frederick Webb Hodge, Herbert J. Spinden, and Oliver La Farge. New York, 1931.

Izikowitz, Karl Gustav
    Musical and Other Sound Instruments of the South American Indians. Göteborg, 1935.

[51] Jade, correspondence on, with Harvard Geological Museum, Cambridge, and J. L. Kraft, Chicago.
Jenness, D.
    Editor, The American Aborigines. A compilation. Toronto, 1933.
Jockelson, W.
    Archaeological Investigations in the Aleutian Islands. Washington, 1925.
Johnson, Frederick
    [52] Linguistic Map of Mexico and Central America in "The Maya and their Neighbors," *q.v.*
[53] *Journal de la Société des Américanistes,* 1916, miscellaneous short notes in.
Joyce, Thomas Athol
    [54] South American Archaeology. London, 1912.
    Ancient American Mosaic in *Burlington Magazine,* 1914.
    Mexican Archaeology. New York and London, 1914.
    Central American and West Indian Archaeology. London, 1916.
    Guide to the Maudslay Collection of Maya Sculptures. London, 1923.
    [55] An Example of Cast Goldwork Discovered at Palenque by Waldeck. *Proc. 25th Internat. Cong. of Americanists,* The Hague, 1924.
    Maya and Mexican Art. London, 1927.
    A Maya Jadeite Carving from Central America in *The British Museum Quarterly,* 1929.
    [56] The Gann Jades in *The British Museum Quarterly,* 1938.
Judd, Neil M.
    Dating Our Prehistoric Pueblo Ruins. Washington, 1930.
    The Excavation and Repair of Betatakin. Washington, 1930.

Kelemen, Pál
    [57] Battlefield of the Gods. London, 1937.
    Pre-Columbian Jades in *Parnassus,* 1939.
    Some pre-Columbian Gold Pieces in *Parnassus,* 1940.
    [58] The Stephens Centenary in *El Palacio,* 1941.
Kelly, Eoghan John
    Pedro de Alvarado Conquistador. Princeton, 1932.
Kelsey, Vera, and Osborne, Lilly deJongh
    [59] Four Keys to Guatemala. New York, 1939.
Kidder, Alfred, II
    [60] South American Penetrations in Middle America in "The Maya and their Neighbors," *q.v.*
    See also Strong, William Duncan

BIBLIOGRAPHY

Kidder, Alfred V.
    [61] An Introduction to the Study of Southwestern Archaeology. New Haven,
        1924.
    The Pottery of Pecos. Vol. I. Andover, Mass., 1931.
    Archaeological Problems of the Highland Maya in "The Maya and their
        Neighbors," q.v.

Kidder, Alfred V., and Shepard, Anna O.
    The Pottery of Pecos. Vol. II. New Haven, 1936.

Kidder, Alfred V., and Thompson, J. Eric
    The Correlation of Maya and Christian Chronologies. Washington, 1938.

Kluckhohn, Clyde
    The Conceptual Structure in Middle American Studies in "The Maya and their
        Neighbors," q.v.

Krickeberg, Walter
    Die Totonaken. Berlin, 1925.

Kroeber, A. L.
    Archaeological Explorations in Peru. Chicago, 1926.
    Culture Stratifications in Peru in *American Anthropologist*, 1926.
    Coast and Highland in Prehistoric Peru in *American Anthropologist*, 1927.
    Conclusions: The Present Status of Americanistic Problems in "The Maya and
        their Neighbors," q.v.
    See also O'Neale, Lila M.

La Farge, Oliver
    Maya Ethnology: The Sequence of Cultures in "The Maya and their Neigh-
        bors," q.v.
    Editor, "The Changing Indian," q.v.
    Co-editor, "Introduction to American Indian Art," q.v.
    See also Blom, Frans, and Byers, D. S.

Lago, Roberto, and Cueto, Lola
    [62] Mexican Folk Puppets. Birmingham, Mich., 1941.

Landa, Diego de. *See* Gates, William, and Tozzer, Alfred M.

Larsen, Helge
    [63] The Monolithic Rock Temple of Malinalco in *Ethnos,* 1938.

Las Casas, Bartolomé de
    Historia de las Indias. Mexico, 1877.

Lehmann, Heinz
    Les Styles des Vases de Nazca in *Journal de la Société des Américanistes,* 1934.

Lehmann, Walter
    [64] Ergebnisse und Aufgaben der Mexikanistischen Forschung. Braunschweig,
        1907.
    Die Sprachen Zentralamerikas. Berlin, 1920.

Lehmann, Walter, and Doering, Heinrich
    Kunstgeschichte des Alten Peru. Berlin, 1924.

Lilly, Eli
    Prehistoric Antiquities of Indiana.   Indianapolis, 1937.

Lincoln, J. Steward
    The Maya Calendar of the Ixil of Guatemala in *CIW Contrib. to Am. Anthro. and Hist.*   Washington, 1942.

Lines, Jorge A.
    Una Huaca en Zapandi.   San José, Costa Rica, 1936.
    [65] Notes on the Archaeology of Costa Rica.   San José, Costa Rica, 1939.

Linné, S.
    † Archaeological Researches at Teotihuacan, Mexico.   London, 1934.
    † Zapotecan Antiquities.   Stockholm, 1938.

Linton, Ralph L.
    North American Maize Culture in *American Anthropology,* 1924.
    Use of Tobacco among North American Indians.   Chicago, 1924.
    Study of Man.   New York, 1936.
    [66] Crops, Soils, and Culture in America in "The Maya and their Neighbors," *q.v.*
    Primitive Art in *The Kenyon Review,* 1941.
    Land Tenure in Aboriginal America in "The Changing Indian," *q.v.*

Los Angeles County Museum
    Pre-Columbian Art.   Catalogue.   1940.

Lothrop, Samuel Kirkland
    [67] Tulum, an Archaeological Study of the East Coast of Yucatan.   Washington, 1924.
    Pottery of Costa Rica and Nicaragua.   New York, 1926.
    Pottery Types and their Sequence in El Salvador.   New York, 1927.
    [68] Sculptured Fragments from Palenque in *Journal of the Royal Anthropological Institute,* 1929.
    Sculptured Pottery of the Maya and Pipil in *Maya Research,* 1936.
    [69] Zacualpa.   Washington, 1936.
    [70] † Coclé.   Cambridge, 1937.
    Gold and Silver from Southern Peru and Bolivia in *Journal of the Royal Anthropological Institute,* 1937.
    [71] Inca Treasure as Depicted by Spanish Historians.   Los Angeles, 1938.
    The Southeastern Frontier of the Maya in *American Anthropologist,* 1939.
    South America as Seen from Middle America in "The Maya and their Neighbors," *q.v.*

Lowie, Robert H.
    American Culture History in *American Anthropologist,* 1940.
    Editor, "Essays in Anthropology," *q.v.*

Lummis, Charles F.
    [72] Mesa, Cañon and Pueblo.   New York and London, 1925.

MacCurdy, George Grant
    A Study of Chiriquian Antiquities.   New Haven, 1911.
    Editor, "Early Man," *q.v.*

McGregor, John C.
    [73] †Southwestern Archaeology. New York, 1941.

Madariaga, Salvador de
    Christopher Columbus. New York, 1940.

Maler, Teobert
    [74] Researches in the Central Portion of the Usumatsintla Valley. Cambridge, 1901.
    [75] Explorations in the Department of Peten, Guatemala. Tikal. Cambridge, 1908–11.

Marett, R. H. K.
    [76] Archaeological Tours from Mexico City. New York, 1934.

Markham, Clements R.
    [77] A History of Peru. Chicago, 1892.
    [78] The Incas of Peru. London, 1910.
    Translator and *editor,* Reports of the Discovery of Peru. London, 1872.
    See also Vega, Garcilaso de la

Marquina, Ignacio
    Estudio Arquitectónico Comparativo de los Monumentos Arqueológicos de México. Mexico, 1928.

Marshall, J.
    Mohenjo-Daro and the Indus Civilization. London, 1931.

Martin, Paul S.
    Archaeology of North America. Chicago, 1933.
    Lowry Ruin in Southwestern Colorado. Chicago, 1936.

Mason, J. Alden
    Use of Tobacco in Mexico and South America. Chicago, 1924.
    Turquoise Mosaics from Northern Mexico in *The Museum Journal,* Philadelphia, 1929.
    [79] A Maya Carved Stone Lintel from Guatemala in *The University Museum Bulletin,* Philadelphia, 1931.
    [80] Collections from Santarem in *The University Museum Bulletin,* 1935.
    Three Inca Wood Cups in *The University Museum Bulletin,* 1935.
    Observations on the Present Status and Problems of Middle American Archaeology in *American Antiquity,* 1938.
    See also Gordon, G. B.

Maudslay, Alfred Percival
    [81] Biologia Centrali-Americana. London, 1889–1902.

Maudslay, Alfred P., and Maudslay, Anne Cary
    A Glimpse at Guatemala. London, 1899.

†"The Maya and their Neighbors." A compilation. New York, 1940. *Ed.* by Clarence L. Hay, Ralph L, Linton, Samuel K. Lothrop, Harry L. Shapiro, and George C. Vaillant.

Mead, Charles W.
    [82] Old Civilizations of Inca Land. New York, 1932.

< 397 >

Means, Philip Ainsworth
  Some Comments on the Inedited Manuscript of Poma de Ayala in *American Anthropologist,* 1923.
  [83] Peruvian Textiles.   Metropolitan Museum of Art, New York, 1930.
  [84] †Ancient Civilizations of the Andes.   New York, 1931.
  [85] A Study of Peruvian Textiles.   Museum of Fine Arts, Boston, 1932.
  Fall of the Inca Empire.   New York, 1932.
  The Philosophic Interrelationship between Middle American and Andean Religions in "The Maya and their Neighbors," *q.v.*
  †Pre-Columbian Art and Culture in the Andean Area in *Bulletin of the Museum of Art,* Providence, R.I., 1940.
  Pre-Columbian Andean Art in *Magazine of Art,* 1940–41.

Mena, Ramón
  [86] Catálogo de la Colección de Objetos de Jade.   Museo Nacional, Mexico, 1927.

Mera, H. P.
  Observations on the Archaeology of the Petrified Forest National Monument.   Santa Fé, 1934.
  The "Rain Bird."   Santa Fé, 1937.   (forthcoming Dover reprint)

Merrill, E. D.
  [87] Domesticated Plants in Relation to the Diffusion of Culture in "Early Man," *q.v.*

Merwin, Raymond E., and Vaillant, G. C.
  The Ruins of Holmul, Guatemala.   Cambridge, 1932.

Michigan, University of
  Latin-American and Pre-Columbian Art.   Catalogue.   Ann Arbor, Mich., 1939.

Mills, C. William
  Certain Mounds and Village Sites in Ohio.   Columbus, 1916.

Mimenza Castillo, Ricardo
  La Civilización Maya.   Barcelona, 1929.

Minnesota, University of
  Primitive Art.   Catalogue.   Minneapolis, 1940.

Montell, Gösta
  Dress and Ornaments in Ancient Peru.   Göteborg, 1929.

Moorehead, Warren K.
  Explorations of the Etowah Site in Georgia.   New Haven, 1932.

Morant, George S. de
  [88] A History of Chinese Art.   London, 1931.

Morgadanes, Dolores
  [89] Similarity between Mixco and the Yalalag Costumes in *American Anthropologist,* 1940.

Morison, Samuel Eliot
  Admiral of the Ocean Sea.   Boston, 1942.

< 398 >

BIBLIOGRAPHY

Morley, Frances R., and Sylvanus G.
  [90] The Age and Provenience of the Leyden Plate in *CIW Contrib. to Am. Anthro. and Hist.* Washington, 1939.

Morley, Sylvanus Griswold
  An Introduction to the Study of Maya Hieroglyphs. Washington, 1920.
  The Inscriptions at Copan. Washington, 1920.
  Unearthing America's Ancient History in *The National Geographic Magazine,* 1931.
  [91] Guide Book to the Ruins of Quiriguá. Washington, 1935.
  The Inscriptions of Peten. Washington, 1937–38.
  [92] Maya Epigraphy in "The Maya and their Neighbors," *q.v.*
  See also Smith, A. Ledyard

Morris, Earl H.
  [93] The Temple of the Warriors. New York, 1931.

Morris, Earl H., with Charlot, J., and Morris, Ann A.
  [94] The Temple of the Warriors at Chichen Itza, Yucatan. 2 vols. Washington, 1931.

Murdock, George Peter
  [95] Our Primitive Contemporaries. New York, 1934.

Museum of Modern Art
  Twenty Centuries of Mexican Art. Catalogue. New York, 1940.
  See also Cahill, Holger

Nash, Ruth Cutter
  [96] Calendrical Interpretation of a Golden Breastplate from Peru. New York, 1939.

Noguera, Eduardo
  [97] Ruinas de Tizatlán, Tlaxcala. Mexico, 1927.
  Algunas Características de la Cerámica de México in *Journal de la Société des Américanistes,* 1930.
  Ruinas Arqueológicas del Norte de México. Mexico, 1930.
  Extensiones Cronológico—Culturales y Geográficas de las Cerámicas de México. Mexico, 1932.
  [98] Importancia Arqueológica del Descubrimiento en Texmilincan, Guerrero, in *Boletín del Museo Nacional.* Mexico, 1933.
  [99] Guía Morelos. Mexico, 1934.
  [100] Guidebook to the National Museum. Mexico, 1938.
  Excavations at Tehuacan in "The Maya and their Neighbors," *q.v.*

Nordenskiöld, Erland
  The Copper and Bronze Age in South America. Göteborg, 1921.
  The American Indian as an Inventor in *The Journal of the Royal Anthropological Institute,* 1929.

Nordenskiöld, G.
  The Cliff-dwellers of the Mesa Verde. Stockholm, 1893.

Norman, Daniel, and Johnson, W. W. A.
    [101] Note on a Spectrographic Study of Central American and Asiatic Jades in *Journal of the Optical Society of America,* 1941.
Nuttall, Zelia
    Ancient Mexican Feather Work at the Columbian Historical Exposition at Madrid. Washington, 1895.
    The Fundamental Principles of Old and New World Civilizations. Cambridge, 1901.
    [102] The Book of Life of the Ancient Mexicans. Berkeley, 1903.
    A Penitential Rite of the Ancient Mexicans. Cambridge, 1904.

Olsen, R. L.
    [103] The Indians of the Northwest Coast in *Natural History,* 1935.
O'Neale, Lila M.
    [104] Wide-Loom Fabrics of the Early Nazca Period in "Essays in Anthropology," *q.v.*
    Textiles of the Early Nazca Period. Chicago, 1937.
O'Neale, Lila M., and Kroeber, A. L.
    [105] Textile Periods in Ancient Peru. Berkeley, 1930.
Orchard, William C.
    Peruvian Gold and Gold Plating. New York, 1930.
Osborne, Lilly deJongh
    Guatemala Textiles. New Orleans, 1935.
    See also Kelsey, Vera
Osgood, Cornelius
    The Archaeological Problem of Chiriqui in *American Anthropologist,* 1935.

Palacios, Enrique Juan
    Arqueología de México. Mexico, 1937.
    Más Gemas del Arte Maya en Palenque. Mexico, 1937.
Paul, A. J. Drexel, Jr. *See* Strong, William Duncan
Peabody Museum of Archaeology and Ethnology, Harvard University
    Prehistoric Ruins of Copan, Honduras. Cambridge, 1896.
    †An Exhibition of Pre-Columbian Art. Catalogue. Fogg Art Museum, Cambridge, 1940.
Peake, Harold
    Early Steps in Human Progress. London.
Peake, Harold, and Fleure, Herbert John
    [106] Hunters and Artists. Oxford, 1927.
    The Horse and the Sword. Oxford, 1933.
Peñafiel, Antonio
    [107] Monumentos del Arte Mexicano Antiguo. Mexico and Berlin, 1890.
Phillips, Phillip
    [108] Middle American Influences on the Archaeology of the Southeastern United States in "The Maya and their Neighbors," *q.v.*

< 400 >

Pijoán. *See* Cossío-Pijoán

Pleasants, Frederick R.
> Pre-Columbian Art at the Fogg in *Magazine of Art,* 1940.

Pollock, H. E. D.
> [109] Round Structures of Aboriginal Middle America. Washington, 1936.
> Sources and Methods in the Study of Maya Architecture in "The Maya and their Neighbors," *q.v.*

Posnansky, Arthur
> Una Metrópoli en la América del Sud. Berlin, 1914.

Prescott, William H.
> Conquest of Mexico. New York, 1855.
> [110] Conquest of Peru. New York, 1855.

Preuss, K. Th.
> Monumentale Vorgeschichtliche Kunst. Göttingen, 1929.

Priest, Alan
> [111] Chinese Bronzes. Catalogue. Metropolitan Museum of Art, New York, 1938.

Radin, Paul
> Histoire de la Civilisation Indienne. *Tr.* by Eva Métraux. Paris, 1935.

Redfield, Robert
> The Folk Culture of Yucatan. Chicago, 1941.

Reiss, W., and Stuebel, A.
> Das Totenfeld von Ancon in Peru. Berlin, 1880–87.

Reiter, Paul. *See* Alexander, Herbert J.

Richardson, Francis B.
> Non-Maya Monumental Sculpture of Central America in "The Maya and their Neighbors," *q.v.*

Rickards, Constantine George
> The Ruins of Mexico. London, 1910.
> Monograph on Ornaments on Zapotec Funerary Urns in *Journal de la Société des Américanistes,* 1938.

Ricketson, O. G.
> [112] Report on the Excavations at Uaxactun. Washington, 1925.

Ries, Maurice
> Stamping: A Mass-production Printing Method 2000 Years Old in *Middle American Papers.* New Orleans, 1932.
> Ancient American Art. Catalogue. Santa Barbara, Calif., 1942.

Riggs, Arthur Stanley
> [113] The Romance of Human Progress. Indianapolis, 1938.

Riggs, Elmer S.
> [114] The Geological History and Evolution of the Horse. Chicago, 1932.

Rivero, Mariano Eduardo de, and Tschudi, Juan Diego de
> Antigüedades Peruanas. Text and map. Vienna, 1851.

Rivet, Paul, and Verneau, R.
    Ethnographie Ancienne de l'Equateur. Paris, 1912.
Röck, Fritz
    Ein Altindianisches Bilderbuch. Vienna, 1935.
    Kalenderkreise und Kalenderschichten im alten Mexiko und Mittelamerika. Vienna.
    Kunstgewerbe von Mexiko, Mittelamerika und Westindien. Berlin.
    [115] Feder Kopfschmuck des Gottes Quetzalcoatl. Manuscript. Museum für Völkerkunde, Vienna.
Rosny, Leon de
    [116] Les Documents Écrits de l'Antiquité Américaine. Paris, 1882.
Ruppert, Karl
    [117] The Caracol. Washington, 1935.
    A Special Assemblage of Maya Structures in "The Maya and their Neighbors," q.v.
Ruskin, John
    [118] Stones of Venice. London, 1853.

Sachs, Curt
    [119] The History of Musical Instruments. New York, 1940.
Sahagún, Fray Bernardino de
    A History of Ancient Mexico. *Tr.* by Fanny R. Bandelier. Fisk University, Nashville, 1932.
Salaman, R. N.
    Deformities and Mutilations of the Face as Depicted in the Chimu Pottery of Peru in *The Journal of the Royal Anthropological Institute,* 1939.
Sapper, Carl
    Altindianische Ansiedelungen in Guatemala und Chiapas. Berlin, 1895.
Satterthwaite, L., Jr.
    [120] Notes on the Work of the Fourth and Fifth University Museum Expeditions to Piedras Negras, Peten, Guatemala, in *Maya Research,* 1936, and in *The University Museum Bulletin,* Philadelphia, 1933, 1936, 1937.
    Identification of Maya Temple Buildings at Piedras Negras in *Twenty-fifth Anniversary Studies*. Philadelphia Anthropological Society, 1937.
Saville, Marshall H.
    Cruciform Structures near Mitla in *Bulletin,* American Museum of Natural History, 1900.
    The Antiquities of Manabí, Ecuador. New York, 1907 and 1910.
    A Sculptured Vase from Guatemala. New York, 1919.
    [121] The Goldsmith's Art in Ancient Mexico. New York, 1920.
    [122] *Editor,* The Earliest Notices Concerning the Conquest of Mexico by Cortes in 1519. New York, 1920.
    [123] A Golden Breastplate from Cuzco, Peru. New York, 1921.
    [124] Bibliographic Notes on Uxmal. New York, 1921.
    Editor, Reports on the Maya Indians of Yucatan. New York, 1921.

[125] Turquoise Mosaic Art in Ancient Mexico. New York, 1922.
The Gold Treasure of Sigsig, Ecuador. New York, 1924.
[126] The Wood-Carver's Art in Mexico. New York, 1925.
[127] Bibliographic Notes on Palenque, Chiapas. New York, 1928.
Bibliographic Notes on Xochicalco, Mexico. New York, 1928.
[128] Tizoc, Great Lord of the Aztecs. New York, 1929.

Schmidt, Max
Kunst und Kultur von Peru. Berlin, 1929.

Seler, Edward
[129] Gesammelte Abhandlungen zur Amerikanischen Sprach- und Altertumskunde. Berlin, 1902–23.

Shapiro, Harry L.
World Migrations in *Natural History,* 1942.
The Mixed-Blood Indian in "The Changing Indian," *q.v.*

Shepard, Anna O. *See* Kidder, Alfred V.

Shetrone, H. C.
[130] The Mound-Builders. New York, 1930.

Smith, A. Ledyard
Report on the Investigation of Stelae. Washington, 1929.
Excavations at Uaxactun. Washington, 1933.
Uaxactun. Washington, 1935.
[131] The Corbeled Arch in the New World in "The Maya and their Neighbors," *q.v.*

Smith, A. Ledyard, and Morley, Sylvanus G.
[132] Report on Some Excavations at Uaxactun. Washington, 1932.

Smith, Howell
[133] Brief Guide to the Peruvian Textiles. Catalogue. Victoria and Albert Museum. London, 1926.

Smith, Philip S.
[134] Certain Relations between Northwest America and Northeast Asia in "Early Man," *q.v.*

Smith, Robert E.
[135] A Study of Structure A-1 Complex at Uaxactun, Peten, Guatemala, in *CIW Contrib. to Am. Anthro. and Hist.* Washington, 1937.
Ceramics of the Peten in "The Maya and their Neighbors," *q.v.*

Spinden, Ellen S.
[136] Place of Tajin in Totonac Archaeology in *American Anthropologist,* 1933.

Spinden, Herbert J.
[137] †A Study of Maya Art. Cambridge, 1913.
Notes on the Archaeology of Salvador in *American Anthropologist,* 1915.
The Origin and Distribution of Agriculture in America. *Proc. 19th Internat. Cong. of Americanists,* Washington, 1917.
The Reduction of Mayan Dates. Cambridge, 1924.

The Chorotegan Culture Area. *Proc. 21st Internat. Cong. of Americanists.* Göteborg, 1925.

Ancient Civilizations of Mexico and Central America. New York, 1928.

Indian Manuscripts of Southern Mexico. Washington, 1935.

Huaxtec Sculptures and Apotheosis in *The Brooklyn Museum Quarterly,* 1937.

[138] Diffusion of Maya Astronomy in "The Maya and their Neighbors," *q.v.*

Co-editor, "Introduction to American Indian Art," *q.v.*

Squier, E. G.

Nicaragua, its People, Scenery, Monuments and the Proposed Interoceanic Canal. With numerous original maps and illustrations. New York, 1852.

The States of Central America. New York, 1858.

[139] Peru, Incidents of Travel and Exploration in the Land of the Incas. New York, 1877.

Stafford, Cora E.

Paracas Embroideries. New York, 1941.

Stallings, W. S., Jr.

Dating Prehistoric Ruins by Tree-Rings. Santa Fé, 1939.

Stephens, John L.

Incidents of Travel in Central America, Chiapas, and Yucatan. New York, 1841. (forthcoming Dover reprint)

[140] Incidents of Travel in Yucatan. New York, 1843. (Dover reprint)

Stirling, Matthew W.

An Initial Series from Tres Zapotes, Vera Cruz, Mexico. Washington, 1940.

[141] Expedition Unearths Buried Masterpieces in *The National Geographic Magazine,* 1941.

Stirling, Matthew W., and Marion

Finding Jewels of Jade in a Mexican Swamp in *The National Geographic Magazine,* 1942.

Stone, Doris

[142] Masters in Marble. New Orleans.

The Ulua Valley and Lake Yojoa in "The Maya and their Neighbors," *q.v.*

Archaeology of the North Coast of Honduras. Cambridge, 1941.

Strómsvik, Gustav

[143] Substela Caches and Stela Foundations at Copan and Quiriguá in *CIW Contrib. to Am. Anthro. and Hist.* Washington, 1942.

Strong, William Duncan

Anthropological Problems in Central America in "The Maya and their Neighbors," *q.v.*

Indian Religion in the Modern World in "The Changing Indian," *q.v.*

Strong, William Duncan, Kidder, Alfred, II, and Paul, A. J. Drexel, Jr.

Preliminary Report on the Smithsonian Institution-Harvard University Archaeological Expedition to Northwestern Honduras, 1936. Washington, 1938.

BIBLIOGRAPHY

Stuebel, A., and Uhle, Max
> Die Ruinenstätte von Tiahuanaco im Hochlande des Alten Peru. Leipzig, 1892.

[144] "A Survey of Persian Art." *Ed.* by Arthur Upham Pope. London and New York, 1939.

Sydow, Eckart von
> Die Kunst der Naturvölker und der Vorzeit. Berlin, 1923.

Tello, Julio C.
> Introducción a la Historia Antigua del Perú. Lima, 1921.
[145] Los Descubrimientos del Museo de Arqueología Peruana en la Península de Paracas. Rome, 1928.
> Antiguo Perú. Lima, 1929.

[146] Tenayuca. A compilation. Mexico, 1935.

Terry, T. Philip
[147] Terry's Guide to Mexico. Boston, 1931.

Textile Museum of the District of Columbia
> Correspondence and data concerning Peruvian fabrics.

Thausing, M.
[148] Quellenschriften für Kunstgeschichte—Dürers Briefe, Tagebücher und Reime. Wien, 1888.

Thompson, Edward Herbert
> Archaeological Researches in Yucatan. Cambridge, 1904.
[149] People of the Serpent. Boston, 1932.

Thompson, J. Eric S.
[150] The Civilization of the Mayas. Chicago, 1927 and 1942.
> A Correlation of the Mayan and European Calendars. Chicago, 1927.
[151] Mexico before Cortez. New York, 1933.
> Archaeology of South America. Chicago, 1936.
> An Eccentric Flint from Quintana Roo, Mexico, in *Maya Research,* 1936.
[152] Excavations at San José, British Honduras. Washington, 1939.
[153] The Moon Goddess in Middle America in *CIW Contrib. to Am. Anthro. and Hist.* Washington, 1939.
> Archaeological Problems of the Lowland Maya in "The Maya and their Neighbors," *q.v.*
[154] Dating of Certain Inscriptions of non-Maya Origin. Washington, 1941.
> Maya Arithmetic. Washington, 1941.
[155] Critical review and correspondence in reference to this survey.
> *See also* Kidder, Alfred V., and Gann, T. W.

Totten, George Oakley
> Maya Architecture. Washington, 1926.

Tovey, Donald Francis
> The Integrity of Music: A Musician Talks. London, 1941.

< 405 >

Tozzer, Alfred M.

    A Comparative Study of the Mayas and the Lacandones. New York, 1907.

[156] A Preliminary Study of the Prehistoric Ruins of Tikal, Guatemala. Cambridge, 1911.

[157] A Preliminary Study of the Prehistoric Ruins of Nakum, Guatemala. Cambridge, 1913.

    Social Origins and Social Continuities. New York, 1925.

    Time and American Archaeology in *Natural History,* 1927.

    Maya and Toltec Figures at Chichen Itzá. *Proc. 23rd Internat. Cong. of Americanists.* New York, 1930.

    Maya Research in *Maya Research,* 1934.

    Stephens, Prescott, Bancroft and Others in *Los Mayas Antiguos.* Mexico, 1941.

[158] †*Editor,* Landa's Relación de las Cosas de Yucatan. Cambridge, 1941.

Tozzer, Alfred M., and Allen, G. M.

    Animal Figures in the Maya Codices. Cambridge, 1910.

Trik, Aubrey S.

[159] Temple XXII at Copan in *CIW Contrib. to Am. Anthro. and Hist.* Washington, 1939.

Tschudi, Juan Diego de. *See* Rivero, Mariano Eduardo de

Tucker, Mary

    †Books of the Southwest. A General Bibliography. New York.

Uhle, Max

[160] Pachacamac. Philadelphia, 1903.

[161] Explorations at Chincha. Berkeley, 1924.

    See also Stuebel, A.

Vaillant, George C.

[162] Excavations at Zacatenco. New York, 1930.

[163] Artists and Craftsmen in Ancient Central America. New York, 1935.

    Indian Arts in North America. New York, 1939.

    Patterns in Middle American Archaeology in "The Maya and their Neighbors," *q.v.*

    †Aztecs of Mexico. New York, 1941.

    See also Merwin, Raymond E.

Valcárcel, Luis E.

    El Cuzco Precolombino. Cuzco, 1924.

    Ancient Peruvian Art. Lima, 1937.

[164] The Latest Archaeological Discoveries in Peru. Lima, 1938.

    Muestrario de Arte Peruano Precolombino. Lima, 1938.

Vega, Garcilaso de la

    The First Part of the Royal Commentaries of the Yncas. *Tr.* and *ed.* by Clements R. Markham. London, 1871.

Vignaud, Henry
      Toscanelli and Columbus. London, 1902.

Villacorta B., Carlos A.
      Vaso de Guastatoya. Guatemala, 1941.

Villacorta C., J. Antonio
      Arqueología Guatemalteca. Guatemala, 1927.
    [165] Prehistoria e Historia Antigua de Guatemala. Guatemala, 1938.

Waldeck, Frédéric de
    [166] Voyage Pittoresque et Archéologique dans la Province d'Yucatan, pendant les Années 1834 et 1836. Paris, 1838.

Waldeck, Frédéric de, and Brasseur de Bourbourg, C. E.
      Monuments Anciens du Mexique. Paris, 1866.

Wardle, H. Newell
    [167] Guetar Art in Stone in *The University Museum Bulletin,* Philadelphia, 1939.
    [168] Correspondence and data furnished for this survey.

Wauchope, Robert
      Zacualpa. Washington, 1936.

Wiener, Charles
      Pérou et Bolivie. Paris, 1880.

Willard, T. A.
      The City of the Sacred Well. London.

Wissler, Clark
    [169] †The American Indian. New York, 1922.

Woodward, Arthur
    [170] A Shell Bracelet Manufactory in *American Antiquity,* 1936.
    [171] Notes on the Archaeological Specimens from the Grewe Site, Gila Valley, Arizona. Typescript. Los Angeles, 1936.

Wooley, C. Leonard
    [172] Ur Excavations. London and New York, 1934.

Zinsser, Hans
    [173] Rats, Lice and History. New York, 1934.

Zweig, Stefan
      Amerigo. New York, 1942.

< 407 >

ADDENDA TO THE BIBLIOGRAPHY
(For Preface and Plates 307–308)

Adams, Henry
> The Education of Henry Adams. Boston, 1912.

Aveleyra A. de Anda, Luis
> The Second Mammoth at Santa Isabel Iztapan, Mexico, in *American Antiquity,* July 1956.

Bennett, Wendell C.
> The Archaeology of Colombia, in *Handbook of South American Indians,* Vol. 2. Washington, 1946.

Bennett, Wendell C., and Hernandez de Alba, Gregorio
> The Archaeology of San Agustín and Tierradentro, Colombia, in *Handbook of South American Indians,* Vol. 2. Washington, 1946.

Drucker, Philip
> La Venta, Tabasco, a Study of Olmec Ceramics and Art. Washington, 1952.

Ho, Ping-ti
> American Food Plants in China in *American Anthropologist,* April 1955.

Kelemen, Pál
> Pre-Colombian Art and Art History in *American Antiquity,* January 1946.

Perez de Barradas, José
> Orfebrería prehispánica de Colombia. Museo del Oro del Banco de la Republica, Bogotá. Madrid, 1954.

"Report of the Committee on the Visual Arts at Harvard University." Harvard University Press. Cambridge, 1956.

Ruppert, Karl; Thompson, J. Eric S., and others
> Bonampak, Chiapas, Mexico. Washington, 1955.

Stirling, Matthew W.
> Stone Monuments of the Rio Chiquito, Veracruz, Mexico, in *Anthropological Papers,* No. 43, Smithsonian Institution, Washington, 1955.

Thompson, J. Eric S.
> The Rise and Fall of Maya Civilization. Norman, 1954, 1955, 1956.

CHRONOLOGICAL CHART OF TENTATIVE DATES

compiled on the basis of latest publications

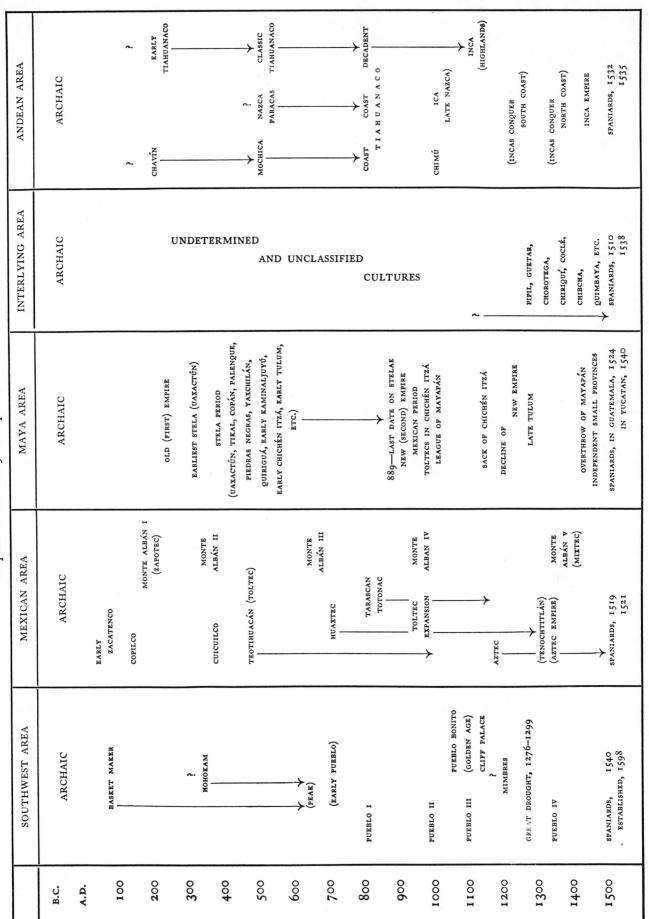

ILLUSTRATIONS

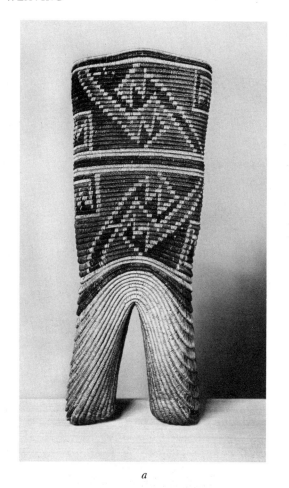

a

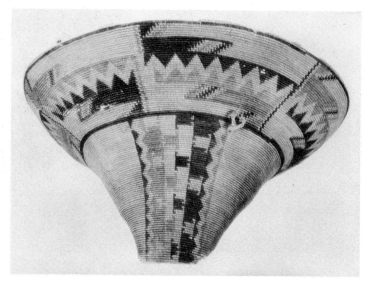

b

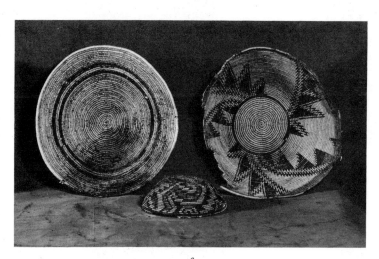

c

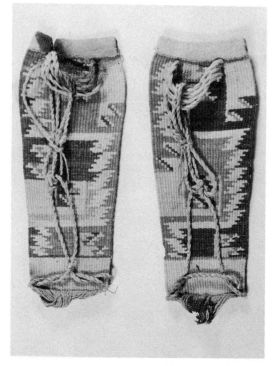

d

PLATE 169. ©. *a*) Cliff-dweller basketry "cradle," Utah, Pueblo III. *b*) Burden basket, Arizona,
Basket Maker III. *c*) Baskets from Arizona: two larger, Basket Maker III; smaller, Pueblo I.
d) Twined sandals, Arizona, Basket Maker III.

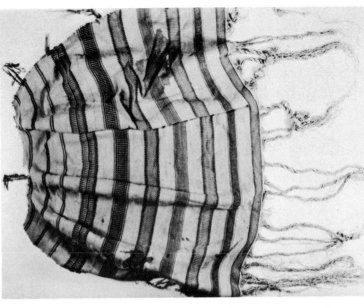

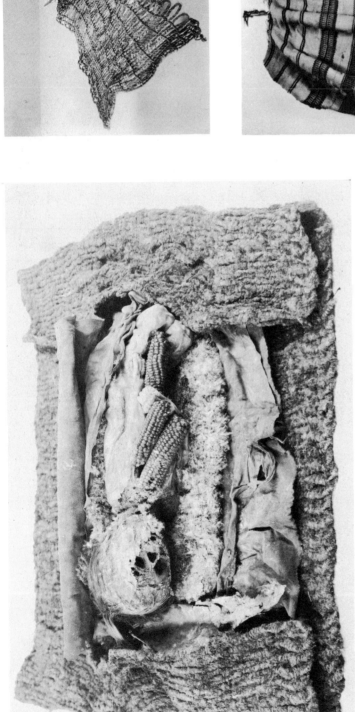

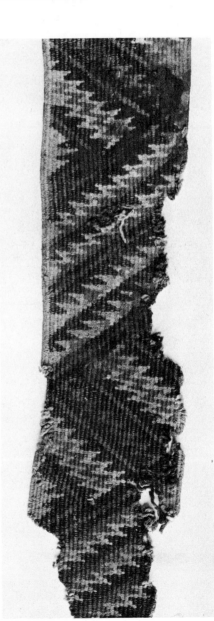

PLATE 170. ©. *a*) Pueblo child's desiccated body wrapped in feather and deerskin blankets, New Mexico. *b*) Yucca fiber foundation for rabbit-skin blanket, Arizona. Basket Maker or Pueblo. *c*) Basket Maker burden strap of yucca, Colorado. *d*) Twined woven fabric, Basket Maker III.

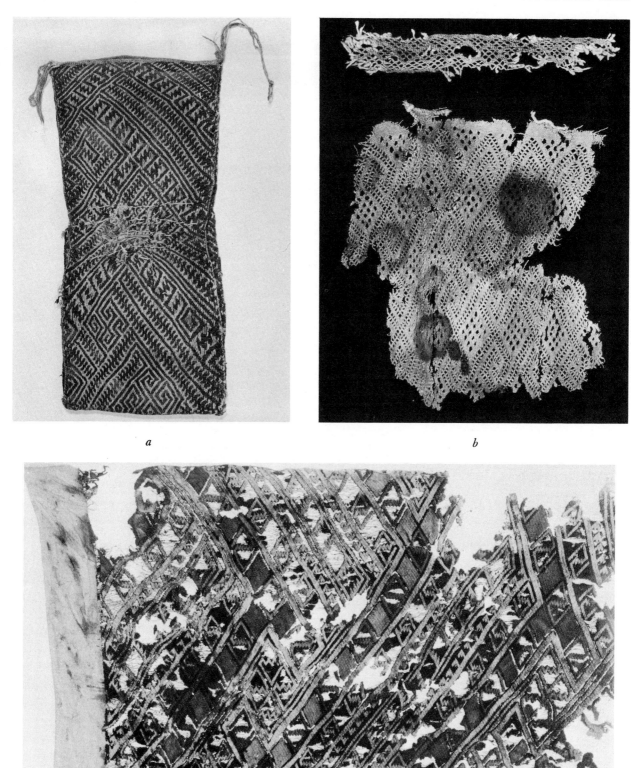

a   *b*

c

PLATE 171. ©. *a*) Pueblo cotton bag woven in damask technique, Arizona. *b*) Lacy openwork
in cotton, New Mexico, Pueblo III. *c*) Fragment of cotton kilt, Utah, Pueblo IV.

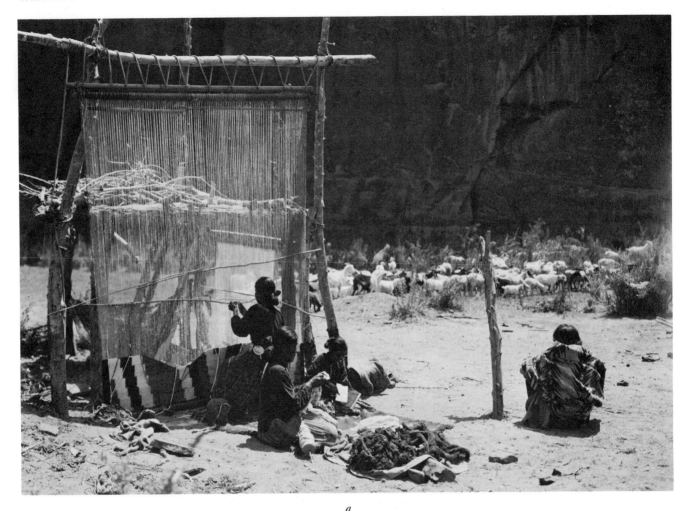

a

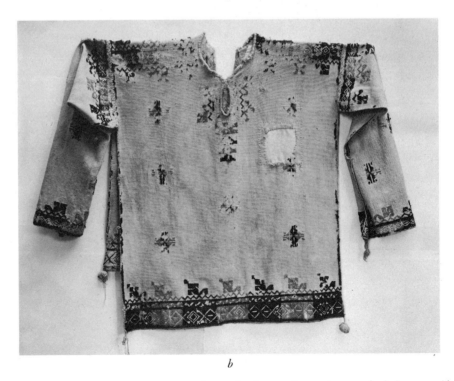

b

PLATE 172. ©. *a*) Navaho women carding, spinning, and weaving wool, Arizona. *b*) Modern
Pueblo embroidered shirt, New Mexico.

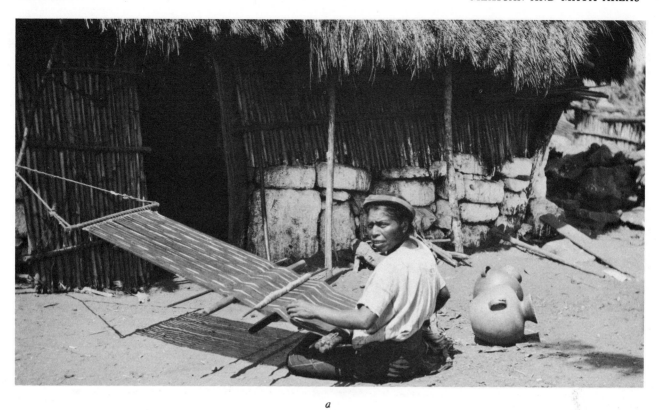

a

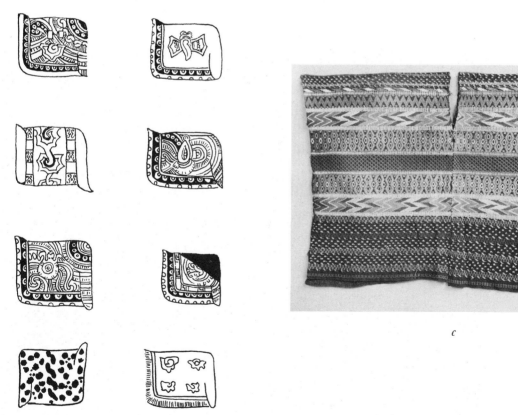

b

c

PLATE 173. ©. *a*) Indian weaver, Guatemalan highlands. *b*) Aztec blankets as represented
in the Tribute Roll of Montezuma. *c*) Girl's modern blouse, Guatemala.

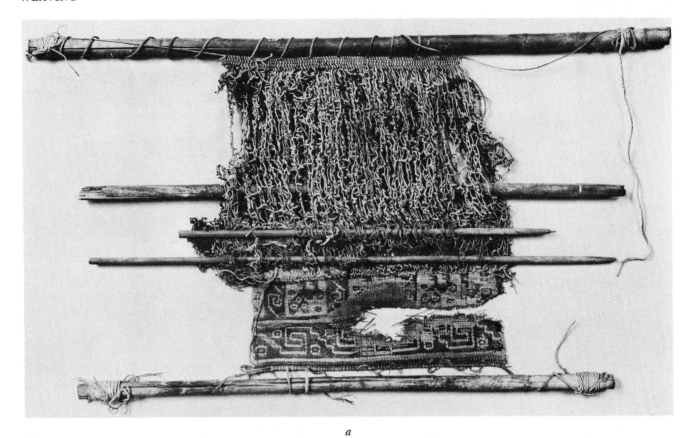

a

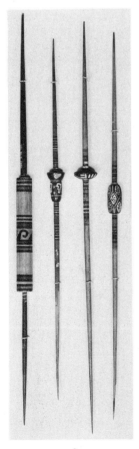

b

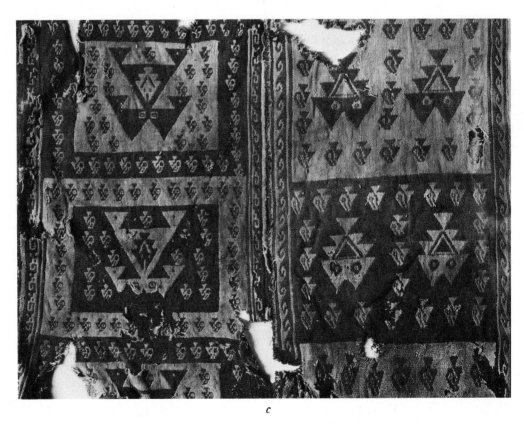

c

PLATE 174.   ©.   *a*) Girdle-back loom with partly woven double cloth, Ica?.   *b*) Spindles and bobbins, Ica?.
c) Double cloth, Ica.

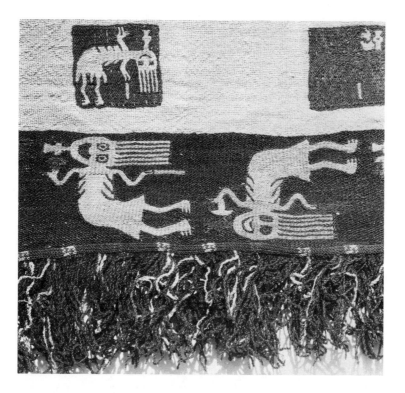

a

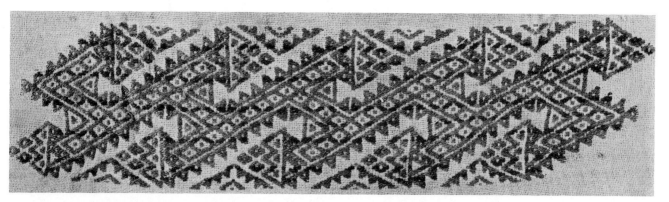

b

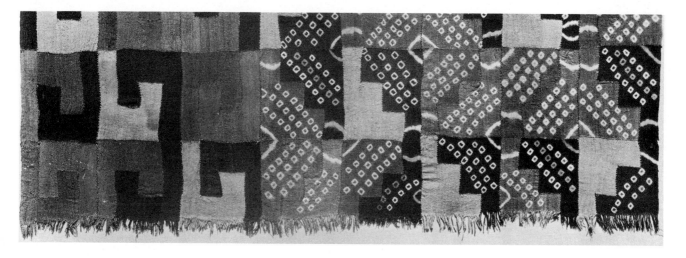

c

PLATE 175. Ⓒ. *a*) Section of fringed shawl with over-all embroidery, Paracas. *b*) Wool
embroidery and brocade on cotton, Nazca. *c*) Interlocking warp (left) and patchwork tie-dye
(right), Coast Tiahuanaco?.

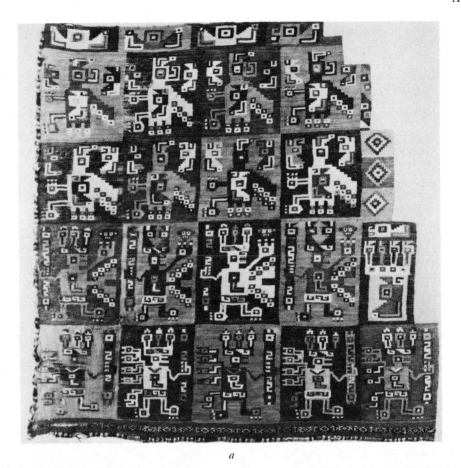

a

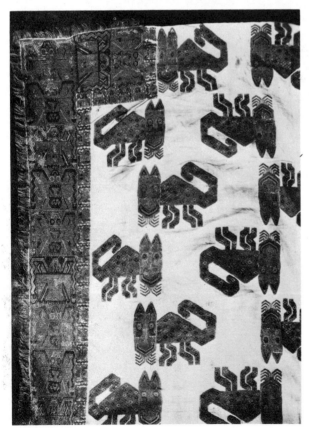

b

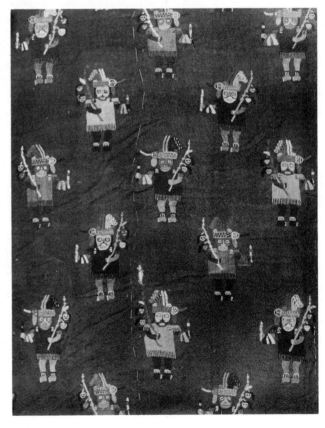

c

PLATE 176. ©.   *a*) Tapestry-like weft pattern, Coast Tiahuanaco. Embroidery: *b* and *c*) Paracas.

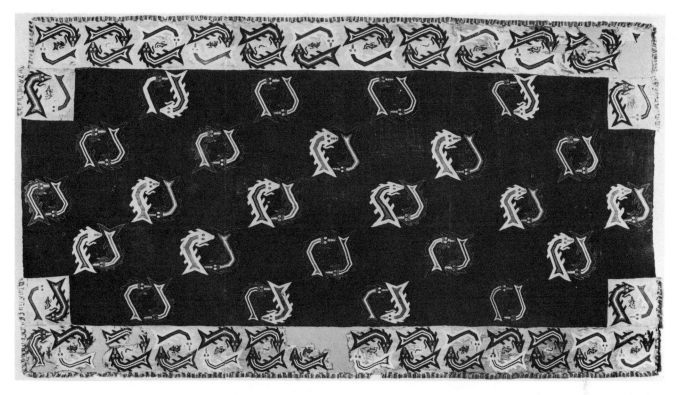

a

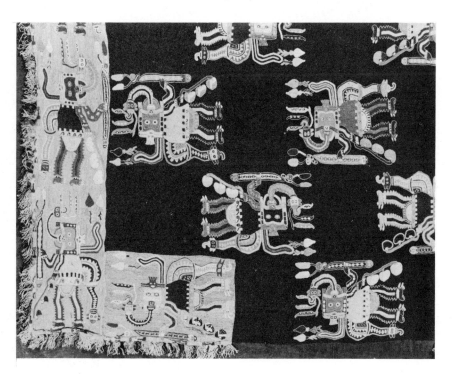

b

PLATE 177.   ©.   Paracas embroidery.

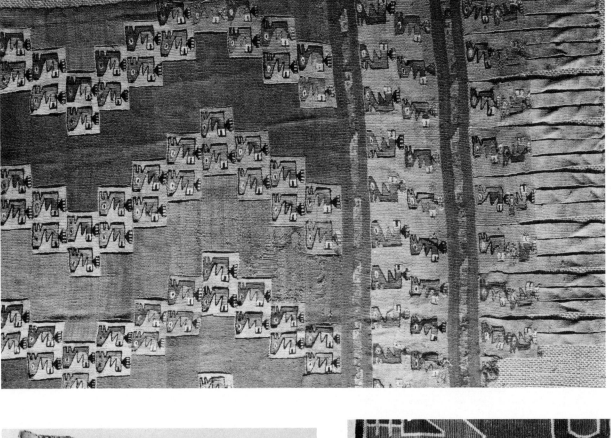

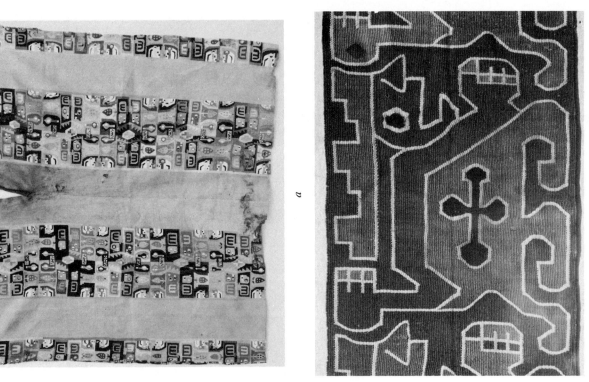

c

a

b

PLATE 178. ©. Coast Tiahuanaco tapestry: *a*) poncho, or shirt; *b*) detail of a band; *c*) section of garment.

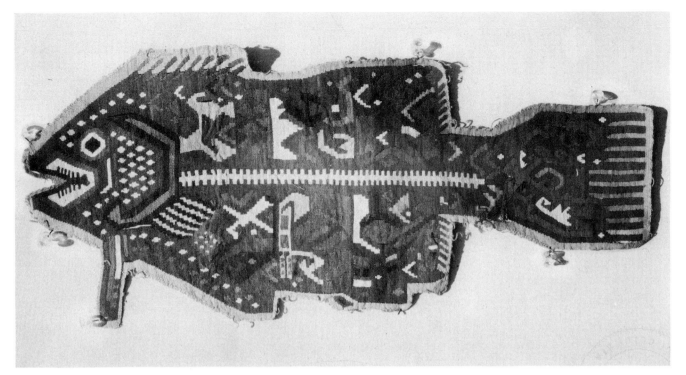

a

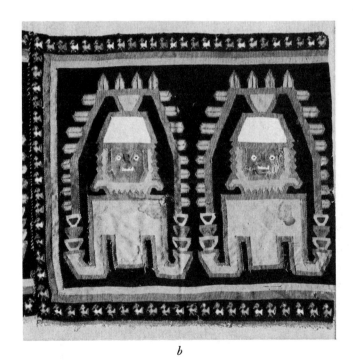

b

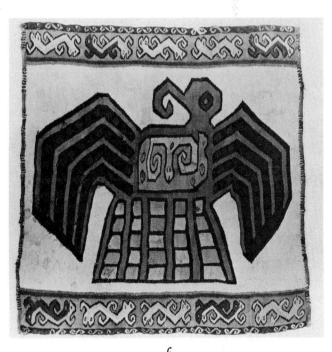

c

PLATE 179. ©. Tapestry: *a*) Chimú?; *b*) Ica; *c*) Coast Tiahuanaco.

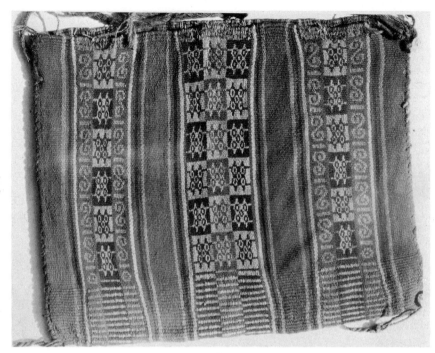

a

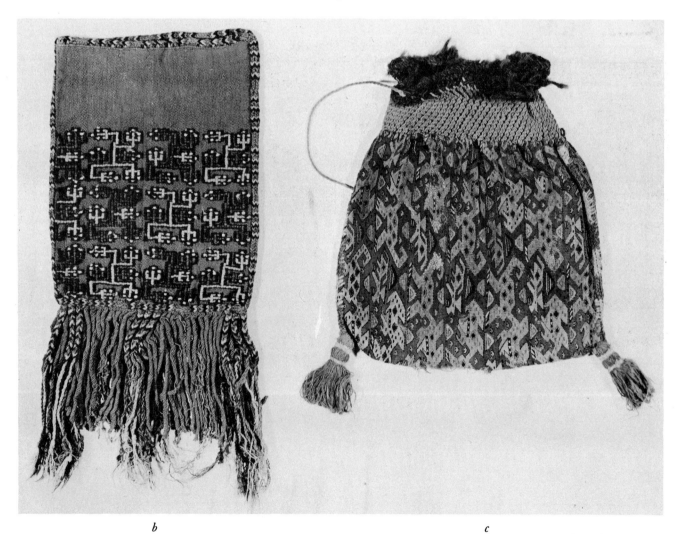

b   *c*

PLATE 180. ©. Bags, or pouches: *a*) Inca; *b*) Late Coast Tiahuanaco; *c*) Coast Tiahuanaco.

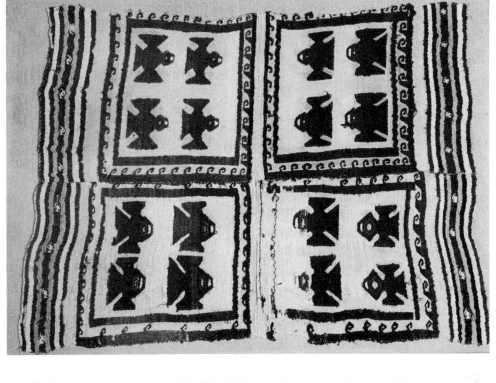

b

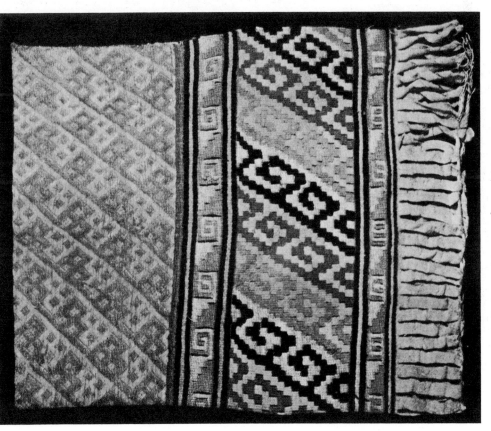

a

PLATE 181. ©. *a*) Brocade with tapestry border, Ica? *b*) Ica brocade, Nazca Valley.

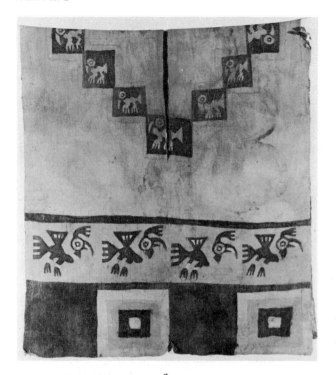

a

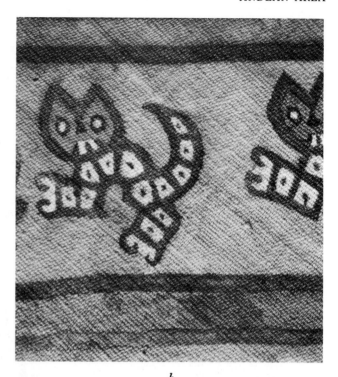

b

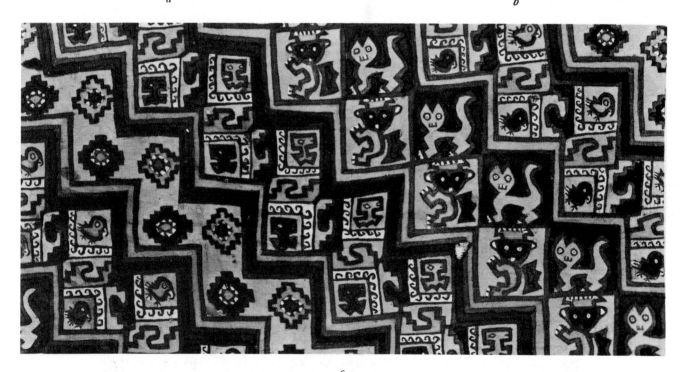

c

PLATE 182. ©. Painted plain-woven cloth: *a*) Chimú?; *b*) Coast Tiahuanaco?; *c*) Late Coast Tiahuanaco?.

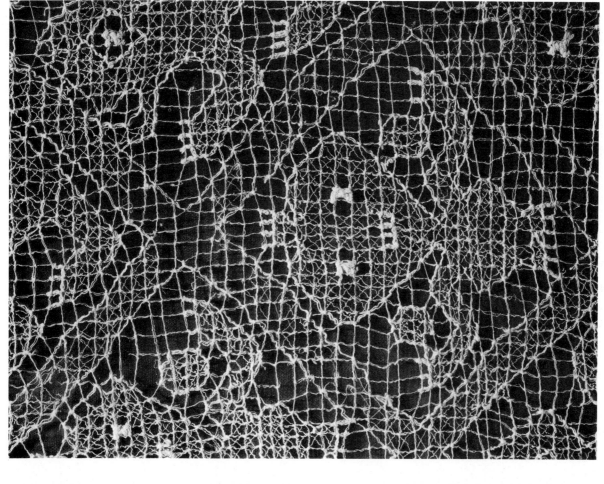

c

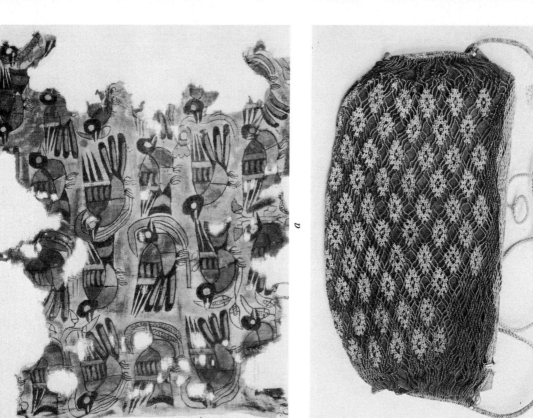

a

b

PLATE 183. © . *a*) Painted cloth, Nazca. *b*) Hairnet of plant fiber, Chimú?. *c*) Embroidered lacelike fabric, Chimú?.

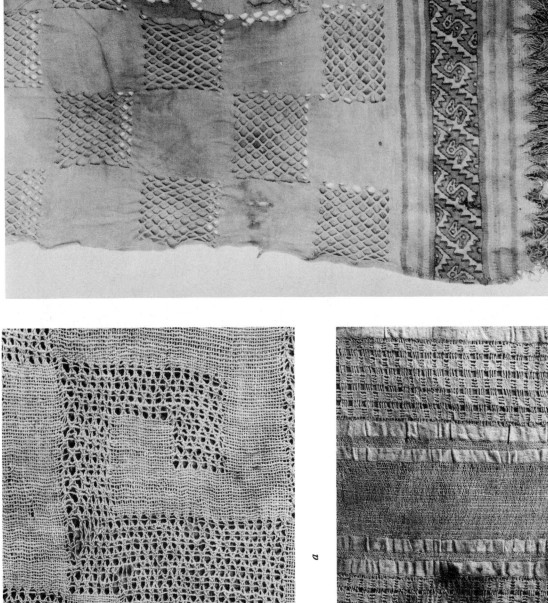

PLATE 184. ©. *a*) Gauze, Nazca. *b*) Gauze with open weave, Chimú?. *c*) Openwork with tapestry border, Ica?.

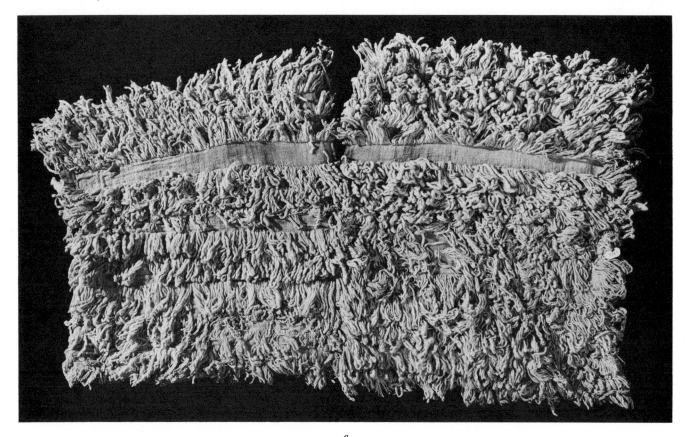

a

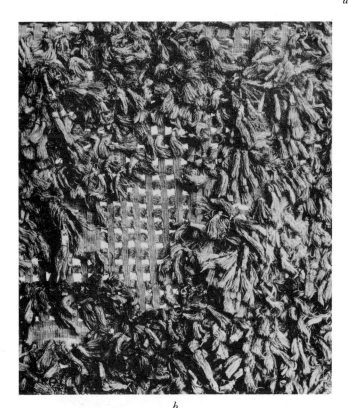

b

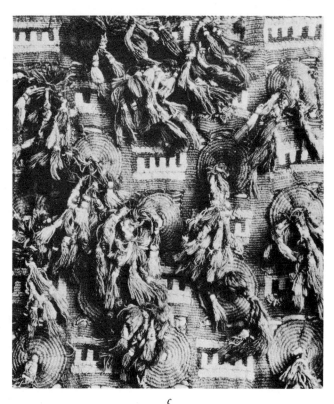

c

PLATE 185. ©.   *a*) Poncho in weft-loop weave.   *b*) Openwork tapestry with tassels.   *c*) Tapestry
with tasseled rosettes.   Chimú?

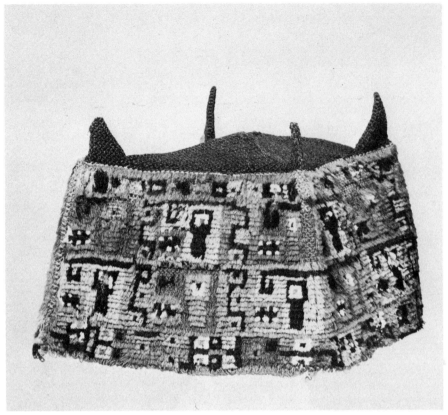

a

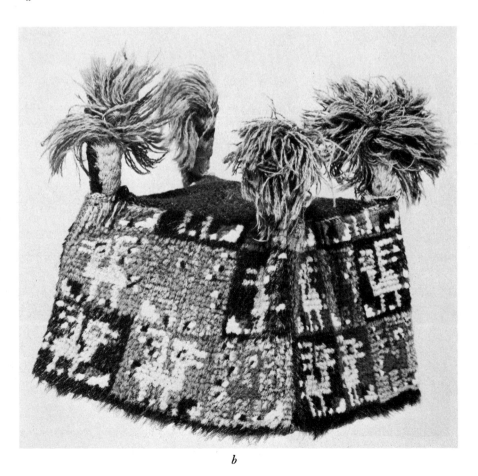

b

PLATE 186. ©. Plush hats, Coast Tiahuanaco.

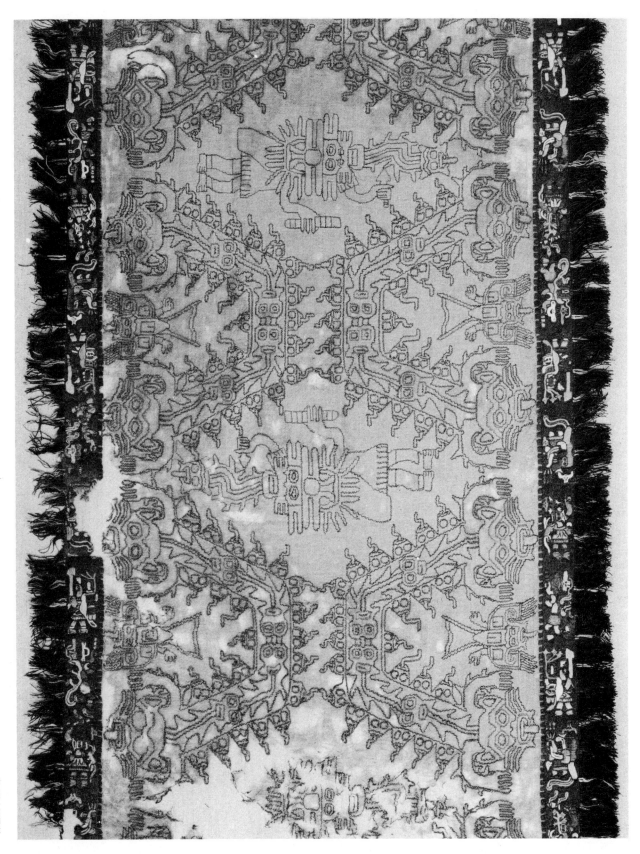

PLATE 187. ⓒ. Section of Paracas embroidered shawl.

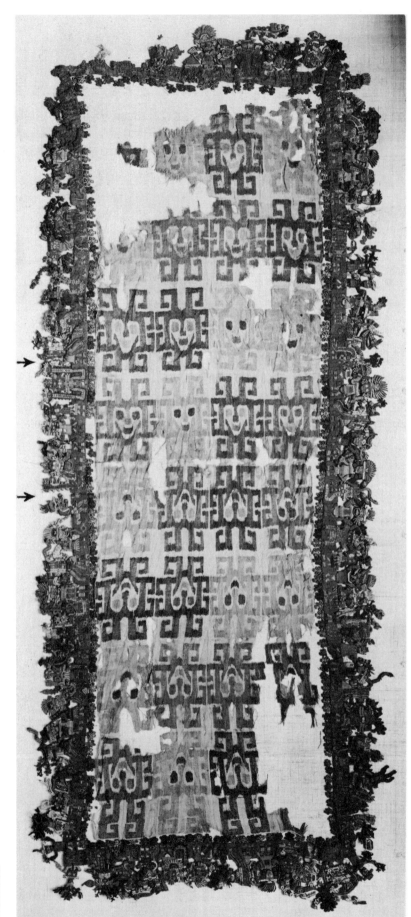

a

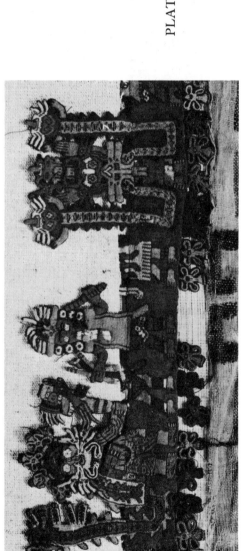

b

PLATE 188. ©. *a*) Paracas mantle with border in three-dimensional knitting. *b*) Detail of border.

WEAVING

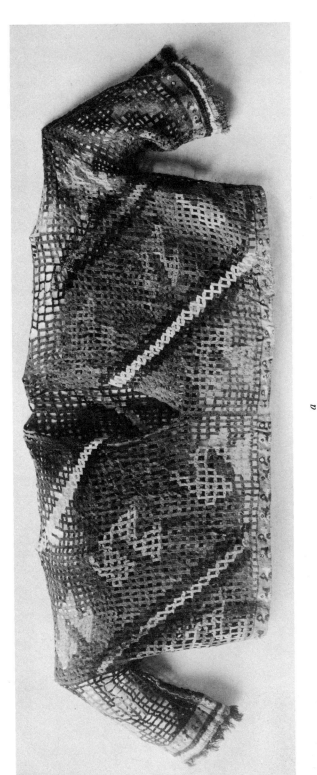

a

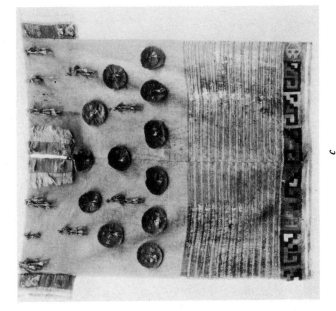

c

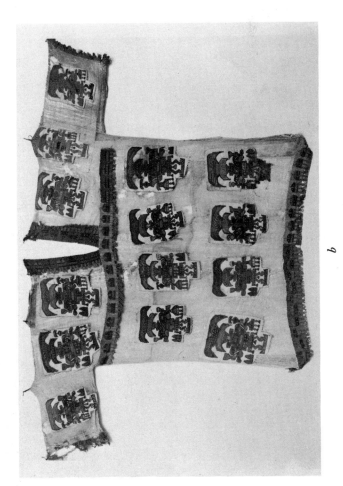

b

PLATE 189. ©. Ponchos: *a)* spaced-warp tapestry, Ica?; *b)* with tapestry medallions, Chimú?; *c)* plain and open weave, with tassels and medallions, Chimú?.

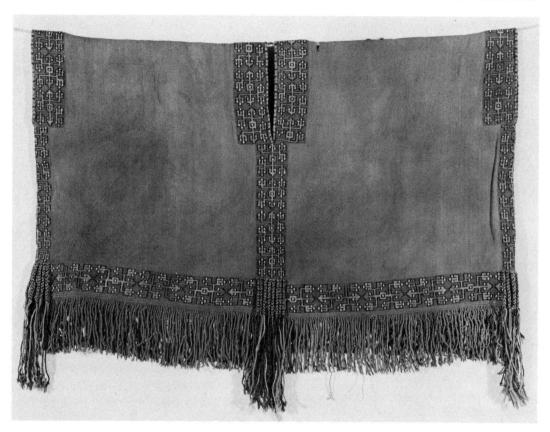

a

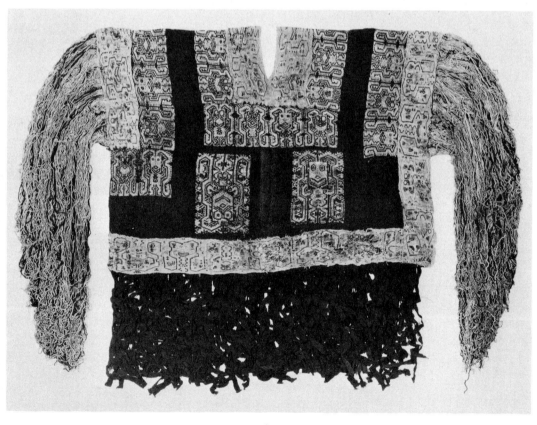

b

PLATE 190. ©. Ponchos: *a*) Late Coast Tiahuanaco?; *b*) Paracas.

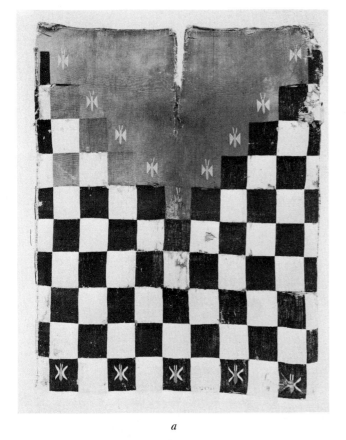

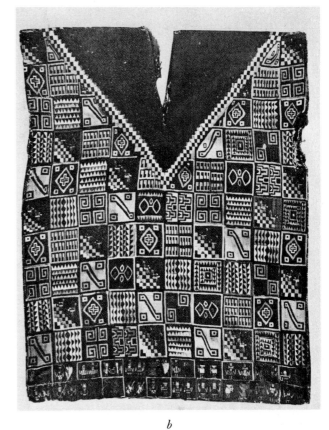

a

b

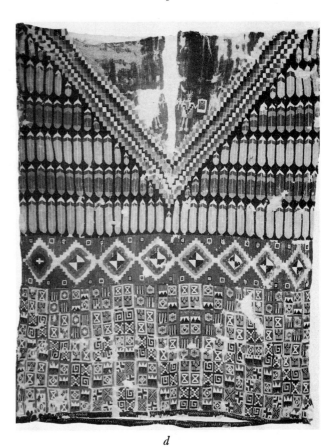

c

d

PLATE 191. ⓒ. Inca tapestry ponchos.

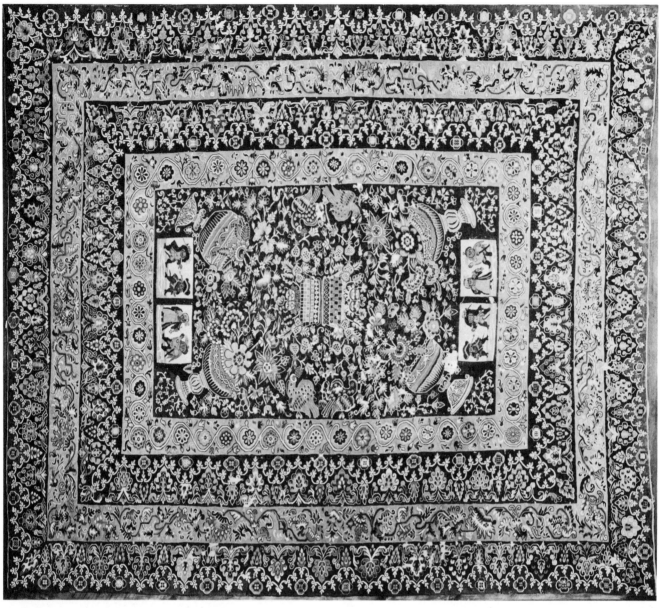

a

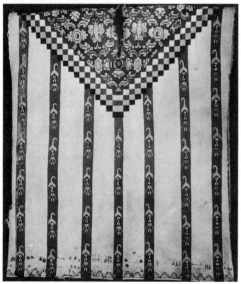

b

PLATE 192. Ⓒ. *a*) Spanish colonial tapestry, Peru, 17th-18th century. *b*) Post-Columbian tapestry poncho, Lake Titicaca, Bolivia, late 16th century.

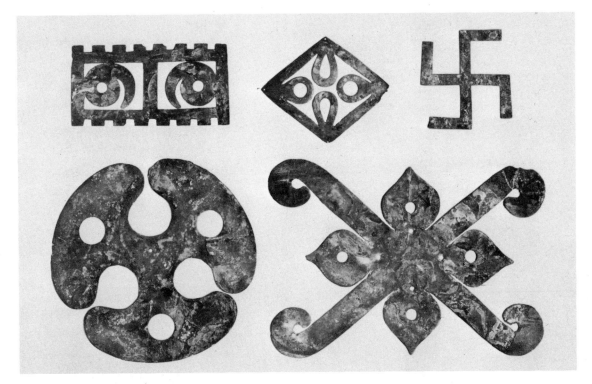

a

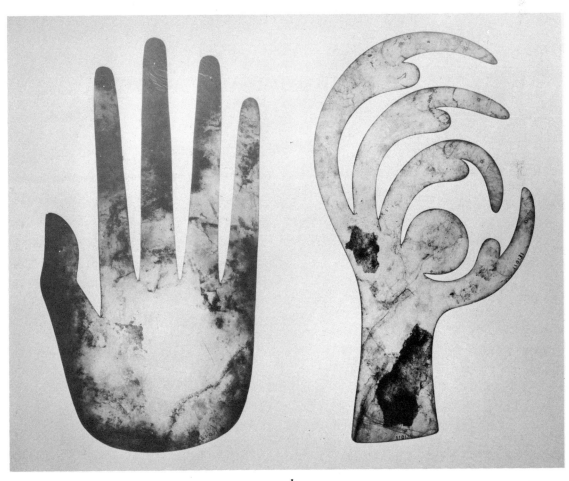

b

PLATE 193. ©. *a*) Copper ornaments for clothing. *b*) Human hand and eagle foot
of mica. Ohio.

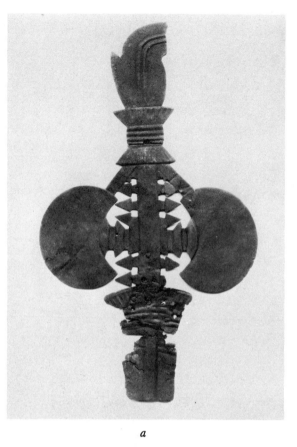

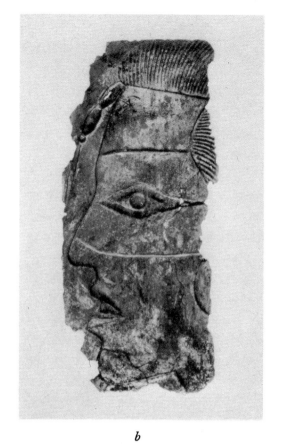

a   *b*

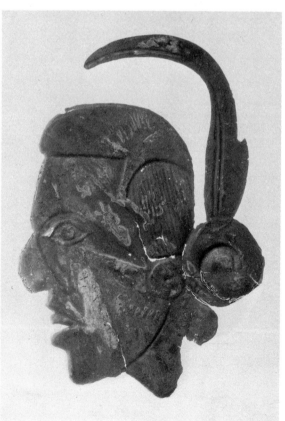

c   *d*

PLATE 194.   ©.   *a*) Copper headdress ornament, Tennessee.   *b, c,* and *d*) Human heads
embossed on sheet copper, Oklahoma.

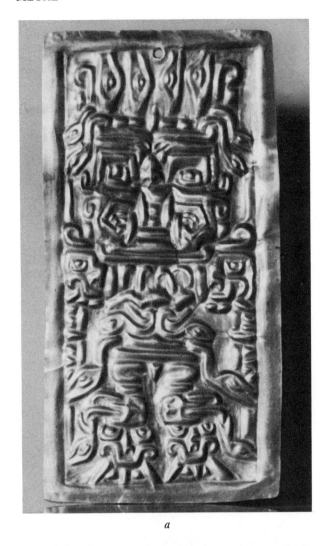

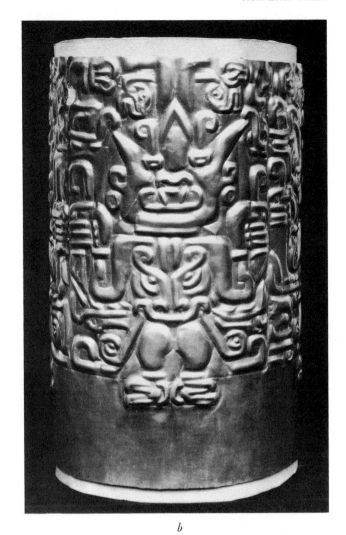

a   *b*

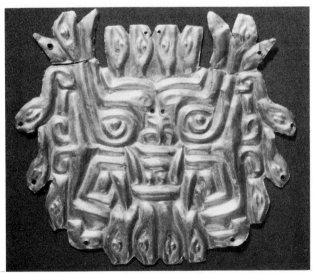

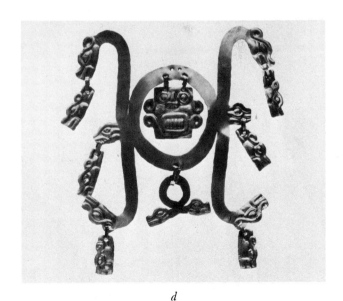

c   *d*

PLATE 195.   ©.   Variations of a Chavin motif in gold, Lambayeque, Peru.

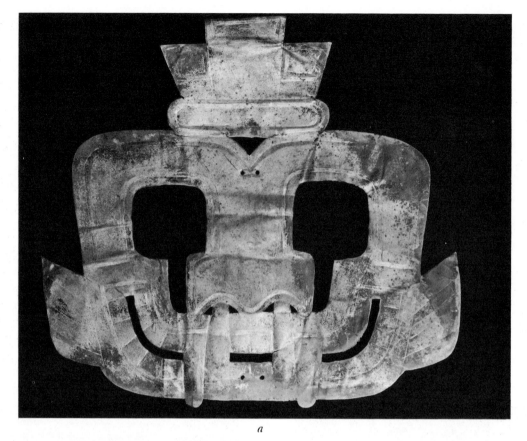

a

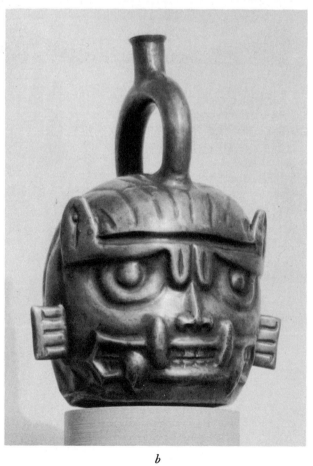

b

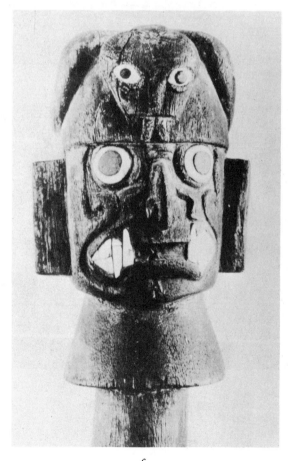

c

PLATE 196.   ©.   Variations of a Chavín motif in silver and wood: *a*) Coast Tiahuanaco;
b) Mochica;   *c*) Late Coast Tiahuanaco.

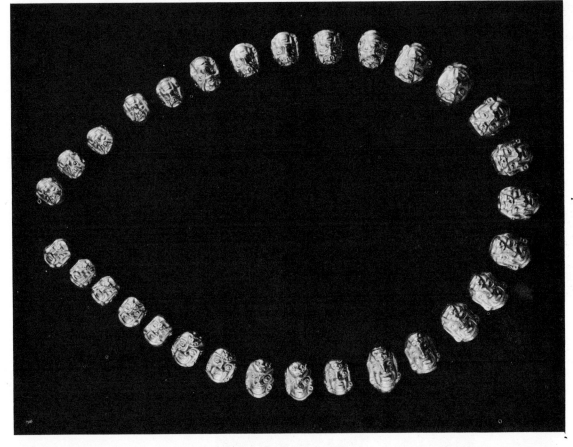

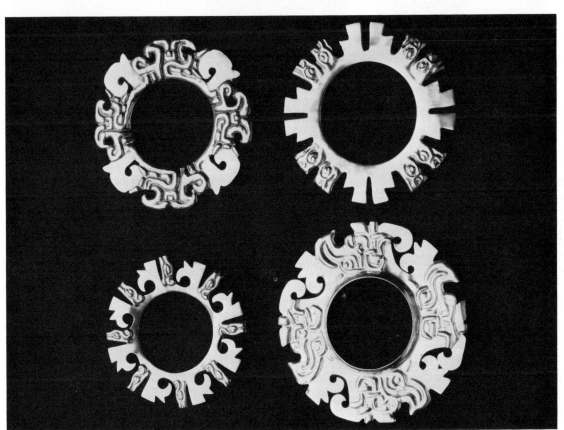

PLATE 197. ⓒ. *a*) Chavín gold ear ornaments, Lambayeque. *b*) Mochica gold necklace embossed with human heads.

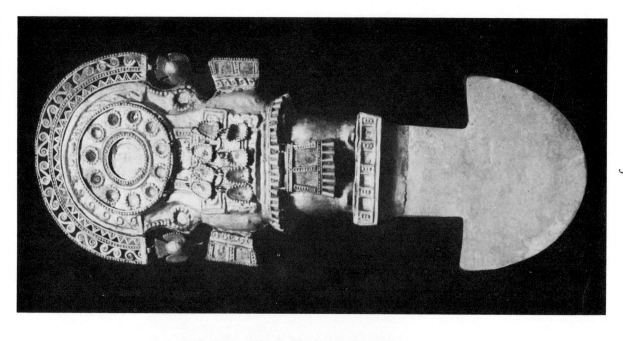

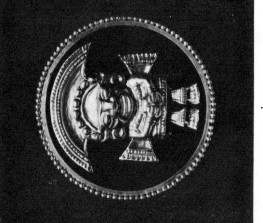

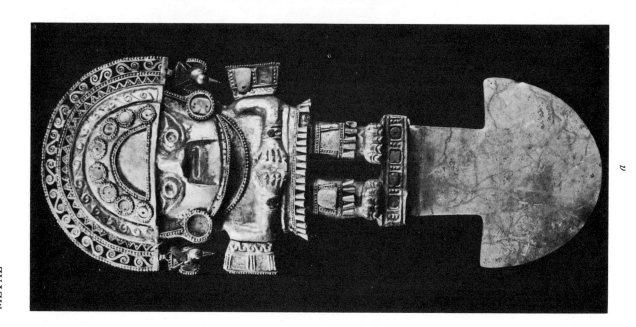

PLATE 198. ©. *a* and *c*) Chimú gold ceremonial knife with turquoise inlay, Illimo, Lambayeque Valley. *b*) Face of Chimú gold earplug showing same figure, Jayanga.

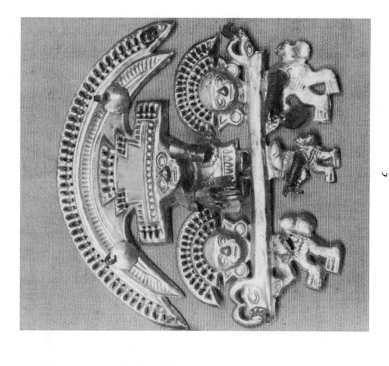

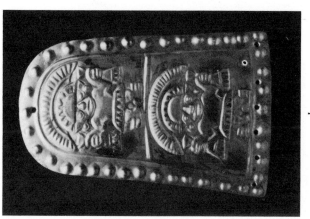

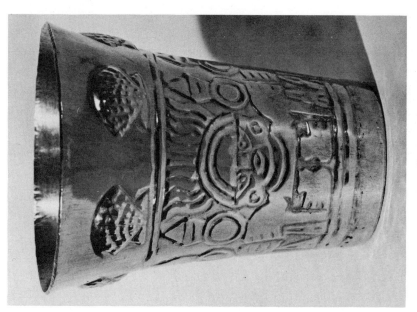

PLATE 199. ©. Chimú gold objects decorated with human figures: *a*) cup; *b*) plaque; *c*) face of earplug.

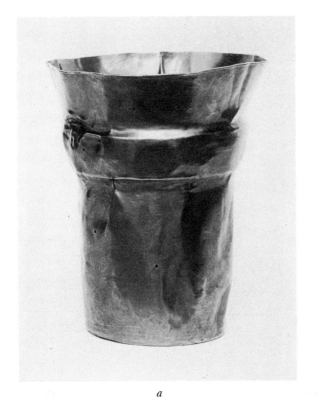

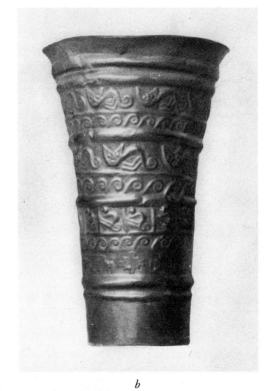

a

b

c

PLATE 200. ©. *a*) Gold cup, Classic Tiahuanaco. *b*) Silver embossed cup, Late Coast
Tiahuanaco. *c*) Gold cups and cup-shaped ear ornaments, Chimú.

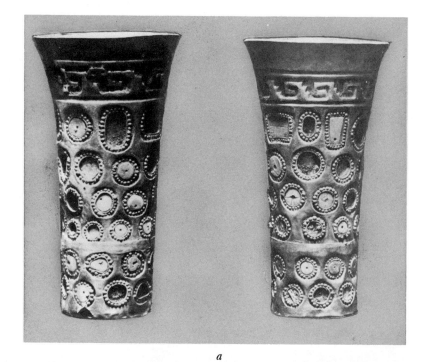

a

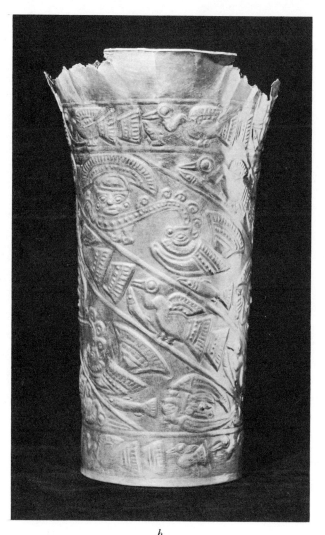

b

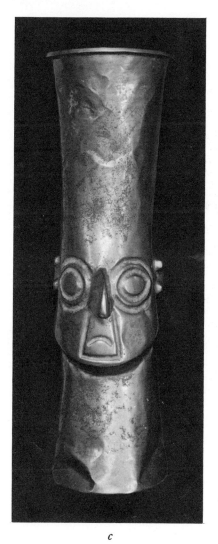

c

PLATE 201. ©. *a*) Chimú gold cups with turquoise incrustation, Illimo. *b*) Chimú silver
cup, embossed, Piura Valley. *c*) Chimú gold goblet in the shape of a human head, Peru.

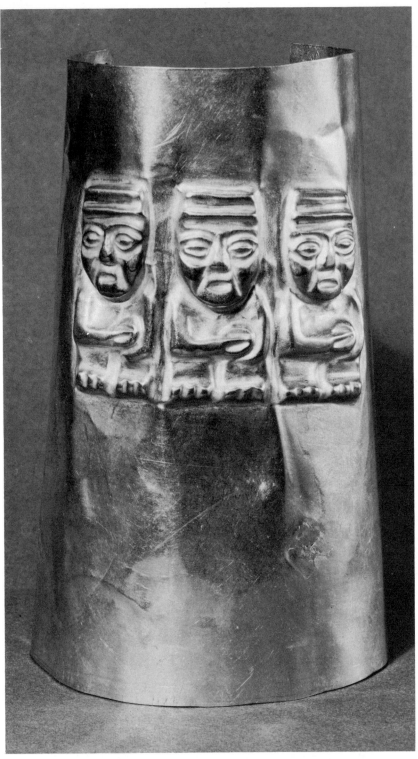

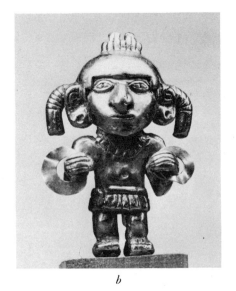

b

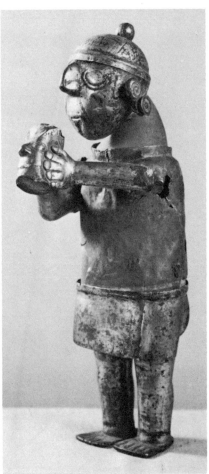

c

a

PLATE 202.   ©.   *a*) Gold cuff, Mochica?.   *b*) Cast gold figure, Chimú.   *c*) Silver doll with
hinged arms, Chimú.

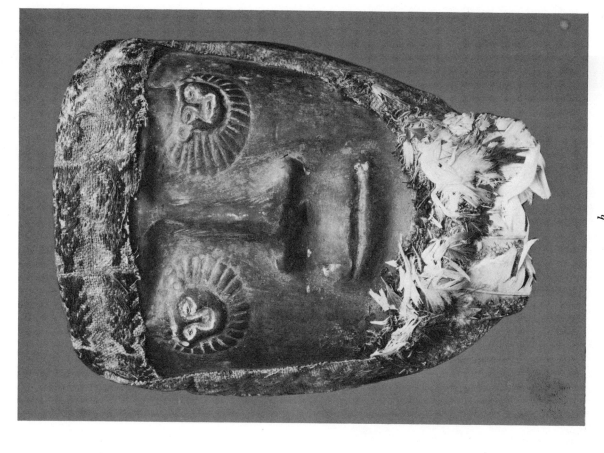

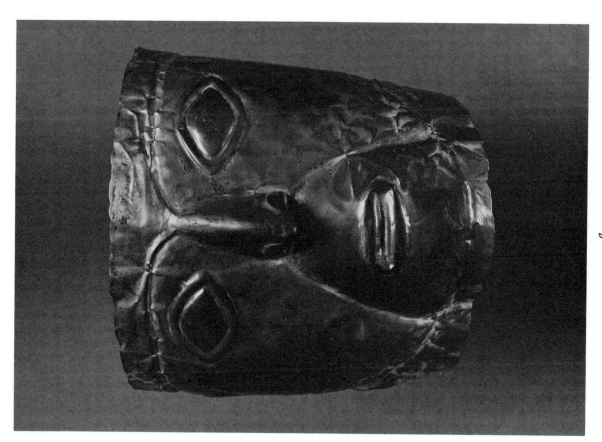

b

a

PLATE 203. ©. Chimú metal masks from mummy packs: *a*) hammered gold; *b*) base silver with textile and feather additions.

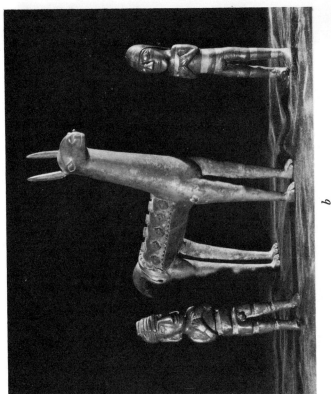

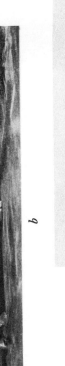

b

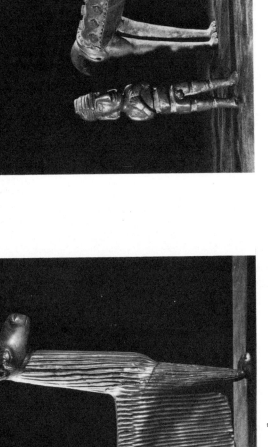

a

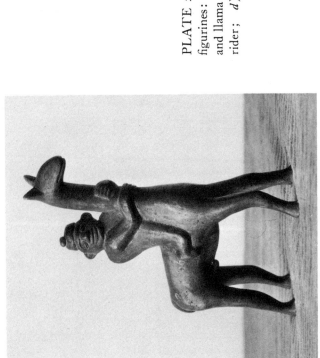

PLATE 204. ©. Inca human and animal figurines: *a*) silver alpaca; *b*) man, woman, and llama of cast silver; *c*) copper llama and rider; *d*) alpaca or guanaco, silver alloy with gold head.

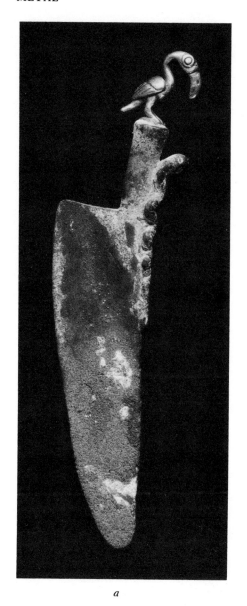

a

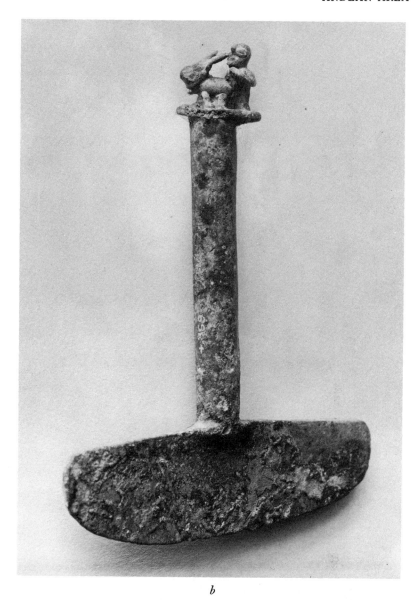

b

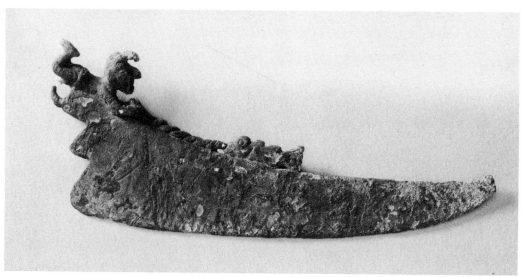

c

PLATE 205.   ©.   Inca bronze knives: *a*) with snake and gold pelican;   *b*) man and llama;   *c*) boy fishing.

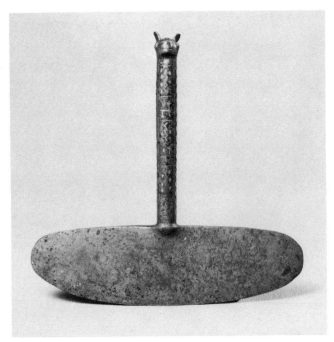

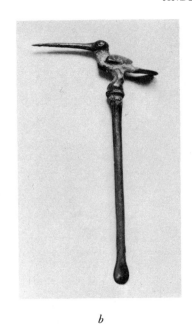

a

b

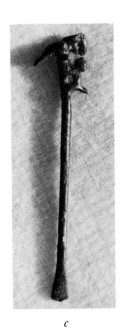

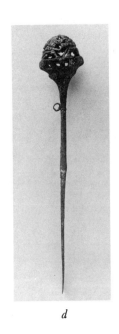

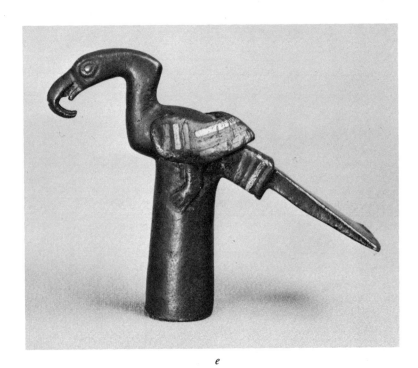

c

d

e

PLATE 206. Ⓒ. Inca implements: *a*) bronze knife with inlaid handle shaped into a llama head; *b*) bronze "spoon" with bird; *c*) bronze tool with parrot and monkey; *d*) copper awl or pin with human figures, Inca or Chimú; *e*) bronze adze in the form of a bird, with copper and silver inlay.

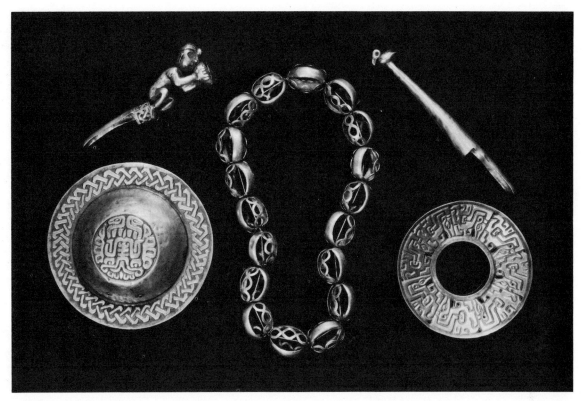

a

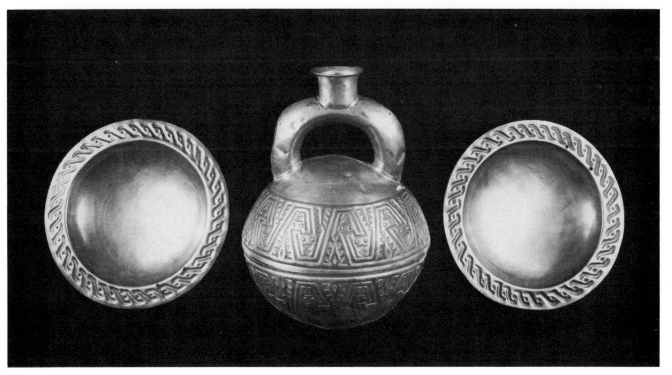

b

PLATE 207.   ©.   *a*) Chavín gold objects for personal use.   *b*) Chimú gold plates and stirrup jar.

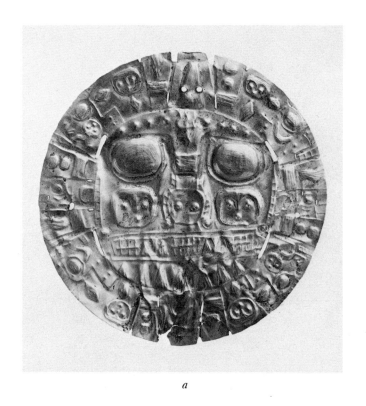

a

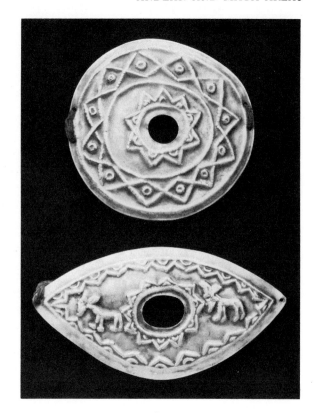

b

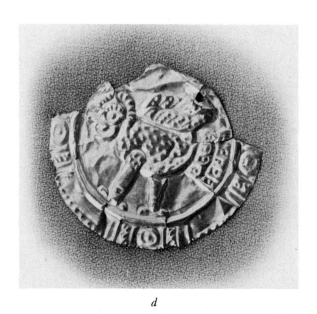

c

d

PLATE 208. ©. *a*) Gold calendar? disk, Peruvian highlands. *b*) Inca? silver ornaments, Cuzco, Peru.
c and *d*) Gold disks found near Zacualpa, Guatemala.

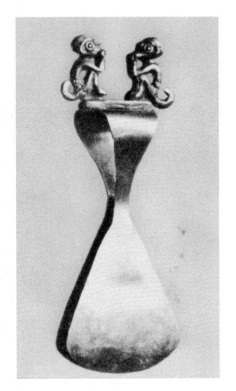

a

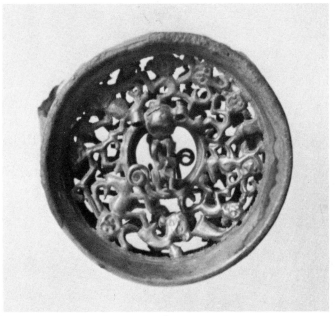

b

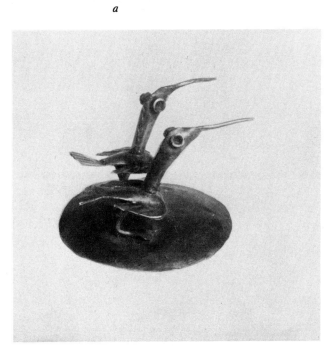

c

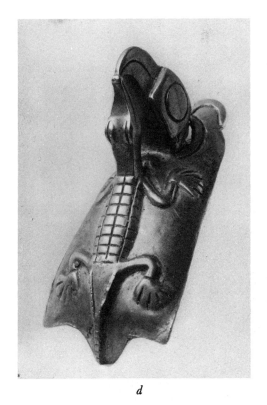

d

PLATE 209. Ⓒ. Gold animal representations of late cultures: *a*) beard-tongs with monkeys,
Chimú?; *b*) earplug with monkeys, Chimú?; *c*) face of earplug with colibris, Ica; *d*) pendant
with bird and alligator, Coast Tiahuanaco?.

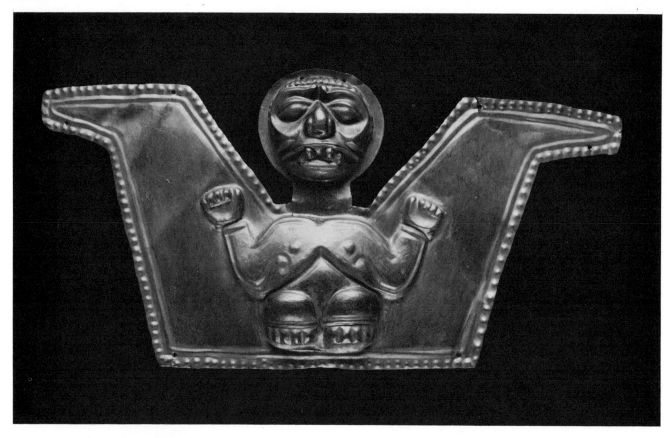

a

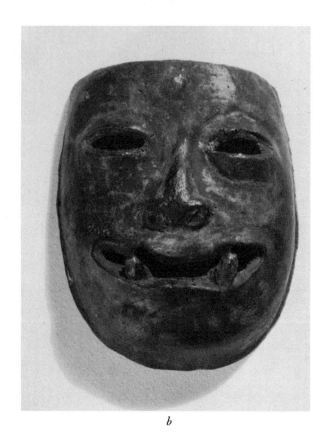

b

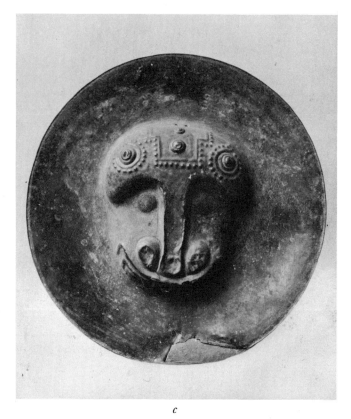

c

PLATE 210. Ⓒ. *a*) Gold breast ornament. *b*) Bronze mask. *c*) Bronze disk. Ecuador.

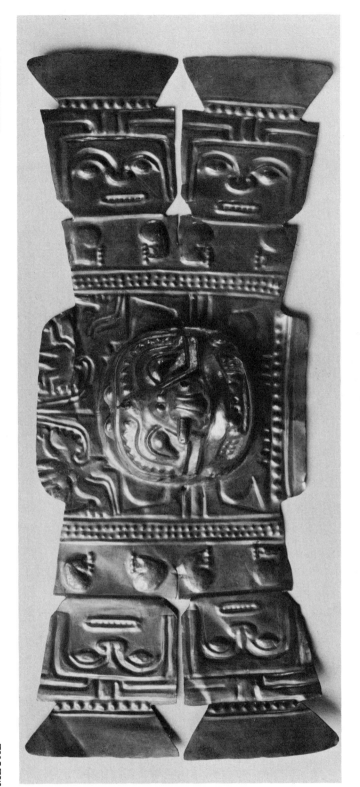

a

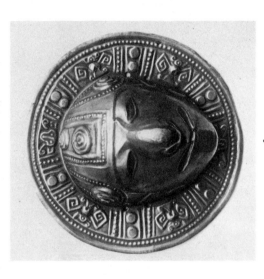

b

PLATE 211. ©. *a*) Gold breastplate. *b*) Small gold mask. Ecuador.

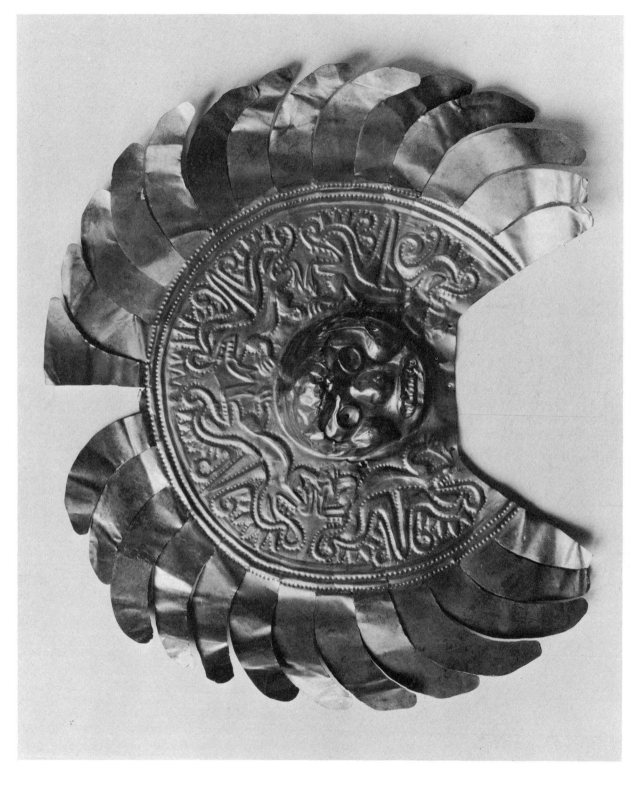

PLATE 212.   ©.   Gold breastplate, Esmeraldas, Ecuador.

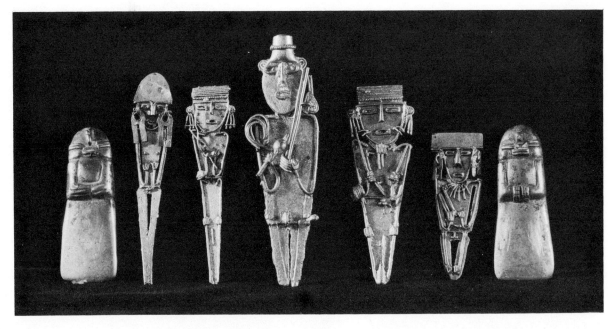

a

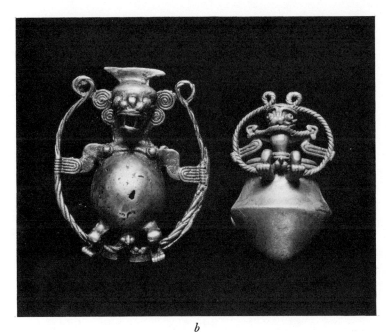

b

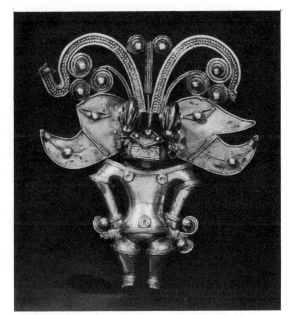

c

PLATE 213.   ©.   *a*) Chibcha gold ornaments, Colombia.   *b*) Gold bells, Colombia.   *c*) Gold anthropomorphic figure, Venezuela.

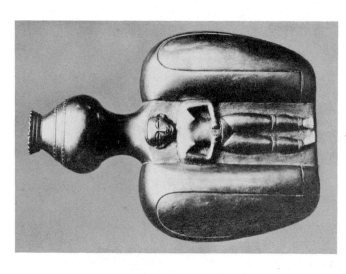

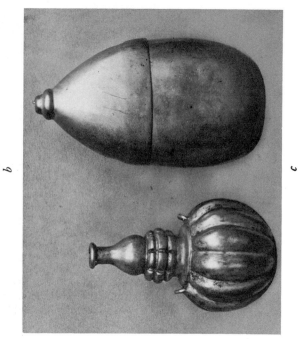

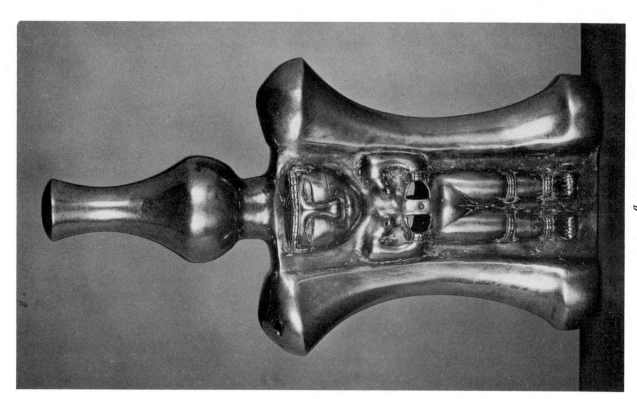

PLATE 214. ©. Quimbaya gold flasks, Antioquia, Colombia.

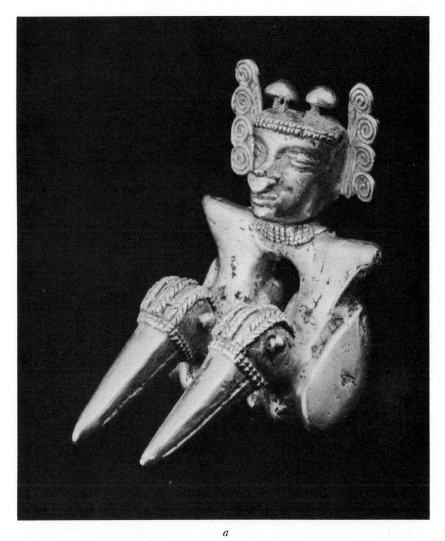

a

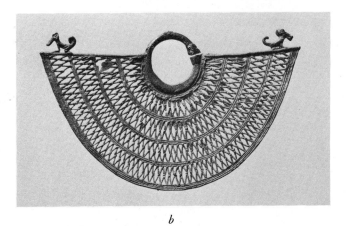

b

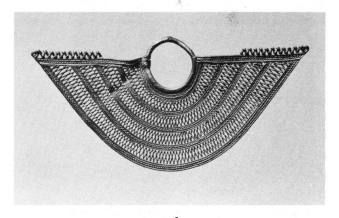

c

PLATE 215. ©. *a*) Quimbaya gold pendant, blending human and bird elements. *b* and *c*) Gold nose ornaments, such as worn by figure above.

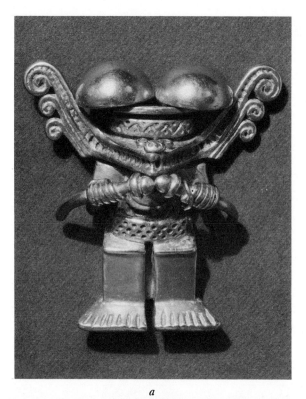

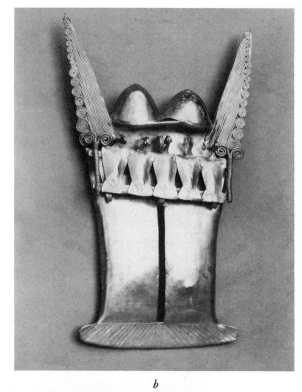

a   *b*

c

PLATE 216.   ⓒ.   Metamorphosis of a Quimbaya figure, Colombia.

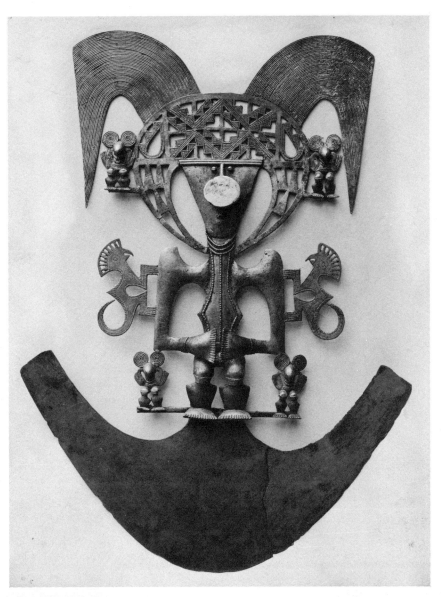

a

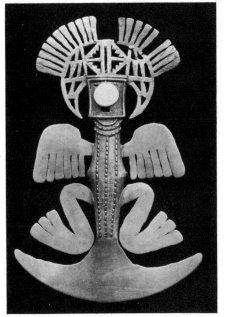

PLATE 217. ©. Versions of
knife-shaped pendants, Colombia.

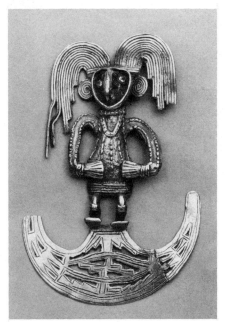

b

c

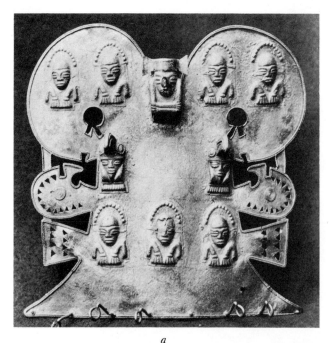

a

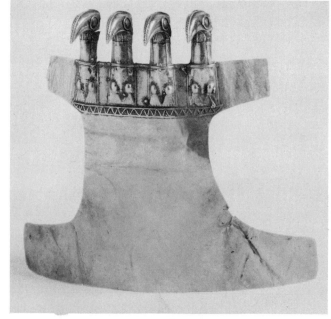

b

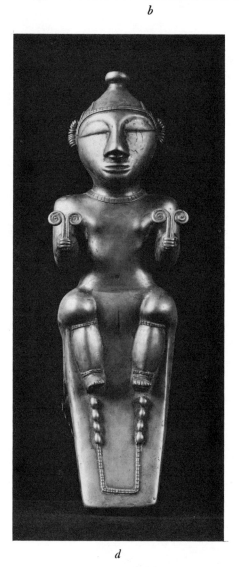

c   *d*

PLATE 218. ©. Gold plaques, Colombia: *a*) with human figures; *b*) with birds on a tower; *c* and *d*) Quimbaya female idols in cast gold.

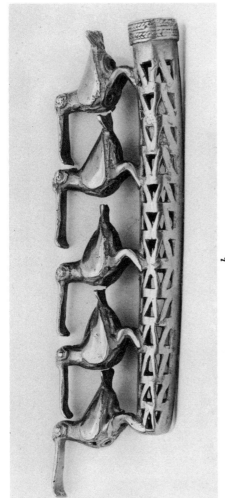

b

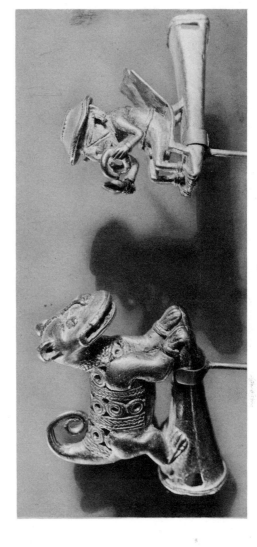

c

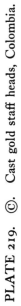

a

PLATE 219. ©. Cast gold staff heads, Colombia.

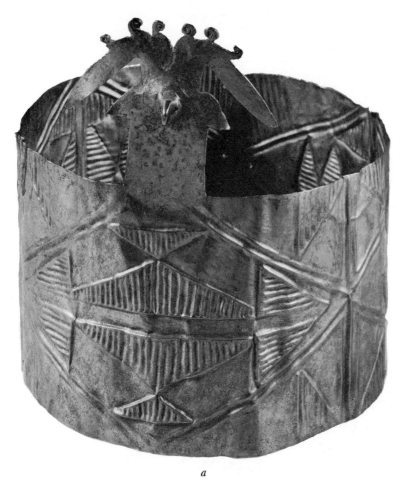

a

b

PLATE 220.   ⓒ.   Quimbaya gold crown and helmet, Colombia.

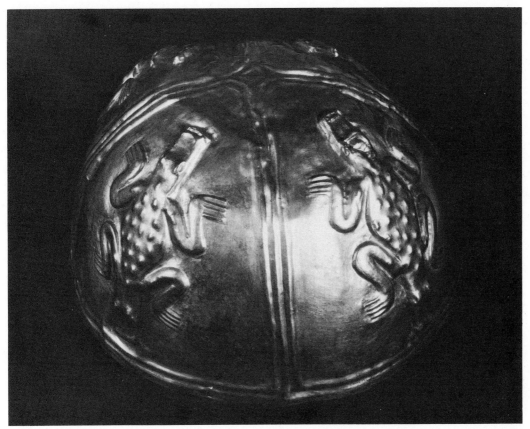

a

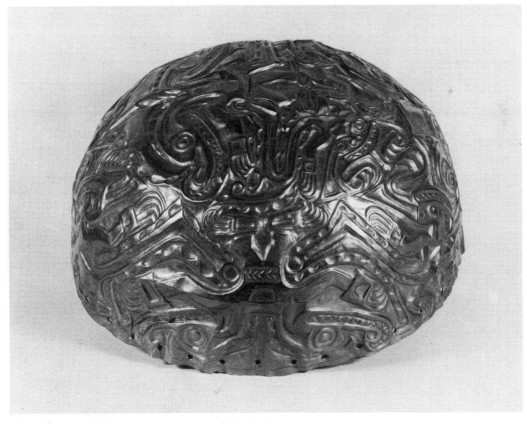

b

PLATE 221. Ⓒ. Gold helmets, Panama.

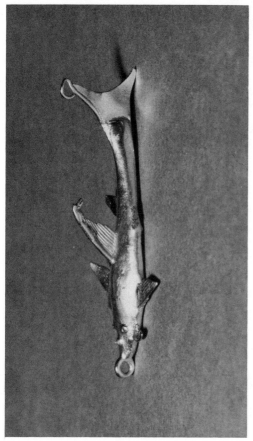

b

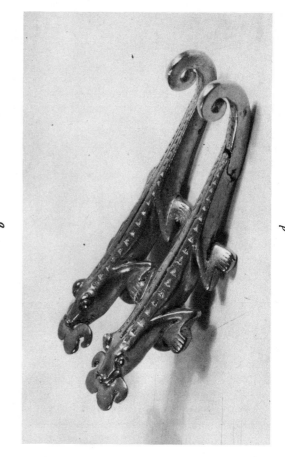

d

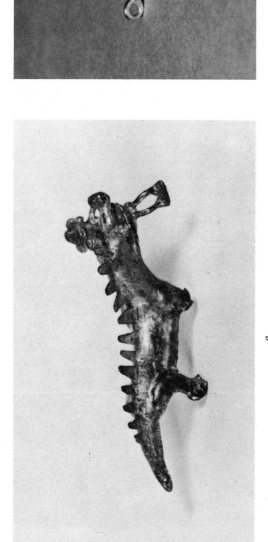

a

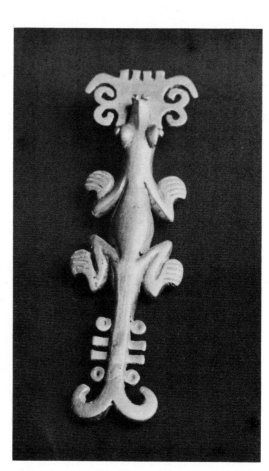

c

PLATE 222. ⓒ. *a*) Gold alligator or crocodile with human prey, Costa Rica. *b*) Gold shark pendant, Chiriquí, Panama. *c* and *d*) Gold alligators carrying conventionalized shapes, Coclé, Panama.

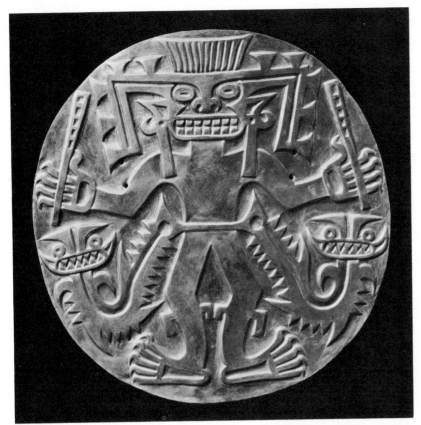

a

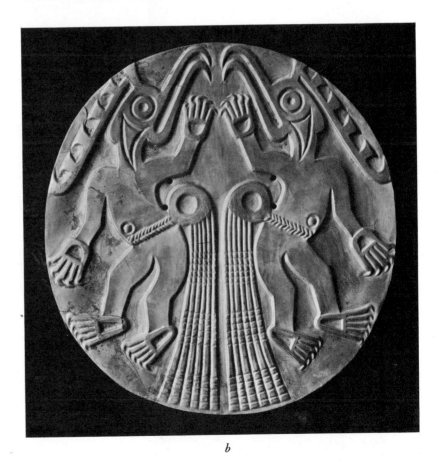

b

PLATE 223. ©. Embossed gold plaques, Coclé, Panama.

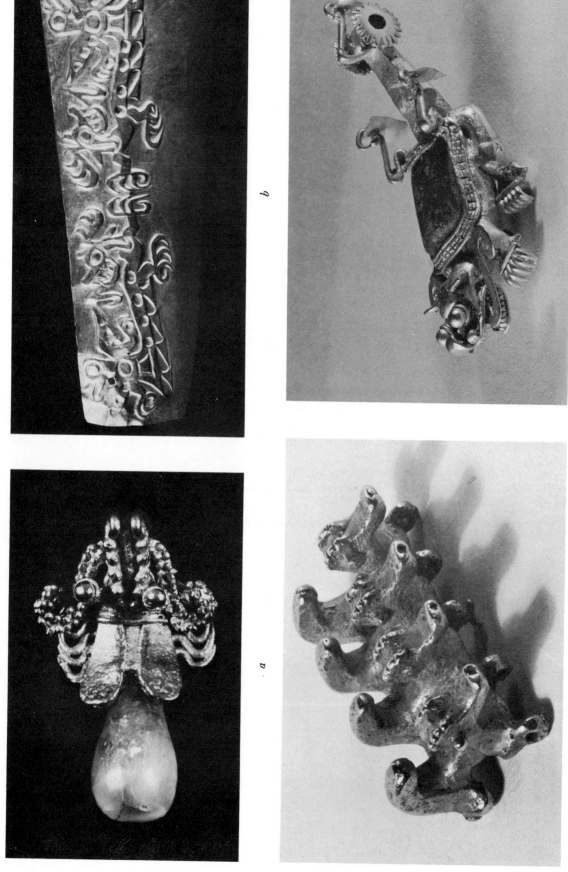

b

a

c

d

PLATE 224. ©. Masterpieces of the jeweler's art, Coclé, Panama: *a*) insect of gold and quartz; *b*) gold cuff with animals in repoussé; *c*) gold dogs or alligator cubs; *d*) gold pendant with inset emerald, in the form of a fantastic animal.

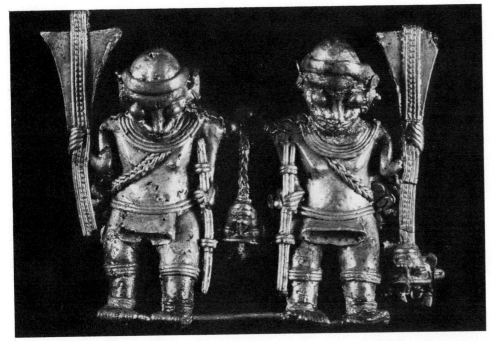

a

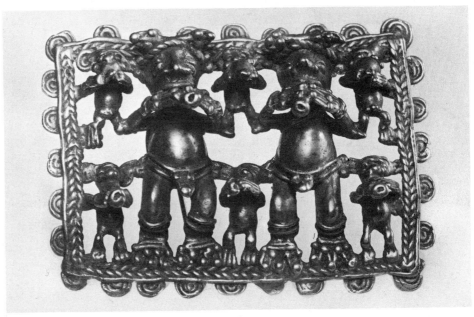

b

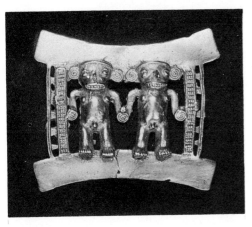

c

PLATE 225. Ⓒ. Pendants with twin figures: *a*) *tumbaga* alloy,
Coclé, Panama; *b*) gold, Chiriquí?, Panama; *c*) gold, Costa Rica.

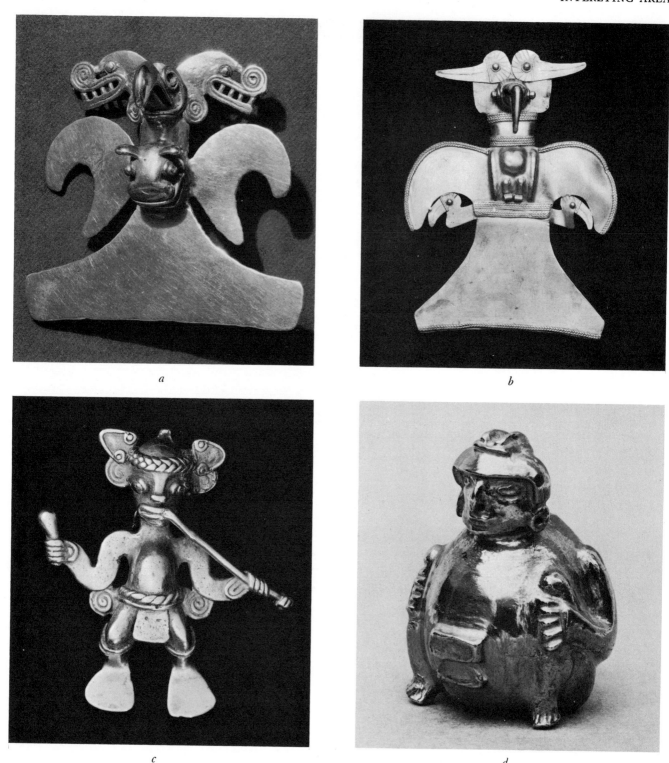

a

b

c

d

PLATE 226. ©. *a* and *b*) Gold bird pendants, Costa Rica and Colombia. *c*) Gold figurine, Panama. *d*) Gold rattle in human shape, Costa Rica.

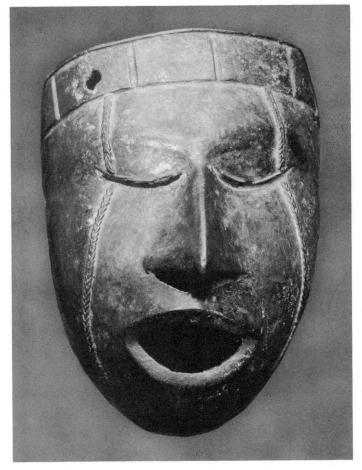

a

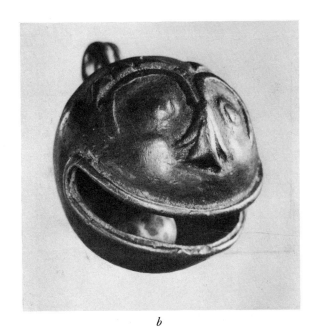

b

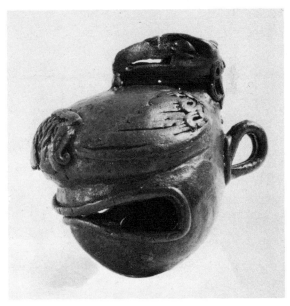

c

PLATE 227.   ©.   *a*) Tarascan copper mask of Xipe-Totec, Mexico.   *b* and *c*) Copper
bells, Honduras and British Honduras.

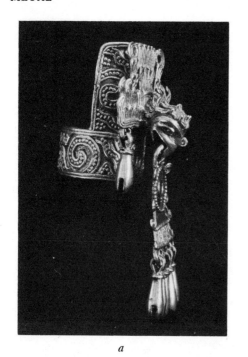

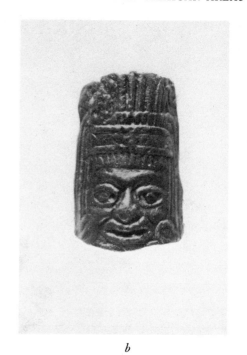

a

b

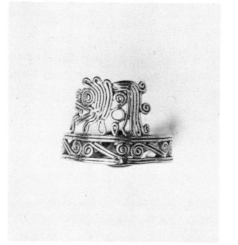

c

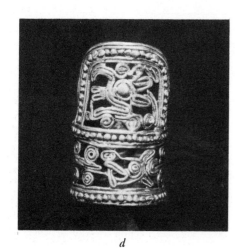

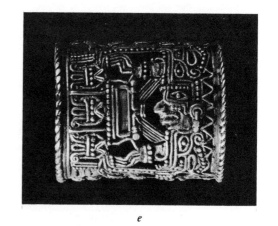

d

e

PLATE 228. ©. Finger rings: *a*) gold with eagle pendant, Oaxaca, Mexico; *b*) copper, with human head, El Salvador; *c*) gold, with feathered serpent, Oaxaca; *d*) gold, with glyphs, Oaxaca; *e*) gold with human profile, Oaxaca.

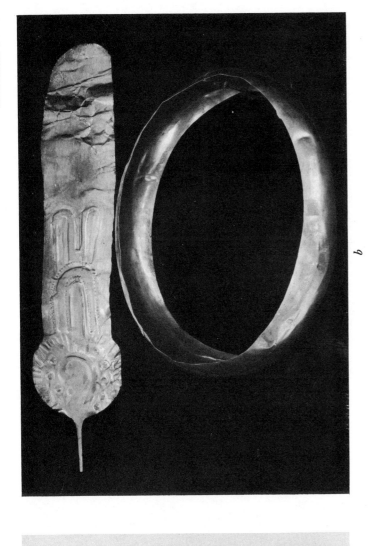

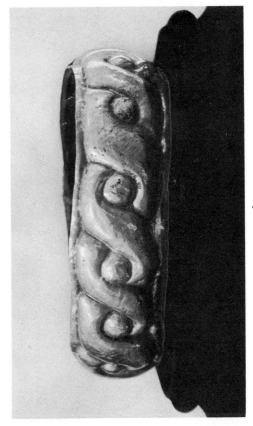

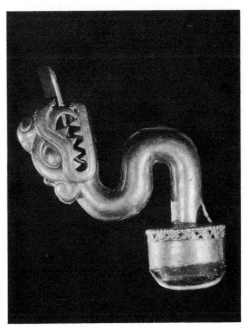

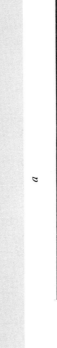

PLATE 229. ©. Gold articles of personal adornment, Oaxaca: *a* and *c*) lipplugs; *b*) diadem with feather; *d*) bracelet.

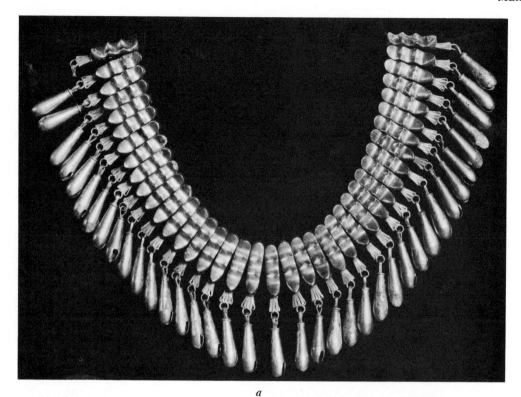

a

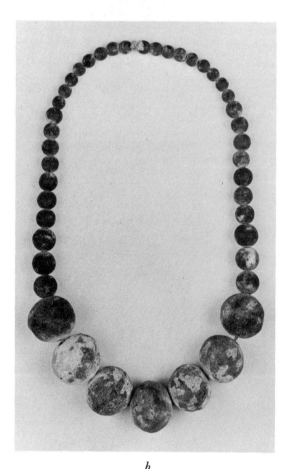

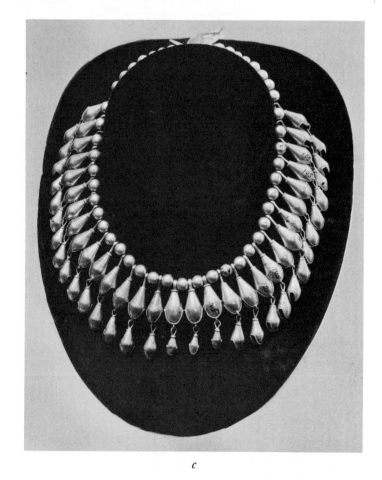

b   *c*

PLATE 230. Ⓒ. Necklaces: *a* and *c*) gold, Tomb 7, Monte Albán, Oaxaca; *b*) silver and copper alloy,
Texcoco, Mexico.

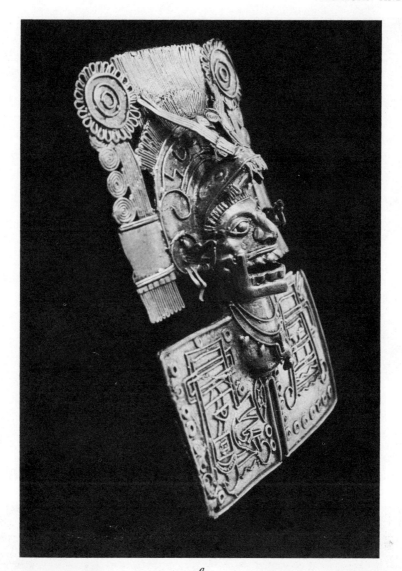

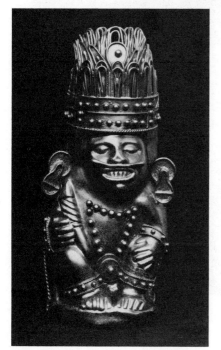

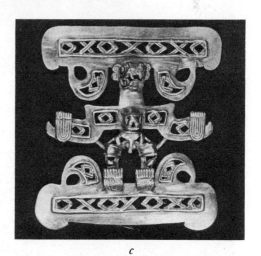

PLATE 231. ©. *a*) Cast gold pectoral of Jaguar-Knight, Tomb 7, Monte Albán, Oaxaca, Mexico. *b*) Gold figure of the Aztec king, Tizoc, Texcoco, Mexico. *c*) Cast gold pectoral with fantastic animal, Costa Rica.

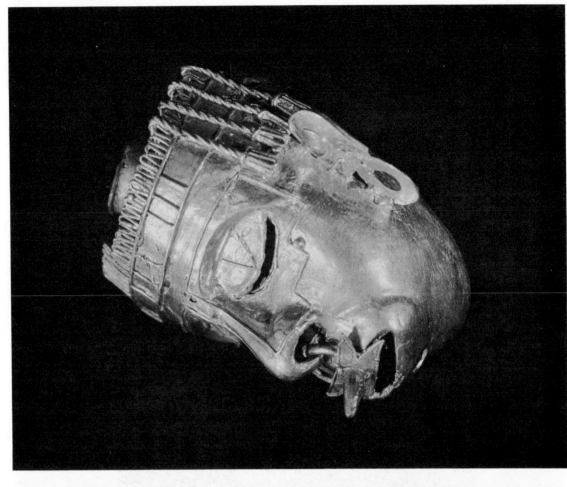

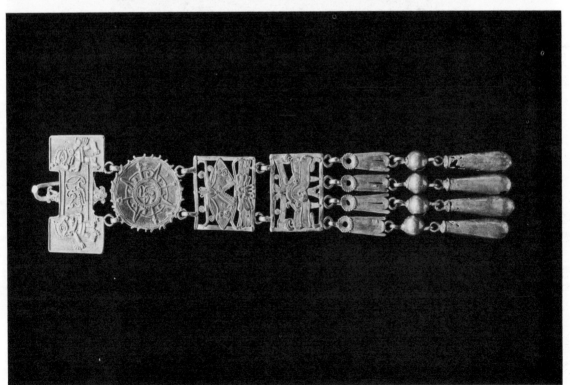

PLATE 232. ©. *a*) Gold pendant made up of seven symbolic elements. *b*) Small gold mask of Xipe-Totec. Tomb 7, Monte Albán.

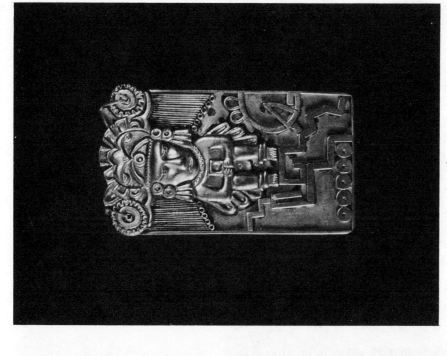

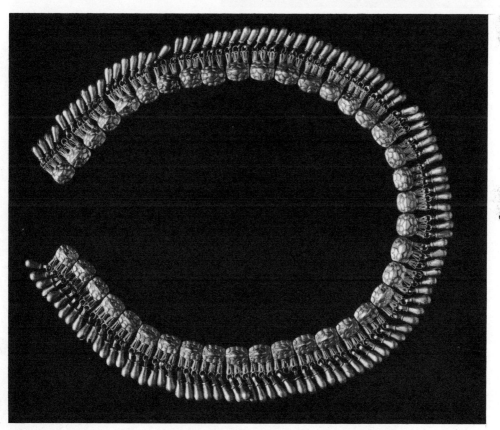

PLATE 233. ©. *a*) Gold necklace, Oaxaca. *b*) Small gold plaque, Vera Cruz.

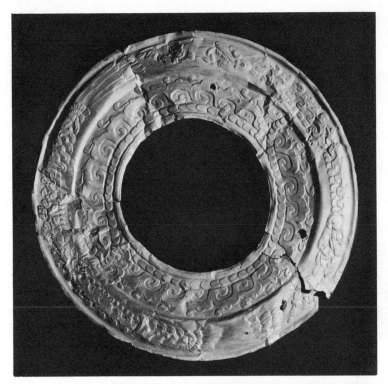

a

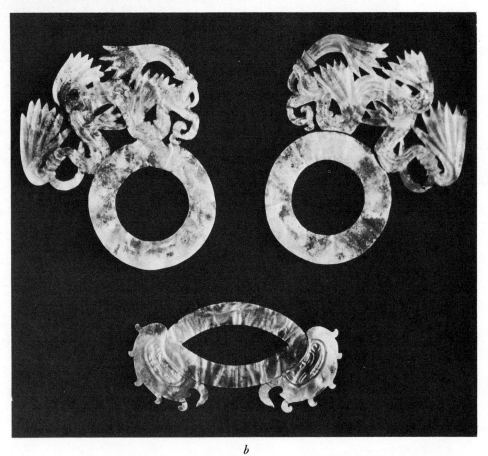

b

PLATE 234.   ©.   *a*) Gold solar disk in repoussé, Texmilincan, Guerrero.   *b*) Gold frames for eyes
and mouth from a mask, Sacred Well, Chichén Itzá.

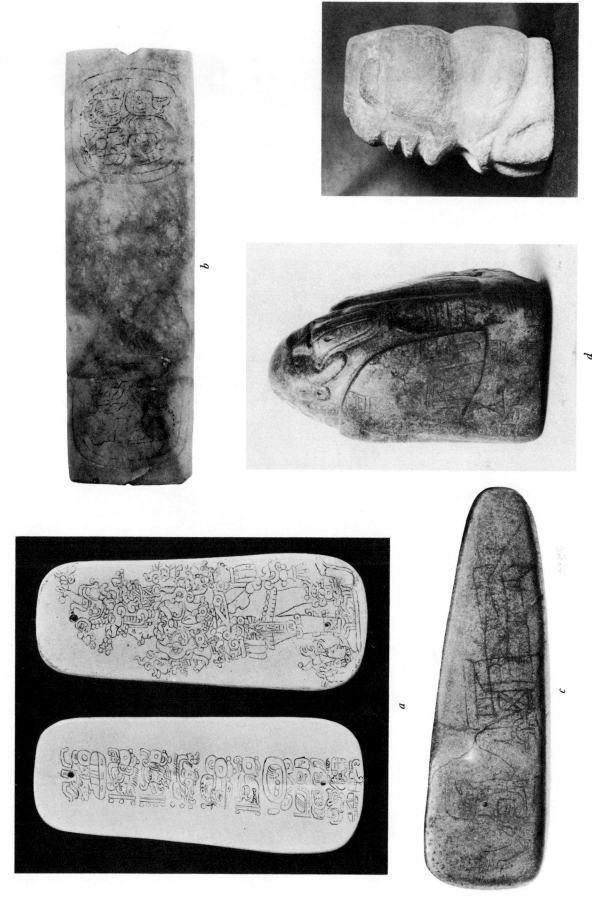

PLATE 235. ©. *a*) The Leyden plaque, Guatemala. *b*) Bar bead with Maya glyphs. *c*) Celt-shaped "palette" with incision, Mexico. *d*) The Tuxtla statuette, Mexico. *e*) Light-colored stone statuette, Guatemala.

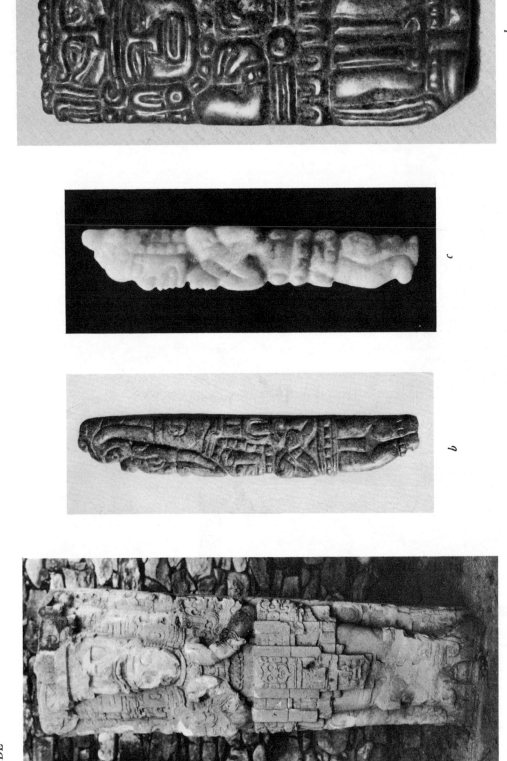

PLATE 236. ©. *a*) Early stone stela (Stela I), Copán, Honduras. *b* and *c*) Bar pectorals with human figures, Kaminaljuyú and Quiriguá, Guatemala. *d*) Plaque showing similarity to *fig. a*, San Salvador.

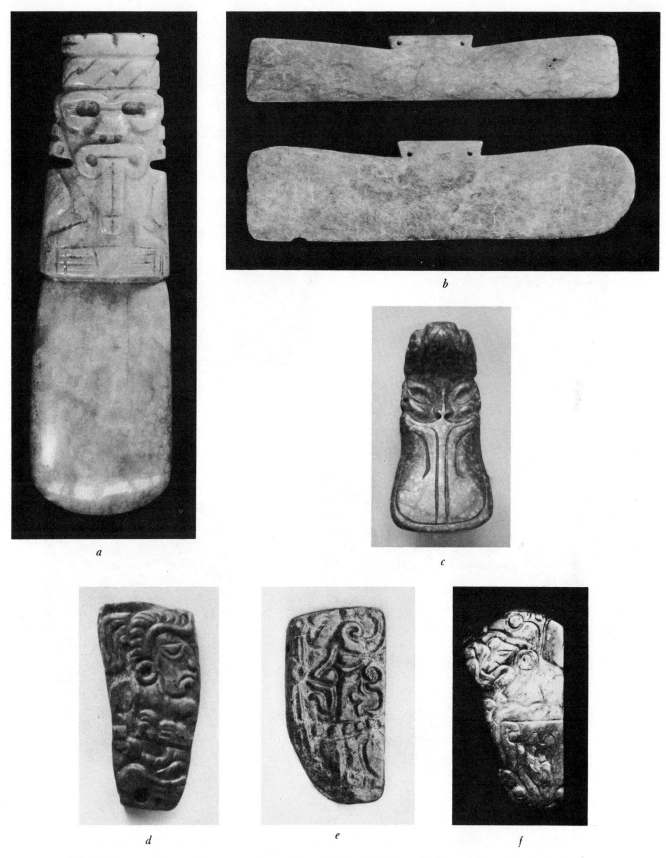

PLATE 237. ©. *a*) Large pendant, Costa Rica. *b*) Pectorals, Venezuela. Small pendants:
c and *d*) provenience unknown; *e*) Zacualpa, Guatemala; *f*) Oaxaca, Mexico.

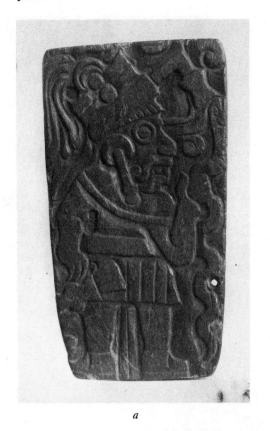

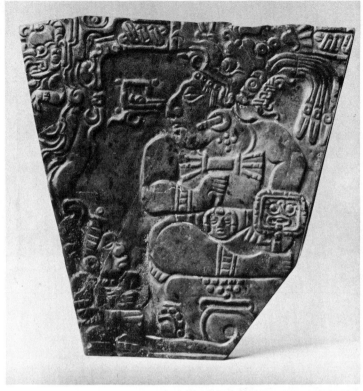

a

b

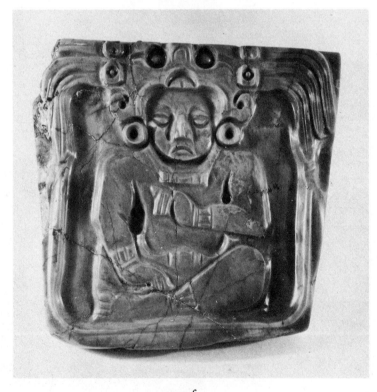

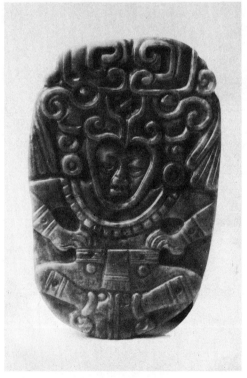

c

d

PLATE 238. ©. *a*) Serpentine plaque representing Tlaloc, Mexico. *b*) Large pendant, found near
Teotihuacán. *c*) Maya plaque. *d*) Mexican pendant.

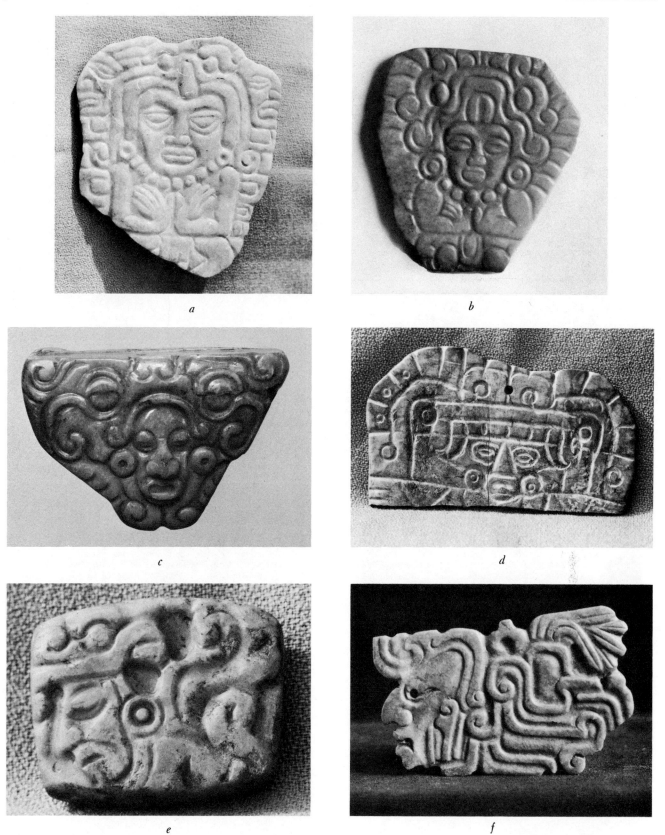

PLATE 239. Ⓒ. Small Mexican pendants showing: *a* and *b*) figures; *c* and *d*) heads in frontal view;
e and *f*) heads in profile.

JADE

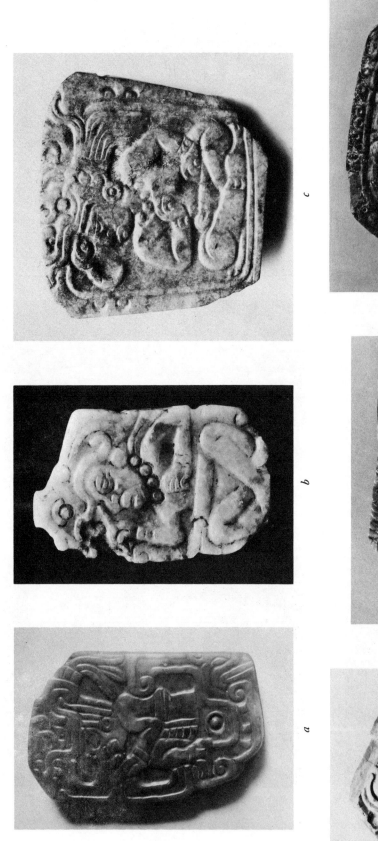

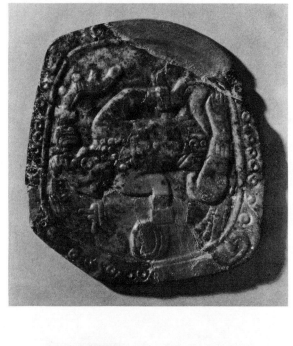

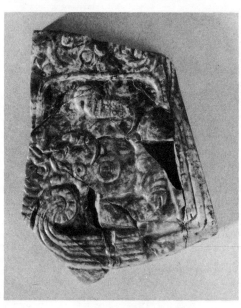

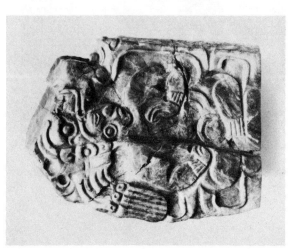

PLATE 240. ©. *a* and *b*) Mexican pendants, with figures engaged in some activity. *c* and *d*) Mayoid plaques, with seated dignitaries. *e* and *f*) Maya plaques, with seated dignitaries.

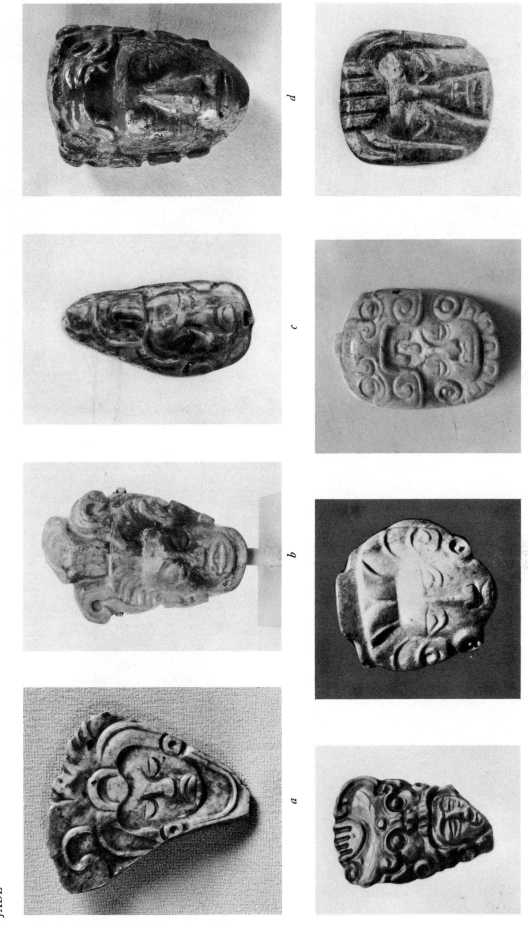

PLATE 241. ©. Small Maya and Mayoid heads: *a*, *e*, and *g*) provenience unknown; *b*) Palenque, Mexico; *c* and *h*) Guatemalan highlands; *d*) Chichén Itzá, Mexico; *f*) Oaxaca?, Mexico.

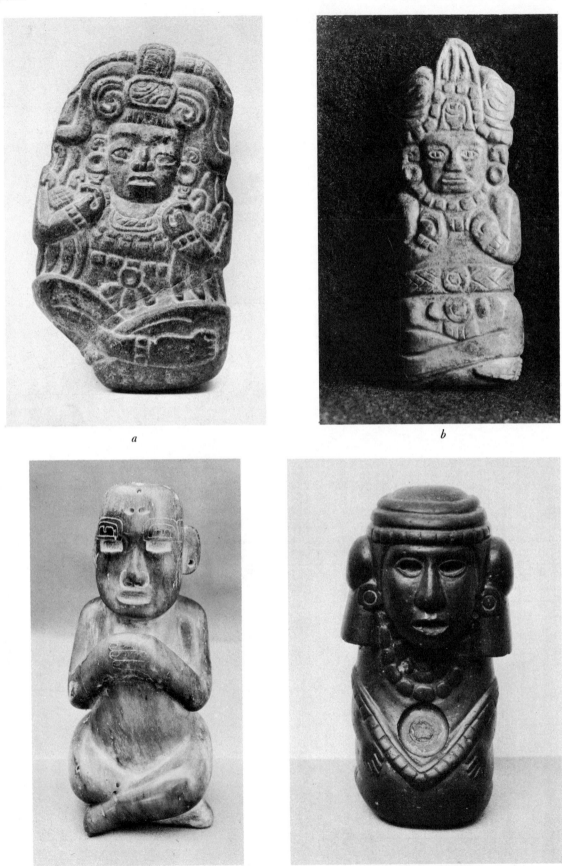

a

b

c

d

PLATE 242. ©. Statuettes: *a* and *b*) Copán, Honduras; *c*) Uaxactún, Guatemala,
by special permission of Carnegie Institution of Washington; *d*) green diorite, Mexico.

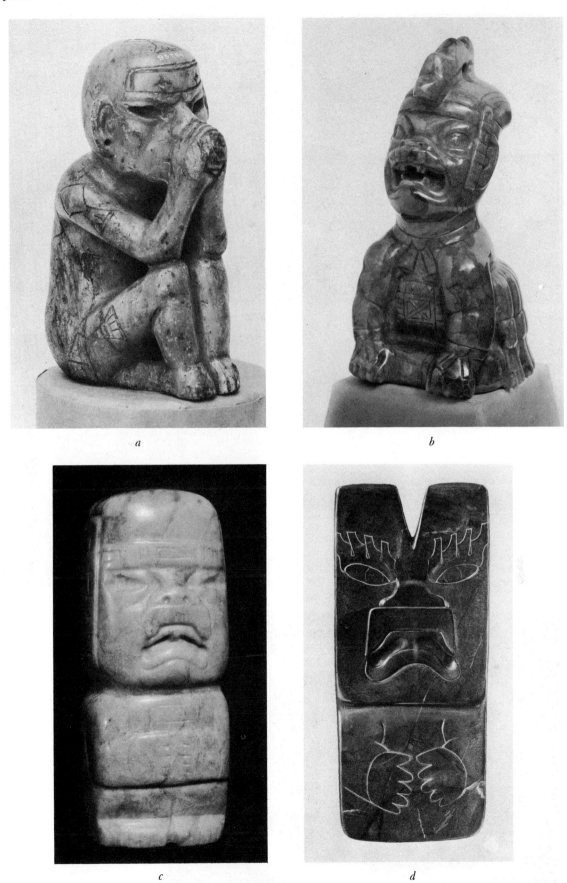

PLATE 243. ©. *a*) Serpentine statuette, Vera Cruz. *b*) Tiger-mouth figure,
Puebla. *c* and *d*) Olmec types.

JADE

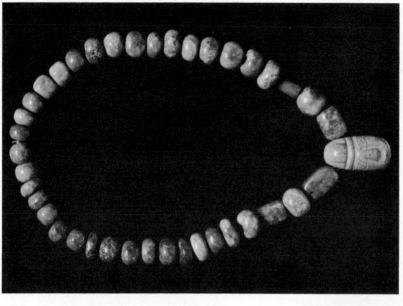

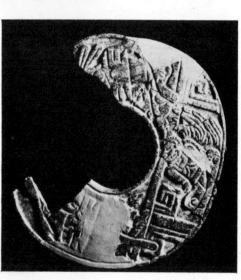

c

b

a

PLATE 244.   ©.   *a* and *b*) Crystal bead necklace and fragment of carved jade disk, Chichén Itzá.   *c*) Jade beads and pendant, Mexico.

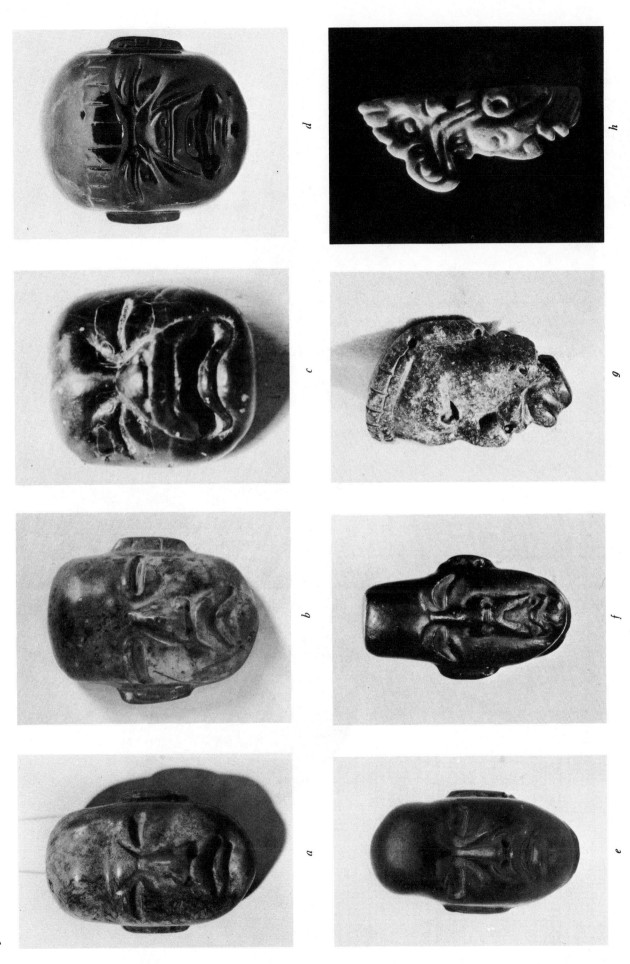

PLATE 245. ©. Small pendants in the form of human heads showing stylistic variations: *a, b, c, d,* and *f*) provenience unknown, Mexico; *e*) Palenque, Mexico; *g*) El Salvador; *h*) Yucatan, Mexico.

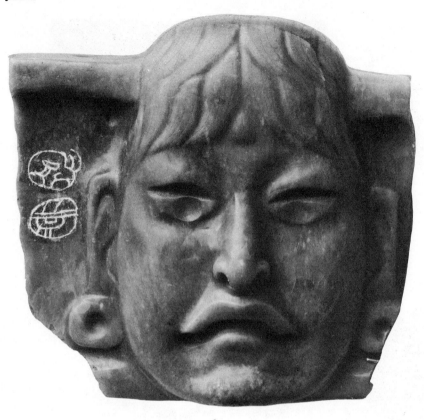

a

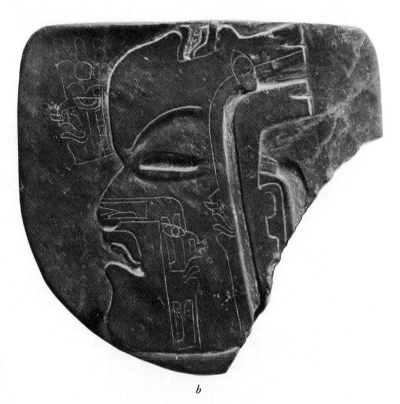

b

PLATE 246. ©. *a*) Olmec pectoral. *b*) Olmec plaque.

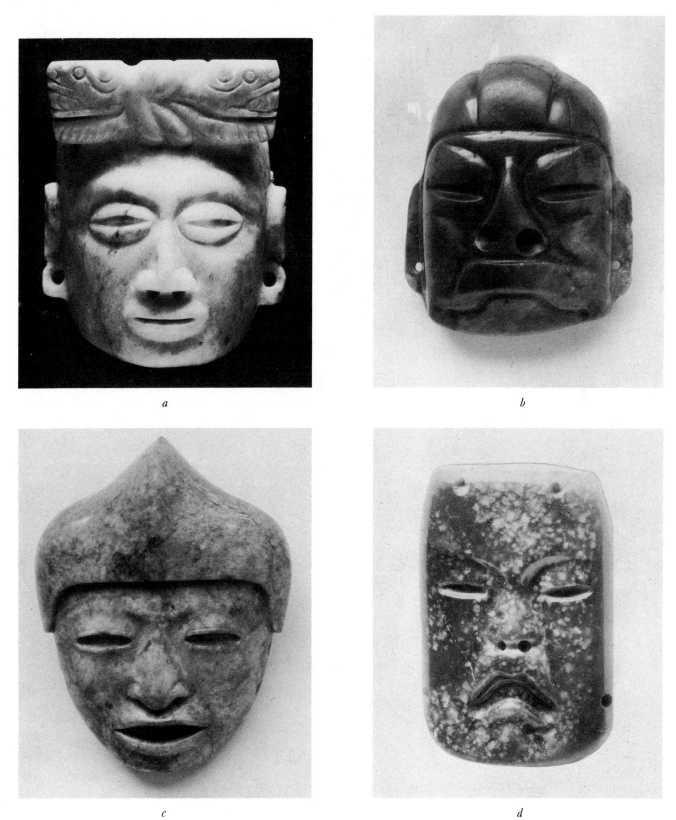

a

b

c

d

PLATE 247. ©. Small heads. Mexico.

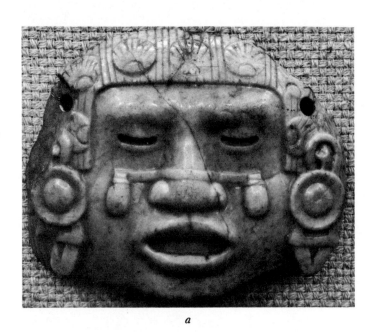

a

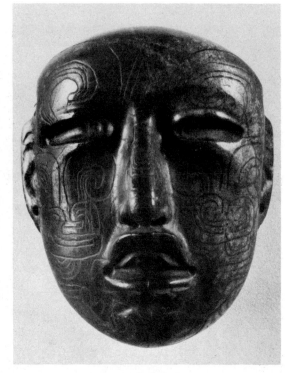

b

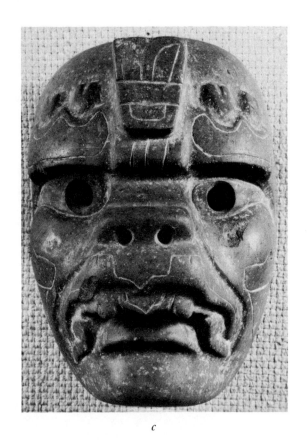

c

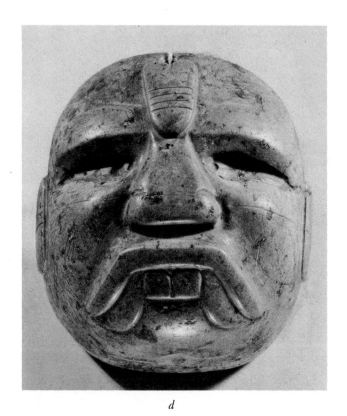

d

PLATE 248. ©. Larger stone masks: a) Aztec; b) Totonac? with Olmec traits; c and d) Totonac.

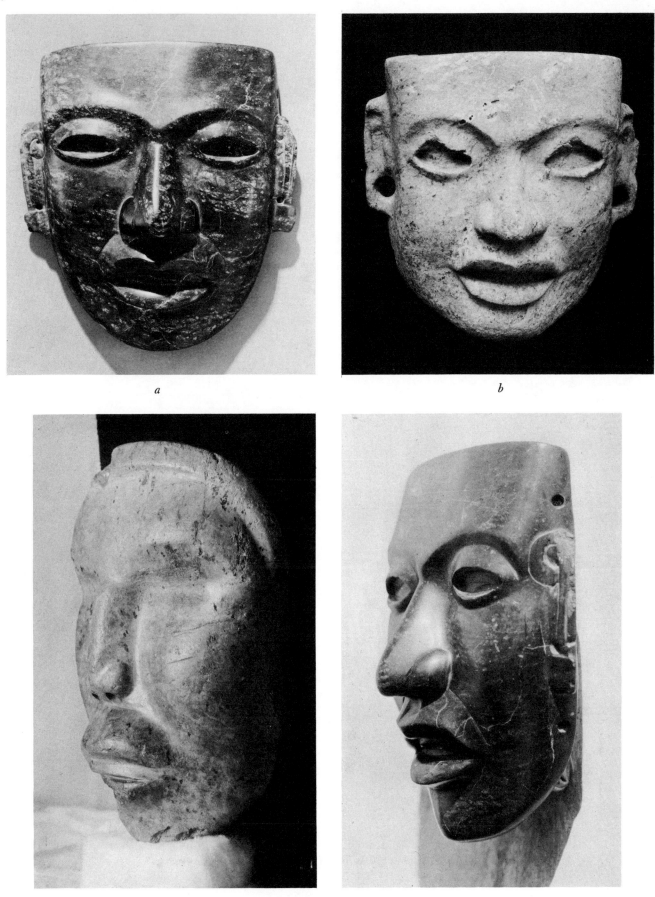

a

b

c

d

PLATE 249. ©. Large stone masks: *a* and *d*) Toltec; *b*) showing Toltec influence; *c*) style indefinite.

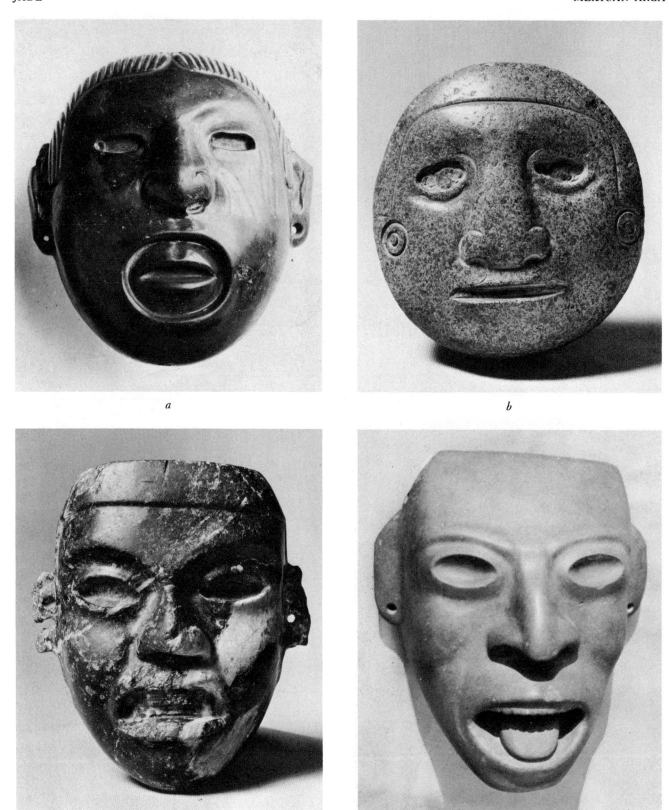

a   *b*

c   *d*

PLATE 250.   ©.   *a*) Black stone mask of Xipe-Totec, Oaxaca.   *b*) Round mask, provenience
unknown.   *c*) Toltec mask.   *d*) Large Toltec? serpentine mask.

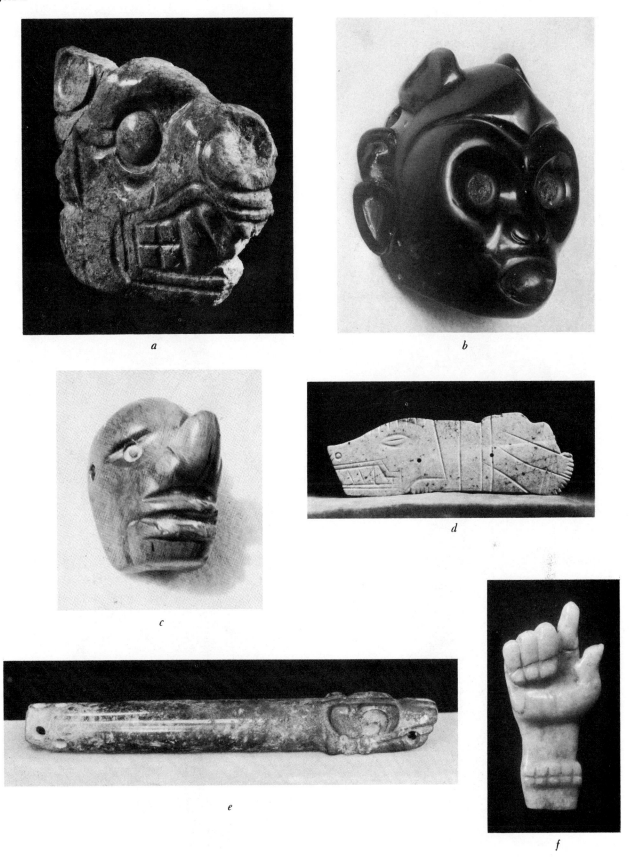

PLATE 251. Ⓒ. *a*) Jaguar head, Piedras Negras, Guatemala. *b*) Obsidian monkey head, Puebla, Mexico. *c*) Small mask, El Salvador. *d*) Amphibian, provenience unknown. *e*) Fan handle, Monte Albán, Mexico. *f*) Hand, Ulúa Valley, Honduras.

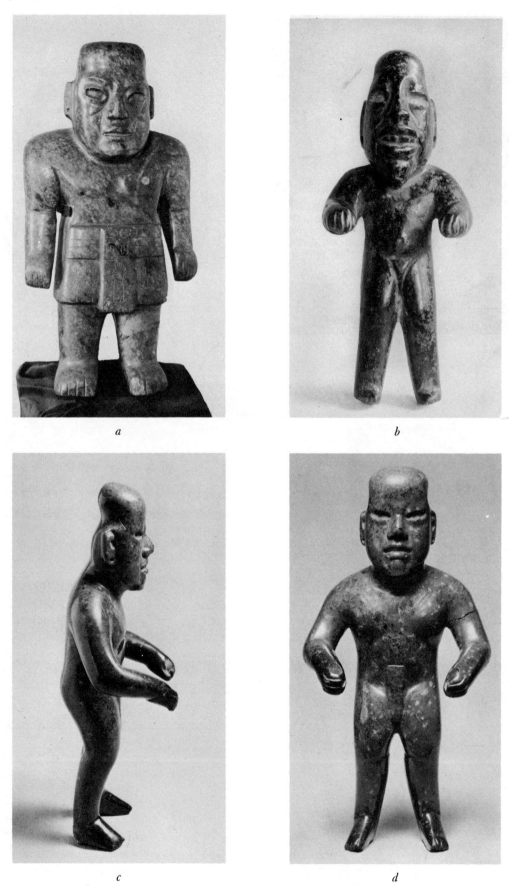

PLATE 252. ©. Standing human figures, Mexico: *a*) Puebla; *b*) dark stone, provenience unknown; *c* and *d*) side and frontal views, light green jade, with Olmec traits, provenience unknown.

MAYA AND MEXICAN AREAS

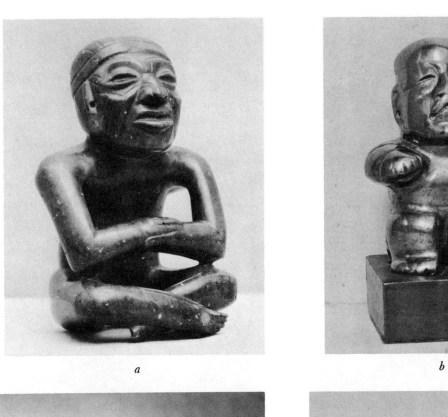

a

b

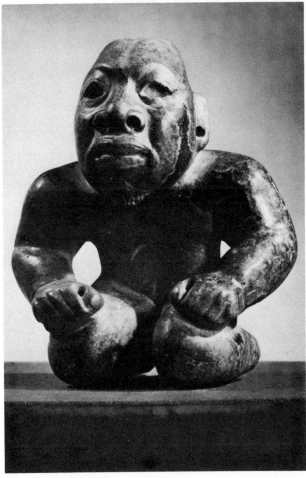

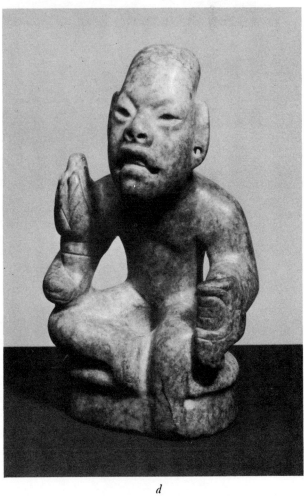

c

d

PLATE 253. ©. Seated human figures: *a*) dark stone, provenience unknown; *b*) pyrite, provenience unknown; *c*) dark jade, Ulúa Valley, Honduras; *d*) light green jade, with Olmec traits, provenience unknown.

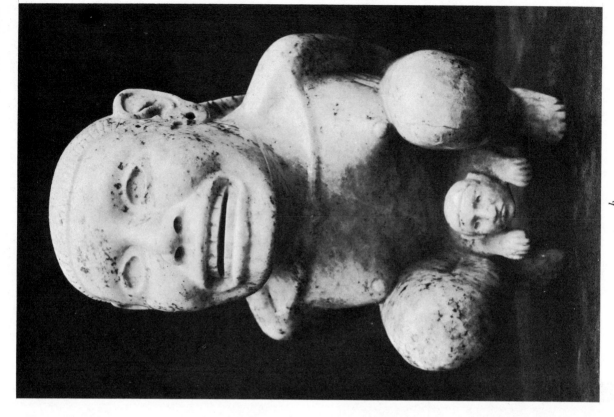

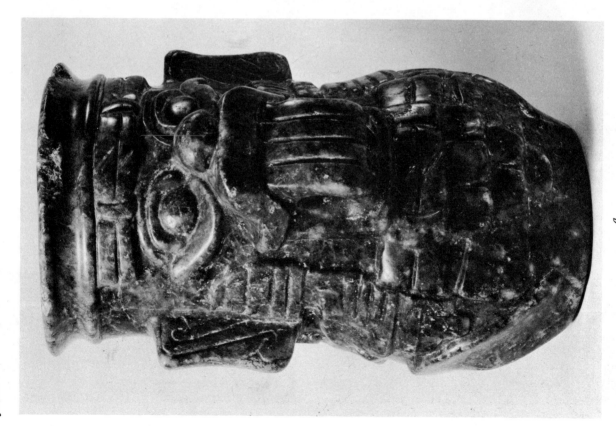

PLATE 254. ⓒ. *a*) Vessel representing Tlaloc, the Rain-god. *b*) Statue of Toci, Mother of the Gods. Mexico.

a

b

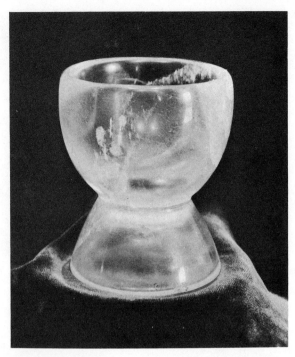

a

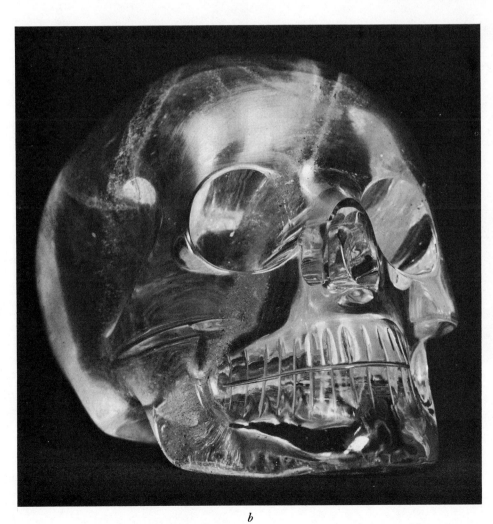

b

PLATE 255. ©. Objects of rock crystal, Mexico: *a*) goblet, Monte Albán; *b*) skull.

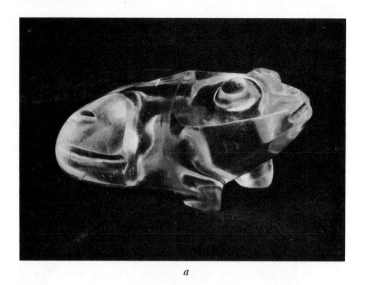

a

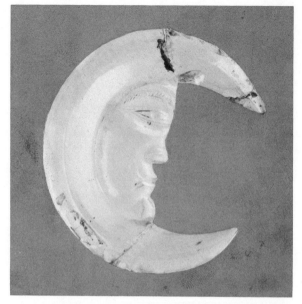

b

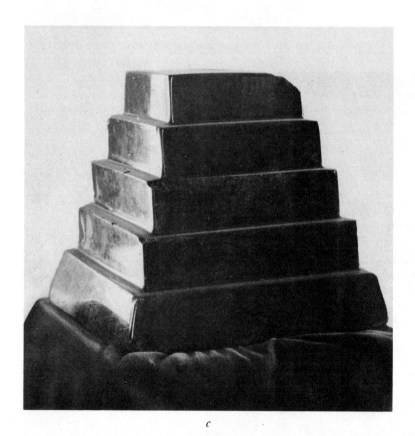

c

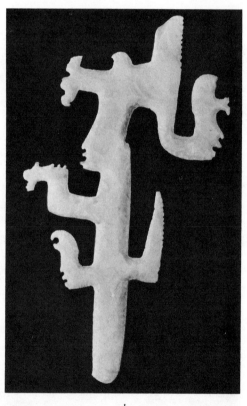

d

PLATE 256. ©. *a*) Rock crystal frog, Mexico. *b*) Rock crystal man in the moon, Mexico. *c*) Obsidian model of a temple-base, Mexico. *d*) Eccentric flint in human shape, Maya?.

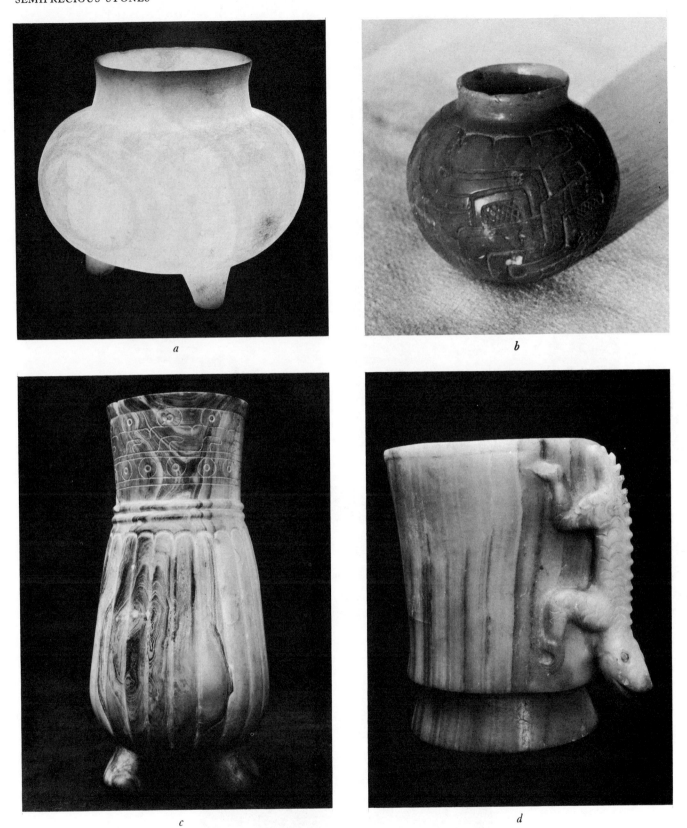

PLATE 257. ©. Onyx vases: *a*) Monte Albán, Mexico; *c* and *d*) Isla de los Sacrificios, Vera Cruz, Mexico. *b*) Small jade vase, El Salvador.

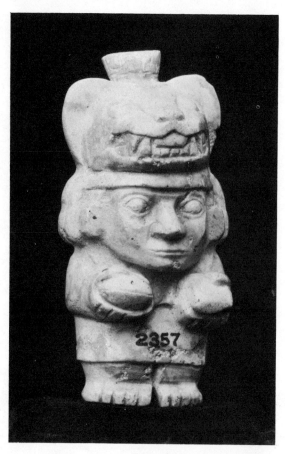

a

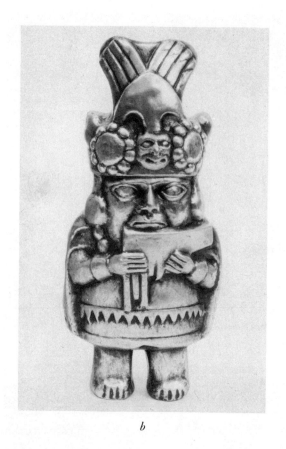

b

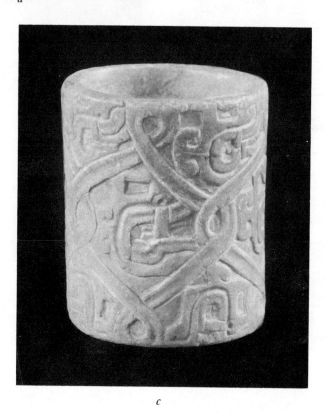

c

PLATE 258. ©. *a* and *b*) Mochica statuettes of turquoise and silver, demonstrating uniformity of iconography, North Coast of Peru. *c*) Small turquoise vase with Chavín traits.

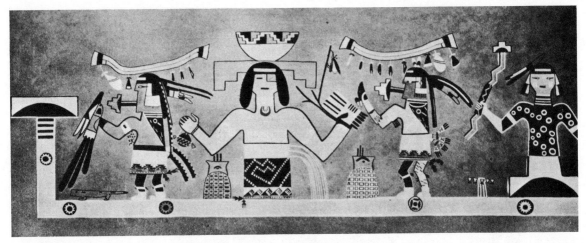

a

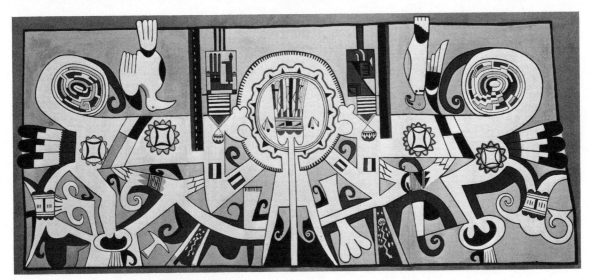

b

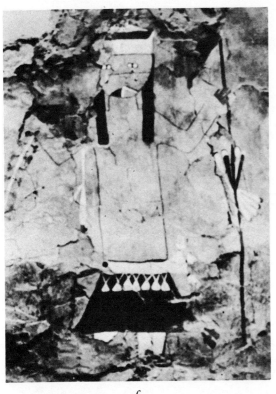

c

PLATE 259. ©. *a* and *b*) Murals, Awatovi, Arizona.
c) Fragment of mural, Kuaua, New Mexico.

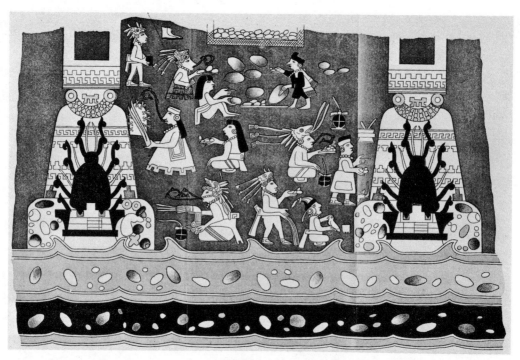

a

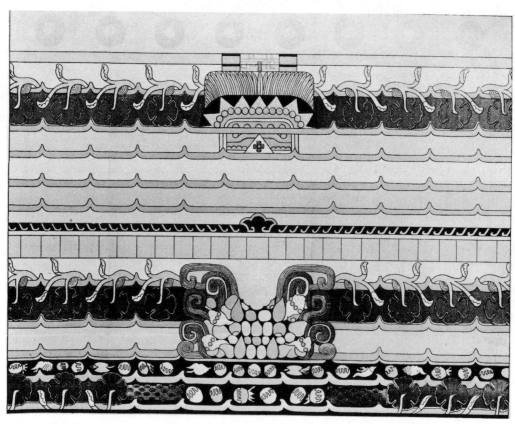

b

PLATE 260.   ©.   Sections of murals in the Temple of Agriculture, Teotihuacán.

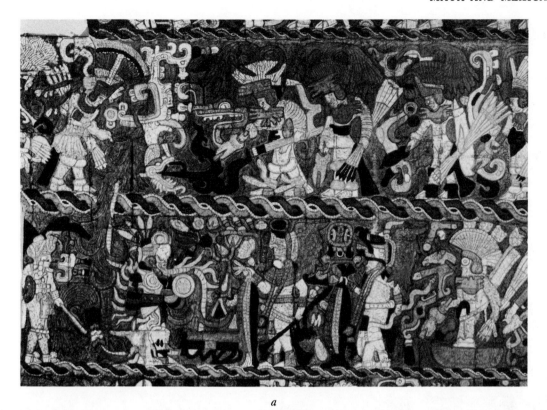

a

b

PLATE 261.   ©.   *a*) Section of a carved and painted wall, Temple of the Bas-Relief, Chichén Itzá.
b) Mural, Altar A, Tizatlán.   Mexico.

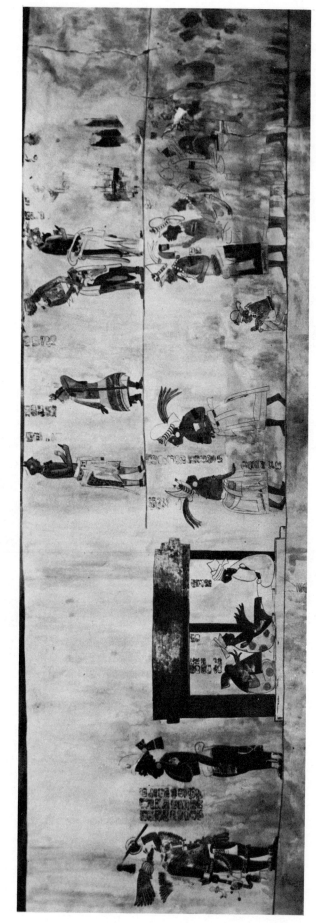

a

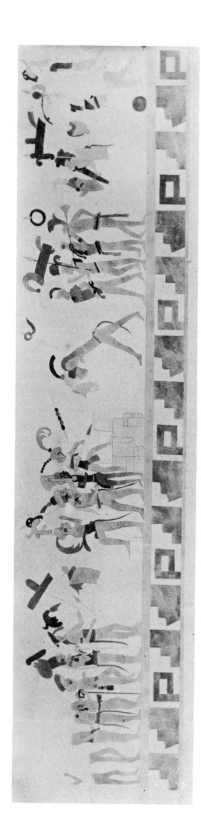

b

PLATE 262. ©. *a*) Wall-painting from early Maya structure B-XIII, Uaxactún, Guatemala. *By special permission of Carnegie Institution of Washington and A. Ledyard Smith.* *b*) Wall-painting from Edifice 3, Chacmultun, Yucatan, Mexico. Note stylistic differences in these pure Maya murals when compared with the fragments below from the Mexican period of Chichén Itzá.

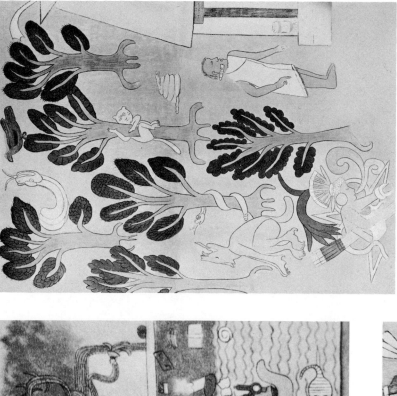

b

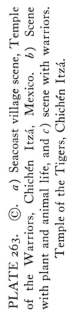

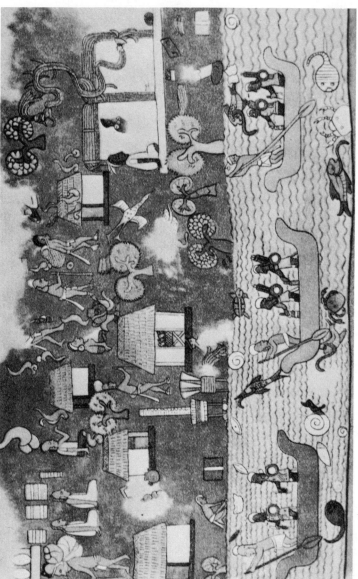

a

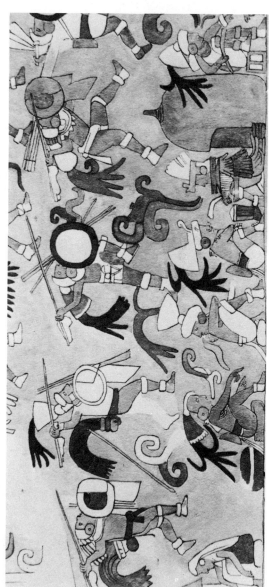

c

PLATE 263. ©. *a*) Seacoast village scene, Temple of the Warriors, Chichén Itzá, Mexico. *b*) Scene with plant and animal life, and *c*) scene with warriors. Temple of the Tigers, Chichén Itzá.

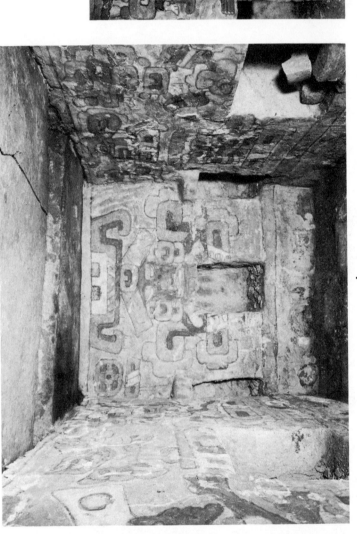

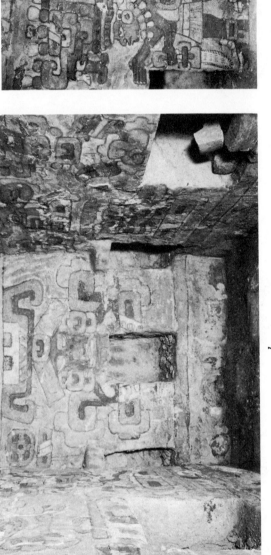

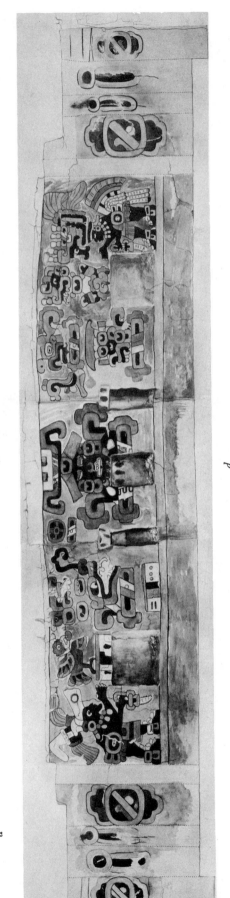

PLATE 264. ©. *b*) Interior of Zapotec Tomb 104, Monte Albán. *a* and *c*) Details. Figures of Xipe-Totec and the Maize-god. *d*) Unrolled design of entire mural.

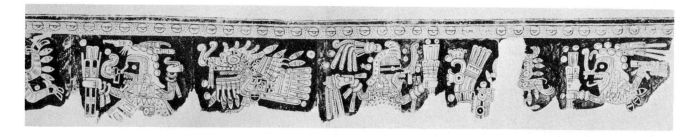

a

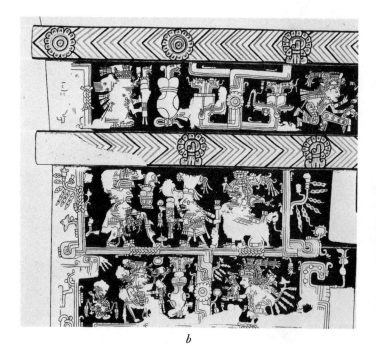

b

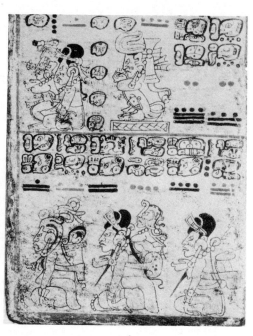

c

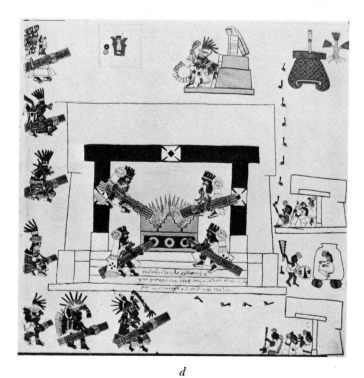

d

PLATE 265. ©. *a* and *b*) Details of murals at Mitla, Oaxaca, and Tulum, Quintana Roo, Mexico. *c*) Section of Maya codex (Dresdensis). *d*) Section of Aztec codex (Borbonicus).

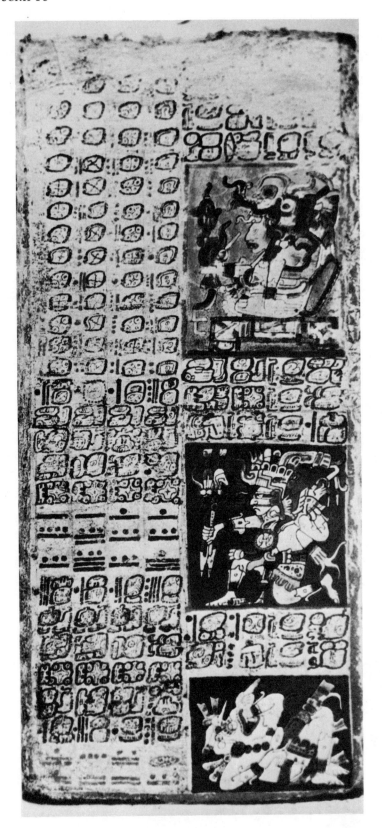

PLATE 266. ©. Page from the Maya Codex Dresdensis.

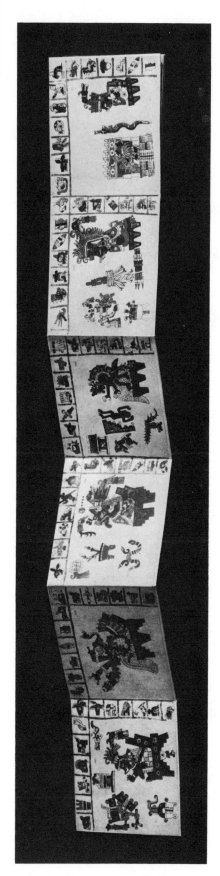

a

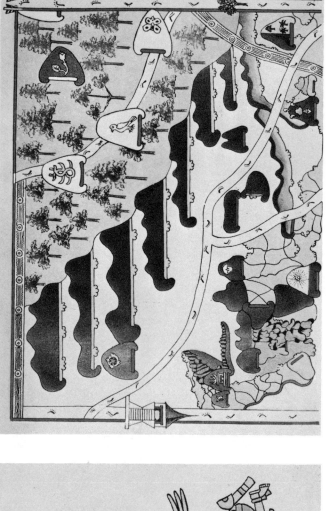

c

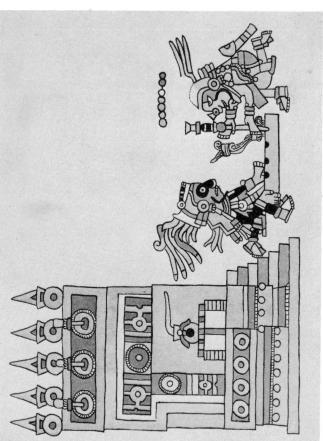

b

PLATE 267. ©. *a*) Unfolded pages of Aztec codex (Vaticanus B). *b*) Detail from Zapotec codex (Colombino). *c*) Section of Aztec map.

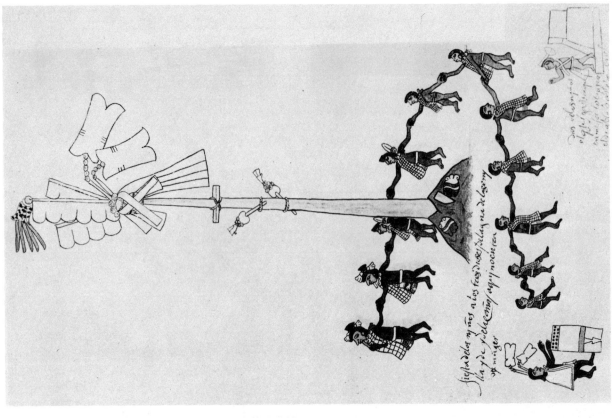

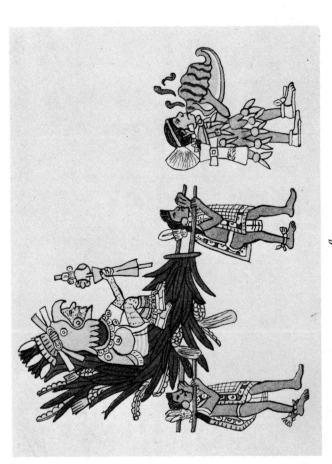

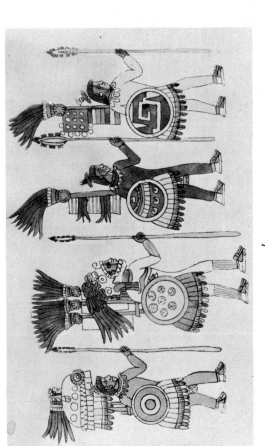

PLATE 268. ©. *a*) Scene from post-Columbian Aztec codex (Magliabecchiano). *b*) Detail from post-Columbian Aztec codex (Mendoza). *c*) Fiesta scene from pre-Columbian Aztec codex (Borbonicus)

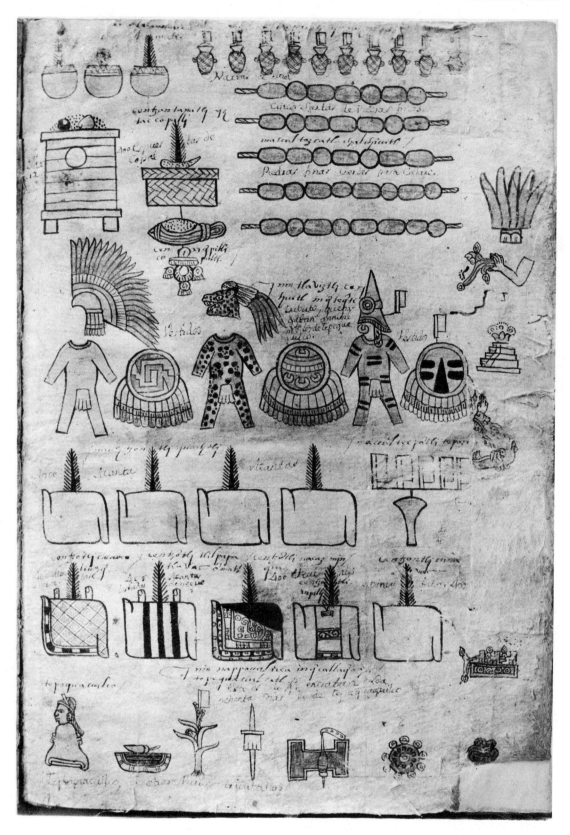

PLATE 269.   ©.   Page from the Tribute Roll of Montezuma.

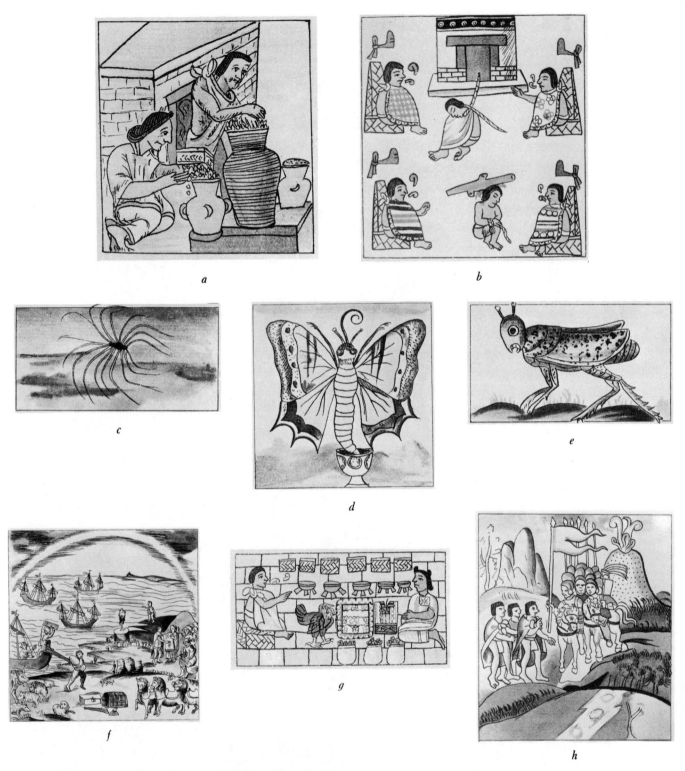

PLATE 270. ©. Vignettes from Sahagún's codex (Florentino): *a*) farmers storing corn; *b*) four judges supervising execution of malefactors by noose and club—note different fabrics; *c, d,* and *e*) spider, butterfly, and grasshopper; *f*) Spaniards landing at Vera Cruz—note delineation of animals; *g*) market scene; *h*) the *conquistadores* on their way to the capital meeting a native deputation—note volcanoes in the background.

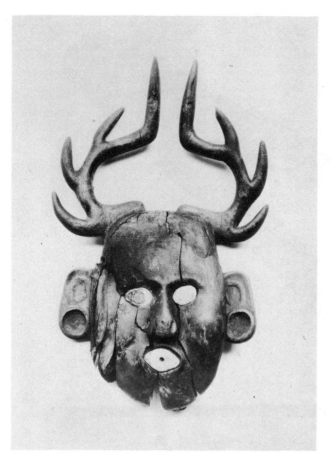

a

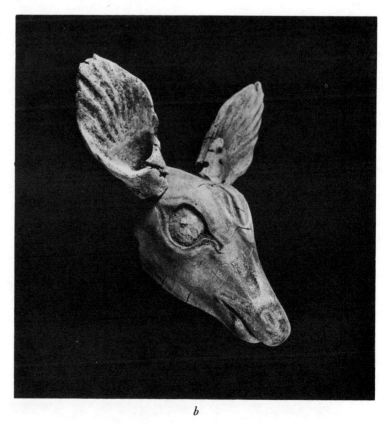

b

PLATE 271.   ©.   *a*) Wooden mask representing antlered human head, Oklahoma.
b) Wooden mask of a doe, Florida.

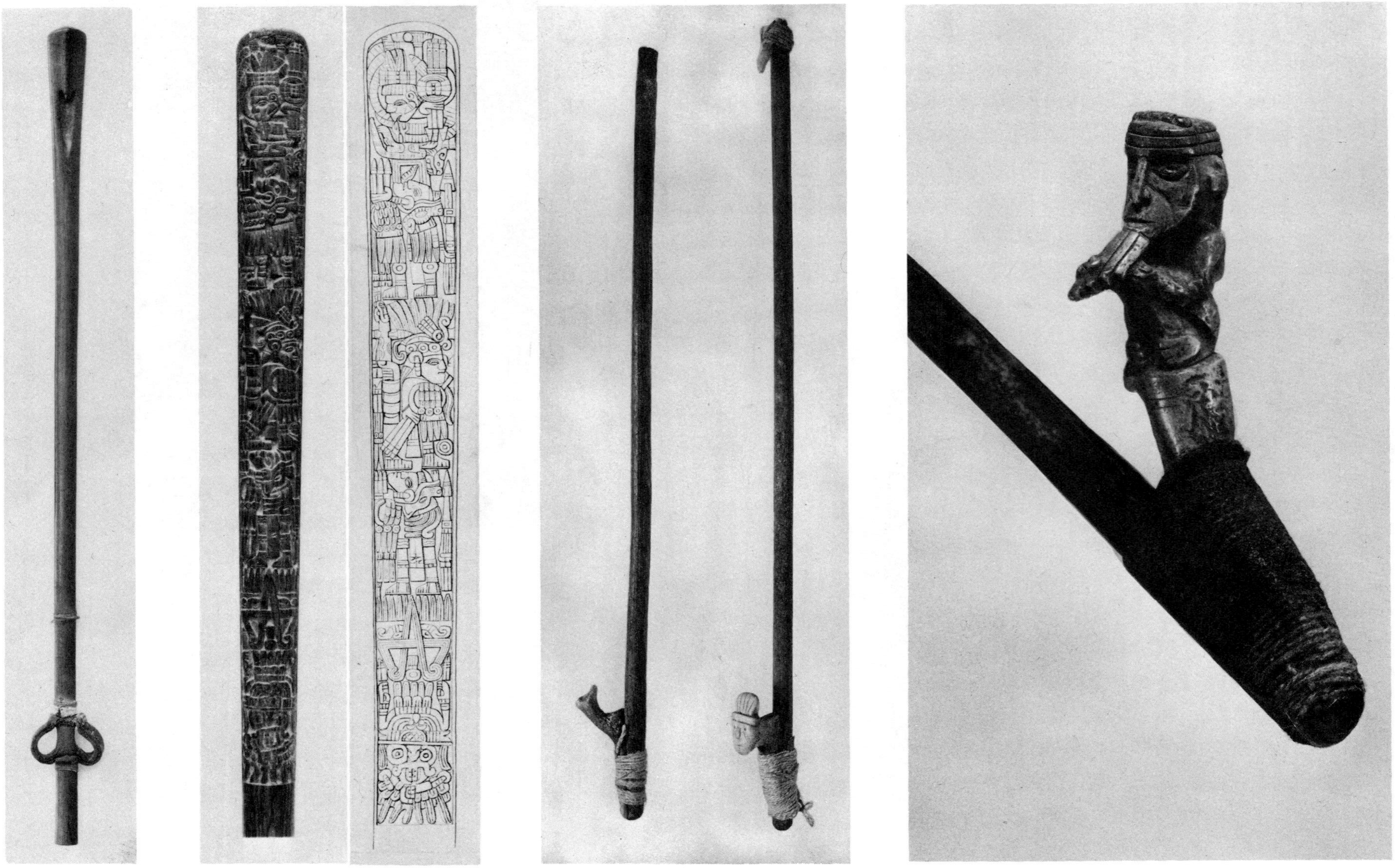

a b c d e

PLATE 272. ©. Wooden spear-throwers, or *atlatls*: *a*) Southwest; *b*) Mexico; *c*) copy of design; *d*) Peru; *e*) detail of hand grip, with bone figure playing panpipes, Peru.

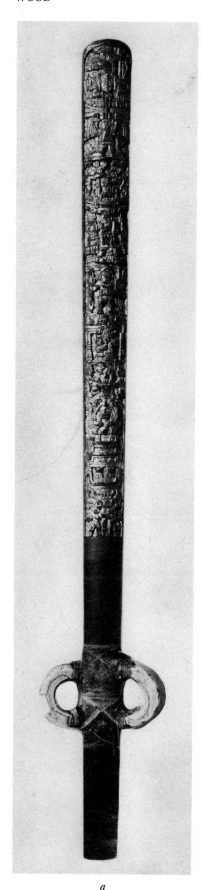

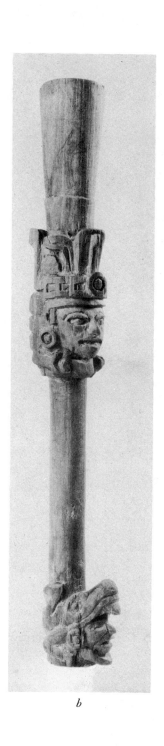

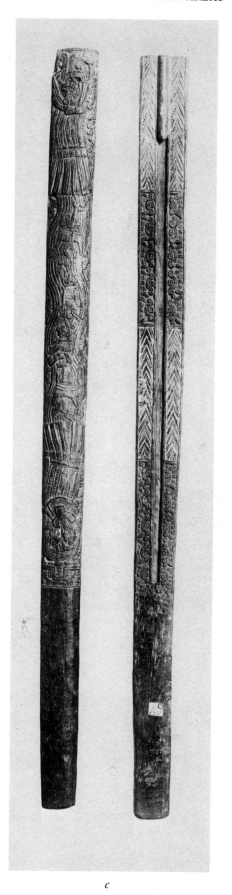

a											*b*											*c*

PLATE 273. ⓒ. *a*) Carved and gilded ceremonial *atlatl*, Mexico. *b*) Top of wooden
ceremonial staff, Sacred Well, Chichén Itzá. *c*) Carved and painted *atlatls*, Oaxaca.

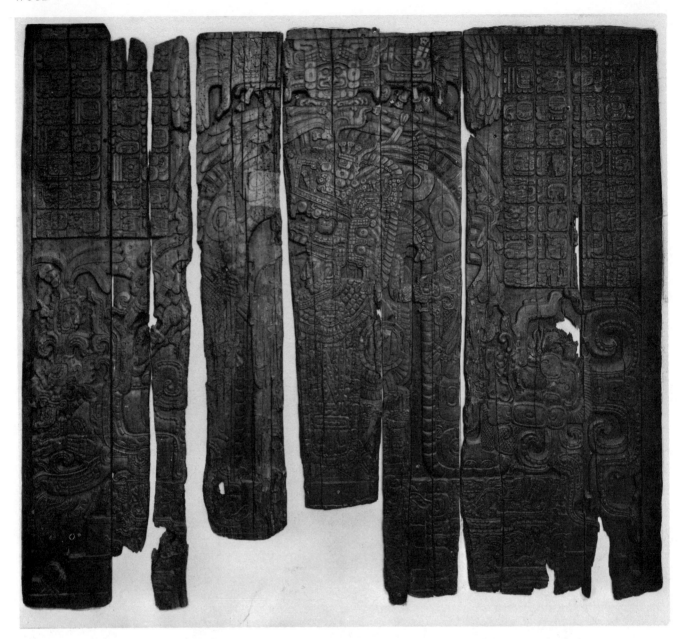

PLATE 274. Ⓒ. Carved wood lintel, Tikal, Guatemala.

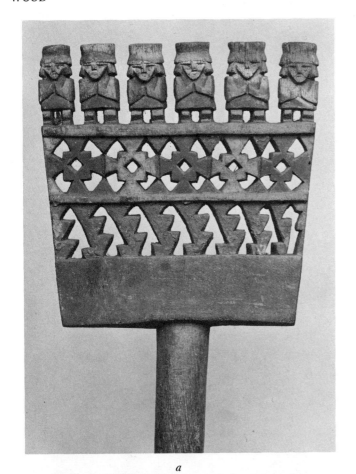

a

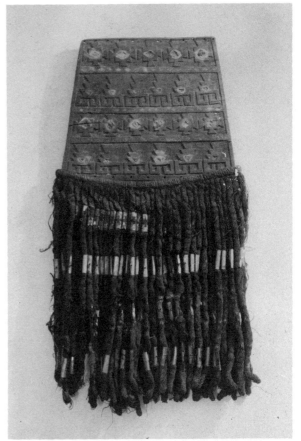

b

c

PLATE 275. ⓒ. *a*) Carved top of staff or paddle, Ica. *b*) Pendant of a coca bag, Ica. *c*) Wooden spoons with carved handles, Coast Tiahuanaco.

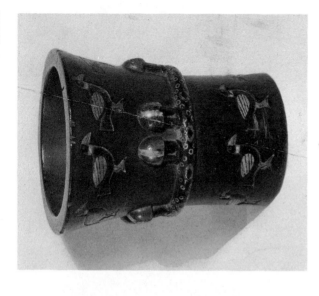

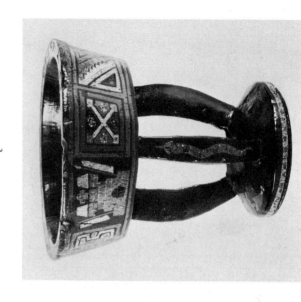

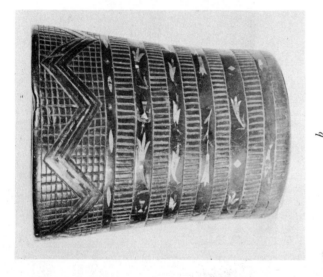

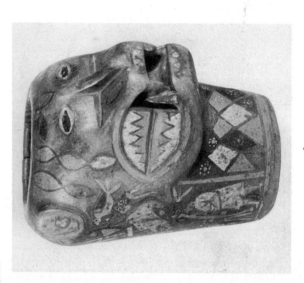

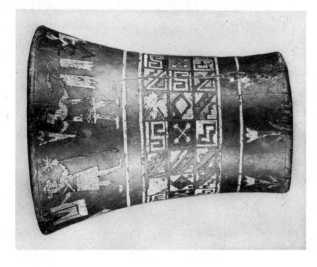

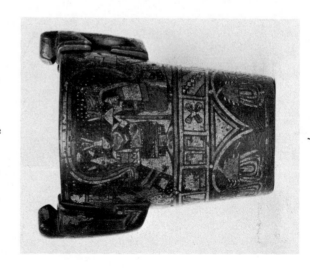

PLATE 276. ©. *Keros,* or wooden cups with lacquer-like finish, late Inca and post-Conquest.

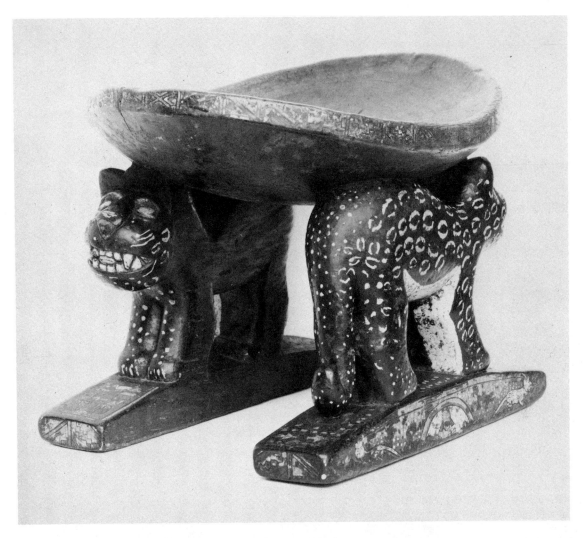

a

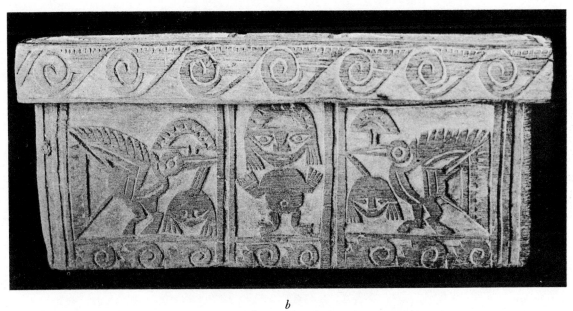

b

PLATE 277.   ©.   *a*) Seat supported by jaguars, lacquer-like finish, Inca.   *b*) Carved
beam of a scale, Chimú?.

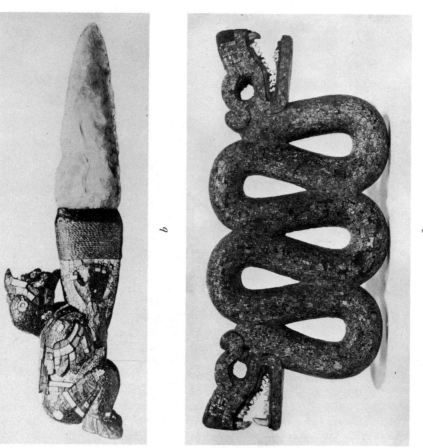

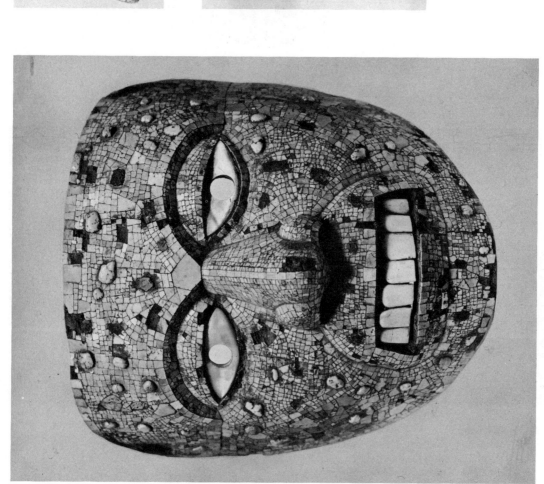

PLATE 278. ©. Objects incrusted with turquoise mosaic, Mexico: *a*) mask of Quetzalcóatl?; *b*) ceremonial knife with Eagle Knight; *c*) ornament with double-headed serpent.

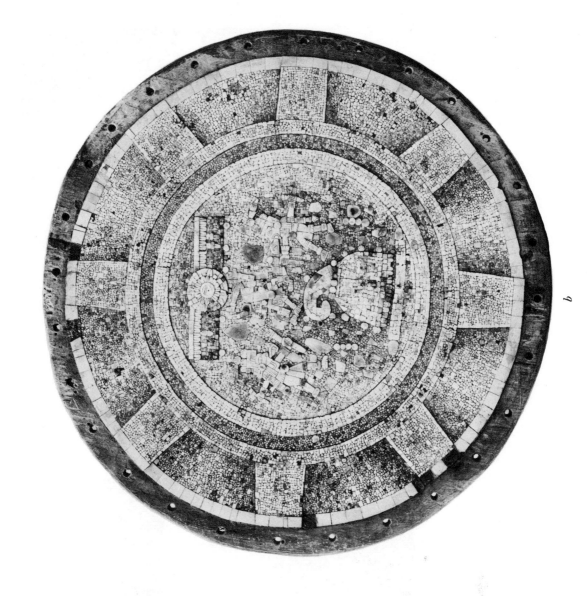

b

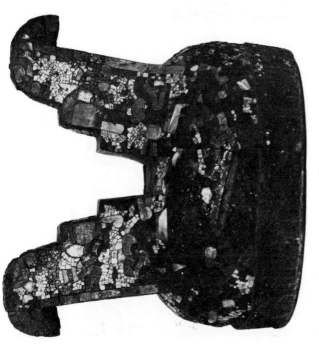

a

PLATE 279. ©. *a*) Wooden helmet with mosaic
incrustation. *b*) Wooden shield with ceremonial scene
in turquoise. Mexico.

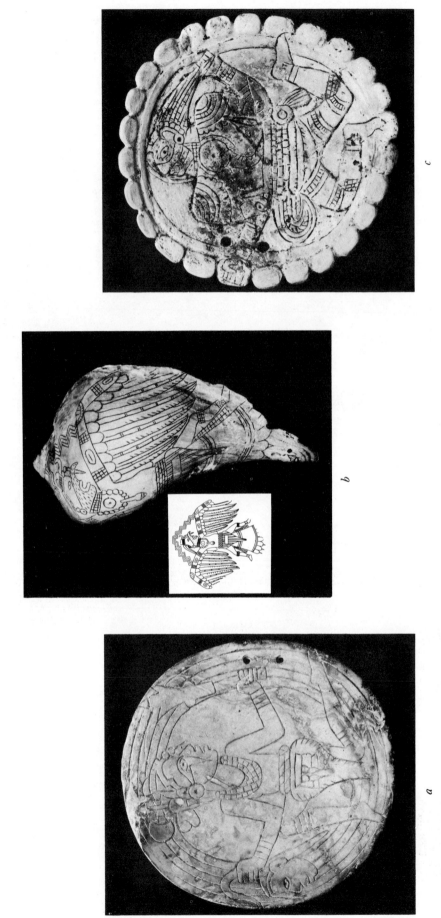

PLATE 280. ©. Shell gorgets: *a*) Tennessee; *c*) Oklahoma. *b*) Conch with incised decoration and inset showing bird-man design, Oklahoma.

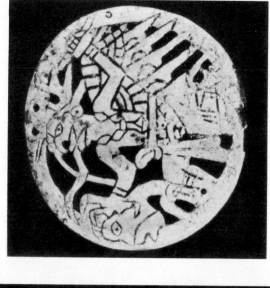

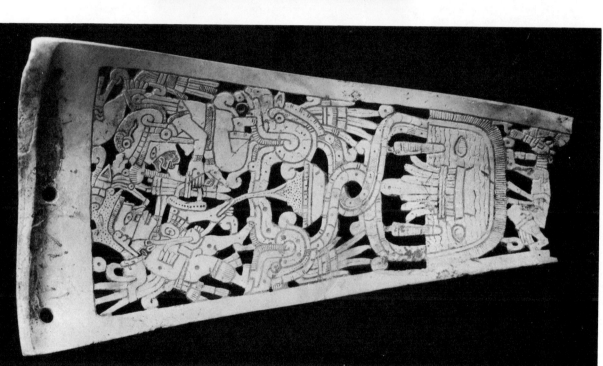

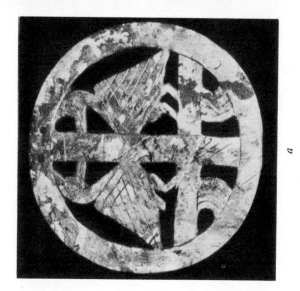

PLATE 281. ©. *a* and *c*) Perforated shell gorgets, Georgia. *b*) Perforated shell ornament, Vera Cruz, Mexico.

a

b

c

SHELL

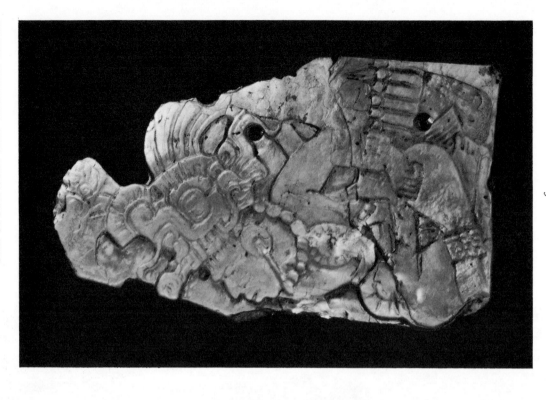

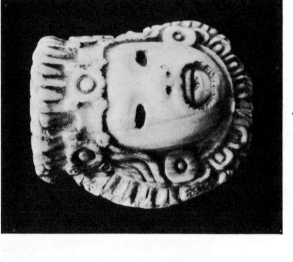

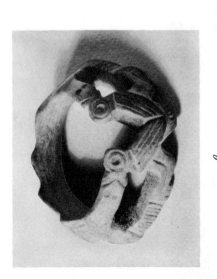

PLATE 282. ©. *a*) Hohokam ring of glycimeris shell, Arizona. *b*) Xipe-Totec mask of reddish shell, Mexico. *c*) Mother-of-pearl pendant with seated Maya warrior, Tula, Mexico.

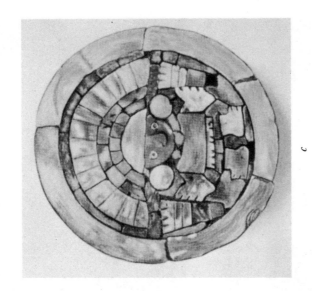

c

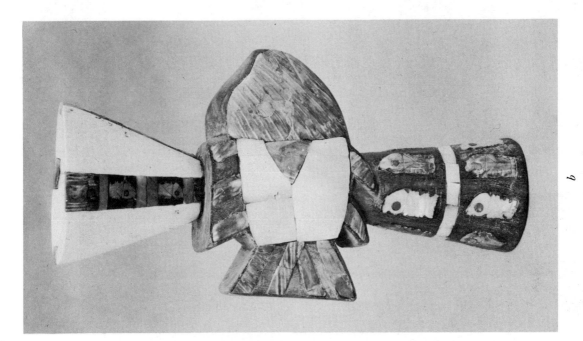

b

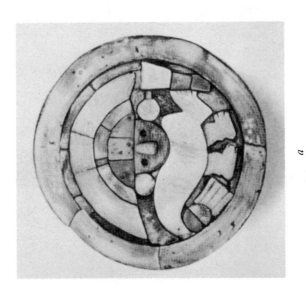

a

PLATE 283. ⓒ. Chimú shell mosaic-work: *a* and *c*) earplugs; *b*) cup with wooden base.

BONE

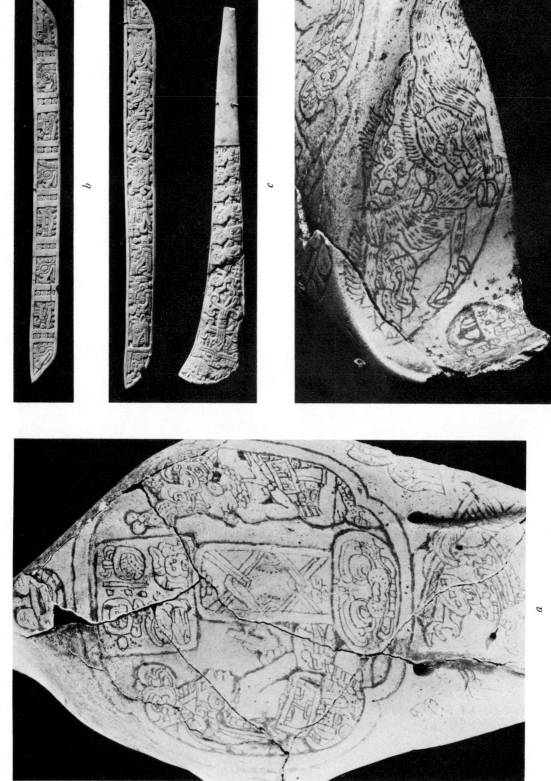

PLATE 284. ©. *a* and *d*) Details of an incised peccary skull, Copán, Honduras.   *b* and *c*) Jaguar bone with glyphic carving,
Monte Albán, Mexico.

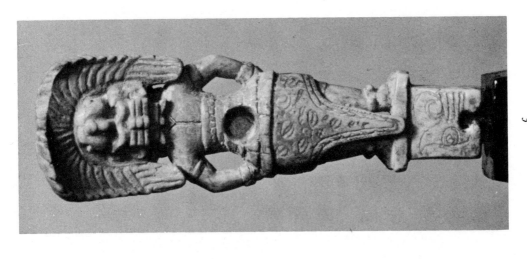

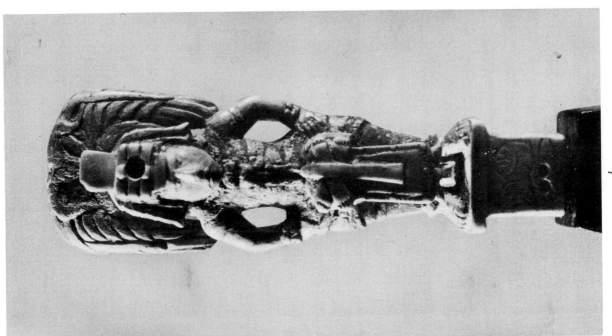

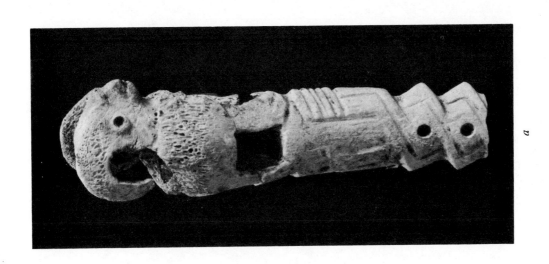

PLATE 285. ⓒ. *a*) Hohokam bone awl handle with mountain sheep, Arizona. *b*) Maya priest carved of jaguar bone, probably top of a staff, provenience unknown. *c*) Back of figure.

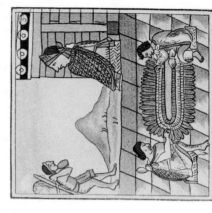

b

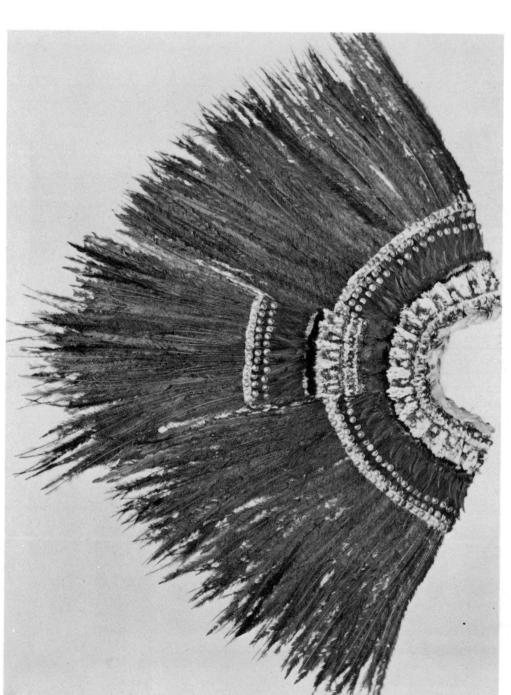

a

PLATE 286. © *a*) Aztec feather headdress or cloak, gift from Mexico to Charles V. *b*) Vignette from Sahagún's codex (Florentino) showing craftsmen making feather-work.

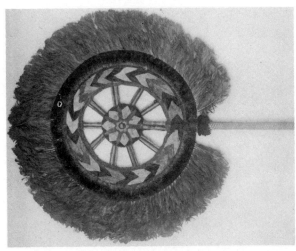

c

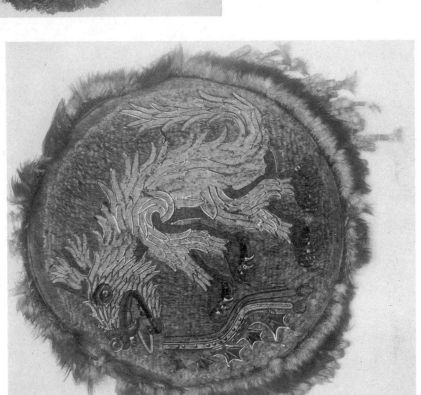

b

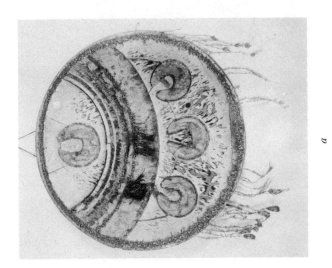

a

PLATE 287. ©. *a*) Aztec feather shield mounted on jaguar skin. *b*) Aztec ceremonial shield of feathers with gold outlining, showing the coyote Fire-god, and *c*) Aztec feather standard with fire-flower, both gifts from Mexico to Charles V.

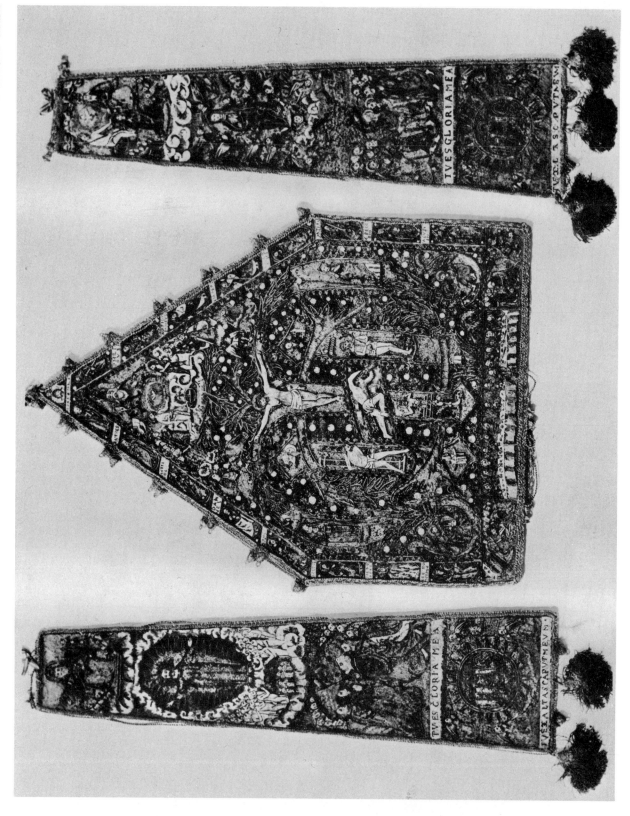

PLATE 288.   Ⓒ.   Mitre and infula of Mexican feather-work, post-Columbian.

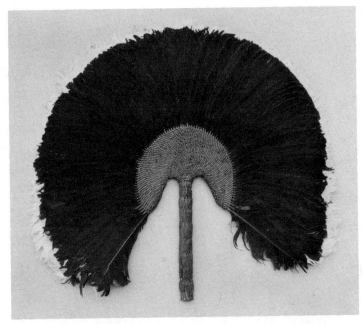

a

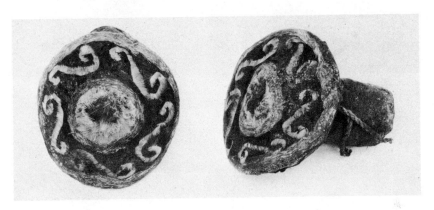

b

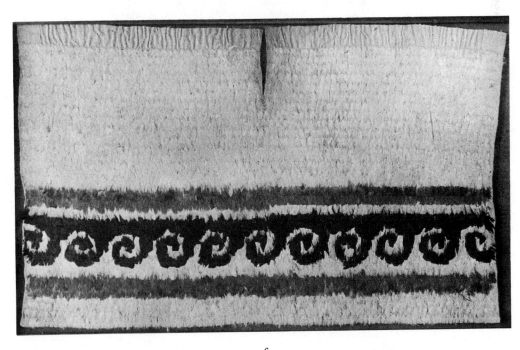

c

PLATE 289. ©. *a*) Feather fan with woven framework, Central Coast? of Peru.
b) Pair of earplugs decorated with feather-work, Ica. *c*) Feather poncho, Chimú.

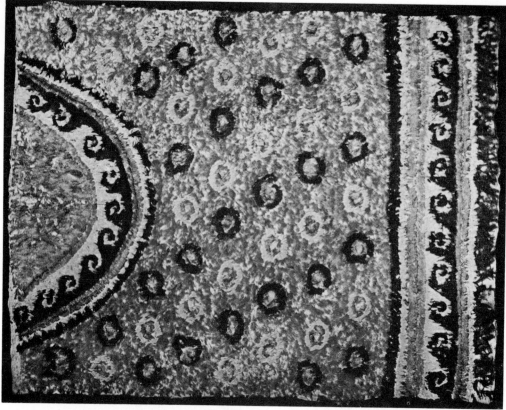

b

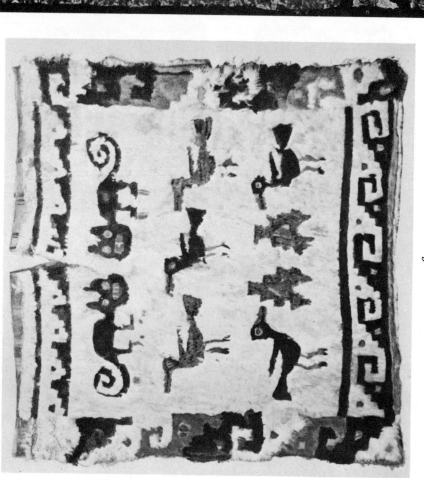

a

PLATE 290. ©. *a*) Feather poncho with birds and feline figures, Ica. *b*) Feather poncho with geometric design, Chimú.

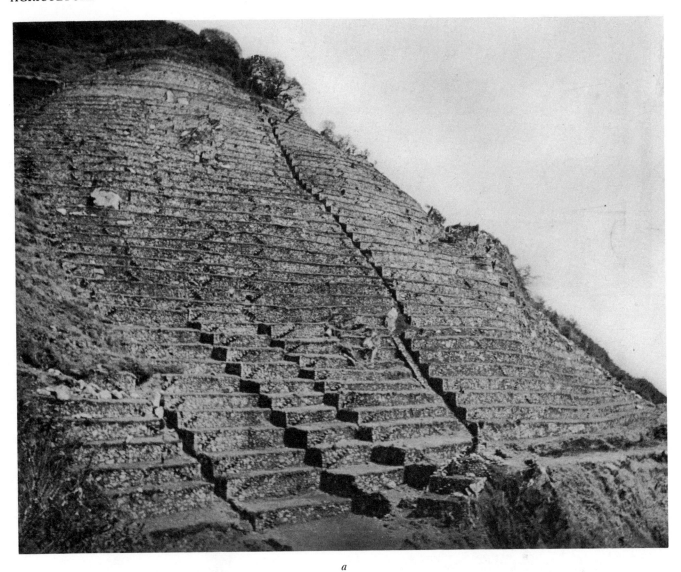

a

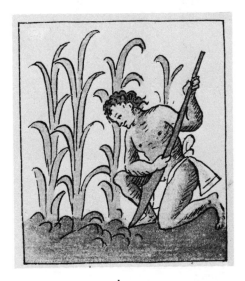

b

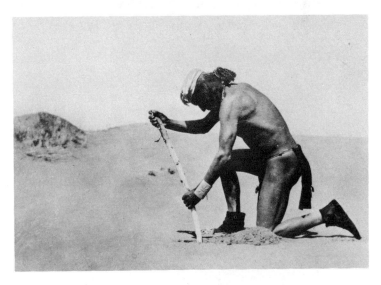

c

PLATE 291. ©. *a*) Agricultural terraces, Andean highlands, Peru. *b*) Vignette from Sahagún's codex (Florentino), showing cultivation of corn with planting stick, Mexico. *c*) Modern Hopi Indian planting corn, using similar implement, Arizona.

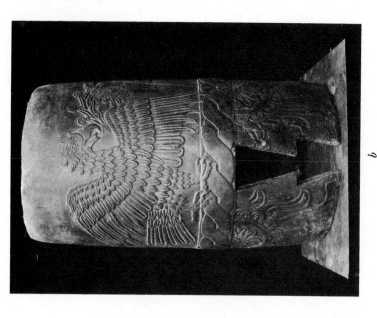

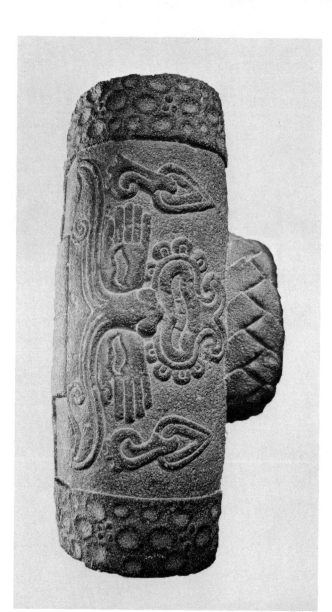

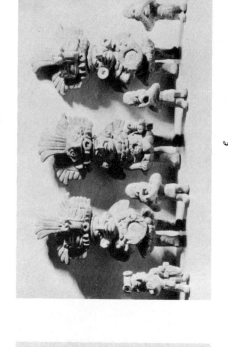

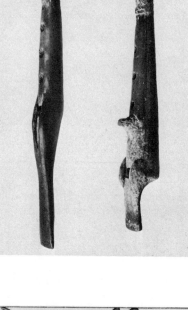

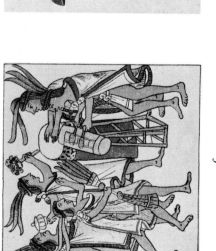

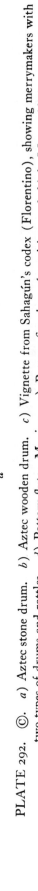

PLATE 292. ©. *a*) Aztec stone drum. *b*) Aztec wooden drum. *c*) Vignette from Sahagún's codex (Florentino), showing merrymakers with two types of drums and rattles. *d*) Pottery flutes, Mexico. *e*) Pottery figurines of musicians and chiefs, Monte Albán.

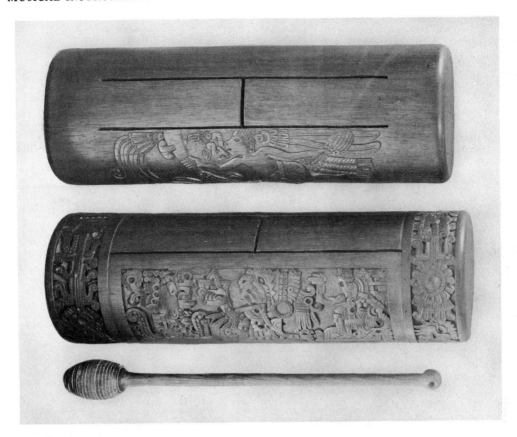

a

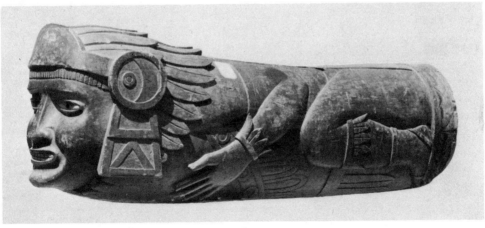

b

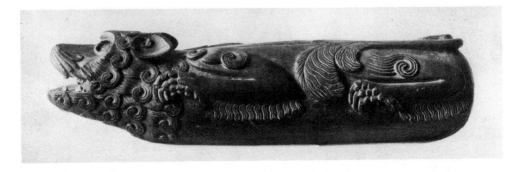

c

PLATE 293. ©. *a*) Wooden *teponaztlis,* or two-toned drums, carved in
relief, and drumstick. *b* and *c*) Same type of instrument, carved in human and
animal shapes. Mexico.

MUSICAL INSTRUMENTS

ANDEAN AND INTERLYING AREAS

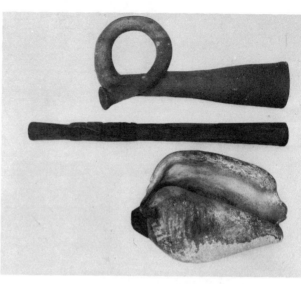

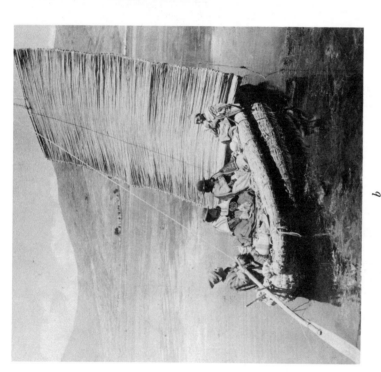

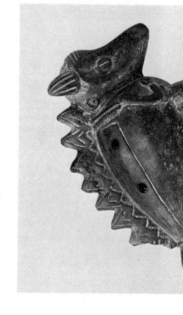

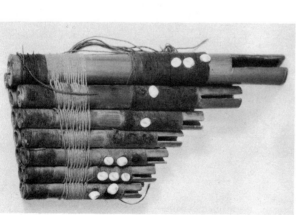

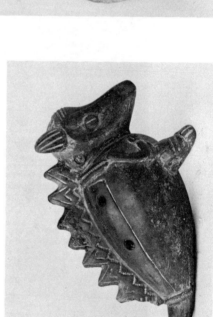

PLATE 294. ©. *a* and *c*) Peruvian panpipes of reed and stone. *b*) Natives in *balsa*, or reed boat, Lake Titicaca, Andean highlands—note the man in prow playing the same ancient type of panpipe. *d*) Mochica pottery vessels, with panpipe player and drummer. *e*) Bulbous flute (ocarina type) in animal shape, Ica? wooden flute, Mochica clay trumpet. *f*) Chimú conch trumpet, Costa Rica.

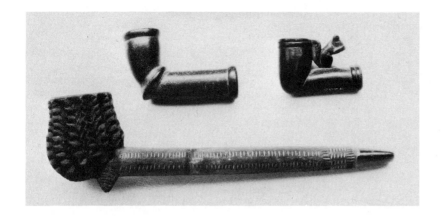

a

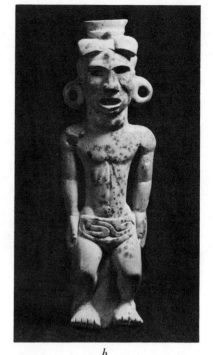

b

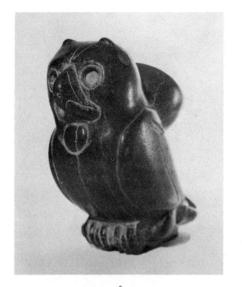

c

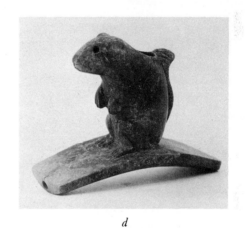

d

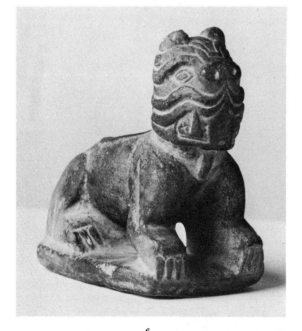

e

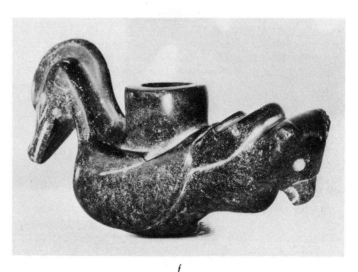

f

PLATE 295. ©. *a*) Universal types of pipes: top row, stone, Georgia; corncob shape, pottery, Mexico. Mound Builder stone effigy pipes: *b*) human, Ohio; *c*) owl, Illinois; *d*) squirrel, Ohio; *e*) monster, Alabama; *f*) duck and owl, Virginia.

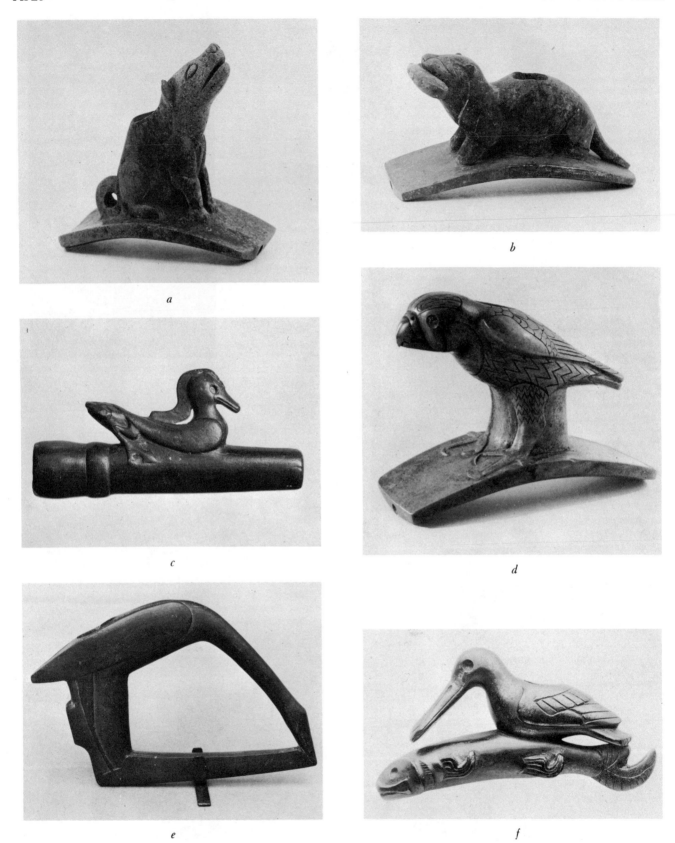

PLATE 296. ©. Mound Builder stone effigy pipes: *a*) dog; *b*) otter with fish; *d*) hawk; *e*) crane; *f*) duck on back of fish. All from Ohio. *c*) Swimming duck, Kentucky.

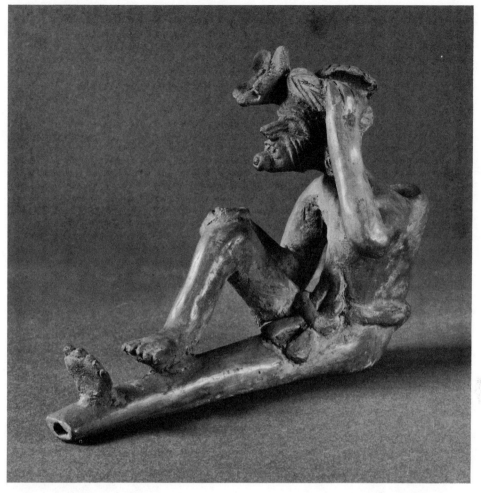

a

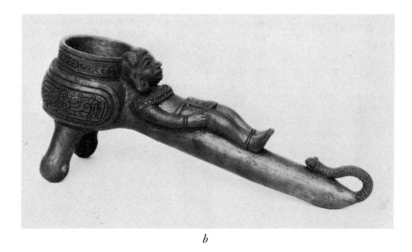

b

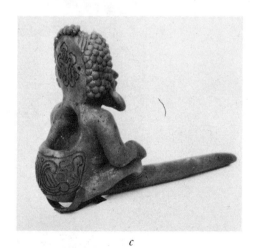

c

PLATE 297.   ©.   *a* and *c*) Pottery effigy pipes in human shape.   *b*) Pottery incense burner, with human figure used for decoration.   Mexico.

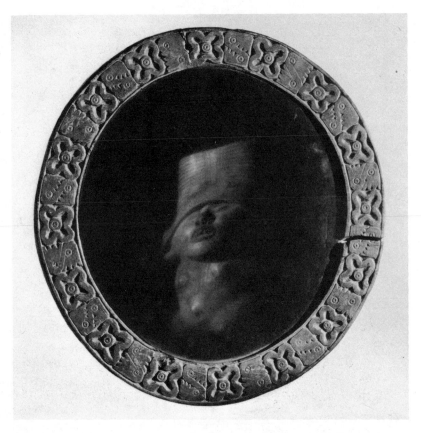

a

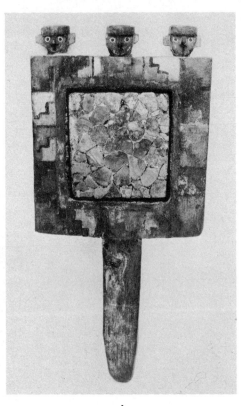

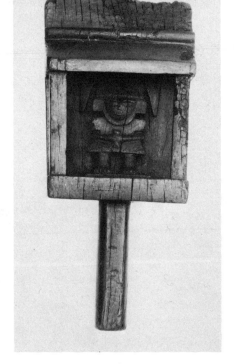

b   *c*

PLATE 298. ©. *a*) Obsidian mirror with gilded wood frame, showing reflection of
effigy vessel, Vera Cruz?, Mexico. *b*) Chimú? pyrite mirror with carved and painted
wood frame, coast of Peru. *c*) Carved and painted wood back of a Chimú mirror,
Lambayeque, Peru.

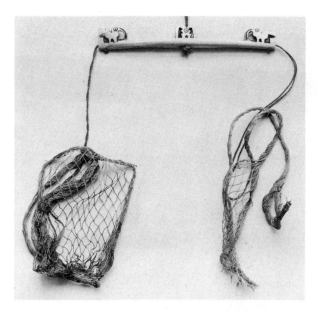

a

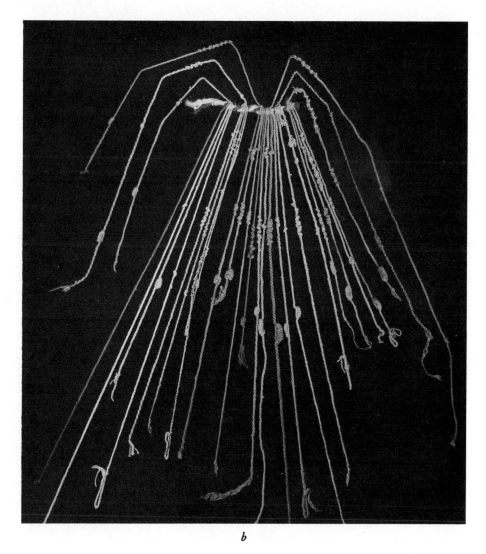

b

PLATE 299. Ⓒ. *a*) Chimú balance scale with beam of carved bone and netted bags. *b*) *Quipu,* or
knot record, Chancay.   Peru.

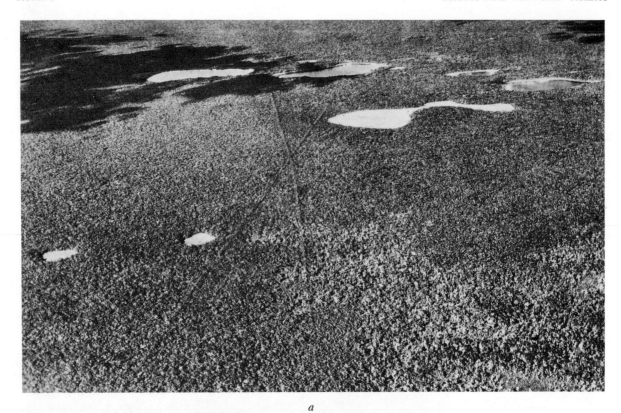

a

b

PLATE 300.   ©.   *a*) Airview of jungle bush, showing the course of two intersecting Maya roads, Yucatan, Mexico.   *b*) Airview of remnants of Chimú highways and ruin in coastal sands, Chicama Valley, Peru.

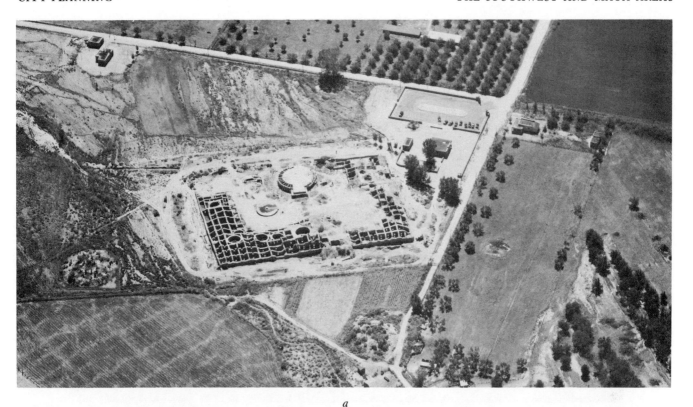

a

b

PLATE 301. ©. *a*) Airview of Pueblo ruins, Aztec, New Mexico. *b*) Airview of ancient Maya
walled seacoast city, Tulum, Mexico.

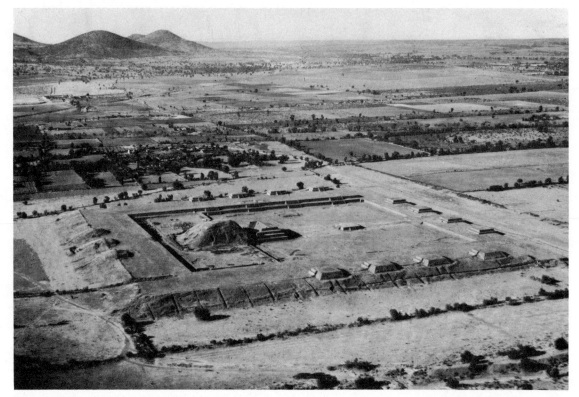

a

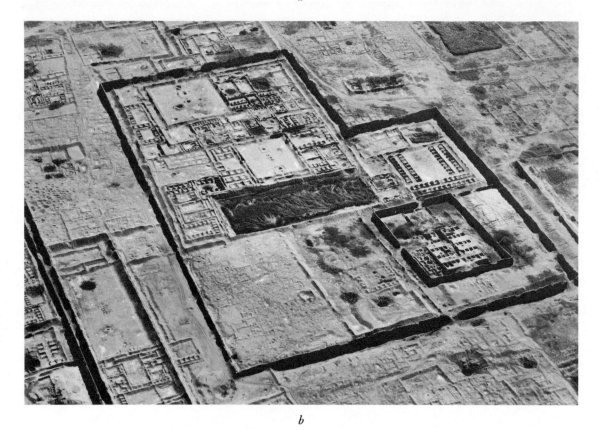

b

PLATE 302.   ©.   *a*) Airview of the Citadel, with Quetzalcóatl Temple, Teotihuacán, Mexico.   *b*) Airview of a section of the ancient Chimú capital, Chan-Chan, Peru.

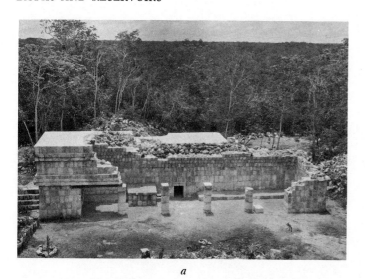

a

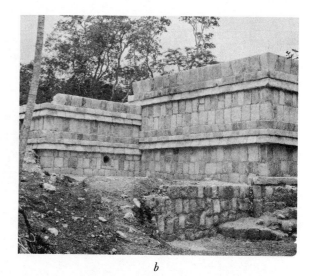

b

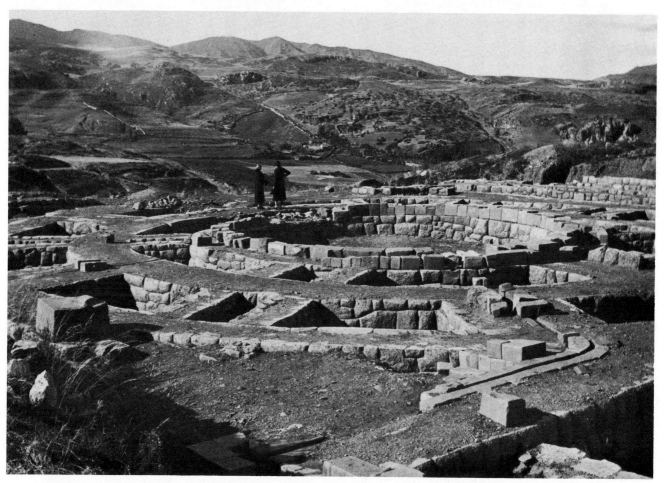

c

PLATE 303. ©. *a*) Partly restored antechamber and entrance to Maya sweat bath, Chichén Itzá, Mexico. *b*) Restored section, showing vapor vent. *c*) Ruins of an Inca reservoir and water distributing system, Sacsahuamán, Peru.

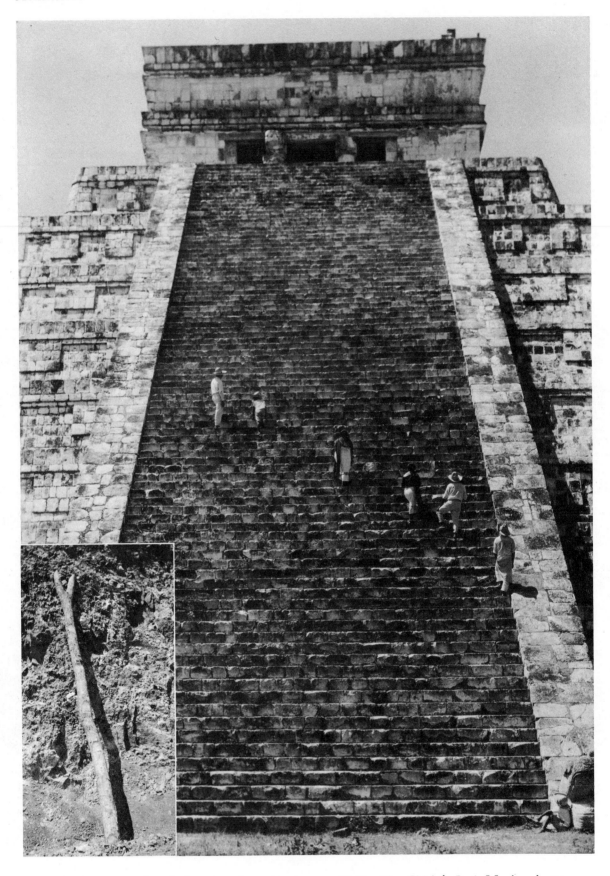

PLATE 304. ©. Stairway to the main entrance, El Castillo, Chichén Itzá, Mexico; inset: wooden pole with hewn footholds, a primitive ladder still in use, border region of Guatemala and El Salvador.

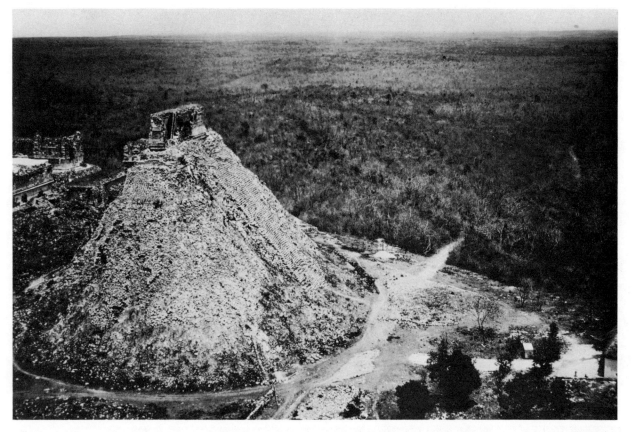

a

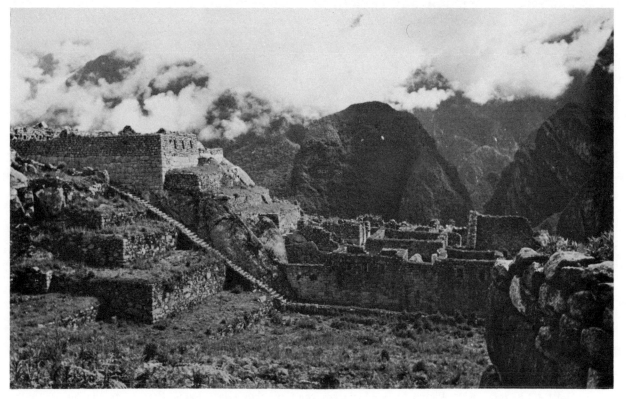

b

PLATE 305.   ©.   *a*) Ruined east stairway, Temple of the Dwarf, Uxmal, Mexico.   *b*) Stairway
connecting different levels, Machu Picchu, Peru.

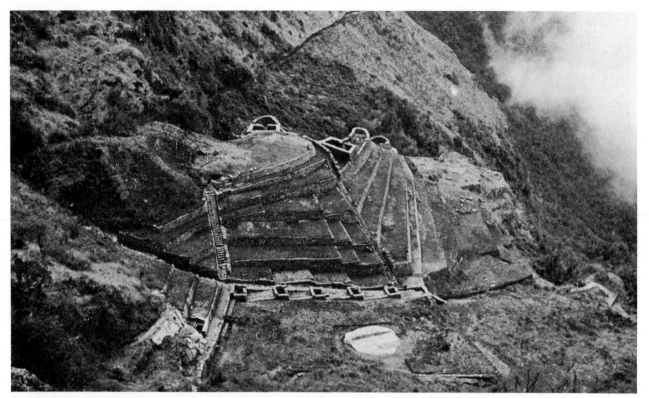

a

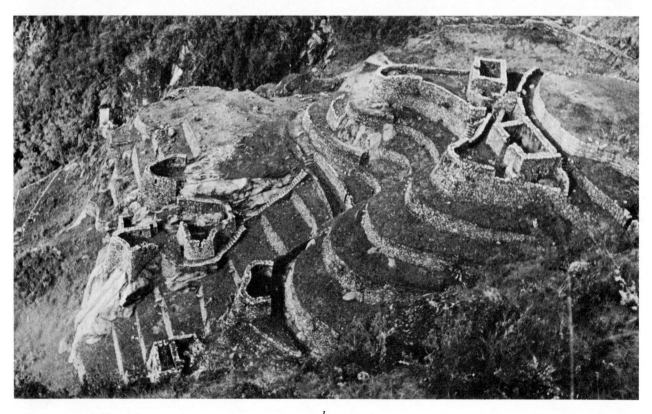

b

PLATE 306. ⓒ. Phuyu Pata Marka, or the City above the Clouds, Peru, near Machu Picchu: *a*) view from the northeast, showing water channels and basins in foreground; *b*) view from the northwest.

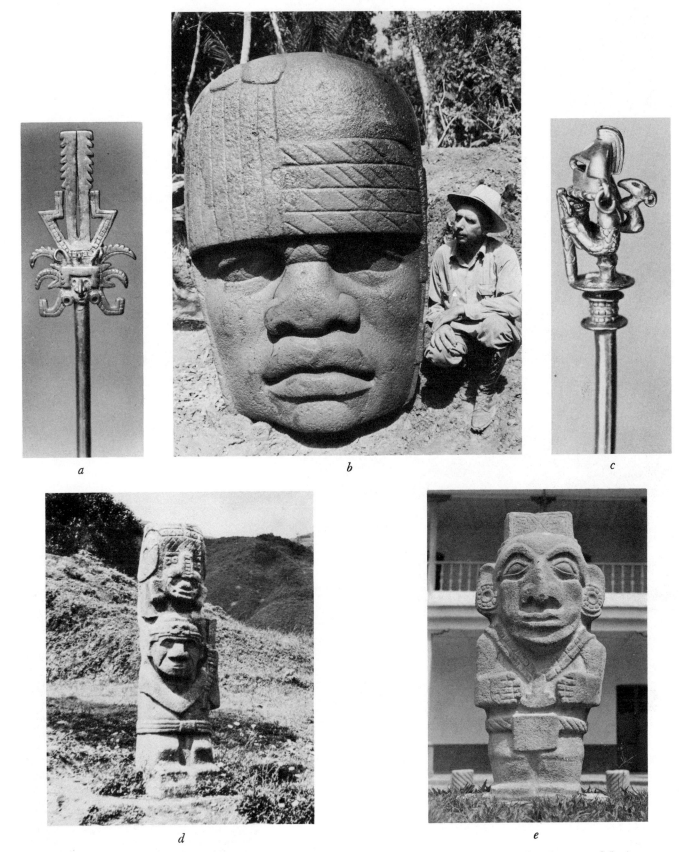

PLATE 307. ©. a and c) Quimbaya gold pins, Colombia. b) Olmec stone head, San Lorenzo, Mexico.
d and e) Stone statues, San Agustín and Moscopán, Colombia.

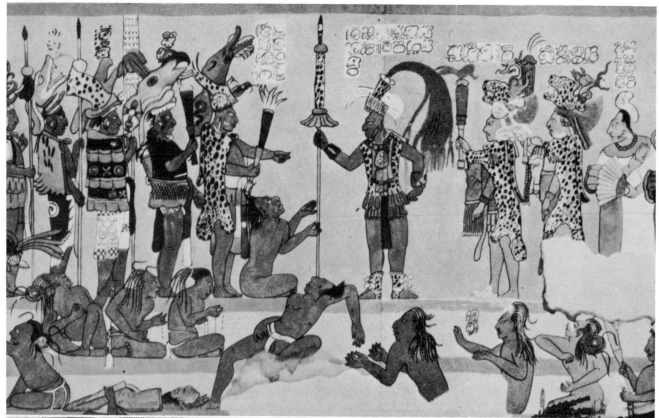

a

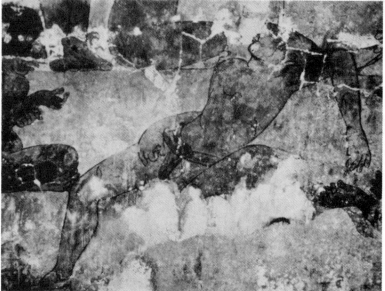

b

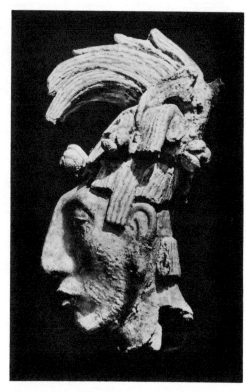

PLATE 308. ©. *a*) Maya wall-painting. *b*) Detail of same.
Bonampak. *c*) Maya stucco head, Palenque. Mexico.

c

Index

Italic numbers refer to plates

< 411 >

INDEX

< 413 >

INDEX

< 416 >

INDEX

< 418 >

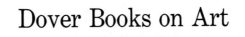
Dover Books on Art

THE FOUR BOOKS OF ARCHITECTURE, Andrea Palladio. A compendium of the art of Andrea Palladio, one of the most celebrated architects of the Renaissance, including 250 magnificently-engraved plates showing edifices either of Palladio's design or reconstructed (in these drawings) by him from classical ruins and contemporary accounts. 257 plates. xxiv + 119pp. 9½ x 12¾.   21308-0   Clothbound $10.00

150 MASTERPIECES OF DRAWING, A. Toney. Selected by a gifted artist and teacher, these are some of the finest drawings produced by Western artists from the early 15th to the end of the 18th centuries. Excellent reproductions of drawings by Rembrandt, Bruegel, Raphael, Watteau, and other familiar masters, as well as works by lesser known but brilliant artists. 150 plates. xviii + 150pp. 5⅜ x 11¼.   21032-4   Paperbound $2.00

MORE DRAWINGS BY HEINRICH KLEY. Another collection of the graphic, vivid sketches of Heinrich Kley, one of the most diabolically talented cartoonists of our century. The sketches take in every aspect of human life: nothing is too sacred for him to ridicule, no one too eminent for him to satirize. 158 drawings you will not easily forget. iv + 104pp. 7⅜ x 10¾.

20041-8   Paperbound $1.85

THE TRIUMPH OF MAXIMILIAN I, 137 Woodcuts by Hans Burgkmair and Others. This is one of the world's great art monuments, a series of magnificent woodcuts executed by the most important artists in the German realms as part of an elaborate plan by Maximilian I, ruler of the Holy Roman Empire, to commemorate his own name, dynasty, and achievements. 137 plates. New translation of descriptive text, notes, and bibliography prepared by Stanley Appelbaum. Special section of 10pp. containing a reduced version of the entire Triumph. x + 169pp. 11⅛ x 9¼.   21207-6   Paperbound $3.00

PAINTING IN ISLAM, Sir Thomas W. Arnold. This scholarly study puts Islamic painting in its social and religious context and examines its relation to Islamic civilization in general. 65 full-page plates illustrate the text and give outstanding examples of Islamic art. 4 appendices. Index of mss. referred to. General Index. xxiv + 159pp. 6⅝ x 9¼.   21310-2   Paperbound $2.50

THE MATERIALS AND TECHNIQUES OF MEDIEVAL PAINTING, D. V. Thompson. An invaluable study of carriers and grounds, binding media, pigments, metals used in painting, al fresco and al secco techniques, burnishing, etc. used by the medieval masters. Preface by Bernard Berenson. 239pp. 5⅜ x 8.

20327-1   Paperbound $2.00

THE HISTORY AND TECHNIQUE OF LETTERING, A. Nesbitt. A thorough history of lettering from the ancient Egyptians to the present, and a 65-page course in lettering for artists. Every major development in lettering history is illustrated by a complete aphabet. Fully analyzes such masters as Caslon, Koch, Garamont, Jenson, and many more. 89 alphabets, 165 other specimens. 317pp. 7½ x 10½.   20427-8   Paperbound $2.25

200 DECORATIVE TITLE-PAGES, edited by A. Nesbitt. Fascinating and informative from a historical point of view, this beautiful collection of decorated titles will be a great inspiration to students of design, commercial artists, advertising designers, etc. A complete survey of the genre from the first known decorated title to work in the first decades of this century. Bibliography and sources of the plates. 222pp. $8\frac{3}{8}$ x $11\frac{1}{4}$.

21264-5 Paperbound $2.75

ON THE LAWS OF JAPANESE PAINTING, H. P. Bowie. This classic work on the philosophy and technique of Japanese art is based on the author's first-hand experiences studying art in Japan. Every aspect of Japanese painting is described: the use of the brush and other materials; laws governing conception and execution; subjects for Japanese paintings, etc. The best possible substitute for a series of lessons from a great Oriental master. Index. xv + 117pp. + 66 plates. $6\frac{1}{8}$ x $9\frac{1}{4}$.

20030-2 Paperbound $2.25

A HANDBOOK OF ANATOMY FOR ART STUDENTS, Arthur Thomson. This long-popular text teaches any student, regardless of level of technical competence, all the subtleties of human anatomy. Clear photographs, numerous line sketches and diagrams of bones, joints, etc. Use it as a text for home study, as a supplement to life class work, or as a lifelong sourcebook and reference volume. Author's prefaces. 67 plates, containing 40 line drawings, 86 photographs—mostly full page. 211 figures. Appendix. Index. xx + 459pp. $5\frac{3}{8}$ x $8\frac{3}{8}$. 21163-0 Paperbound $3.00

WHITTLING AND WOODCARVING, E. J. Tangerman. With this book, a beginner who is moderately handy can whittle or carve scores of useful objects, toys for children, gifts, or simply pass hours creatively and enjoyably. "Easy as well as instructive reading," N. Y. Herald Tribune Books. 464 illustrations, with appendix and index. x + 293pp. $5\frac{1}{2}$ x $8\frac{1}{8}$.

20965-2 Paperbound $1.75

ONE HUNDRED AND ONE PATCHWORK PATTERNS, Ruby Short McKim. Whether you have made a hundred quilts or none at all, you will find this the single most useful book on quiltmaking. There are 101 full patterns (all exact size) with full instructions for cutting and sewing. In addition there is some really choice folklore about the origin of the ingenious pattern names: "Monkey Wrench," "Road to California," "Drunkard's Path," "Crossed Canoes," to name a few. Over 500 illustrations. 124 pp. $7\frac{7}{8}$ x $10\frac{3}{4}$. 20773-0 Paperbound $2.00

ART AND GEOMETRY, W. M. Ivins, Jr. Challenges the idea that the foundations of modern thought were laid in ancient Greece. Pitting Greek tactile-muscular intuitions of space against modern visual intuitions, the author, for 30 years curator of prints, Metropolitan Museum of Art, analyzes the differences between ancient and Renaissance painting and sculpture and tells of the first fruitful investigations of perspective. x + 113pp. $5\frac{3}{8}$ x $8\frac{3}{8}$. 20941-5 Paperbound $1.50

Dover Books on Art

PRINCIPLES OF ART HISTORY, H. Wölfflin. This remarkably instructive work demonstrates the tremendous change in artistic conception from the 14th to the 18th centuries, by analyzing 164 works by Botticelli, Dürer, Hobbema, Holbein, Hals, Titian, Rembrandt, Vermeer, etc., and pointing out exactly what is meant by "baroque," "classic," "primitive," "picturesque," and other basic terms of art history and criticism. "A remarkable lesson in the art of seeing," SAT. REV. OF LITERATURE. Translated from the 7th German edition. 150 illus. 254pp. 6⅛ x 9¼. 20276-3 Paperbound $2.25

FOUNDATIONS OF MODERN ART, A. Ozenfant. Stimulating discussion of human creativity from paleolithic cave painting to modern painting, architecture, decorative arts. Fully illustrated with works of Gris, Lipchitz, Léger, Picasso, primitive, modern artifacts, architecture, industrial art, much more. 226 illustrations. 368pp. 6⅛ x 9¼. 20215-1 Paperbound $2.50

METALWORK AND ENAMELLING, H. Maryon. Probably the best book ever written on the subject. Tells everything necessary for the home manufacture of jewelry, rings, ear pendants, bowls, etc. Covers materials, tools, soldering, filigree, setting stones, raising patterns, repoussé work, damascening, niello, cloisonné, polishing, assaying, casting, and dozens of other techniques. The best substitute for apprenticeship to a master metalworker. 363 photos and figures. 374pp. 5½ x 8½. T183 Clothbound $8.50

SHAKER FURNITURE, E. D. and F. Andrews. The most illuminating study of Shaker furniture ever written. Covers chronology, craftsmanship, houses, shops, etc. Includes over 200 photographs of chairs, tables, clocks, beds, benches, etc. "Mr. & Mrs. Andrews know all there is to know about Shaker furniture," Mark Van Doren, NATION. 48 full-page plates. 192pp. 7⅞ x 10¾. 20679-3 Paperbound $2.50

LETTERING AND ALPHABETS, J. A. Cavanagh. An unabridged reissue of "Lettering," containing the full discussion, analysis, illustration of 89 basic hand lettering styles based on Caslon, Bodoni, Gothic, many other types. Hundreds of technical hints on construction, strokes, pens, brushes, etc. 89 alphabets, 72 lettered specimens, which may be reproduced permission-free. 121pp. 9¾ x 8. 20053-1 Paperbound $1.50

THE HUMAN FIGURE IN MOTION, Eadweard Muybridge. The largest collection in print of Muybridge's famous high-speed action photos. 4789 photographs in more than 500 action-strip-sequences (at shutter speeds up to 1/6000th of a second) illustrate men, women, children—mostly undraped—performing such actions as walking, running, getting up, lying down, carrying objects, throwing, etc. "An unparalleled dictionary of action for all artists," AMERICAN ARTIST. 390 full-page plates, with 4789 photographs. Heavy glossy stock, reinforced binding with headbands. 7⅞ x 10¾. 20204-6 Clothbound $10.00

AFRICAN SCULPTURE, Ladislas Segy. 163 full-page plates illustrating masks, fertility figures, ceremonial objects, etc., of 50 West and Central African tribes—95% never before illustrated. 34-page introduction to African sculpture. "Mr. Segy is one of its top authorities," NEW YORKER. 164 full-page photographic plates. Introduction. Bibliography. 244pp. 6⅛ x 9¼.

20396-4 Paperbound $2.25

CALLIGRAPHY, J. G. Schwandner. First reprinting in 200 years of this legendary book of beautiful handwriting. Over 300 ornamental initials, 12 complete calligraphic alphabets, over 150 ornate frames and panels, 75 calligraphic pictures of cherubs, stags, lions, etc., thousands of flourishes, scrolls, etc., by the greatest 18th-century masters. All material can be copied or adapted without permission. Historical introduction. 158 full-page plates. 368pp. 9 x 13.   20475-8 Clothbound $10.00

PRINTED EPHEMERA, edited and collected by John Lewis. This book contains centuries of design, typographical and pictorial motives in proven, effective commercial layouts. Hundreds of the most striking examples of labels, tickets, posters, wrappers, programs, menus, and other items have been collected in this handsome and useful volume, along with information on the dimensions and colors of the original, printing processes used, stylistic notes on typography and design, etc. Study this book and see how the best commercial artists of the past and present have solved their particular problems. Most of the material is copyright free. 713 illustrations, many in color. Illustrated index of type faces included. Glossary of technical terms. Indexes. 288pp. 9¼ x 12.   22284-5, 22285-3 Clothbound $15.00

DESIGN FOR ARTISTS AND CRAFTSMEN, Louis Wolchonok. Recommended for either individual or classroom use, this book helps you to create original designs from things about you, from geometric patterns, from plants, animals, birds, humans, landscapes, manmade objects. "A great contribution," N. Y. Society of Craftsmen. 113 exercises with hints and diagrams. More than 1280 illustrations. xv + 207pp. 7⅞ x 10¾.

20274-7 Paperbound $2.75

HANDBOOK OF ORNAMENT, F. S. Meyer. One of the largest collections of copyright-free traditional art: over 3300 line cuts of Greek, Roman, Medieval, Renaissance, Baroque, 18th and 19th century art motifs (tracery, geometric elements, flower and animal motifs, etc.) and decorated objects (chairs, thrones, weapons, vases, jewelry, armor, etc.). Full text. 300 plates. 3300 illustrations. 562pp. 5⅜ x 8.   20302-6 Paperbound $2.75

THREE CLASSICS OF ITALIAN CALLIGRAPHY, Oscar Ogg, ed. Exact reproductions of three famous Renaissance calligraphic works: Arrighi's OPERINA and IL MODO, Tagliente's LO PRESENTE LIBRO, and Palatino's LIBRO NUOVO. More than 200 complete alphabets, thousands of lettered specimens, in Papal Chancery and other beautiful, ornate handwriting. Introduction. 245 plates. 282pp. 6⅛ x 9¼. 20212-7 Paperbound $2.75

ART ANATOMY, Dr. William Rimmer. One of the few books on art anatomy that are themselves works of art, this is a faithful reproduction (rearranged for handy use) of the extremely rare masterpiece of the famous 19th century anatomist, sculptor, and art teacher. Beautiful, clear line drawings show every part of the body—bony structure, muscles, features, etc. Unusual are the sections on falling bodies, foreshortenings, muscles in tension, grotesque personalities, and Rimmer's remarkable interpretation of emotions and personalities as expressed by facial features. It will supplement every other book on art anatomy you are likely to have. Reproduced clearer than the lithographic original (which sells for $500 on up on the rare book market.) Over 1,200 illustrations. xiii + 153pp. 7¾ x 10¾.

20908-3 Paperbound $2.50

THE CRAFTSMAN'S HANDBOOK, Cennino Cennini. The finest English translation of IL LIBRO DELL' ARTE, the 15th century introduction to art technique that is both a mirror of Quatrocento life and a source of many useful but nearly forgotten facets of the painter's art. 4 illustrations. xxvii + 142pp. D. V. Thompson, translator. 5⅜ x 8. 20054-X Paperbound $1.75

THE BROWN DECADES, Lewis Mumford. A picture of the "buried renaissance" of the post-Civil War period, and the founding of modern architecture (Sullivan, Richardson, Root, Roebling), landscape development (Marsh, Olmstead, Eliot), and the graphic arts (Homer, Eakins, Ryder). 2nd revised, enlarged edition. Bibliography. 12 illustrations. xiv + 266 pp. 5⅜ x 8.

20200-3 Paperbound $2.00

THE STYLES OF ORNAMENT, A. Speltz. The largest collection of line ornament in print, with 3750 numbered illustrations arranged chronologically from Egypt, Assyria, Greeks, Romans, Etruscans, through Medieval, Renaissance, 18th century, and Victorian. No permissions, no fees needed to use or reproduce illustrations. 400 plates with 3750 illustrations. Bibliography. Index. 640pp. 6 x 9. 20577-6 Paperbound $3.00

THE ART OF ETCHING, E. S. Lumsden. Every step of the etching process from essential materials to completed proof is carefully and clearly explained, with 24 annotated plates exemplifying every technique and approach discussed. The book also features a rich survey of the art, with 105 annotated plates by masters. Invaluable for beginner to advanced etcher. 374pp. 5⅜ x 8. 20049-3 Paperbound $2.75

OF THE JUST SHAPING OF LETTERS, Albrecht Dürer. This remarkable volume reveals Albrecht Dürer's rules for the geometric construction of Roman capitals and the formation of Gothic lower case and capital letters, complete with construction diagrams and directions. Of considerable practical interest to the contemporary illustrator, artist, and designer. Translated from the Latin text of the edition of 1535 by R. T. Nichol. Numerous letterform designs, construction diagrams, illustrations. iv + 43pp. 7⅞ x 10¾. 21306-4 Paperbound $1.25

Dover Books on Art

LANDSCAPE GARDENING IN JAPAN, Josiah Conder. A detailed picture of Japanese gardening techniques and ideas, the artistic principles incorporated in the Japanese garden, and the religious and ethical concepts at the heart of those principles. Preface. 92 illustrations, plus all 40 full-page plates from the Supplement. Index. xv + 299pp. 8⅜ x 11¼.

21216-5 Paperbound $3.50

DESIGN AND FIGURE CARVING, E. J. Tangerman. "Anyone who can peel a potato can carve," states the author, and in this unusual book he shows you how, covering every stage in detail from very simple exercises working up to museum-quality pieces. Terrific aid for hobbyists, arts and crafts counselors, teachers, those who wish to make reproductions for the commercial market. Appendix: How to Enlarge a Design. Brief bibliography. Index. 1298 figures. x + 289pp. 5⅜ x 8½.

21209-2 Paperbound $2.00

THE STANDARD BOOK OF QUILT MAKING AND COLLECTING, M. Ickis. Even if you are a beginner, you will soon find yourself quilting like an expert, by following these clearly drawn patterns, photographs, and step-by-step instructions. Learn how to plan the quilt, to select the pattern to harmonize with the design and color of the room, to choose materials. Over 40 full-size patterns. Index. 483 illustrations. One color plate. xi + 276pp. 6¾ x 9½.

20582-7 Paperbound $2.50

LOST EXAMPLES OF COLONIAL ARCHITECTURE, J. M. Howells. This book offers a unique guided tour through America's architectural past, all of which is either no longer in existence or so changed that its original beauty has been destroyed. More than 275 clear photos of old churches, dwelling houses, public buildings, business structures, etc. 245 plates, containing 281 photos and 9 drawings, floorplans, etc. New Index. xvii + 248pp. 7⅞ x 10¾.

21143-6 Paperbound $3.00

A HISTORY OF COSTUME, Carl Köhler. The most reliable and authentic account of the development of dress from ancient times through the 19th century. Based on actual pieces of clothing that have survived, using paintings, statues and other reproductions only where originals no longer exist. Hundreds of illustrations, including detailed patterns for many articles. Highly useful for theatre and movie directors, fashion designers, illustrators, teachers. Edited and augmented by Emma von Sichart. Translated by Alexander K. Dallas. 594 illustrations. 464pp. 5⅛ x 7⅛.

21030-8 Paperbound $3.00

Dover publishes books on commercial art, art history, crafts, design, art classics; also books on music, literature, science, mathematics, puzzles and entertainments, chess, engineering, biology, philosophy, psychology, languages, history, and other fields. For free circulars write to Dept. DA, Dover Publications, Inc., 180 Varick St., New York, N.Y. 10014.